A HISTORY

OF

EPIDEMICS IN BRITAIN.

A HISTORY

OF

EPIDEMICS IN BRITAIN

from A.D. 664 to the Extinction of Plague

BY

CHARLES CREIGHTON, M.A., M.D.,

FORMERLY DEMONSTRATOR OF ANATOMY IN THE UNIVERSITY OF CAMBRIDGE.

CAMBRIDGE:
AT THE UNIVERSITY PRESS.
1891

CAMBRIDGE UNIVERSITY PRESS
Cambridge, New York, Melbourne, Madrid, Cape Town,
Singapore, São Paulo, Delhi, Mexico City

Cambridge University Press
The Edinburgh Building, Cambridge CB2 8RU, UK

Published in the United States of America by Cambridge University Press, New York

www.cambridge.org
Information on this title: www.cambridge.org/9781107621930

© Cambridge University Press 1891

First published 1891
First paperback edition 2013

A catalogue record for this publication is available from the British Library

ISBN 978-1-107-62193-0 Paperback

PREFACE.

THE title and contents-table of this volume will show sufficiently its scope, and a glance at the references in the several chapters will show its sources. But it may be convenient to premise a few general remarks under each of those heads. The date 664 A.D. has been chosen as a starting-point, for the reason that it is the year of the first pestilence in Britain recorded on contemporary or almost contemporary authority, that of Beda's 'Ecclesiastical History.' The other limit of the volume, the extinction of plague in 1665–66, marks the end of a long era of epidemic sickness, which differed much in character from the era next following. At or near the Restoration we come, as it were, to the opening of a new seal or the outpouring of another vial. The history proceeds thenceforth on other lines and comes largely from sources of another kind; allowing for a little overlapping about the middle of the seventeenth century, it might be continued from 1666 almost without reference to what had gone before. The history is confined to Great Britain and Ireland, except in Chapter XI. which is occupied with the first Colonies and the early voyages, excepting also certain sections of other chapters, where the history has to trace the antecedents of some great epidemic sickness on a foreign soil.

C.   *b*

The sources of the work have been the ordinary first-hand sources of English history in general. In the medieval period these include the monastic histories, chronicles, lives, or the like (partly in the editions of Gale, Savile, Twysden, and Hearne, and of the English Historical Society, but chiefly in the great series edited for the Master of the Rolls), the older printed collections of State documents, and, for the Black Death, the recently published researches upon the rolls of manor courts and upon other records. From near the beginning of the Tudor period, the Calendars of State Papers (Domestic, Foreign, and Colonial), become an invaluable source of information for the epidemiologist just as for other historians. Also the Reports of the Historical Manuscripts Commission, together with its Calendars of private collections of papers, have yielded a good many facts. Many exact data, relating more particularly to local outbreaks of plague, have been found in the county, borough, and parish histories, which are of very unequal value for the purpose and are often sadly to seek in the matter of an index. The miscellaneous sources drawn upon have been very numerous, perhaps more numerous, from the nature of the subject, than in most other branches of history.

Medical books proper are hardly available for a history of English epidemics until the Elizabethan period, and they do not begin to be really important for the purpose until shortly before the date at which the present history ends. These have been carefully sought for, most of the known books having been met with and examined closely for illustrative facts. In the latter part of the seventeenth century the best English writers on medicine occupied themselves largely with the epidemics of their own time, and the British school of epidemiology, which took a distinguished start with Willis, Sydenham and Morton, was worthily continued by many writers throughout the eighteenth century; so that the history subsequent to the period here treated of becomes more and more dependent upon medical sources, and of more special interest to the profession itself.

Reference has been made not unfrequently to manuscripts; of which the more important that have been used (for the first time) are a treatise on the Sweating Sickness of 1485 by a contemporary physician in London, two original London plague-bills of the reign of Henry VIII., and a valuable set of tables of the weekly burials and christenings in London for five years (almost complete) from 1578 to 1583, among the Cecil papers—these last by kind permission of the Marquis of Salisbury.

Collecting materials for a British epidemiology from these various sources is not an easy task; had it been so, it would hardly have been left to be done, or, so far as one knows, even attempted, for the first time at so late a period. Where the sources of information are so dispersed and casual it is inevitable that some things should have been overlooked: be the omissions few or many, they would certainly have been more but for suggestions and assistance kindly given from time to time by various friends.

The materials being collected, it remained to consider how best to use them. The existing national epidemiologies, such as that of Italy by Professor Corradi or the older 'Epidemiologia Española' of Villalba, are in the form of Annals. But it seemed practicable, without sacrificing a single item of the chronology, to construct from the greater events of sickness in the national annals a systematic history that should touch and connect with the general history at many points and make a volume supplementary to the same. Such has been the attempt; and in estimating the measure of its success it may be kept in mind that it is the first of the kind, British or foreign, in its own department. The author can hardly hope to have altogether escaped errors in touching upon the general history of the country over so long a period; but he has endeavoured to go as

little as possible outside his proper province and to avoid
making gratuitous reflections upon historical characters and
events. The greater epidemic diseases have, however, been
discussed freely—from the scientific side or from the point of
view of their theory.

It remains to acknowledge the liberality of the Syndics of
the Cambridge University Press in the matter of publication,
and the friendly interest taken in the work by their Chairman,
the Master of Peterhouse.

November, 1891.

CONTENTS.

CHAPTER I.

CHAPTER II.

CHAPTER III.

CHAPTER IV.

ENGLAND AFTER THE BLACK DEATH, WITH THE EPIDEMICS TO 1485.

CHAPTER V.

THE SWEATING SICKNESS, 1485–1551.

CHAPTER VI.

PLAGUE IN THE TUDOR PERIOD.

CHAPTER VII.

GAOL FEVERS, INFLUENZAS, AND OTHER FEVERS IN THE TUDOR PERIOD.

CHAPTER VIII.

THE FRENCH POX.

CHAPTER IX.

SMALLPOX AND MEASLES.

CHAPTER X.

PLAGUE, FEVER AND INFLUENZA FROM THE ACCESSION OF JAMES I. TO THE RESTORATION.

CHAPTER XI.

SICKNESSES OF EARLY VOYAGES AND COLONIES.

CHAPTER XII.

THE GREAT PLAGUE OF LONDON, AND THE LAST OF PLAGUE IN ENGLAND.

ERRATA.

At p. 28 line 4, *for* "for" *read* "at." At p. 126 line 2 *for* "1351" *read* "1350;" same change at p. 130, lines 6 and 9. At p. 185 note 1 *read* "Ochenkowski." At p. 264 line 18, and at p. 554 line 11 from bottom, read "*pathognomonicum.*" At p. 401, note 3 *for* "1658" *read* "1558." At p. 420, line 17, *for* "Henry IV.," *read* "Henry V." At p. 474, line 4, *for* "more" *read* "less." At p. 649 line 22 *omit* "Hancock."

CHAPTER I.

PESTILENCES PREVIOUS TO THE BLACK DEATH, CHIEFLY
FROM FAMINES.

THE Middle Age of European history has no naturally fixed
beginning or ending.   The period of Antiquity may be taken as
concluded by the fourth Christian century, or by the fifth or by
the sixth; the Modern period may be made to commence in
the fourteenth, or in the fifteenth or in the sixteenth.   The
historian Hallam includes a thousand years in the medieval
period, from the invasion of France by Clovis to the invasion of
Italy by Charles VIII. in 1494.   We begin, he says, in darkness
and calamity, and we break off as the morning breathes upon us
and the twilight reddens into the lustre of day.   To the epidemiologist the medieval period is rounded more definitely.   At
the one end comes the great plague in the reign of Justinian,
and at the other end the Black Death.   Those are the two greatest
pestilences in recorded history; each has no parallel except in
the other.   They were in the march of events, and should not
be fixed upon as doing more than their share in shaping the
course of history.   But no single thing stands out more clearly
as the stroke of fate in bringing the ancient civilization to an
end than the vast depopulation and solitude made by the plague
which came with the corn-ships from Egypt to Byzantium in
the year 543; and nothing marks so definitely the emergence
of Europe from the middle period of stagnation as the other
depopulation and social upheaval made by the plague which
came in the overland track of Genoese and Venetian traders

C.

I

from China in the year 1347. While many other influences were in the air to determine the oncoming and the offgoing of the middle darkness, those two world-wide pestilences were singular in their respective effects : of the one, we may say that it turned the key of the medieval prison-house ; and of the other, that it unlocked the door after eight hundred years.

The Black Death and its after-effects will occupy a large part of this work, so that what has just been said of it will not stand as a bare assertion. But the plague in the reign of Justinian hardly touches British history, and must be left with a brief reference. Gibbon was not insensible of the part that it played in the great drama of his history. " There was," he says, " a visible decrease of the human species, which has never been repaired in some of the fairest countries of the globe." After vainly trying to construe the arithmetic of Procopius, who was a witness of the calamity at Byzantium, he agrees to strike off one or more ciphers, and adopts as an estimate "not wholly inadmissible," a mortality of one hundred millions. The effects of that depopulation, in part due to war, are not followed in the history. So far as Gibbon's method could go, the plague came for him into the same group of phenomena as comets and earthquakes ; it was part of the stage scenery amidst which the drama of emperors, pontiffs, generals, eunuchs, Theodoras, and adventurers proceeded. Even of the comets and earthquakes, he remarks that they were subject to physical laws ; and it was from no want of scientific spirit that he omitted to show how a plague of such magnitude had a place in the physical order, and not less in the moral order.

A new science of epidemiology has sprung up since the time of Gibbon, who had to depend on the writings of Mead, a busy and not very profound Court physician. More particularly the Egyptian origin of the plague of the sixth century, and its significance, have been elucidated by the brilliant theory of Pariset, of which some account will be given at the end of the chapter on the Black Death. For the present, we are concerned with it only in so far as it may have a bearing upon the pestilences of Britain. The plague of the sixth century made the greatest impression, naturally, upon the oldest civilized countries of

Europe; but it extended also to the outlying provinces of the empire, and to the countries of the barbarians. It was the same disease as the Black Death of the fourteenth century, the bubo-plague; and it spread from country to country, and lasted from generation to generation, as that more familiar infection is known to have done[1].

Renewals of it are heard of in one part of Europe or another until the end of the sixth century, when its continuity is lost. But it is clear that the seeds of pestilence were not wanting in Rome and elsewhere in the centuries following. Thus, about the year 668, the English archbishop-elect, Vighard, having gone to Rome to get his election confirmed by the Pope Vitalianus, was shortly after his arrival cut off by pestilence, with almost all who had gone with him[2]. Twelve years after, in 680, there was another severe pestilence in the months of July, August and September, causing a great mortality at Rome, and such panic at Pavia that the inhabitants fled to the mountains[3]. In 746 a pestilence is said to have advanced from Sicily and Calabria, and to have made such devastation in Rome that there were houses without a single inhabitant left[4]. The common name for all such epidemics is *pestis* or *pestilentia* or *magna mortalitas*, so that it is open to contend that some other type than bubo-plague, such as fever or flux, may have been at least a part of them; but no type of infection has ever been so mortal as the bubo-plague, and a mortality that is distinguished by a chronicler as causing panic and devastation was presumably of that type.

---

[1] The references to the Justinian plague by contemporary and later historians have been collected, together with partly irrelevant matter about portents and earthquakes, by Val. Seibel, *Die grosse Pest zur Zeit Justinian's I.* Dillingen, 1857. The author, a layman, throws no light upon its origin.

[2] Beda, *Hist. Eccles.* Eng. Hist. Society's ed. p. 243: "qui ubi Romam pervenit, cujus sedi apostolicae tempore illo Vitalianus praeerat, postquam itineris sui causam praefato papae apostolico patefecit, non multo post et ipse et omnes pene, qui cum eo advenerant, socii, pestilentia superveniente, deleti sunt."

[3] *Flores Histor.* by Roger of Wendover. Eng. Hist. Society's ed. I. 180.

[4] *Ibid.* I. 228.

Pestilence in England and Ireland in the Seventh Century.

It is more than a century after the first great wave of pestilence had passed over Europe in the reign of Justinian, before we hear of a great plague in England and Ireland. Dr Willan, the one English writer on medicine who has turned his erudition to that period, conjectures that the infection must have come to this country from the continent at an earlier date. From the year 597, he says, the progress of conversion to the Christian religion " led to such frequent intercourse with Italy, France and Belgium, that the epidemical and contagious disease prevailing on the continent at the close of the sixth century must necessarily be communicated from time to time through the Heptarchy[1]." Until we come to the *Ecclesiastical History* of Beda, the only authorities are the Irish annals ; and in them, the first undoubted entry of a great plague corresponds in date with that of Beda's history, the year 664. It is true, indeed, that the Irish annals, or the later recensions of them, carry the name that was given to the plague of 664 (*pestis ictericia* or *buide connaill*) back to an alleged mortality in 543, or 548, and make the latter the " first *buide connaill* " ; but the obituary of saints on that occasion is merely what might have occurred in the ordinary way, and it is probable, from the form of entry, that it was really the rumour of the great plague at Byzantium and elsewhere in 543 and subsequent years that had reached the Irish annalist[2].

The plague of 664 is the only epidemic in early British annals that can be regarded as a plague of the same nature, and on the same great scale, as the devastation of the continent of

[1] *Miscellaneous Works of the late Robert Willan, M.D., F.R.S., F.A.S.* Edited by Ashby Smith, M.D. London, 1821. 'An Enquiry into the Antiquity of the Smallpox etc.' p. 108.

[2] *Annals of the Four Masters*, ed. O'Donovan, Dublin, 1851, I. 183. "A.D. 543. There was an extraordinary universal plague through the world, which swept away the noblest third part of the human race."

p. 187. "A.D. 548. Of the mortality which was called Cron Chonaill—and that was the first Buide Chonaill [*flava ictericia*],—these saints died," several names following. The entries of that plague are under different years in the various original Annals.

Europe more than a century earlier, whether it be taken to be a late offshoot of that or not. The English pestilence of 664 is the same that was fabled long after in prose and verse as the great plague "of Cadwallader's time." It left a mark on the traditions of England, which may be taken as an index of its reality and its severity; and with it the history of epidemics in Britain may be said to begin. It was still sufficiently recent to have been narrated by eyewitnesses to Beda, whose *Ecclesiastical History* is the one authentic source, besides the entry in the Irish annals, of our information concerning it.

The pestilence broke out suddenly in the year 664, and after "depopulating" the southern parts of England, seized upon the province of Northumbria, where it raged for a long time far and wide, destroying an immense multitude of people[1]. In another passage Beda says that the same mortality occurred also among the East Saxons, and he appears to connect therewith their lapse to paganism[2].

The epidemic is said to have entered Ireland at the beginning of August, but whether in 664 or 665 is not clear. According to one of those vague estimates which we shall find again in connexion with the Black Death, the mortality in Ireland was so vast that only a third part of the people were left alive. The Irish annals do, however, contain a long list of notables who died in the pestilence[3].

Beda follows his general reference to the plague by a story of the monastery of Rathmelsigi, identified with Melfont in

[1] " Eodem anno dominicae incarnationis sexcentesimo sexagesimo quarto, facta erat eclipsis solis die tertio mensis Maii, hora circiter decima diei; quo etiam anno subita pestilentiae lues, depopulatis prius australibus Brittaniae plagis, Nordanhymbrorum quoque provinciam corripiens, atque acerba clade diutius longe lateque desaeviens, magnam hominum multitudinem stravit. Qua plaga praefatus Domini sacerdos Tuda raptus est de mundo, et in monasterio, quod dicitur Paegnalaech, honorifice sepultus. Haec autem plaga Hiberniam quoque insulam pari clade premebat. Erant ibidem eo tempore multi nobilium simul et mediocrium de gente Anglorum, qui tempore Finani et Colmani episcoporum, relicta insula patria, vel divinae lectionis, vel continentioris vitae gratia, illo secesserant......Erant inter hos duo juvenes magnae indolis, de nobilibus Anglorum, Aedilhun et Ecgberct," etc. Beda's *Hist. Eccles.* ed. Stevenson. Engl. Hist. Soc. I. p. 231.

[2] *Ibid.* p. 240.

[3] *Annals of the Four Masters*, I. 275.

Meath, which he heard many years after from the chief actor in it. Egbert, an English youth of noble birth, had gone to Ireland to lead the monastic life, like many more of his countrymen of the same rank or of the middle class. The plague in his monastery had been so severe that all the monks either were dead of it or had fled before it, save himself and another, who were both lying sick of the disease. Egbert's companion died; and he himself, having vowed to lead a life of austerity if he were spared, survived to give effect to his vow and died in the year 729 with a great name for sanctity at the age of ninety.

The plague of 664 is said, perhaps on constructive evidence[1], to have continued in England and Ireland for twenty years; and there are several stories told by Beda of incidents in monasteries which show, at least, that outbreaks of a fatal infection occurred here or there as late as 685. Several of these relate to the new monastery of Barking in Essex, founded for monks and nuns by a bishop of London in 676. First we have a story relating to many deaths on the male side of the house[2], and then two stories in which a child of three and certain nuns figure as dying of the pestilence[3]. Another story appears to relate to the plague in a monastery on the Sussex coast, seemingly Selsea[4]. Still another, in which Beda

[1] Thorpe, in his edition of Florence of Worcester, for the Eng. Hist. Society, I. 25.

[2] The first of Beda's incidents of the Barking monastery relates to a miraculous sign in the heavens showing where the cemetery was to be. It begins: "Cum tempestas saepe dictae cladis, late cuncta depopulans, etiam partem monasterii hujus illam qua viri tenebantur, invasisset, et passim quotidie raperentur ad Dominum."

[3] "Erat in eodem monasterio [Barking] puer trium circiter, non amplius annorum, Æsica nomine, qui propter infantilem adhuc aetatem in virginum Deo dedicatarum solebat cella nutriri, ibique medicari. Hic praefata pestilentia tactus ubi ad extrema pervenit clamavit tertio unam de consecratis Christo virginibus, proprio eam nomine quasi praesentem alloquens 'Eadgyd, Eadgyd, Eadgyd'; et sic terminans temporalem vitam intravit aeternam. At virgo illa, quam moriens vocabat, ipso quo vocata est die de hac luce subtracta, et illum qui se vocavit ad regnum coeleste secuta est." Beda, p. 265. Then follows the story of a nun dying of the pestilence in the same monastery.

[4] Beda, Lib. IV. cap. 14. In addition to the instances in the text, which I have collected from Beda's *Ecclesiastical History*, I find two mentioned by Willan in his "Inquiry into the Antiquity of the Smallpox," (*Miscell. Works*, London, 1821,

himself is supposed to have played a part, is told of the monastery of Jarrow, the date of it being deducible from the context as the year 685.

Of the two Northumbrian monasteries founded by Benedict, that of Wearmouth lost several of its monks by the plague, as well as its abbot Easterwine, who is otherwise known to have died in March, 685. The other monastery of Jarrow, of which Ceolfrith was abbot, was even more reduced by the pestilence. All who could read, or preach, or say the antiphonies and responses were cut off, excepting the abbot and one little boy whom Ceolfrith had brought up and taught. For a week the abbot conducted the shortened services by himself, after which he was joined by the voice of the boy ; and these two carried on the work until others had been instructed. Beda, who is known to have been a pupil of Ceolfrith's at Jarrow, would then have been about twelve years old, and would correspond to the boy in the story[1].

The nature of these plagues, beginning with the great invasion of 664, can only be guessed. They have the look of having been due to some poison in the soil, running hither and thither, as the Black Death did seven centuries after, and re-

pp. 109, 110) : "About the year 672, St Cedda, Bishop of the East Saxons, being on a visitation to the monastery of Lestingham, was infected with a contagious distemper, and died on the seventh day. Thirty monks, who came to visit the tomb of their bishop, were likewise infected, and most of them died" (*Vita S. Ceddae,* VII. Jan. p. 375. Cf. Beda, IV. 3). Again : "In the course of the year 685, the disease re-appeared at Lindisfarne, (Holy Island), St Cuthbert's abbacy, and in 686 spread through the adjoining district, where it particularly affected children" (*Vita S. Cuthberti,* cap. 33). Willan's erudition has been used in support of a most improbable hypothesis, that the pestilence of those years, in monasteries and elsewhere, was smallpox.

[1] *Historia Abbatum Gyrvensium, auctore anonymo,* §§ 13 and 14. (App. to vol. II. of Beda's works. Eng. Hist. Society's edition, p. 323.)

§ 13. Qui dum transmarinis moraretur in locis [Benedict] ecce subita pestilentiae procella Brittaniam corripiens lata nece vastavit, in qua plurimi de utroque ejus monasterio, et ipse venerabilis ac Deo dilectus abbas Eosterwini raptus est ad Dominum, quarto ex quo abbas esse coeperat anno.

§ 14. Porro in monasterio cui Ceolfridus praeerat omnes qui legere, vel praedicare, vel antiphonas ac responsoria dicere possent ablati sunt excepto ipso abbate et uno puerulo, qui ab ipso nutritus et eruditus.

In the Article "Baeda," *Dict. Nat. Biog.,* the Rev. W. Hunt points out that the boy referred to in the above passage would have been Beda himself.

maining in the country to break out afresh, not universally as at first, but here and there, as in monasteries. The hypothesis of a late extension to England and Ireland of the great European invasion of bubo-plague in 543, would suit the facts so far as we know them. The one medical detail which has been preserved, on doubtful authority, that the disease was a *pestis ictericia*, marked by yellowness of the skin, and colloquially known in the Irish language as *buide connaill*, is not incompatible with the hypothesis of bubo-plague, and is otherwise unintelligible[1].

For the next seven centuries, the pestilences of Britain are mainly the results of famine and are therefore of indigenous origin. So strongly is the type of famine-pestilence impressed upon the epidemic history of medieval England that the chroniclers and romancists are unable to dissociate famine from their ideas of pestilence in general. Thus Higden, in his reference to the outbreak of the Justinian plague at Constantinople, associates it with famine alone[2]; and the metrical romancist, Robert of Brunne, who had the great English famine of 1315–16 fresh in his memory, describes circumstantially the plague of 664 or the plague of Cadwallader's time, as a famine-pestilence, his details being taken in part from the account given by Simeon of Durham of the harrying of Yorkshire by William the Conqueror, and in part, doubtless, from his own recent experience of a great English famine[3]. But before we come to these typical famine-pestilences of Britain, which fill the medieval interval between the foreign invasion of plague in Beda's time and the foreign invasion of 1348, it remains to dispose in this place of those outbreaks on English soil which do not bear the marks of famine-sickness, but, on the other hand, the marks of a virulent infection arising at particular spots probably from a tainted soil. These have to be collected from casual notices in the most

---

[1] The history of the name *pestis flava ictericia* is given by O'Donovan in a note to the passage in the *Annals of the Four Masters*, I. 275 : "Icteritia vel aurigo, id est abundantia flavae bilis, per corpus effusae, hominemque pallidum reddentis," is the explanation of P. O'S. Beare. The earliest mention of "yellow plague" appears to have been in an ancient life of St Gerald of Mayo, in Colgan's *Acta Sanctorum*, at the calendar date of 13th March.

[2] *Polychronicon*, Rolls edition, v. 250.

[3] *The Story of England*, Rolls series, ed. Furnivall, II. 569.

unlikely corners of monastic chronicles; but it is just the casual nature of the references that makes them credible, and leads one to suppose that the recorded instances are only samples of epidemics not altogether rare in the medieval life of England.

Early Epidemics not connected with Famine.

The earliest of these is mentioned in the annals of the priory of Christ Church, Canterbury.   In the year 829, all the monks save five are said to have died of pestilence, so that the monastery was left almost desolate.   The archbishop Ceolnoth, who was also the abbot of the monastery, filled up the vacancies with secular clerks, and he is said to have done so with the consent of the five monks "that did outlive the plague."   The incident comes into the Canterbury MS. of the Anglo-Saxon Chronicle[1] under the year 870, in connexion with the death of Ceolnoth and the action of his successor in expelling the seculars and completing the original number of regulars.   So far as the records inform us, that great mortality within the priory of Christ Church two centuries after it was founded by Augustine, was an isolated event; the nearest general epidemic to it in the Anglo-Saxon Chronicle was a great mortality of man and beast about the year 897 following the Danish invasion which Alfred at length repelled.

That such deadly intramural epidemics in monasteries were not impossible is conclusively proved by the authentic particulars of a sudden and severe mortality among the rich monks of Croyland at a much more recent date—between the years 1304 and 1315.   In the appendix to the chronicle of Ramsey Abbey[2] there is printed a letter from Simon, abbot of Croyland, without date but falling between the years above given, addressed to his neighbours the abbots of Ramsey, Peterborough and Thorney, and the prior of Spalding.   The letter is to ask their prayers on the occasion of the sudden death of thirteen of the monks of Croyland and the sickness of others; that large number of the

---

[1] Rolls series, ed. Thorpe, I. 136, 137 (Transl. II. 60).   Also in Gervase of Canterbury, Rolls series, ed. Stubbs, II. 348.

[2] *Chronicon Abbatiae Ramesiensis,* Rolls ed. 1886, p. 397.

brethren had been cut off within fifteen days—"potius violenter rapti quam fataliter resoluti[1]." The letter is written from Daddington, whither abbot Simon had doubtless gone to escape the infection.

These are two instances of deadly epidemics within the walls of English monasteries. In the plague-years 664—685, and long after in the Black Death, the mortalities among the monks were of the same degree, only there was an easy explanation of them, in one if not in both cases, as being part of an imported infection universally diffused in English soil. What the nature of the occasional outbreaks in earlier times may have been, we can only guess: something almost as deadly, we may say, as the plague itself, and equally sudden. The experience was not peculiar to England. An incident at Rome almost identical with that of Vighard in 668 is related in a letter sent home in 1188, by Honorius the prior of Canterbury, who had gone with others of the abbey on a mission to Rome to obtain judgment in a dispute between the archbishop and the abbey, that the whole of his following was stricken with sickness and that five were dead. John de Bremble, who being also abroad was ordered to go to the help of the prior, wrote home to the abbey that when he reached Rome only one of the brethren was alive, and he in great danger, and that the first thing he had to do on his arrival was to attend the cook's funeral[2].

There is no clue to the type of these fatal outbreaks of sickness within monastic communities. One naturally thinks of a soil-poison fermenting within and around the monastery walls, and striking down the inmates by a common influence as if at one blow. There are in the medieval history previous to the Black Death a few instances of local pestilences among the common people also, which differ from the ordinary famine-sicknesses of the time. The most significant of these is a story told by William of Newburgh at the end of his chronicle and

---

[1] According to an inquisition of 2 Edward III., the abbey of Croyland contained in 1328, forty-one monks, besides fifteen "corrodiarii" and thirty-six servitors. *Chronicle of Croyland* in Gale, I. 482.

[2] *Epistolae Cantuarienses*, Rolls series, No. 38, ed. Stubbs, Epist. CCLXXII. p. 254, and Introduction, p. lxvii.

probably dating from the corresponding period, about the year 1196[1]. For several years there had been, as we shall see, famine and fever in England; but the particular incident does not relate to the famine, although it may join on to it. It is the story of a ghost walking, and it comes from the village of Annan on the Solway, having been related to the monk of Newburgh in Yorkshire by one who had been an actor in it. A man who had fled from Yorkshire and taken refuge in the village under the castle of Annan, was killed in a quarrel about the woman whom he had married, and was buried without the rites of the church. His unquiet ghost walked, and his corpse tainted the air of the village; pestilence was in every house, so that the place which had been populous looked as if deserted, those who escaped the plague having fled. William of Newburgh's informant had been in the midst of these calamities, and had taken a lead in mitigating them; he had gone to certain wise men living "in sacra dominica quae Palmarum dicitur," and having taken counsel with them, he addressed the people: " Let us dig up that pestilence and let us burn it with fire" (*effodiamus pestem illam et comburamus igni*). Two young men were, accordingly, induced to set about the task. They had not far to dig: " repente cadaver non multa humo egesta nudaverunt, enormi corpulentia distentum, facie rubenti turgentique supra modum."

The story, like others of the kind with a mixture of legend in them, is more symbolical than real. The wise men of Annan may have been in error in tracing the plague of their village to a single corpse, but they were probably on the right lines of causation. It is curious to observe in another chronicler of the same period, Ralph of Coggeshall in Essex, and in a part of his chronicle which relates to the last years of Richard I., and first years of John, a comment upon the action of Pope Innocent III. (about 1200 A.D.) in interdicting all Christian rites save baptism by the clergy in France: " O how horrible...to refuse the Christian rite of burial to the bodies of the dead, so that they infected the air by their foetor and struck horror into the souls of the living by their ghastly looks[2]." The same pope's interdict

---

[1] William of Newburgh, Rolls ed. p. 481.
[2] Ralph of Coggeshall, Rolls series, No. 66, p. 112.

of decent burial and of other clerical rites extended to England in 1208, the famous Interdict of the reign of John. It was the papal method of checkmating the kingdoms of this world; that it was subversive of traditional decency and immemorial sanitary precaution was a small matter beside the assertion of the authority of Peter.

Rightly or wrongly, taught by experience or misled by fancy, the medieval world firmly believed that the formal and elaborate disposal of the dead had a sanitary aspect as well as a pious. The infection of the air, of which we shall hear much more in connexion with the plague, was a current notion in England for several centuries before the Black Death. Especially does the dread of it find expression where corpses were unburied after a battle, massacre, or calamity of nature. The exertions made in these circumstances to bury the dead, even when all pious and domestic feeling was hardened to the barest thought of self-preservation, are explained in set terms as instigated by the fear of breeding a pestilence. The instinct is as wide as human nature, and there is clear evidence in our own early writers that its sanitary meaning was recognised. One such instance may be quoted from the St Albans annalist of the time of John and first years of Henry III.[1] In the year 1234, an unusually savage raid was made by the Welsh as far as Shrewsbury; they laid waste the country by fire and sword; wayfarers were horrified at the sight of naked and unburied corpses without number by the road sides, preyed on by ravenous beasts and birds; the foetor of so much corruption infected the air on all sides, so that even the dead slew the living. The chronicler's language, "quod etiam homines sanos mortui peremerunt," is marked by the perspicacity or correctness which distinguishes him. When the bubo-plague came to be domesticated in English soil more than a century later, the disposal of the dead became a sanitary question of obvious importance. But even in the centuries before the Black Death, and most of all in the times when the traditional practices of decent burial were interdicted by Popes or turned to mercenary

---

[1] Roger of Wendover, III. 72.

purposes by clergy[1], we shall perhaps not err in looking for one, at least, of the causes of localised outbreaks of pestilence in the tainting of the soil and the air by the corruption of corpses insufficiently buried and coffined.

There still remains, before we come to famine-sickness as the common type of pestilence in medieval England, to discover from the records any evidence of pestilence due to war and invasion. The domestic history from first to last is singularly free from such calamities. The whole history of Mohammedan conquest and occupation is a history of infection following in the train of war; and in Western Europe, at least from the invasion of Italy by Charles VIII., when the medieval period (according to Hallam) closes, the sieges, battles, and campaigns are constantly associated with epidemic sickness among the people as well as among the troops. There is only one period in the history of England, that of the civil wars of the Parliament and the Royalists, in which the people had a real taste of the common continental experience. The civil wars of York and Lancaster, as we shall see, touched the common people little, and appear to have bred no epidemics.

Apart from civil war, there were invasions, by the Welsh and Scots on the western and northern marches, and by the Danes. One instance of pestilence following a Welsh raid in the thirteenth century has been given from Roger of Wendover. A single instance is recorded in the history of the Danish invasions. It has been preserved by several independent chroniclers, with some variation in details; and it appears to have been distinguished by so much notice for the reason that it illustrates the magnanimity, sanctity, and miraculous power of St Elphege, archbishop of Canterbury.

In the year 1010 (or 1011 according to some), the Danes had stormed Canterbury, burnt the fair city, massacred the inhabitants, or carried them captive to their ships at Sandwich.

[1] In the Life of St Hugh of Lincoln, who died in 1200, or eight years before the Papal Interdict, there is a clear reference to difficulties thrown by the priests in the way of burial, especially for the poor, and perhaps in a time of epidemic sickness such as the years 1194—6. See *Vita S. Hugonis Lincolnensis*, Rolls series, No. 37, pp. 228—233.

The archbishop Elphege was put on board a small vessel and taken (doubtless by the inland channel which was then open from the Stour to the Thames) to Greenwich, where he was imprisoned for seven months[1]. A council had assembled in London for the purpose of raising forty thousand pounds to buy off the invaders. According to the account used by Higden[2], Elphege refused to sanction the payment of a ransom of three thousand pounds for his own person : he was accordingly taken from prison, and on the 13th of the Calends of May, 1010, was stoned to death by the Danes disappointed of his ransom. Therefore a pestilence fell upon the invaders, a *dolor viscerum*, which destroyed them by tens and twenties so that a large number perished. The earlier narrative of William of Malmesbury[3] is diversified by the introduction of a miracle, and is otherwise more circumstantial. While the archbishop was held in durance, a deadly sickness broke out among the Danes, affecting them in troops (*catervatim*), and proving so rapid in its effects that death ensued before they could feel pain. The stench of their unburied bodies so infected the air as to bring a plague upon those of them who had remained well. As the survivors were thrown into a panic, " sine numero, sine modo," Elphege appeared upon the scene, and having administered to them the consecrated bread, restored them to health and put an end to the plague.

Disregarding what is fabulous, we may take these narratives to establish the fact that a swift and fatal pestilence did break out among the Danes in Kent. It had consisted probably of the same forms of camp sickness, including dysentery (as the name *dolor viscerum* implies), which have occurred in later times. It is the only instance of the kind recorded in the early history.

---

[1] Eadmer, *l.c.*

[2] *Polychronicon*, Rolls ed. VII. 90.

[3] *Gesta Pontificum*, Rolls ed. p. 171. Another narrator of the story of St Elphege and the Danes is Henry of Huntingdon (Rolls ed. p. 179) ; he says nothing of the pestilence, but describes the sack of Canterbury. Eadmer also (*Historia Novorum in Anglia*, Rolls ser. 81, p. 4) omits the pestilence.

Medieval Famine-pestilences.

The foregoing are all the instances of pestilence in early English history, unconnected with famine, that have been collected in a search through the most likely sources. The history of English epidemics, previous to the Black Death, is almost wholly a history of famine sicknesses; and the list of such famines with attendant sickness, without mentioning the years of mere scarcity, is a considerable one.

TABLE OF FAMINE-PESTILENCES IN ENGLAND.

Year	Character	Authority
679	Three years' famine in Sussex from droughts	Beda, *Hist. Eccles.* § 290
793	General famine and severe mortality	Anglo-Saxon Chronicle, *sub anno.* Roger of Howden. Simeon of Durham
897	Mortality of men and cattle for three years during and after Danish invasion	Anglo-Saxon Chronicle. Florence of Worcester. Annales Cambriae (*anno* 896)
962	Great mortality: "the great fever in London"	Anglo-Saxon Chronicle
976	Famine	Anglo-Saxon Chronicle. Roger of Howden
984 986 987	Famine. Fever of men and murrain of cattle	Anglo-Saxon Chronicle. Roger of Howden. Simeon of Durham. Malmesbury. *Gest. Pontif. Angl.* p. 171. Flor. of Worcester. Roger of Wendover, *Flor. Hist.* Bromton (in Twysden). Higden
1005	Desolation following expulsion of Danes	Henry of Huntingdon
1036 1039	Famine	Anglo-Saxon Chronicle. Henry of Huntingdon
1044	Famine	Anglo-Saxon Chronicle
1046	Very hard winter; pestilence and murrain	Anglo-Saxon Chronicle
1048 1049	Great mortality of men and cattle	Anglo-Saxon Chronicle (*sub anno* 1049). Roger of Howden. Simeon of Durham (*sub anno* 1048)

Year	Character	Authority
1069	Wasting of Yorkshire	Simeon of Durham, ii. 188
1086 1087	Great fever-pestilence. Sharp famine	Anglo-Saxon Chronicle. Malmesbury. Henry of Huntingdon, and most annalists
1091	Siege of Durham by the Scots	Simeon of Durham, ii. 339
1093 1095 1096 1097	Floods; hard winter; severe famines; universal sickness and mortality	Anglo-Saxon Chronicle. Annals of Winchester. William of Malmesbury. Henry of Huntingdon. Annals of Margan. Matthew Paris, and others
1103 1104 1105	General pestilence and murrain	Anglo-Saxon Chronicle. Roger of Wendover
1110 1111	Famine	Anglo-Saxon Chronicle. Roger of Wendover
1112	" Destructive pestilence"	Anglo-Saxon Chronicle. Annals of Osney. Annales Cambriae
1114	Famine in Ireland; flight or death of people	Annals of Margan
1125	Most dire famine in all England; pestilence and murrain	Anglo-Saxon Chronicle. William of Malmesbury, *Gest. Pont.* p. 442. Henry of Huntingdon. Annals of Margan. Roger of Howden.
[1130	Great murrain	Annals of Margan. Anglo-Saxon Chronicle (*sub anno* 1131)]
1137 1140	Famine from civil war; mortality	Anglo-Saxon Chronicle. Annals of Winchester. Henry of Huntingdon (1138)
1143	Famine and mortality.	Gesta Stephani, p. 98. William of Newburgh. Henry of Huntingdon
1171	Famine in London in Spring	Stow, *Survey of London*
1172	Dysentery among the troops in Ireland	Radulphus de Diceto, *Imag. Hist.* i. 348
1173	" Tussis quaedam mala et inaudita"	Chronica de Mailros
1175	Pestilence; famine	Benedict of Peterborough. Roger of Howden

Year	Character	Authority
1189	Famine and mortality	Annals of Margan. Giraldus Cambrensis, *Itin. Walliae*
1194 1195 1196 1197	Effects of a five years' scarcity; great mortality over all England	Annals of Burton. William of Newburgh. Roger of Howden iii. 290. Rigord. Bromton (in Twysden col. 1271). Radulphus de Diceto (*sub anno* 1197)
1201	Unprecedented plague of people and murrain of animals	Chronicon de Lanercost (probably relates to 1203)
1203	Great famine and mortality	Annals of Waverley. Annals of Tewkesbury. Annals of Margan. Ralph of Coggeshall (*sub anno* 1205)
1210	Sickly year throughout England	Annals of Margan
1234	Third year of scarcity; sickness	Roger of Wendover. Annals of Tewkesbury
1247	Pestilence from September to November; dearth and famine	Matthew Paris. Higden Annales Cambriae (*sub anno* 1248)
1257 1258 1259	Bad harvests; famine and fever in London and the country	Matthew Paris. Annals of Tewkesbury. Continuator of M. Paris (1259). Rishanger
1268	Probably murrain only. ("Lungessouth")	Chronicon de Lanercost
1271	Great famine and pestilence in England and Ireland	Continuator of William of Newburgh ii. 560 [doubtful]
[1274	Beginning of a great imported murrain among sheep	Rishanger (also *sub anno* 1275). Contin. Fl. of Worcester *sub anno* 1276]
1285	Deaths from heat and drought	Rishanger
1294	Great scarcity; epidemics of flux	Rishanger. Continuator of Florence of Worcester p. 405. Trivet
1315 1316	General famine in England; great mortality from fever, flux &c.; murrain	Trokelowe. Walsingham, *Hist. Angl.* i. 146. Contin. Trivet, pp. 18, 27. Rogers, *Hist. of Agric. and Prices*
1322	Famine and mortality in Edward II.'s army in Scotland; scarcity in London	Higden. Annales Londinenses

C.

The period covered by this long list is itself a long one; and the intervals between successive famine-pestilences are sometimes more than a generation. A history of epidemics is necessarily a morbid history. In this chapter of it, we search out the lean years, saying nothing of the fat years; and by exclusively dwelling upon the dark side we may form an entirely wrong opinion of the comforts or hardships, prosperity or adversity, of these remote times. English writers of the earliest period, when they use generalities, are loud in praise of the advantages of their own island; until we come to the fourteenth century poem of 'The Vision of Piers the Ploughman' we should hardly suspect, from their usual strain, that England was other than an earthly paradise, and every village an Auburn, "where health and plenty cheered the labouring swain." There is a poem preserved in Higden's *Polychronicon* by one Henricus, who is almost certainly Henry archdeacon of Huntingdon in the time of Henry I., although the poem is not included among the archdeacon's extant verse. The subject is 'De Praerogativis Angliae,' and the period, be it remarked, is one of the early Norman reigns, when the heel of the conquering race is supposed to have been upon the neck of the English. Yet this poem contains the famous boast of 'Merry England,' and much else that is the reverse of unhappy:—

> "Anglia terra ferax et fertilis angulus orbis.
> Anglia plena jocis, gens libera, digna jocari;
> Libera gens, cui libera mens et libera lingua:
> Sed lingua melior liberiorque manus.
> Anglia terrarum decus et flos finitimarum,
> Est contenta sui fertilitate boni.
> Externas gentes consumptis rebus egentes,
> Quando fames laedit, recreat et reficit.
> Commoda terra satis mirandae fertilitatis
> Prosperitate viget, cum bona pacis habet[1]."

Or, to take another distich, apparently by Alfred of Beverley,

> "Insula praedives, quae toto non eget orbe,
> Et cujus totus indiget orbis ope."

[1] Quoted by Higden, *Polychronicon*, Rolls ed. II. 18. This may have been one of Henry of Huntingdon's poems which were extant in Leland's time, but are now lost.

Or, in Higden's own fourteenth century words, after quoting these earlier estimates : " Prae ceteris gulae dedita, in victu et vestitu multum sumptuosa[1]. "

On the other hand there is a medieval proverbial saying which places England in a light strangely at variance with this native boast of fertility, plenty, and abundance overflowing to the famished peoples abroad : " Tres plagae tribus regionibus appropriari solent, Anglorum fames, Gallorum ignis, Normannorum lepra"—three afflictions proper to three countries, famine to England, St Anthony's fire to France, leprosy to Normandy[2]. Whatever the " lepra Normannorum" may refer to, there is no doubt that St Anthony's fire, or ergotism from the use of bread containing the grains of spurred rye, was a frequent scourge of some parts of France ; and, in common repute abroad, famine seems to have been equally characteristic of England. Perhaps the explanation of England's evil name for famines is that there were three great English famines in the medieval history, before the Black Death, separated by generations, no doubt, but yet of such magnitude and attended by so disgraceful circumstances that the rumour of them must have spread to foreign countries and made England a by-word among the nations. These were the famines of 1194–96, 1257–59, and 1315–16. Of the first we have a tolerably full account by William of Newburgh, who saw it in Yorkshire ; of the second we have many particulars and generalities by Matthew Paris of St Albans, who died towards the end of it ; and of the third we have an account by one of his successors as historiographer at St Albans, John Trokelowe. All other references to famine in England are meagre beside the narratives of these competent observers, although there were probably two or three famines in the Norman period equally worthy of the historian's pen. For the comprehension of English famine-pestilences in general, we ought to take the best recorded first ; but it will be on the whole

---

[1] *Polychronicon*, II. 166.

[2] Marchand, *Étude sur quelques épidémies et endémies du moyen âge* (Thèse), Paris, 1873, p. 49, with a reference to Fuchs, " Das heilige Feuer im Mittelalter " in Hecker's *Annalen*, vol. 28, p. 1, which journal I have been unable to consult.

more convenient to observe the chronological order, and to introduce, as occasion offers, some generalities on the types of disease which famine induced, the extent of the mortalities, and the conditions of English agriculture and food-supply which made possible occasional famines of such magnitude.

From the great plague "of Cadwallader's time," which corresponds in history to the foreign invasion of pestilence in 664, until nearly the end of the Anglo-Saxon rule, there is little recorded of famines and consequent epidemic sickness. It does not follow that the period was one of plenty and prosperity for the people at large. The Anglo-Saxon Chronicle is at no period detailed or circumstantial on the subject of famines and pestilences; and although the entries become more numerous in the last hundred years before the Chronicle came to an end in 1137, their paucity in the earlier period probably means no more than the imperfection of the record. Some of the generalities of Malthus might be applied to help the imagination over a period of history which we might otherwise be disposed to view as the Golden Age. One of these, originally written for the South Sea Islands, is applicable to all romantic pictures of "rude plenty," such as the picture of the Anglo-Saxon household in *Ivanhoe.* It has been remarked of Scott as a novelist that he always feeds everyone well; but the picture, grateful to the imagination though it be, is probably an illusion. "In a state of society," says Malthus, "where the lives of the inferior order of the people seem to be considered by their superiors as of little or no value, it is evident that we are very liable to be deceived with regard to the appearances of abundance"; and again: "We may safely pronounce that among the shepherds of the North of Europe, war and famine were the principal checks that kept the population down to the level of their scanty means of subsistence." The history of English agriculture is known with some degree of accuracy from the thirteenth century, and it is a history of prices becoming steadier and crops more certain. It is not to be supposed that tillage was more advanced before the Conquest than after it. On the other hand the probabilities are that England had steadily emerged from a pastoral state. It would be unfair to judge of the state of rural England at any time by the state of Wales in the twelfth century, as it is described by Giraldus Cambrensis, or by the condition of Ireland as described from the same traveller's observations. But in the absence of any concrete view of primitive England itself, the picture of the two neighbouring provinces may be introduced here.

Ireland, says Giraldus, closely following Beda, is a fertile land neglected; it had no agriculture, industries or arts; its inhabitants were rude and inhospitable, leading a purely pastoral life, and living more upon milk than upon meat. At the same time there was little sickness; the island had little need of physicians; you will hardly ever find people ill unless they be at the extremity of death; between continuous good health and final dissolution there was no middle term. The excessive number of children born blind, or deaf, or deformed, he ascribes to incestuous unions and other sexual laxities[1].

The picture of Wales is that of a not less primitive society[2]. The Welsh do not congregate in towns, or in villages, or in fortified places, but live solitary in the woods; they build no sumptuous houses of stone and lime, but only ozier booths, sufficient for the year, which they run up with little labour or cost. They have neither orchards nor gardens, and little else than pasture land. They partake of a sober meal in the evening, and if there should be little or nothing to eat at the close of day, they wait patiently until the next evening. They do not use table-cloths nor towels; they are more natural than neat (*naturae magis student quam nitori*). They lie down to sleep in their day clothes, all in one room, with a coarse covering drawn over them, their feet to the fire, lying close to keep each other warm, and when they are sore on one side from lying on the hard floor, they turn over to the other. There are no beggars among this nation. It is of interest, from the point of view of the "positive checks" of Malthus, to note that Giraldus more than hints at the practice of a grosser form of immorality than he had charged the Irish with. Spinning and weaving were of

---

[1] Giraldus Cambrensis, *Topographia Hiberniae*, in Rolls edition of his works; No. 21, vol. v.

[2] "Itinerarium Walliae" and "Descriptio Kambriae," *Opera*, vol. vi.

course not unknown, for the hard and rough blanket mentioned above was a native product. By the time that Higden wrote (about 1340), he has to record a considerable advance in the civilization of Wales. Having used the description of Giraldus, he adds: "They now acquire property, apply themselves to agriculture, and live in towns[1]." But in the reign of Henry II., it was found easy to bring the rebellious Welsh to terms by stopping the supplies of corn from England, upon which they were largely dependent[2].

Of the condition of Scotland in the twelfth century we have no such sketch as Giraldus has left for Wales and Ireland. Uncivilized compared with England, the northern part of the island must certainly have been, if we may trust the indignant references by Simeon of Durham and Henry of Huntingdon to the savage practices of the Scots who swarmed over the border, with or without their king to lead them, or the remark by William of Malmesbury concerning the Scots who went on the Crusade leaving behind them the insects of their native country.

Giraldus intended to have written an itinerary or topography of England also, but his purpose does not appear to have been fulfilled. Higden, his immediate successor in that kind of writing a century and a half later, is content, in his section on England, to reproduce the generalities of earlier authors from Pliny downwards. Of these, we have already quoted the 'Prerogatives of England' by Henry of Huntingdon, from which one might infer that the British Isles, under the Norman yoke, were the Islands of the Blest. On the other hand, the impression made by the details of the Domesday survey upon a historian of the soundest judgment, Hallam, is an impression of poor cultivation and scanty sustenance. "There cannot be a more striking proof," he says, "of the low condition of English agriculture in the eleventh century than is exhibited in Domesday book. Though almost all England had been partially cultivated, and we find nearly the same manors, except in the north, which exist at present, yet the value and extent of cultivated ground are inconceivably small. With every allowance

---

[1] *Polychronicon*, I. 410.

[2] William of Newburgh, *sub anno* 1157, I. 107.

for the inaccuracies and partialities of those by whom that famous survey was completed, we are lost in amazement at the constant recurrence of two or three carucates in demesne, with folkland occupied by ten or a dozen villeins, valued all together at forty shillings, as the return of a manor which now would yield a competent income to a gentleman [1]."

Whether the population at the Domesday survey were nearer two millions than one, the people were almost wholly on the land. Of the size of the chief towns, as the Normans found them, we may form a not incorrect estimate from the Domesday enumeration of houses held of the king or of other superiors [2]. London, Winchester and Bristol do not come at all into the survey. Besides these, the towns of the first rank are Norwich, York, Lincoln, Thetford, Colchester, Ipswich, Gloucester, Oxford, Cambridge,.and Exeter.

Norwich had 1320 burgesses in the time of Edward the Confessor ; in the borough were 665 English burgesses rendering custom, and 480 bordarii rendering none on account of their poverty ; there were also more than one hundred French households. Lincoln had 970 inhabited houses in King Edward's time, of which 200 were waste at the survey. Thetford had 943 burgesses before the Conquest, and at the survey 720, with 224 houses vacant. York was so desolated just before the survey that it is not easy to estimate its ordinary population ; but it may be put at about 1200 houses. Gloucester had 612 burgesses. Oxford seems to have had about 800 houses ; and for Cambridge we find an enumeration of the houses in nine of the ten wards of the town in King Edward's time, the total being about 400. Colchester appears to have had some 700 houses, Ipswich 538 burgesses, with 328 houses "waste" so far as tax was concerned. Exeter had 300 king's houses, and an uncertain number more. Next in importance come such places as Southampton, Wallingford, Northampton, Leicester, Warwick, Shrewsbury, Nottingham, Coventry, Derby, Canterbury, Yarmouth, Rochester, Dover, Sandwich (about 400 houses), and Sudbury. In a third class may be placed towns like Dorchester, Ilchester, Bridport, Wareham, Shaftesbury, Bath, Chichester, Lewes, Guildford, Hythe, Romney, Pevensey, Windsor, Bath, Chester, Worcester, Hereford, Huntingdon, Stamford, Grantham, Hertford, St Albans, Torchesey, Maldon, each with from 100 to 200 burgesses. Dover and Sandwich each supplied twenty ships, with crews of twenty-four men, for King Edward's service during fifteen days of the year. In Hereford there were six smiths, each rendering one penny a year for his forge, and making 120 nails of the king's iron. Many of these houses were exceedingly small, with a frontage of seven feet ; the poorest

---

[1] *Europe during the Middle Ages*, chap. IX.
[2] I have used for this purpose Merewether and Stephens' *History of Boroughs*, 3 vols. 1835.

class were mere sheds, built in the ditch against the town wall, as at York and Canterbury.

It would be within the mark to say that less than one-tenth of the population of England was urban in any distinctive sense of the term. After London, Norwich, York, and Lincoln, there were probably no towns with five thousand inhabitants. There were, of course, the simpler forms of industries, and there was a certain amount of commerce from the Thames, the East Coast, and the Channel ports. The fertile soil of England doubtless sustained abundance of fruit trees and produced corn to the measure of perhaps four or six times the seed. There were flocks of sheep, yielding more wool than the country used, herds of swine and of cattle. The exports of wool, hides, iron, lead, and white metal gave occasion to the importation of commodities and luxuries from Flanders, Normandy, and Gascony. If there was "rude plenty" in England, it was for a sparse population, and it was dependent upon the clemency of the skies. A bad season brought scarcity and murrain, and two bad seasons in succession brought famine and pestilence.

Of the general state of health we may form some idea from the Anglo-Saxon leechdoms, or collections of remedies, charms and divinations, supposed to date from the eleventh century[1]. The maladies to which the English people were liable in these early times correspond on the whole to the everyday diseases of our own age. There were then, as now, cancers and consumptions, scrofula or "kernels," the gout and the stone, the falling sickness and St Vitus' dance, apoplexies and palsies, jaundice, dropsies and fluxes, quinsies and anginas, sore eyes and putrid mouth, carbuncles, boils and wildfire, agues, rheums and coughs. Maladies peculiar to women occupy a chief place, and there is evidence that hysteria, the outcome of hardships, entered largely into the forms of sickness, as it did in the time of Sydenham. Among the curiosities of the nosology may be mentioned wrist-drop, doubtless from working in lead. One great chapter in disease, the sickness and mortality of infants

---

[1] *Leechdoms, Wort-cunning and Starcraft of Early England.* Edited by Cockayne for the Rolls Series, 3 vols. 1864–66.

and children, is almost a complete blank. It ought doubtless to have been the greatest chapter of all. The population remained small, for one reason among others, that the children would be difficult to rear. There is no direct evidence ; but we may infer from analogous circumstances, that the inexpansive population meant an enormous infant mortality. The sounds which fell on the ear of Æneas as he crossed the threshold of the nether world may be taken as prophetic, like so much else in Virgil, of the experience of the Middle Ages :

> " Continuo auditae voces, vagitus et ingens
> Infantumque animae flentes, in limine primo :
> Quos dulcis vitae exsortes, et ab ubere raptos,
> Abstulit atra dies, et funere mersit acerbo."

We come, then, to the chronology of famine-pestilences, and first in the Anglo-Saxon period. The years from 664 to 685 are occupied, as we have seen, by a great plague, probably the bubo-plague, which returned in 1348 as the Black Death, affecting, like the latter, the whole of England and Ireland on its first appearance, and afterwards particular monasteries, such as Barking and Jarrow. But it is clear that famine-sickness was also an incident of the same years. The metrical romancist of the fourteenth century, Robert of Brunne, was probably mistaken in tracing the great plague of "Cadwaladre's time" to famine in the first instance ; there is no such suggestion in the authentic history of Beda. But that historian does make a clear reference to famine in Sussex about the year 679 [1]. Describing the conversion of Sussex to Christianity by Wilfrid, he says that the province had been afflicted with famine owing to three seasons of drought, that the people were dying of hunger, and that often forty or fifty together, "inedia macerati," would proceed to the edge of the Sussex cliffs, and, joining hands, throw themselves into the sea. But on the very day when the people accepted the Christian baptism, there fell a plenteous

---

[1] It is illustrative of the confusion which arises from careless copying by later compilers of history that Roger of Wendover, in his *Flores Historiarum* (Eng. Hist. Society's edition I. 159), takes Beda's Sussex reference to famine and makes it do duty, under the year 665, for the great general plague of 664, having apparently overlooked Beda's entirely distinct account of the latter.

rain, the earth flourished anew, and a glad and fruitful season ensued [1].

The anarchy in Northumbria which followed the death of Beda (in 735), with the decline of piety and learning in the northern monasteries, is said to have led to famine and plague [2]. It is not until the year 793 that an entry of famine and mortality occurs in the Anglo-Saxon Chronicle. It is in keeping with the disappointing nature of all these early records that Simeon of Durham and Roger of Howden, the two compilers who had access to lost records, are more particular in enumerating the portents that preceded the calamity than in describing its actual circumstances. Then a whole century elapses (but for a vague entry under the year 822) until we come to the three calamitous years, with 897 as the centre, which followed Alfred's famous resistance to the Danes. In that mortality, many of the chief thanes died, and there was a murrain of cattle, with a scarcity of food in Ireland. Two generations pass before the chronicle contains another entry of the kind: in 962 there was a great mortality, and the "great fever" was in London. At no long intervals there are two more famines, in 976 and 986. That of 986 (or 987) would appear to have been severe; the church plate at Winchester was melted for the benefit of the starving [3], and there was "a fever of men and a murrain of cattle [4]." After the expulsion of the Danes in 1005, says Henry of Huntingdon, there was such desolation of famine as no one

---

[1] *Hist. Eccles.* § 290 :—" Siquidem tribus annis ante adventum ejus in provinciam, nulla illis in locis pluvia ceciderat, unde et fames acerbissima plebem invadens inopia nece prostravit. Denique ferunt quia saepe quadraginta simul aut quinquaginta homines inedia macerati procederent ad praecipitium aliquod sive ripam maris, et junctis misere manibus pariter omnes aut ruina perituri, aut fluctibus absorbendi deciderent. Verum ipso die, quo baptisma fidei gens suscepit illa, descendit pluvia serena sed copiosa, refloruit terra, rediit viridantibus arvis annus laetus et frugifer."

[2] Green, *Short History of the English People*, p. 39 : "The very fields lay waste, and the land was scourged by famine and plague." I have missed this reference to plague in the original authorities. A passage in Higden's *Polychronicon* (v. 258) may relate to that period, although it is referred to the mythical time of Vortigern.

[3] Stow, in enumerating the instances of public charity in his *Survey of London*, ascribes the melting of the church plate to Ethelwald, bishop of Winchester in the reign of King Edgar, about the year 963.

[4] The murrain was a flux, *anglicé* "scitha" (Roger of Howden) or "schitta" (Bromton).

remembered. Then in 1010 or 1011 comes the incident of St Elphege, already given. From 1036 to 1049 we find mention of four, or perhaps five, famines, those of the years 1046 and 1049 being marked by a great mortality of men and murrain of cattle.

Except in Yorkshire, the Norman Conquest had no immediate effects upon the people of England in the way of famine and pestilence. From the last great mortality of 1049, a period of nearly forty years elapses until we come to the great pestilence and sharp famine in the last year of the Conqueror's reign (1086–7). The harrying of Yorkshire, however, is too important a local incident to be passed over in this history. Of these ruthless horrors in the autumn of 1069 we have some particulars from the pen of Simeon of Durham, who has contemporary authority. There was such hunger, he says, that men ate the flesh of their own kind, of horses, of dogs, and of cats. Others sold themselves into perpetual slavery in order that they might be able to sustain their miserable lives on any terms (like the Chinese in later times). Others setting out in exile from their country perished before their journey was ended. It was horrible to look into the houses and farm-yards, or by the wayside, and see the human corpses dissolved in corruption and crawling with worms. There was no one to bury them, for all were gone, either in flight or dead by the sword and famine. The country was one wide solitude, and remained so for nine years. Between York and Durham no one dwelt, and travellers went in great fear of wild beasts and of robbers[1]. William of Malmesbury says that the city of York was so wasted by fire that an old inhabitant would not have recognized it; and that the country was still waste for sixty miles at the time of his writing (1125)[2]. In the Domesday survey we find that there were 540 houses so waste that they paid nothing, 400 houses "not inhabited," of which the better sort pay one penny and others less, and only 50 inhabited houses paying full dues.

The same local chronicler who has left particulars of the

[1] Simeon of Durham, in Rolls series, II. 188. As to fugitives, see Chr. Evesham, p. 91.

[2] *Gesta Pontif. Angl.* p. 208.

devastation of 1069—70, has given also a picture of the siege
of Durham by Malcolm Canmore in 1091, which may serve
to realize for us what a medieval siege was, and what the
Scots marches had to endure for intervals during several
centuries :—

> Malcolm advancing drives the Northumbrians before him, some into the
> woods and hills, others into the city of Durham ; for there have they always
> a sure refuge. Thither they drive their whole flocks and herds and carry
> their furniture, so that there is hardly room within the town for so great a
> crowd. Malcolm arrives and invests the city. It was not easy for one to go
> outside, and the sheep and cattle could not be driven to pasture : the
> churchyard was filled with them, and the church itself was scarcely kept
> clear of them. Mixed with the cattle, a crowd of women and children
> surrounded the church, so that the voices of the choristers were drowned by
> the clamour. The heat of summer adds to the miseries of famine. Every-
> where throughout the town were the sounds of grief, 'et plurima mortis
> imago,' as in the sack of Troy. The siege is raised by the miraculous
> intervention of St Cuthbert[1].

The wasting of Yorkshire by William and the five incursions
of the Scots into Northumberland and Durham in the reign of
Malcolm Canmore had the effect of reducing a large part of the
soil of England to a comparatively unproductive state. The
effacement of farms (and churches) in Hampshire, for the planting of the New Forest, had the same effect in a minor degree.
The rigorous enforcement of the forest laws in the interests of
the Norman nobles must have served also to remove one considerable source of the means of subsistence from the people.
Whether these things, together with the general oppression of
the poor, contributed much or little to what followed, it is the
fact that the long period from the last two years of William
to the welcomed advent of Henry II. to the throne in 1154,
is filled with a record of famines, pestilences, and other national
misfortunes such as no other period of English history shows.

The first general famine and pestilence under Norman rule
was in the years 1086 and 1087, the last of the Conqueror's reign.
It is probable from the entries in the Anglo-Saxon Chronicle
that the aggravation (for which we must always look in order
to explain a historical famine and pestilence) was due to two

---

[1] Simeon of Durham, " On the Miracles of St Cuthbert," *Works,* II. 338–40.

bad harvests in succession. The year 1086 was "heavy, toilsome and sorrowful," through failure of the corn and fruit crops owing to an inclement season, and through murrain of cattle[1]. Some form of sickness appears to have been prevalent between that harvest and the next. Almost every other man, says the Anglo-Saxon Chronicle, was stricken with fever, and that so sharply that many died of it. "Alas! how miserable and how rueful a time was then! when the wretched men lay driven almost to death, and afterwards came the sharp famine and destroyed them quite." It is probably a careless gloss upon that, by a historian of the next generation[2], when he says that "a promiscuous fever destroyed more than half the people," and that famine, coming after, destroyed those whom the fever had spared[3]. But there can be no question that this was one of those great periodic conjunctions of famine and fever ($\lambda\iota\mu\grave{o}\nu$ $\acute{o}\mu o\hat{v}$ $\kappa\alpha\grave{\iota}$ $\lambda o\iota\mu\acute{o}\nu$), of which we shall find fuller details in the chronicles of the twelfth, thirteenth and fourteenth centuries. It is easy to understand that England, with all her wealth of fruits and corn in a good season, had no reserve for the poor at least, and sometimes not even for the rich, to get through two or more bad seasons with. How much the corn crop in those days depended on the season is clear from the entry in the chronicle two years after (1089), that reaping was still in progress at Martinmas (11 November) and even later. Fields cultivated to yield an average of only four or six times the seed were, of course, more at the mercy of the seasons than the highly cultivated corn-land of our own time.

The next famine with pestilence in England, seven years later, or in the seventh year of William Rufus, introduces us to a new set of considerations. It was the time when the exactions of tribute for the king's wars in Normandy, or for the satisfaction of his greed and that of his court, were severely felt both by the church and the people. England, says one[4], was

---

[1] Anglo-Saxon Chronicle. Malmesbury adds "a mortality of men."

[2] William of Malmesbury, *Gest. Reg.* Eng. Hist. Soc. II. 452.

[3] Malmesbury's construction is repeated by Henry of Huntingdon, Rolls ed. p. 209. Florence of Worcester merely says: "primo febribus, deinde fame."

[4] Henry of Huntingdon, p. 232.

suffocated and unable to breathe. Both clergy and laity, says another[1], were in such misery that they were weary of life. But the most remarkable phraseology is that of William of Malmesbury, the chief historian of the period, who seldom descends from the region of high political and ecclesiastical affairs to take notice of such things as famine and pestilence. In the 7th year of Rufus, he says, "agriculture failed" on account of the tributes which the king had decreed from his position in Normandy. The fields running to waste, a famine followed, and that in turn was succeeded by a mortality so general that the dying were left untended and the dead unburied[2]. The phrase about the lack of cultivation is a significant and not incredible statement, which places the England of Rufus in the same light as certain belated feudal parts of India within recent memory.

In the villages of Gujerat, when the festival comes round early in May, the chief of a village collects the cultivators and tells them that it is time for them to commence work. They say : "No ! the assessment was too heavy last year, you lay too many taxes upon us." However, after much higgling, and presents made to the more important men, a day is fixed for cultivation to begin, and the clearing and manuring of the fields proceeds as before[3]. But while Gujerat was still possessed by hundreds of petty feudal chiefs under the Mahratta rule, previous to the establishment of the British Agency in 1821, the exactions of tribute by the Baroda government were so extreme, and enforced by so violent means[4], that cultivation was almost neglected ; the towns and villages swarmed with idlers, who subsisted upon milk and ghee from their cows, while indolence and inactivity affected the whole community[5]. A dreadful famine had "raged with destructive fury" over Gujerat and Kattiwar for more than one year about 1812–13–14, which was followed, not by a contagious fever, but by the true bubo-plague.

If the English historian's language, "agricultura defecit," with

---

[1] Annals of Winchester, *sub anno* 1096.

[2] "Septimo anno propter tributa quae rex in Normannia positus edixerat, agricultura defecit ; qua fatiscente fames e vestigio ; ea quoque invalescente mortalitas hominum subsecuta, adeo crebra ut deesset morituris cura, mortuis sepultura." *Gest. Reg.* II. 506. Copied in the Annals of Margan, Rolls ed. II. 506.

[3] *Râs Mâlâ*, by A. Kinloch Forbes, 2nd ed. p. 543.

[4] *Ibid.*

[5] Thomas Whyte, "Report on the disease which prevailed in Kattywar in 1819–20." *Trans. Med. Phys. Soc. Bombay,* I. (1838), p. 169. See also Gilder, *ibid.* p. 192 ; Frederick Forbes *ibid.* II. 1, and Thesis on Plague, Edin. 1840.

reference to the tribute exacted by Rufus, have that fitness which we have reason to expect from him,—Higden varies it to " ita ut agricultura cessaret et fames succederet,"—then the famine and mortality about the years 1094-5 were due to no less remarkable a cause than a refusal to cultivate the land.   It is not to be supposed that the incubus of excessive tribute passed away with the accession of Henry I.   The Anglo-Saxon Chronicle repeats the complaint of heavy taxation in connexion with bad harvests and murrains in 1103, 1105 and 1110[1].   Severe winters, or autumn floods, with murrains and scarcity, are recorded also for the years 1111, 1115, 1116, 1117, 1124 and 1125, the famine of 1125 having been attended with a mortality, and having been sufficiently great and general to be mentioned by several chroniclers[2].   In the midst of these years of scarcity and its effects upon the population, there occurs one singular entry of another kind in the Anglo-Saxon Chronicle, under the year 1112: "This was a very good year, and very abundant in wood and in field; but it was a very sad and sorrowful one, through a most destructive pestilence[3]."   Under the year 1130, the annalist of the Welsh monastery of Margan, who is specially attentive to domestic events, records a murrain of cattle all over England, which lasted several years so that scarcely one township escaped the pest, the pigsties becoming suddenly empty, and whole meadows swept of their cattle.   It is to the same murrain that the Anglo-Saxon Chronicle refers under the year 1131: in towns where there had been ten or twelve ploughs going there was not one left, and the man who had 200 or 300 swine had not one left; after that died the domestic fowls.

These things happened from time to time in the comparatively prosperous reign of Henry I.   But with the death of Henry in 1135, there began a state of misery and lawlessness lasting

[1] In 1110 the tax was for the dower of the king's daughter on her marriage. That also was parallel with a feudal right in Gujerat : " When a chief has to portion a daughter, or to incur other similar necessary expense, he has the right of imposing a levy upon the cultivators to meet it." A. Kinloch Forbes, *Rás Málá*, 2nd ed. p. 546.   Refusal to plough, *temp.* Henry I. is stated by Pearson, I. 442.

[2] Malmesbury, *Gest. Pont.* p. 442 ; H. of Huntingdon ; Annals of Margan ; Roger of Howden.

[3] Also in the Annals of Osney : " Mortalitas maxima hominum in Anglia."

almost to the accession of Henry II. in 1154, beside which the former state of England was spoken of as "most flourishing[1]." Besides the barbarities of the Scots and the Welsh on the northern and western marches[2], there were the civil wars of the factions of King Stephen and the Empress Maud, and the cruelties and predations of the unruly nobles under the walls of a thousand newly-built strongholds. A graphic account of the condition of England remains to us from the pen of an eyewitness, the observant author of the *Gesta Stephani*[3]. Under the year 1143 he writes that there was most dire famine in all England; the people ate the flesh of dogs and horses or the raw garbage of herbs and roots. The people in crowds pined and died, or another part entered on a sorrowful exile with their whole families. One might see houses of great name standing nearly empty, the residents of either sex and of every age being dead. As autumn drew near and the fields whitened for the harvest, there was no one to reap them, for the cultivators were cut off by the pestilent hunger which had come between. To these home troubles was added the presence of a multitude of barbarous adventurers, without bowels of pity and compassion, who had flocked to the country for military service. The occasion was one of those which cause the archdeacon of Huntingdon to break out into his elegiac verse:

"Ecce Stygis facies, consimilisque lues[4]."

"And in those days," says another, "there was no king in Israel[5]." The Anglo-Saxon Chronicle, which comes to an end in this scene of universal gloom, describes how one might go a day's journey and never find a man sitting in a town, or the land

---

[1] "Attenuata est Anglia, ut ex regno florentissimo infelicissimum videretur." William of Newburgh, Rolls ed. p. 39.

[2] Henry of Huntingdon, *sub anno* 1138.

[3] *Gesta Stephani*, Rolls series, No. 82, vol. III. p. 99. The author is conjectured to have been a foreigner in the service of the bishop of Winchester, brother of the king.

[4] " Affluit ergo fames; consumpta carne gementes
Exhalant animas ossa cutisque vagas.
Quis tantos sepelire queat coetus morientium?
Ecce Stigis facies, consimilisque lues."

[5] William of Newburgh, *sub anno* 1149.

tilled, and how men who once were rich had to go begging their bread, concluding with the words, "And they said openly that Christ and His saints slept."

Among the penances of Henry II. after the murder of Becket, there is recorded his charity in feeding during a dearth ten thousand persons daily from the first of April, 1171, until the harvest[1]. But, apart from a reference to a flux among the troops in Ireland in 1172, from errors of diet[2], the long reign of Henry II. is marked by only one record of general pestilence. It is recorded by the best contemporary writer, Benedict of Peterborough, and it is the first instance in which the number of burials in a day (perhaps at Peterborough) is given. In the year 1175, he says, there was in England and the adjacent regions a pestilential mortality of men, such that on many days seven or eight corpses were carried out to be buried. And immediately upon that pestilential mortality there followed a dire famine[3]. It is to be observed that the famine is explicitly stated to have come after the pestilence, just as in the great mortality of 1087 ; and, as in the latter case, it may be that a hard winter, with scarcity of food, brought a general sickness, and that the scarcity had been raised to famine point by a second bad harvest. The entry in the chronicle of Melrose for 1173 may refer to Scotland only : a bad kind of cough, unheard of before, affected almost everyone far and wide, whereof, "or from which pest," many died. This is perhaps the only special reference to "tussis" as epidemic until the influenzas of the seventeenth century.

The comparative freedom of the long reign of Henry II. from famines and national distress probably arose as much from good government as from the clemency of the seasons. The country was growing rich by foreign trade. In 1190 the two leading Jews of York, Joyce and Benedict, were occupying residences in the heart of the town like royal palaces in size and in the sumptuousness of their furniture. The same historian, William of Newburgh,

---

[1] Stow's *Survey of London*, Popular ed. (1890) p. 116.

[2] "Recentium esus carnium et haustus aquae, tam insolitus quam incognitus, plures de regis exercitu panis inedia laborantes, fluxu ventris afflixit in Hybernia." Radulphus de Diceto, *Imagines Historiar.* I. 350.

[3] Benedict of Peterborough, I. 104, and, in identical terms, in Roger of Howden.

who records the king's protection of these envied capitalists, mentions also his protection of " the poor, the widows and the orphans," and his liberal charities.   That the king's protection of his poorer subjects was not unneeded, would be obvious if we could trust the extraordinary account of the keen traders of London which is put by Richard of Devizes into the mouth of a hostile witness[1]. The peoples of all nations, it appears, flocked to London, each nationality contributing to the morals of the capital its proper vices and manners.   There was no righteous person in London, no, not one; there were more thieves in London than in all France[2]. In the entirely different account, of the same date, by an enthusiastic Londoner, the monk Fitz-Stephen, the only " plagues" of London are said to be " the immoderate drinking of fools and the frequency of fires."   The city and suburbs had one hundred and twenty-six small parish churches, besides thirteen greater conventual churches; and it was a model to all the world for religious observances.   " Nearly all the bishops, abbots, and magnates of England are, as it were, citizens and freemen of London; having there their own splendid houses, to which they resort, where they spend largely when summoned to great councils by the king or by their metropolitan, or drawn thither by their own private affairs[3]."   The archdeacon of London, of the same date, Peter of Blois, in a letter to the pope, Innocent III., concerning the extent of his duties and the smallness of his stipend, gives the parish churches in the city at one hundred and twenty, and the population at forty thousand[4].

---

[1] The speaker is represented as a Jew in France. It is significant that the massacre of the Jews at Lynn in 1190 is stated by William of Newburgh to have been instigated by the *foreign* traders.

[2] Ricardus Divisiensis. Eng. Hist. Society's ed. p. 60.

[3] Description of London, prefixed to Fitzstephen's Life of Becket.   Reproduced in Stow's *Survey of London.*

[4] *Petri Blesensis omnia opera*, ed. Giles, Epist. CLI.   The number of churches may seem large for the population; but it should be kept in mind that these city parish churches were mere chapels or oratories, like the side-chapels of a great church. Indeed, at Yarmouth, they were actually built along the sides of the single great parish church; whereas, at Norwich, there were sixty of them standing each in its own small parish area, the Cathedral, as well as the other conventual churches, being the greater places of worship.   Lincoln is said to have had 49 of these small churches, and York 40.   An example of them remains in St Peter's at Cambridge.

The Germans who came in the train of Richard I. on his return to England in 1194, after his release from the hands of the emperor, were amazed at the display of wealth and finery which the Londoners made to welcome back the king; if the emperor had known the riches of England, they said, he would have demanded a heavier ransom[1]. The ransom, all the same, required a second, or even a third levy before it was raised, owing, it was said, to peculation; and the ecclesiastics, who held a large part of the soil, appear to have had so little in hand to pay their share that they had to pledge the gold and silver vessels of the altar[2].

The year of Richard's accession, 1189, is given by the annalist of the Welsh monastery of Margan, as a year of severe famine and of a mortality of men.   Probably it was a local famine, and it may well have been the same in which Giraldus Cambrensis says that he himself saw crowds of poor people coming day after day to the gates of the monastery of Margan, so that the brethren took counsel and sent a ship to Bristol for corn[3].   The great and general famine with pestilence in Richard's time was in the years 1193, 1194, 1195, 1196 and 1197, and it appears to have been felt in France, in the basin of the Danube, and over all Europe, as well as in England.   Of the pestilence which came with it in England we have an exceptionally full account from the pen of William of Newburgh.   The monastery in which William wrote his history was situated among woods by the side of a stream under the Hambledon hills in Yorkshire, on the road between York and the mouth of the Tees; so that when he says of this famine and pestilence, "we speak what we do know, and testify what we have seen," he may be taken as recording the experience of a sufficiently typical region of rural England.

---

[1] William of Newburgh, p. 431.

[2] *Ibid.*

[3] " His quoque nostris diebus, ingruente famis inedia, et maxima pauperum turba quotidie ad januam jacente, de communi patrum consilio, ad caritatis explendae sufficientiam, propter bladum in Angliam navis Bristollum missa est." *Itiner. Walliae,* Rolls ed. VI. 68. The itinerary of Bishop Baldwin, which the author follows, was in 1188; but the "his quoque nostris diebus" clearly refers to a later date, which may have been the year after, or may have been the more severe famine of 1195-7 or of 1203.

His narrative of the pestilence[1] is given under the year 1196, which was the fourth year of the scarcity or famine : After the crowds of poor had been dying on all sides of want, a most savage plague ensued, as if from air corrupted by dead bodies of the poor.   This pestilence showed but little respect even for those who had abundance of food ; and as to those who were in want, it put an end to their long agony of hunger.   The disease crept about everywhere, always of one type, namely that of an acute fever.   Day after day it seized so many, and finished so many more, so that there were scarcely to be found any to give heed to the sick or to bury the dead.   The usual rites of burial were omitted, except in the case of some nobler or richer person ; at whatever hour anyone died the body was forthwith committed to the earth, and in many places great trenches were made if the number of corpses was too great to afford time for burying them one by one.   And as so many were dying every day, even those who were in health fell into low spirits, and went about with pale faces, themselves the living picture of death.   In the monasteries alone was this pestilence comparatively unfelt.   After it had raged on all sides for five or six months, it subsided when the winter cold came.

Those lean years were doubtless followed by seven fat years ; for it is not until 1203, the fourth year of John, that we again meet with the records of famine and pestilence.   From various monasteries, from Waverley in Sussex, Tewkesbury in Gloucester and Margan in Glamorgan, we have the same testimony—"fames magna et mortalitas," " fames valida, et saeva mortalitas multitudinem pauperum extinguit," " maxima fames."   The monks of Waverley had to leave their own house and disperse themselves through various monasteries.   Two years after, 1205, there came so hard a season that the winter-sown seed was almost killed by frost.   The Thames was crossed on the ice, and there was no ploughing for many weeks.   An Essex annalist says there was a famine, and quotes the famine prices : a quarter of wheat was sold for a pound in many parts of England, although in Henry II.'s time it was often as low as twelve pence ; a quarter of beans

---

[1] *Histor. Rer. Angl.*, Rolls series, No. 82, vol. I. pp. 460, 484.

ten shillings; a quarter of oats forty pence, which used to be four pence[1]. The annalist at Margan enters also the year 1210 as a sickly one throughout England[2].

We are now come to the period when we can read the succession of these events in the domestic life of the people from the more trustworthy records of the St Albans school of historians. Of the scarcity and sickness among the poor in 1234 we have some suggestive particulars by Roger of Wendover[3], and for the series of famines and epidemics from 1257 to 1259 we have a comparatively full account by his famous successor in the office of historiographer to the abbey, Matthew Paris[4]. The next St Albans *scriptorius*, Rishanger[5], notes the kind of harvest every year from 1259 to 1305, and for only one of those years after the scarcity of 1259 was past, namely the year 1294, does he speak of the people dying of hunger. His successor, John Trokelowe[6], carries on the annals to 1323, and gives us some particulars, not without diagnostic value, of the great famine-sickness of 1315–16, and of the succession of dear years of which the epidemic was an incident. It is on these contemporary accounts by the St Albans school, together with the record for the year 1196 by William of Newburgh, that our knowledge of the famine-pestilences of England must be based.

With the harvest of 1259 begins the tabulation of agricultural prices from farm-bailiffs' accounts, by Professor Thorold Rogers, a work of vast labour in which the economic history of the English people is written in indubitable characters, and by means of which we are enabled to check the more general and often rhetorical statements of the contemporary historians.

Although the history of the last year or two of John and of the earlier years of Henry III. is full of turbulence and rapine, yet we hear of no general distress among the cultivators of the soil. The contemporary authority, Roger of Wendover, has no

[1] Ralph of Coggeshall, *sub anno*.
[2] " Variis infirmitatibus homines per Angliam vexantur et quamplures moriuntur," Annals of Margan, Rolls series, No. 36.
[3] Roger of Wendover, *Fl. Hist.* Rolls ed.
[4] Matthew Paris, *Chronica Majora*, Rolls series, No. 57, ed. Luard, vol. v.
[5] Rishanger in *Chron. Monast. S. Albani*, Rolls series, No. 28.
[6] John Trokelowe, *ibid.*

entry of the kind until 1234, excepting a single note under the
year 1222, that wheat rose to twelve shillings the quarter. We
hear of king John and his following as plundering the rich
churchmen and laymen all the way from St Albans to Nottingham, of William Longspée, earl of Salisbury, carrying on the same
practices in the counties of Essex, Middlesex, Hertford, Cambridge and Huntingdon, of the spoliation of the Isle of Ely, and
of the occupation of towns and villages in Essex, Suffolk and
Norfolk by Louis, Dauphin of France, the king-elect, or broken
reed, on whom the Barons of Magna Charta thought for a time
to lean[1]. But the whole of that period, and of the years following
until 1234, is absolutely free from any record of wide-spread
distress among the lower class. We are reminded of the
observation by Philip de Comines, with the civil wars of York
and Lancaster in his mind, a saying which is doubtless true of
all the struggles in England for the settlement of the respective
claims of king and aristocracy: "England has this peculiar
grace," says the French statesman, "that neither the country,
nor the people, nor the houses are wasted or demolished; but
the calamities and misfortunes of the war fall only upon the
soldiers and especially the nobility, of whom they are more than
ordinarily jealous: for nothing is perfect in this world." That
cannot apply of course to the barbarous incursions of the Scots
and the Welsh; for the northern marches were often reduced to
desolation during a period of three hundred years after the
Conquest and were never more desolate than in the reign of
Richard II.; while the marches of Wales were subject to not
less ruthless spoliations until the concessions to the Welsh
by Edward I. Nor is the immunity of the peasantry from the
troubles of civil war to be taken as absolute; for we find
under the year 1264, when Simon de Montfort was in the field
against the king, an explicit statement that the small peasantry
were plundered even to the poor furniture of their cottages. But
on the whole we may take it that the paralysing effect of civil
war seldom reached to the English lower classes in the medieval
period, that the tenour of their lives was seldom disturbed except

---

[1] Wendover, II. 162, 171, 190, 205.

by famine or plague, and that kings and nobles were left to fight it out among themselves.

We become aware, however, from the time of the Great Charter, and during the steady growth of the country's prosperity, of a widening chasm between the rich and the poor within the ranks of the commons themselves, and that too, not only in the centres of trade (as we shall see), but also in country districts. The claims of feudal service did not prevent some among the villagers from adding house to house, and field to field, thereby marking in every parish the interval between the thriving and comfortable and a residuum of *pauperes* composed of the less capable or the less fortunate. A curious story, told by Roger of Wendover of the village of Abbotsley near St Neots, will serve as an illustration of a fact which we might be otherwise well assured of from first principles[1].

The year 1234 was the third of a succession of lean years. So sharp was the famine before the harvest of that year, that crowds of the poor went to the fields in the month of July, and plucked the unripe ears of corn, rubbing them in their hands and eating the raw grain. The St Albans monk is full of indignation against the prevailing spirit of avarice which reduced some of the people to that sad necessity: Alms had everywhere gone out of fashion; the rich, abounding in all manner of temporal goods, were so smitten with blind greed that they suffered Christian men, made in the image of God, to die for want of food. Some, indeed, were so impious as to say that their wealth was due to their own industry, and not to the gift of God. Of that mind seem to have been the more prosperous cultivators of the village of Abbotsley "who looked on the needy with an eye of suspicion[2]."

The following story is told of them. Seeing the poor making free with their corn in the ear, they assembled in the parish church on a Sunday in August, and assailed the parson with their clamours, demanding that he would forthwith pronounce the ban of the Church upon those who helped themselves to the ears of corn. The parson, notwithstanding a well-known precedent in the Gospels, was about to yield to their insistence, when a man

[1] Wendover, III. 95, 98.

[2] " Qui ex avaritia inopiam semper habent suspectam."

of religion and piety rose in the congregation and adjured the priest, in the name of God and all His saints, to refrain from the sentence, adding that those who were in need were welcome to help themselves to his own corn. The others, however, insisted, and the parson was just beginning to ban the pilferers, when a thunderstorm suddenly burst, with hail and torrents of rain. When the storm had passed, the peasants went out to find their crops destroyed,—all but that one simple and just man who found his corn untouched.

We have only to recall the minute subdivisions of the common field, or fields, of the parish into half-acre strips separated by balks of turf, and the fact that no two half-acres of the same cultivator lay together, to realize how nice must have been the discrimination[1].

But the moral of the story is obvious. It is an appeal to the teaching and the sanction of the Gospels, against the rooted belief of the natural man that he owes what he has to his own industry and thrift, and that it is no business of his to part with his goods for the sustenance of a helpless and improvident class.

The spirit of avarice, according to Wendover, permeated all classes at this period, from high ecclesiastics downwards. Walter, archbishop of York, had his granaries full of corn during the scarcity, some of it five years old. When the peasants on his manors asked to be supplied from these stores in the summer of 1234, the archbishop instructed his bailiffs to give out the old corn on condition of getting new for it when the harvest was over. It need not be told at length how the archbishop's barns at Ripon were found on examination to be infested with vermin, how the corn had turned mouldy and rotten, and how the whole of it had to be destroyed by fire[2]. Of the same import are the raids upon the barns of the alien or Italian clergy in 1228, in the diocese of Winchester and elsewhere, and the ostentatious distribution by the raiders of doles to the poor[3].

[1] Alboldslea, or Abbotsley, was the parish of which the famous Grosseteste, bishop of Lincoln, was rector (perhaps non-resident) down to 1231, or to within three years of the date of the above anecdote. The existing church is of great age, and may well have been the actual edifice in which the scene was enacted.

[2] Wendover, III. 96.

[3] *Ibid.* III. 19, 27.

The somewhat parallel course of public morality in the centres of trade, or, as Wendover would call it, the prevalence of avarice, demands a brief notice for our purpose.

In every state of society, there will of course be rich and poor. But a class of *pauperes* seems to emerge more distinctly in the life of England from about the beginning of the thirteenth century. The period corresponds to the appearance on the scene of St Francis and his friars. Doubtless St Francis was inspired by a true sense of what the time needed, even if it be open to contend that his ministrations of charity brought out, consolidated, and kept alive a helpless class who would have been less heard of if they had been left to the tender mercies of economic principles. The mission of the friars was not merely to the poor; it was also to the rich, whether of the church or of the world, "to soften the hardness of their hearts by the oil of preaching[1]." It was one of these interpositions, ever needed and never wanting, to reduce the inequalities of the human lot, not by preaching down-right theoretical communism, but, more by force of rhetoric than of logic, to extort from the strong some concessions to the weak, to mitigate the severity of the struggle for existence, and to bring the respectable vices of greed and sharp practice to the bar of conscience.

As early as 1196 there is the significant incident, in the city of London, of the rising of the poorer class and the middling class, headed by Fitzosbert Longbeard, himself one of the privileged citizens, against an assessment in which the class represented by the mayor and aldermen were alleged to have been very tender of their own interests[2]. Longbeard was hailed as "the friend of the poor," and, having lost his life in their cause (whether in the street before Bow Church, or on a gallows at Tyburn, or at the Smithfield elms, the narratives are not agreed), he is celebrated by the sympathetic Matthew Paris as "the martyr of the poor[3]." That historian continues, after the

[1] Wendover, III. 381.

[2] William of Newburgh, *sub anno* 1196.

[3] On the other hand John Stow seems to have acquired, from some unstated source, an extraordinary prejudice against him.

manner of his predecessor Wendover, to speak of Londoners as on the one hand the "mediocres, populares et plebei," and on the other hand the "divites." In 1258 the latter class over-reached themselves: they were caught in actual vulgar pecu-lation of money raised by assessment for repairing the city walls; some of them were thrown into prison and only escaped death through the royal clemency at the instance of the no-torious pluralist John Mansel, and on making restitution of their plunder; but one of them, the mayor, never recovered the blow to his respectability, and died soon after of grief[1]. Whether it meant a wide-spread spirit of petty fraud, or some unadjusted change in value, the young king in 1228, during a journey from York to London, took occasion along his route to destroy the "false measures" of corn, ale and wine, to substitute more ample measures, and to increase the weight of the loaf.

The scarcity or famine of 1234, to which the Abbotsley incident belongs, was accompanied, says the St Albans annalist, by a mortality which raged cruelly everywhere. On the other hand the annalist of Tewkesbury may be credited when he says that, although the year was one of scarcity, corn being at eight shillings, yet "by the grace of God the poor were better sustained than in other years[2]."

There was an epidemic in 1247, but it is not clear whether it was due to famine. Although Higden, quoting from some unknown record, says that there was dearth in England in that year, wheat being at twelve shillings the quarter, yet he does not mention sickness at all; and Matthew Paris, who was then living, is explicit that the harvest of 1247 was an abundant one, and that the mortality did not begin until September of that year. There does appear, however, to have been a sharp famine in Wales; and it is recorded that the bishop of Norwich, "about the year 1245," in a time of great dearth, sold all his plate and distributed it to the poor[3]. All that we know of this epidemic is the statement of Matthew Paris, that it began in September and lasted for three months; and that as many

---

[1] Matthew Paris, *Chron. Maj.* ed. Luard, v. 663, 675.
[2] Annals of Tewkesbury in *Annales Monastici*, Rolls series, No. 36.
[3] *Chronica Majora*, IV. 647; Stow, *Survey of London*.

as nine or ten bodies were buried in one day in the single churchyard of St Peter's at Saint Albans[1].

Matthew Paris notes the quality of the harvest and the prices of grain every year, and his successor Rishanger continues the practice. The prices noted appear, from comparison with those tabulated by Thorold Rogers from actual accounts, to have been the lowest market rates of the year. The harvest of 1248 was plentiful, and wheat sold at two shillings and sixpence a quarter. In 1249 and 1250 it was at two shillings, oats being at one shilling. But those years of exceptional abundance were followed at no long interval by a series of years of scarcity or famine, which brought pestilential sickness of the severest kind.

The scarcity or famine in the years 1256–59 was all the more acutely felt owing to the dearth of money in the country. The burden of the history of Matthew Paris before he comes to the famine is that England had been emptied of treasure by the exactions of king and pope. Henry III. was under some not quite intelligible obligation of money to his brother, the earl of Cornwall. The English earl was a candidate for the Imperial crown, and had got so far towards the dignity of emperor as to have been made king of the Germans. It was English money that went to pay his German troops, and to further his cause with the electoral princes; but the circulating coin of England does not appear to have sufficed for these and domestic purposes also. The harvest of 1256 had been spoiled by wet, and the weather of the spring of 1257 was wretched in the extreme. All England was in a state of marsh and mud, and the roads were impassable. Many sowed their fields over again; but the autumn proved as wet as the rest of the year. "Whatever had been sown in winter, whatever had germinated in spring, whatever the summer had brought forward—all was drowned in the floods of autumn." The want of coins in circulation caused unheard-of poverty. At the end of the year the fields lay untilled, and a multitude of people were dead of famine. At Christmas wheat rose to ten shillings a quarter. But the year 1257 appears to have had "lethal fevers" before the loss of the

[1] *Chron. Maj.* IV. 654.

harvest of that year could be felt. Not to mention other places, says the St Albans historian, there was at St Edmundsbury in the dog-days so great a mortality that more than two thousand bodies were buried in its spacious cemetery[1].

The full effects of the famine were not felt until the spring of 1258. So great was the pinch in London from the failure of the crops and the want of money that fifteen thousand[2] are said to have died of famine, and of a grievous and wide-spread pestilence that broke out about the feast of the Trinity (19 May).

The earl of Cornwall (and king of Germany) who had relieved the country of a great part of its circulating coin, took the opportunity to buy up corn in Germany and Holland for the supply of the London market. Fifty great ships, says Matthew Paris, arrived in the Thames laden with wheat, barley, and other grain. Not three English counties had produced as much as was imported. The corn was for such as could buy it ; but the king interposed with an edict that, whereas greed was to be discouraged, no one was to buy the foreign corn in order to store it up and trade in it. Those who had no money, we are expressly told, died of hunger, even after the arrival of the ships ; and even men of good position went about with faces pinched by hunger, and passed sleepless nights sighing for bread. No one had seen such famine and misery, although many would have remembered corn at higher prices. The price quoted about this stage of the narrative, although not with special reference to the foreign wheat, is nine shillings the quarter. Elsewhere the price is said to have mounted up to fifteen shillings, which may have been the rate before the foreign supply came in. But such was the scarceness of money, we are told, that if the price of the quarter of wheat had been less, there would hardly have been found anyone to buy it.

[1] *Chr. Maj.* v. 660. Other details occur here and there to the end of the chronicle.

[2] This is the number given by Matthew Paris. It suggests a larger population in the capital than we might have been disposed to credit. The same writer says that London was so full of people when the parliament was sitting the year before (1257) that the city could hardly hold them all in her ample bosom. The Annals of Tewkesbury put the whole mortality from famine and fever in London in 1258 at 20,000. But the whole population did not probably exceed 40,000.

Even those who were wont to succour the miserable were now reduced to perish along with them. It is difficult to believe that the historian has not given way to the temptations of rhetoric, and it is pleasing to be able to give the following complement to his picture. After some 15,000 had died in London, mostly of the poorer sort, one might hear a crier making proclamation to the starving multitude to go to a distribution of bread by this or that nobleman, at such and such a place, mentioning the name of the benefactor and the place of dole.

In other passages, which may be taken as picturing the state of matters in the country, the historian says that the bodies of the starved were found swollen and livid, lying five or six together in pig-sties, or on dungheaps, or in the mud of farm-yards. The dying were refused shelter and succour for fear of contagion, and scarcely anyone would go near the dead to bury them. Where many corpses were found together, they were buried in capacious trenches in the churchyards.

We come now to the harvest of 1258. After a bleak and late spring the crops had come forward well under excessive heat in summer, and the harvest was an unusually abundant, although a late one. Rains set in before the corn could be cut, and at the feast of All Saints (1 November) the heavy crops had rotted until the fields were like so many dungheaps. Only in some places was any attempt made to carry the harvest home, and then it was so spoiled as to be hardly worth the trouble. Even the mouldy grain sold as high as sixteen shillings a quarter. The famishing people resorted to various shifts, selling their cattle and reducing their households. How the country got through the winter, we are not told. Matthew Paris himself died early in 1259, and the annalist who added a few pages to the *Chronica Majora* after his death, merely mentions that the corn, the oil and the wine turned corrupt, and that as the sun entered Cancer a pestilence and mortality of men began unexpectedly, in which many died. Among others Fulk, the bishop of London, died of pestilence in the spring of 1259; and, to say nothing of many other places, at Paris —— thousand (the number is left blank) were buried.

The vagueness of the last statement reminds us that we are now deprived of the comparatively safe guidance of Matthew Paris. His successor in the office of annalist at St Albans, Rishanger, is much less trustworthy. He sums up the year 1259 in a paragraph which repeats exactly the facts of the notorious year 1258, and probably applies to that alone; for the year 1260 his summary is that it was more severe, more cruel and more terrible to all living things than the year before, the pestilence and famine being intolerable. There is, however, no confirmation of that in the authentic prices of the year collected by Thorold Rogers. Parcels of wheat of the harvest of 1259 were sold at about five and six shillings, and of the harvest of 1260 at from three shillings and sixpence to six shillings. For a number of years, corresponding to the Barons' war and the war in Wales, the price is moderate or low, the figures of extant bailiffs' accounts agreeing on the whole with Rishanger's summary statements about the respective harvests[1]. The years from 1271 to 1273 were dear years, and for the first of the series we find a doubtful record by the

[1] The year 1274 was the beginning of so exceptional a murrain of sheep that it deserves mention here, although murrains do not come within the scope of the work. It is recorded by more than one contemporary. Rishanger (p. 84) says: " In that year a disastrous plague of sheep seized upon England, so that the sheep-folds were everywhere emptied through the spreading of it. It lasted for twenty-eight years following, so that no farm of the whole kingdom was without the infliction of that misery. Many attributed the cause of this disease, which the inhabitants had not been acquainted with before, to a certain rich man of the Frankish nation, who settled in Northumberland, having brought with him a certain sheep of Spanish breed, the size of a small two year old ox, which was ailing and contaminated all the flocks of England by handing on its disease to them." Under the year following, 1275, he enters it again, using the term "scabies." Thorold Rogers (*Hist. of Agric. and Prices,* I. 31) has found " scab " of sheep often mentioned in the bailiffs' accounts from about 1288; it is assumed to have become permanent from the item of tar occurring regularly in the accounts; but tar was used ordinarily for marking. It may have been sheep-pox, which Fitzherbert, in his *Book of Husbandry* (edition of 1598), describes under the name of " the Poxe," giving a clear account of the way to deal with it by isolation. For murrains in general, the reader may consult Fleming's *Animal Plagues,* 2 vols. 1871—1884, a work which is mostly compiled (with meagre acknowledgment for " bibliography " only) from the truly learned work of Heusinger, *Recherches de Pathologie Comparée,* Cassel, 1844. Fleming has used only the "pièces justificatives," and has not carried the history beyond the point where Heusinger left it.

Yorkshire continuator of William of Newburgh that there was
" a great famine and pestilence in England and Ireland[1]." The
harvest of 1288 was so abundant that the price of wheat in the
bailiffs' accounts is mostly about two shillings, ranging from
sixteen pence to four and eightpence. Rishanger's prices for
the year are sufficiently near the mark: in some places wheat
sold at twenty pence the quarter, in others at sixteen pence,
and in others at twelve pence. From that extremely low point,
a rise begins which culminates in 1294. The chronicler's statement for 1289, that in London the bushel of wheat rose from
threepence to two shillings, is not borne out by the bailiffs'
accounts, which show a range of from two shillings and eightpence to six shillings the quarter. But these accounts confirm
the statement that the years following were dear years, and
that 1294 was a year of famine prices, wheat having touched
fourteen shillings at Cambridge, in July. Rishanger's two notes
are that the poor perished of hunger, and that the poor died of
hunger on all sides, afflicted with a looseness (*lienteria*)[2]. The
two years following are also given as hard for the poor, but
not as years of famine or sickness; the country was at the
same time heavily taxed for the expenses of the war which
Edward I. was waging against the Scots. Ordinary prosperity
attends the cultivators of the soil until the end of Rishanger's
chronicle in 1305; and from the beginning of Trokelowe's in
1307, the year of Edward II.'s accession, there is nothing for
our purpose until we come to the great famine of 1315[3].

It is clear, however, that prices were high in every year from
1309 until that famine, with the single exception of the harvest
of 1311. At the meeting of Parliament in London before

---

[1] Continuation of Wm. of Newburgh, Rolls series No. 82, vol. II. p. 560 :
" Facta est magna fames per universam Angliam et maxime partibus occidentalibus.
In Hibernia vero tres pestes invaluerunt, sc. mortalitas, fames, et gladius : per guerram
mortalem praevalentibus Hybernicis et Anglicis succumbentibus. Qui vero gladium
et famem evadere potuerunt, peste mortalitatis praeventi sunt, ita ut vivi mortuis
sepeliendis vix sufficere valerent."

[2] See also the continuation of the chronicle of Florence of Worcester, Bohn's
series, p. 405.

[3] Rishanger's annals, 1259–1305, and Trokelowe's, 1307–1323, are printed in the
volumes of *Chronica Monast. S. Albani*, No. 28 of the Rolls series.

Easter in 1315, the dearth was a subject of deliberation, and a King's writ was issued attempting to fix the prices at which fat oxen, cows, sheep, pigs, geese, fowls, capons, chickens, pigeons and eggs should be sold on demand, subject to confiscation if the sale were refused. The statute was ineffective (it was repealed the year after), and provisions became dearer than ever. The quarter of wheat, beans and peas sold for twenty shillings, of oats for ten shillings, and of salt for thirty-five. When the king stopped at St Albans at the feast of St Lawrence, says Trokelowe, it was hardly possible to buy bread for the use of his household. The scarcity was most felt from the month of May until the harvest. With the new crop, ruined as it was by rains and floods, the scarcity lessened somewhat, but not before many had felt the pinch of hunger, and others were seen (as the St Albans annalist says he saw them) lying squalid and dead in the villages and by the road-sides. At Midsummer, 1316, wheat rose to thirty shillings, and after that as high as forty shillings (the highest price found by Thorold Rogers is twenty-six shillings and eightpence at Leatherhead in July). The various forms of famine-sickness are mentioned :— dysentery from corrupt food, affecting nearly everyone, an acute fever which killed many, or a putrid sore throat (*pestis guttu-ruosa*). To show the extremities to which England was reduced, Trokelowe specially inserts the following: Ordinary flesh was not to be had, but horse-flesh was eaten, fat dogs were stolen to eat, and it was rumoured abroad that in many places both men and women secretly ate the flesh of their own children, or of the children of others. But the detail which Trokelowe justly thinks posterity will be most horrified to read, is that prisoners in gaols set upon the thieves newly brought in and devoured them alive.

It is probably the same famine and pestilence that we find worked into the metrical romance of Robert of Brunne (1338), under the guise of the plague 'in Cadwaladre's time,' that is, the pestilence recorded by Beda for the year 664. The Lincoln-shire romancist must have seen the famine and pestilence of 1315–16, for he was then in the prime of life, and probably he transferred his own experiences of famine and pestilence to the remote episode of the seventh century, to which he devotes thirty-eight lines of his romance. In Cadwaladre's time the corn fails and there is great hunger. A man may go for three days before he can buy any food in burgh, or in city, or in upland; he may indeed catch wild creatures, or fishes, or gather leaves and roots. Worse still, a plague comes, from rotten air and wicked winds, so that hale men fall down suddenly and die; gentle and bondmen all go, hardly any are left to till the land, the living cannot bury the dead, those who try fall dead in the grave. Men leave house and land, and few are left in the country. Eleven years does Britain lie waste with but few folk to till the land[1].

After the famine of 1315–16, the third and last of the great and, one may say, disgraceful famines which gave rise to the by-word "Anglorum fames," prices continued at their ordinary level for several years. But from 1320 to 1323 they again came to a height. To that period probably belongs a mortality which is entered, in a chronicle of the next century[2], under the year 1325. On the contemporary authority of Higden we know that, in 1322, the king went to Scotland about the feast of St Peter ad Vincula, "and though he met not with resistance, lost many of his own by famine and disease." After that period of scarcity comes a long succession of cheap years, covering the interval to the next great event in the annals of pestilence that concerns us, the arrival of the Black Death in the autumn of 1348. With that great event the history of English epidemics enters upon a new chapter. There were, of course, years of dearth and scarcity in the centuries following, but there were no great famine-pestilences like those of 1196, 1258 and 1315.

The period of the great famines ought not to be left without another reference to the widening gulf between the rich and the poor, and the keenness of traders which led them sometimes to incur the restraints of government and the punishments of justice.

On 26 March, 1269, was issued one of those ordinances against forestalling, of which many more followed for several

---

[1] Furnivall's ed. Rolls series, No. 87, vol. II. 569, 573.

[2] Chronicle of William Gregory, Camden Society, ed. Gairdner, 1876.

centuries: no citizen to go outside the city of London, either by road or river, to meet victuals coming to market. In the 7th year of Edward I., clipping or debasing the coinage was carried on so systematically that nearly three hundred persons, mostly of the Hebrew race, were drawn and hanged for it. In the 11th year of Edward I. (1283) a statute had been directed against cheating by bakers and millers. Meanwhile the nobility retaliated by plundering the traders and merchants at Boston fair, and the king settled the account with these marauding nobles by hanging them. A statute of 1316, the second year of the famine, to fix the price of ale, has an interest on account of its motive—"ne frumentum ulterius per potum consumeretur." The proportion of the corn of the country turned into malt, or the amount diverted from bread to beer, may be guessed from the fact that in London, for which the beer ordinance was first made, there were in 1309, brewhouses to the number of 1334, and taverns to the number of 354[1]. In the very year of great famine, 1316, an ordinance was issued (in French, dated from King's Langley) against extravagant housekeeping[2]. In the year of great scarcity and mortality, 1322, there was such a crowd for a funeral dole at Blackfriars (for the soul of Henry Fingret) that fifty-five persons, children and adults, were crushed to death in the scramble[3]. At the same time the prior of Christ Church, Canterbury, was sitting down to dinners of seventeen dishes, the cellarer had thirty-eight servants under him, the chamberlain and sacrist had large numbers of people employed as tailors, furriers, launderers and the like, and the servants and equipages of the one hundred and forty brethren were numerous and splendid[4]. The monasteries, on which the relief of the poor mostly depended, have been thus characterized:

"From the end of the twelfth century until the Reformation," says Bishop Stubbs, "from the days of Hubert Walter to those of Wolsey, the monasteries remained magnificent hostelries: their churches were splendid chapels for noble patrons; their inhabitants were bachelor country gentlemen, more polished and charitable, but little more learned or more pure in life

[1] *Annales Londonienses*, Rolls series, No. 76, ed. Stubbs. Introduction, p. lxxvi.
[2] *Ibid.* (*Annales Paulini*), p. 238.
[3] *Ibid.* p. 304.
[4] *Epistolae Cantuarienses*, Rolls series, No. 38, II. Introduction by Stubbs, p. xxxii.

than their lay neighbours ; their estates were well managed, and enjoyed great advantages and exemptions ; they were, in fact, an element of peace in a nation that delighted in war. But, with a few noble exceptions, there was nothing in the system that did spiritual service[1]."

There is little to be said, at this period, of the profession most directly concerned with sickness, epidemic or other, namely the medical. We become aware of its existence on rare occasions: as in the account of the death of William the Conqueror at Rouen on 9 September, 1087, of the illness and death of Hubert, archbishop of Canterbury, on 13 July, 1205, at one of his manors on a journey to Rochester[2], or in the reference by William of Newburgh, to the noted Jewish physician of King's Lynn, whose honourable repute among the citizens for skill and modesty did not save him from the murderous fanaticism against his race in 1190[3], or in occasional letters of the time[4]. There were doubtless benevolent men among the practitioners of medicine, then as now ; but the profession has never been one in which individuals could rise conspicuously above the level of their age, and the moral standard of those centuries was a poor one. It is not surprising, then, that John of Salisbury, indulging a taste for epigram, should have characterized the profession of medicine in the twelfth century as follows: "They have only two maxims which they never violate, 'Never mind the poor ; never refuse money from the rich'[5]."

The one English physician whose writings have come down to us from the period that we are still engaged with, is John of Gaddesden. There is every reason to think that he was practising at the time of the famine and pestilence of 1315–16 ; but it is not from his bulky treatise on medicine that we learn the nosological types of the epidemic maladies of those years. Some account of his *Rosa Anglica* will be found in the

[1] *Epistolae Cantuarienses*, Rolls series, No. 38, II. Introduction by Stubbs, p. cxix.

[2] Ralph of Coggeshall, Rolls series, No. 66, p. 156.

[3] He might have been, and probably was, the prototype of the physician Nathan Ben Israel, in the 35th Chapter of *Ivanhoe*.

[4] Adam de Marisco to Grosseteste, *Mon. Francisc.* ed. Brewer, I. 113.

[5] I have not succeeded in finding this in the author's writings, and quote it at second hand.

chapter on Smallpox; it must suffice to say here that he was
a verbalist compiler from other books, themselves not altogether
original, and that, according to Dr Freind, he displays no great
knowledge of his profession.

It is nothing strange, therefore, that Gaddesden throws no
light upon the famine-pestilences of England, such as those of
1315–16, which he lived through. Dysentery and lientery, he
treats of almost in the very words of Gilbertus Anglicus; but
those maladies might have been among the dwellers in another
planet, so far as native experience comes in. He reproduces
whole chapters from his predecessors, on *synochus* and *synocha*,
without a hint that England ever witnessed such scenes of
hunger-typhus as the St Albans chroniclers have recorded for
us from their own observation. The reference by Trokelowe to
the prevalence of *pestis gutturuosa* in 1316, is one that a medical
writer of the time might well have amplified; but Gaddesden
missed the opportunity of perhaps anticipating Fothergill's description of putrid sore-throat by more than four hundred years.

Epidemics of St Anthony's Fire, or Ergotism.

One form of epidemic malady, intimately connected with
bad harvests and a poor state of agriculture, namely Ergotism,
from the mixture of poisoned grains in the rye or other corn, is
conspicuously missed from English records of the medieval
period, although it plays a great part in the history of French
epidemics of the Middle Ages, under such names as *ignis sacer*,
ignis S. Antonii, or *ignis infernalis*. According to the proverbial saying already quoted, France was as notorious for *ignis*
as England for famine, and Normandy for lepra: "Tres plagae
tribus regionibus appropriari solent, Anglorum fames, Gallorum
ignis, Normannorum lepra[1]." The malady was of a nature to
attract notice and excite pity; it is entered by chroniclers, and
is a frequent topic in French legends of the Saints. Its occurrence in epidemic form can be traced in France, with a degree

[1] Quoted, without date, by Marchand, *Étude historique et nosographique sur quelques épidémies et endémies du moyen âge.* Paris, 1873.

of probability, as far back as 857 (perhaps to 590); six great outbreaks are recorded in the tenth century, seven in the eleventh, ten in the twelfth, and three in the thirteenth, the medieval series ending with one in the year 1373. The estimates of mortality in the several epidemics of ergotism over a larger or smaller area of France, range as high as 40,000, and 14,000, which numbers may be taken to be the roughest of guesses; but in later times upwards of 500 deaths from ergotism have been accurately counted in a single outbreak within a limited district. The epidemics have been observed in particular seasons, sometimes twenty years or more elapsing without the disease being seen; they have occurred also in particular provinces—in the basin of the Loire, in Lorraine, and, since the close of the medieval period, especially in the Sologne. The disease has usually been traced to a spoiled rye crop; but there is undoubted evidence from the more recent period that a poison with corresponding effects can be produced in some other cereals, even in wheat itself.

In a field of rye, especially after a wet sowing or a wet season of growth, a certain proportion of the heads bear long brown or purple corns, one or more upon a head, projecting in the shape of a cock's spur, whence the French name of ergot. The spur appears to be, and probably is, an overgrown grain of rye; it is grooved like a rye-corn, occupies the place of the corn between the two chaff-coverings, and contains an abundant whitish meal. Microscopic research has detected in or upon the spurred rye the filaments of a minute parasitic mould; so that it is to the invasion by a parasite that we may trace the enormous overgrowth of one or more grains on an ear, and it is probably to the ferment-action of the fungus that we should ascribe the poisonous properties of the meal. The proportion of all the stalks in a field so affected will vary considerably, as well as the proportion of grains on each affected head of corn[1]. Rye affected with ergot is apt to be a poor crop at any rate; one or more spurred corns on a head tend to keep the rest of the grains small or unfilled; and if there be many stalks

---

[1] I give this account of the obvious characters of spurred rye from a recent observation of a growing crop of it.

in the field so affected, the spurred grain will bulk considerably in the whole yield. When the diseased grains are ground to meal along with the healthy grains, the meal and the bread will contain an appreciable quantity of the poison of ergot; and if rye-bread were the staple food, there would be a great risk, after an unusually bad harvest, of an outbreak of the remarkable constitutional effects of ergotism. Rye-bread with much ergot in it may be rather blacker than usual; but it is said to have no peculiar taste.

It is almost exclusively among the peasantry that symptoms of ergotism have been seen, and among children particularly. The attack usually began with intense pains in the legs or feet, causing the victims to writhe and scream. A fire seemed to burn between the flesh and the bones, and, at a later stage, even in the bowels, the surface of the body being all the while cold as ice. Sometimes the skin of affected limbs became livid or black; now and then large blebs or blisters arose upon it, as in bad kinds of erysipelas. Gangrene or sloughing of the extremities followed; a foot or a hand fell off, or the flesh of a whole limb was destroyed down to the bones, by a process which began in the deeper textures. The spontaneous separation of a gangrenous hand or foot was on the whole a good sign for the recovery of the patient. Such was the *ignis sacer*, or *ignis S. Antonii* which figures prominently, I am told, in the French legends of the Saints, and of which epidemics are recorded in the French medieval chronicles. Corresponding effects of ergotism may or may not have occurred during the medieval period in other countries of Europe where rye was grown.

The remarkable thing is, that when we do begin in the sixteenth and seventeenth centuries to obtain evidence of agrarian epidemics in Germany, Sweden and Russia, which have eventually come to be identified, in the light of more recent knowledge, with ergotism, the type of the disease is different, not perhaps fundamentally or in the ultimate pathological analysis, but at all events different as being a functional disorder of the nervous system, instead of a disorder, on nervous lines, affecting the nutrition of parts and their structural integrity. This newer form, distinctive of Germany and north-eastern Europe, was known by the name of Kriebelkrankheit, from the creeping or itching sensations in the limbs at the beginning of it; these heightened sensibilities often amounted to acute pain, as in the beginning of the gangrenous form also; but the affection of the sensory nerves, instead of leading to a breakdown in the nutrition of the parts and to gangrene, was followed by disorder of the motor nerves,—by spasms of the hands and arms, feet and legs, very often passing into contractures of the joints which no force could unbend, and in some cases passing into periodic convulsive fits of the whole body like epilepsy, whence the name of convulsive ergotism[1].

Side by side with these German, Swedish and Russian outbreaks of convulsive ergotism, or Kriebelkrankheit (called by Linnaeus in Sweden by the Latin name *raphania*), there had been a renewal or continuance of the medieval epidemics in France, notably in the Sologne; but the French ergotism has retained its old type of *ignis* or gangrene. It was not until the eighteenth century that the learned world became clear as to the connexion between either of those forms of disease among the peasantry and a damaged rye-crop, although the country people themselves, and the observant medical practitioners of the affected districts, had put this and that together long before. Thus, as late as 1672–75, there were communications made to the Paris Academy of Medicine[2] by observers in the Sologne and especially around Montargis, in which ergot of rye is clearly described, as well as the associated symptoms of gangrenous disease in the peasantry; but the connexion between the two was still regarded as open to doubt, and as a question that could only be settled by experiment; while there is not a hint given that these modern outbreaks were of the same nature as the notorious medieval *ignis sacer*. According to Häser, it was not until the French essay of Read (Strasbourg, 1771) that the

---

[1] One of the greatest epidemics was in Westphalia and the Cologne district in 1596 and 1597. It fell to be described by two learned writers, Sennert and Horst, of whose accounts a summary is given by Short, *Air, weather, seasons, etc.* I. 275–285.

[2] Translated into the *Philosophical Transactions*, No. 130, vol. XII. p. 758 (14 Dec. 1676) from the *Journal des Sçavans*.

identity of the old *ignis* with the modern gangrenous ergotism was pointed out.

The result of the modern study of outbreaks of ergotism, including the minute record of individual cases, has been to show that there is no hard and fast line between the gangrenous and convulsive forms, that the French epidemics, although on the whole marked by the phenomena of gangrene, have not been wanting in functional nervous symptoms, and that the German or northern outbreaks have often been of a mixed type. Thus, in the French accounts of 1676, "malign fevers accompanied with drowsiness and raving," are mentioned along with "the gangrene in the arms but mostly in the legs, which ordinarily are corrupted first."

Again, the observations of Th. O. Heusinger[1] on an outbreak near Marburg in 1855–56, led him decidedly to conclude for the essential sameness of *ignis* and Kriebelkrankheit, and for the existence of a middle type, although undoubtedly the sensory and motor disorders, including hyperaesthesia, pain and anaesthesia on the one hand, and contractures of the joints, choreic movements and convulsions on the other, were more distinctive of the epidemics of ergotism on German or northern European soil.

Thus far the foreign experience of ergotism, both medieval and modern, and of its several types. We shall now be in a position to examine the English records for indications of the same effects of damaged grain.

In the English medieval chronicles an occasional reference may be found to *ignis* or wild fire. The reference to wild fire in Derbyshire in the Anglo-Saxon Chronicle under the year 1049, probably means some meteorological phenomenon, elsewhere called *ignis sylvaticus*: "Eac þ wilde fyr on Deorbyscire micel yfel dyde[2]." Whatever the *ignis sylvaticus* or *ignis aereus* was, which destroyed houses as well as crops, there appears to be no

---

[1] *Studien über den Ergotismus*, Marburg, 1856.

[2] Simeon of Durham and Roger of Howden have the following, under the year 1048: "Mortalitas hominum et animalium multas occupavit Angliae provincias, et ignis aereus, vulgo dictus sylvaticus, in Deorbensi provincia et quibusdam aliis provinciis, villas et segetes multas ustulavit."

warrant for the conclusion of C. F. Heusinger that it was the same as the *ignis sacer* of the French peasantry[1]. An undoubted reference to *ignis infernalis* as a human malady occurs in the *Topography of Ireland* by Giraldus Cambrensis: a certain archer who had ravished a woman at St Fechin's mill at Fore was overtaken by swift vengeance, "igne infernali in membro percussus, usque in ipsum corpus statim exarsit, et nocte eadem exspiravit." Taking the incident as legendary, and the diagnosis as valueless, we may still conclude that the name, at least, of *ignis infernalis* was familiar to English writers. But in all the accounts of English famines and wide-spread sicknesses in the medieval period which have been extracted from the nearest contemporary authorities, I have found no mention of any disease that might correspond to ergotism[2].

The first undoubted instance of ergotism in England belongs to the eighteenth century. On or about the 10th of January, 1762, a peasant's family (father, mother, and six children) of Wattisham in Suffolk, were attacked almost simultaneously with

---

[1] " Je crois qu'ils ont voulu indiquer l'ignis sacer ou de St Antoine, qui dans ces années et surtout 1044 sévit en France." *Recherches de Pathologie Comparée*, vol. II. p. cxlviii.

[2] On the other hand, Short, in his *General Chronological History of the Air, Weather, Seasons, Meteors etc.* (2 vols. London, 1749) says that the epidemic of 1110 consisted of "especially an epidemic erysipelas, whereof many died, the parts being black and shrivelled up ; " and that in 1128, " St Anthony's fire was fatal to many in England." He gives no authority in either case. But the one error is run to earth in a French entry of 1109, "membris instar carbonum nigrescentibus" (Sig. Gembl. auctar. p. 274, Migne) ; the other, most likely, in the *ignis* around Chartres, 1128 (Stephen of Caen, Bouquet, XII. 780).

Perhaps this is the best place to express a general opinion on the work by Short, which is the only book of the kind in English previous to my own. It is everywhere uncritical and credulous, and often grossly inaccurate in dates, sometimes repeating the same epidemic under different years. It appears to have been compiled, for the earlier part, at least, from foreign sources, such as a Chronicle of Magdeburg, and to a large extent from a work by Colle de Belluno (fl. 1631). Many of the facts about English epidemics are given almost as in the original chronicles, but without reference to them. English experience of sickness is lost in the general chronology of epidemics for all Europe, and is dealt with in a purely verbalist manner. So far as this volume extends (1667) I have found Short's book of no use, except now and then in calling my attention to something that I had overlooked. His other work, *New Observations on City, Town and County Bills of Mortality* (London, 1750) shows the author to much greater advantage, and I have used his statistical tables for the sixteenth and seventeenth centuries.

the symptoms of gangrenous ergotism, several of them eventually losing portions of their limbs. The disease began with intense pain in the legs, and contractures of the hands and feet. It was proved that they had not been using rye flour; but their bread for a short time before had been made exclusively from damaged wheat, grown in the neighbourhood and kept apart from the farmer's good corn so as not to spoil his sample. It had been sent to the mill just before Christmas, and had been used by some others besides the family who developed the symptoms of ergotism[1].

In that authentic instance of ergotism (although not from rye), there was one symptom, the contractures of the hands and feet, which is distinctive of the convulsive form; so that the English type may be said to have been a mixture of the French form and of the form special to the north-eastern countries of Europe. With that instance as a type, let us now inquire whether any epidemics in England at earlier periods may not be brought under the head of ergotism. It is to be kept in mind that none of the medieval outbreaks were called by their present name, or traced to their true source, until centuries after; so that our task is, not to search the records for the name of ergotism, but to scrutinize any anomalous outbreak of disease, or any outbreak distinguished in the chronicles by some unusual mark, with a view to discovering whether it suits the hypothesis of ergotism. I shall have to speak of three such outbreaks in the fourteenth century, and of one in Lancashire and Cheshire in 1702[2].

[1] The facts were communicated to the Royal Society by Charlton Wollaston, M.D., F.R.S., then resident in Suffolk, and by the Rev. James Bones. They were referred by Dr G. Baker to Tissot of Lausanne, who replied that they corresponded to typical gangrenous ergotism. See *Phil. Trans.* vol. LII. pt. 2 (1762) p. 523, p. 526, p. 529; and vol. LX. (1768) p. 106.

[2] An erroneous statement as to an epidemic of gangrenous ergotism, or of Kriebel-krankheit, in England in 1676, has somehow come to be current in German books. It has a place in the latest chronological table of ergotism epidemics, that of Hirsch in his *Handbuch der historisch-geographischen Pathologie,* vol. II. 1883 (Engl. Transl. II. p. 206), the reference being to Birch, *Philos. Transact.* This reference to ergotism in England in 1676 is given also in Th. O. Heusinger's table (1856), where it appears in the form of "Schnurrer, nach Birch." On turning to Schnurrer's *Chronik der Seuchen* (II. 210), the reference is found to be, "Birch, *Phil. Trans.* vols. XI. and

The first of these is given by Knighton for a period and a locality that may have been within his own cognizance. In the summer of 1340 there happened in England generally, but especially in the county of Leicester, a certain deplorable and enormous infirmity. It was marked by paroxysms or fits, attended by intolerable suffering; while the fit lasted, the victims emitted a noise like the barking of dogs. A "great pestilence," or perhaps a great mortality, is said to have ensued[1]. In that record the salient points are, firstly the wide or epidemic incidence of the malady, at all events in Leicestershire, which was Knighton's own county; secondly the paroxysmal nature of the attacks, and the strange noises emitted therewith; thirdly the intolerable suffering (*poena*) that attended each fit (*passio*). Except for the clear indication of pain, one might think of the strange hysterical outbreaks, extending, by a kind of psychical contagion, to whole communities, which were observed about the same period in some parts of the continent of Europe. But of these medieval psychopathies, as they are called, there is hardly any trace in England. The Flagellants came over from Zealand to London in 1349, and gave exhibitions at St Paul's, but that pseudo-religious mania does not appear to have taken hold among the English. The epidemic recorded by Knighton had probably a more material cause. To illustrate the somewhat meagre reference by Knighton to the strange epidemic of 1340, I shall proceed at once to the remarkable outbreak in Lancashire and Cheshire in 1702, which was clearly not a psychopathy or hysterical outbreak, and yet had a seemingly hysterical element in it. An account of it was sent to the Royal Society by Dr Charles Leigh " of Lancashire[2]."

XII."; and coming at length to the *Philosophical Transactions*, it appears that vols. x., XI. and XII. are bound up together, that vol. XII. (1676) p. 758, contains an extract from the *Journal des Sçavans* about ergot of rye in certain parts of France, and that there is nothing about ergotism in England in either vol. XI. or vol. XII. So far as concerns Dr Birch, he was secretary to the Royal Society in the next century.

[1] Knighton, *De Eventibus Angliae* in Twysden, col. 2580 : " In aestate scilicet anno Gratiae 1340 accidit quaedam execrabilis et enormis infirmitas in Anglia quasi communis, et praecipue in comitatu Leicestriae adeo quod durante passione homines emiserunt vocem latrabilem ac si esset latratus canum ; et fuit quasi intolerabilis poena durante passione: ex inde fuit magna pestilentia hominum."

[2] *Phil. Trans.* XXIII. p. 1174 (June 26, 1702).

"We have this year [1702] had an epidemical fever, attended with very surprising symptoms. In the beginning, the patient was frequently attacked with the colica ventriculi; convulsions in various parts, sometimes violent vomitings, and a dysentery; the jaundice, and in many of them, a suppression of urine; and what urine was made was highly saturated with choler. About the state of the distemper, large purple spots appeared, and on each side of 'em two large blisters, which continued three or four days: these blisters were so placed about the spots that they might in some measure be term'd satellites or tenders: of these there were in many four different eruptions. But the most remarkable instance I saw in the fever was in a poor boy of Lymm in Cheshire, one John Pownel, about 13 years of age, who was affected with the following symptoms :—

"Upon the crisis or turn of the fever, he was seized with an aphonia, and was speechless six weeks [? days], with the following convulsions : the distemper infested the nerves of both arms and legs which produced the Chorea Sancti Viti, or St Vitus's dance; and the legs sometimes were both so contracted that no person could reduce them to their natural position. Besides these, he had most terrible symptoms, which began in the following manner : [description of convulsions follows]...and then he barked in all the usual notes of a dog, sometimes snarling, barking, and at the last howling like an hound. After this the nerves of the mandibles were convulsed, and then the jaws clashed together with that violence that several of his teeth were beaten out, and then at several times there came a great foam from his mouth...These symptoms were so amazing that several persons about him believed he was possessed. I told them there was no ground for such suppositions, but that the distemper was natural, and a species of an epilepsy, and by the effects I convinced them of the truth of it; for in a week's time I recovered the boy his speech, his senses returned, his convulsions vanished, and the boy is now very cheerful. There have been other persons in this country much after the same manner."

This epidemic of 1702 in Lancashire and Cheshire was recorded as something unusual. It had certain intestinal symptoms such as colic, which may well have followed the use of poisoned food and are indeed described among the symptoms of ergotism; there were also convulsions, large purple spots with blisters coming and going on the skin near them, and, in the single case that is given with details, there were contractures of the legs "so that no person could reduce them to their natural position," and a continuance for several days of painful epileptiform fits attended with noises like the barking of a dog, or the hissing of a goose, "all which different sounds (I take it) proceed from the different contractions of the lungs variously forcing out the air." The remarkable case of the boy, certified by several witnesses, is expressly given as one belonging to the general epidemic of the locality, others having been affected "much after the same manner." Whatever suggestion there may be of ergotism in these particulars, nothing is said of gangrene of the limbs, although the livid spots and blisters are part of the symptoms of gangrenous ergotism, just as the convulsions and contractures are of convulsive ergotism. In the Suffolk cases of 1762 there were both contractures of the limbs and gangrene.

Knighton's mention of the barking noises emitted by the sufferers of 1340 has suggested to Nichols, the author of the *History of Leicestershire*[1], a comparison of them with the cases investigated by Dr Freind in the year 1700, at the village of Blackthorn in Oxfordshire. Having heard a great rumour in the summer of that year that certain girls at that Oxfordshire village were taken with frequent barkings like dogs, Dr Freind made a journey to the place to investigate the cases[2].

He found that this *pestis* or plague had invaded two families in the village, on terms of close intimacy with each other. Two or three girls in each family are specially referred to: they were seized at intervals of a few hours with spasms of the neck and mouth, attended by vociferous cries; the spasmodic movements increased to a climax, when the victims sank exhausted. The fits had kept occurring for several weeks, and had appeared in the second family at a considerable interval after the first. The symptoms, said Freind, were those that had been described by Seidelius—distortion of the mouth, indecorous working of the tongue, and noises emitted like barking. He found nothing in the girls' symptoms that could not be referred to a form of St Vitus' dance or to hysteria, in which maladies, laughter, howling and beating of the breast are occasionally seen as well as the spasmodic working of the neck and limbs.

The question remains whether the cases of 1700 in the Oxfordshire village, assuming Dr Freind's reading of them to be correct, were as illustrative of the outbreak of 1340 as the cases of 1702 in Lancashire and Cheshire, which were probably too numerous and too much complicated with symptoms of

[1] *Op. cit.* I. pt. 2, p. 366.
[2] *Phil. Trans.* XXII. (1700–1701), p. 799, a Letter in Latin from Joh. Freind dated Christ Church, Oxford, 31 March.

material toxic disorder to be explained as hysterical. There is, indeed, a larger question raised, whether the so-called psychopathies of the medieval and more recent periods may not have had a beginning, at least, in some toxic property of the staple food. The imagination readily fixes upon such symptoms as foaming at the mouth and barking noises, exalts these phenomena over deeper symptoms that a physician might have detected, and finds a simple explanation of the whole complex seizure as demoniac possession or, in modern phrase, as a psychopathy. Without questioning the subjective or imitative nature of many outbreaks which have been set down to hysteria, it may be well to use some discrimination before we exclude altogether an element of material poisoning such as ergot in the staple food, more especially in the case of the wide-spread hysterical epidemics of Sweden, a country subject to ergotism also[1].

These eighteenth-century instances have been brought in to illustrate Knighton's account of the epidemic of 1340. The next strange outbreak of the fourteenth century is recorded by the St Albans historian ("Walsingham") under a year between 1361 and 1365, probably the year 1362. Like so many more of the medieval records of epidemic sickness, it is a meagre and confused statement: "Numbers died of the disease of lethargy, prophesying troubles to many; many women also died by the flux; and there was a general murrain of cattle[2]." Along with that enigmatical entry, we may take the last of the kind that here concerns us. At Cambridge, in 1389, there occurred an epidemic of "phrensy;" it is described as "a great and formidable pestilence, which arose suddenly, and in which men were attacked all at once by the disease of phrensy of the mind, dying

---

[1] The earliest religious hysterias of Sweden fall in the years 1668 to 1673, which do not correspond to years of ergotism in that country, although there was ergotism in France in 1670 and in Westphalia in 1672. The later Swedish psychopathies have been in 1841–2, 1854, 1858, and 1866–68, some of which years do correspond closely to periods of ergotism in Sweden.

[2] "Moriebantur etiam plures morbo litargiae, multis infortunia prophetantes; mulieres insuper decessere multae per fluxum, et erat communis pestis bestiarum." Walsingham, *Hist. Angl.*, *sub anno*; and in identical terms in the *Chronicon Angliae a Monacho Sancti Albani*.

without the *viaticum,* and in a state of unconsciousness[1]." The names of phrensy and lethargy occur in the manuscript medical treatises of the time in the chapters upon diseases of the brain and nerves[2]; strictly they are names of symptoms, and not of forms or types of disease, and they may be used loosely of various morbid states which have little in common.   A lethargy would in some cases be a name for coma in fever, or for a paralytic stroke; a phrensy might be actual mania, or it might be the delirium of plague or typhus fever.   The "lethargy" of 1362 is alleged of a number of people as if in an epidemic, whatever the singular phrase "prophetantes infortunia multis" may mean; and the "phrensy of the mind" of which many died suddenly at Cambridge in 1389, does not look as if it had been a symptom of plague or pestilential fever.   The judicious reader will make what he can of these disappointingly meagre details.   But for his guidance it may be added that the French accounts of ergotism in 1676 give one of the poisonous effects as being "to cause sometimes malign fevers accompanied with drowsiness and raving," which terms might stand for lethargy and phrensy; also that it has not always been easy, in an epidemic among the peasantry after a bad harvest, to distinguish the cases of ergotism from the cases of typhus, the contractures of the limbs, which seem so special to ergotism, having been described also for undoubted cases of typhus[3].

Whether these anomalous epidemics in medieval England

[1] "Magna et formidabilis pestilentia extemplo subsecuta est Cantabrigiae, qua homines subito, prout dicebatur, sospites, invasi mentis phrenesi moriebantur, sine viatico sive sensu." Walsingham, *Hist. Angl.* II. 186.   Under the same year, 1389, the continuator of Higden's *Polychronicon* (IX. 216) says that the king being in the south and "seeing some of his prostrated by sudden death, hastened to Windsor."

[2] For example in the Sloane MS. 2420 (the treatise by Constantinus Africanus of Salerno), there are chapters "De Litargia," "De Stupore Mentis," and "De Phrenesi."

[3] Th. O. Heusinger, *Studien über den Ergotismus,* Marburg, 1856, p. 35 : "Es werden freilich in den Beschreibungen einiger früheren Epidemieen öfter typhöse Erscheinungen erwähnt ; die Beschreiber behaupten aber auch dann meist die Contagiosität der Krankheit, und es liegt die Vermuthung nahe, dass die Krankheit dann eigentlich ein Typhus war, bei dem die Erscheinungen des Ergotismus ebenso constant vorkommen, wie sie sonst in vereinzelteren Fällen dem Typhus sich beigesellen " (cf. 'Dorf Gossfelden,' in Appendix).

were instances of convulsive ergotism or not, the English records are on the whole wanting in the evidence of such wide-spread and frequent disasters from a poisoned harvest as distinguish the French annals of the same period. One reason of our immunity may have been that the grain was better grown; another reason certainly is that rye was a comparatively rare crop in England, wheaten bread being preferred, although bread made from beans and barley was not uncommon. Thorold Rogers says: " Rye was scantily cultivated. An occasional crop on many estates, it is habitually sown in few. It is regularly sown in Cambridgeshire and some other of the eastern counties. As the period before us passes on [1259–1400], it becomes still more rare, and as will be seen below, some of the later years of this enquiry contain no entries of its purchase and sale[1]." But it is clear from the entries in chronicles, more particularly about the very period of the fourteenth century to which the three epidemics suggestive of ergotism belong, that the English peasantry suffered from the poisonous effects of damaged food, even if they suffered little from spurred rye. Thus, under the year 1383, in the history known as Walsingham's, there is an unmistakeable reference to many fatalities, as well as serious maladies, caused by the eating of damaged fruit[2]. Again, under 1391, it is stated that this was " a hard and difficult year for the poor owing to a dearth of fruits, which had now lasted two years; whence it happened that at the time of the nuts and apples, many of the poor died of dysentery brought on by eating them; and the pestilence would have been worse had it not been for the laudable diligence of the Mayor of London, who caused corn to be brought to London from over sea[3]."

---

[1] *History of Agriculture and Prices*, I. 27.

[2] " Sed in fructibus arborum suspicio multa fuit, eo quod per nebulas foetentes, exhalationes, aerisque varias corruptiones, ipsi fructus, puta poma, pyra, et hujusmodi sunt infecta; quorum esu multi mortales hoc anno [1383] vel pestem letalem vel graves morbos et infirmitates incurrerunt." Walsingham, *Hist. Angl.* II. 109. The continuator of Higden records under the same year, in one place a " great pestilence in Kent which destroyed many, and spared no age or sex " (IX. 27), and on another page (IX. 21) a great epidemic in Norfolk, which attacked only the youth of either sex between the ages of seven and twenty-two !

[3] Walsingham, II. 203 ; Stow's *Survey of London*, p. 133.

Generalities on Medieval Famines in England.

Summing up the English famine-pestilences of the medieval period, we find that they included the usual forms of such sickness—spotted fever of the nature of typhus, dysentery, lientery or looseness (such as has often subsequently accompanied typhus or famine-fever in Ireland), and putrid sore-throat. That some of these effects were due to spoiled grain and fruits, as well as to absolute want, we may reasonably conclude; for example the harvest of 1258 rotted on the ground, and yet the mouldy corn was sold at famine prices. With all those records of famines and their attendant sicknesses in England, it is significant that there is little indication of ergotism. The immunity of England from ergotism, with such a record of famines as the annals show, can only have been because little rye was grown and little black bread eaten. The standard of living would appear to have been higher among the English peasantry than among the French. A bad harvest, still more two bad harvests in succession, made them feel the pinch of famine more acutely, perhaps, than if they had accommodated themselves to the more sober level of rye bread. Hence the somewhat paradoxical but doubtless true saying of the Middle Ages—"Anglorum fames, Francorum ignis." The saying really means, not that England was a poor country, which would be an absurd repute for foreigners to have fixed upon her; but that the English were subject to alternating periods of abundance and scarcity, of surfeit and starvation. The earliest English work which deals fully and concretely with the social condition of the country is the fourteenth-century poem of "The Vision of Piers the Ploughman." A few passages from that poem will be of use as throwing light upon the famines of England, before we finally leave the period of which they are characteristic.

Langland's poem describes the social state of England in peculiar circumstances, namely, after the upheaval and dislocation of the Great Mortality of 1349; and in that respect it has an interest for our subject which comes into a later chapter. But in so far as it illustrates the alternating periods of abundance

C. 5

and scarcity, the vision of medieval England concerns us here
before we quit the subject of famine-pestilences. The average
industrious ploughman, represented by Piers himself, fares but
soberly until Lammas comes round [1] :—

> "I have no penny, quod Piers, pullets for to buy,
> Ne neither geese nor pigs, but two green cheeses,
> A few cruddes and cream, and an haver-cake,
> And two loaves of beans and bran ybake for my fauntis.
> And yet I say, by my soul, I have no salt bacon,
> Nor no cookeney, by Christ, collops for to maken.
> And I have percil and porettes and many kole-plantes,
> And eke a cow and a calf, and a cart-mare
> To draw afield my dung the while the drought lasteth.
> And by this lyflode me mot live till lammas time ;
> And by that I hope to have harvest in my croft ;
> And then may I digte thy dinner as me dear liketh."

Some are worse off than the ploughman in the slack time
before the harvest:

> "All the poor people tho pesecoddes fetched,
> Beans and baken apples they brought in their lappes,
> Chibolles and chervelles and ripe cherries many,
> And proferred Piers this present to plead with Hunger.
> All Hunger ate in haste, and axed after more.
> Then poor folk for fear fed Hunger eagerlie,
> With green poret and pesen, to poison Hunger they thought.
> By that it nighed near harvest, new corn came to chipping.
> Then was folk fain, and fed Hunger with the best,
> With good ale, as glutton taught, and gerte Hunger go sleep.
> And though would waster not work but wandren about,
> Ne no beggar eat bread that beans in were,
> But of cocket or clerematyn or else of clean wheat :
> Ne no halfpenny ale in none wise drink,
> But of the best and of the brownest that in burgh is to sell.
> Labourers that have no land to live on, but their hands,
> Deigned nought to dine a-day night-old wortes.
> May no penny ale them pay ne no piece of bacon,
> But if it be fresh flesh other fish fried other bake."

The waster being now in his season of plenty falls to abusing
the Statute of Labourers:

[1] The spelling, and a few whole words, have been altered from Skeat's text, so as
to make the meaning clear.

"And then cursed he the king and all his council after,
Such laws to loke, labourers to grieve.
But whiles Hunger was their master there would none of them chide,
Nor strive against *his* statute, so sternly he looked.
And I warn you, workmen, wynneth while ye mowe,
For Hunger hitherward hasteth him fast.
He shall awake with water wasters to chasten.
Ere five year be fulfilled such famine shall arise
Through floods and through foul weathers fruits shall fail.
And so said Saturn, and sent you to warn....
Then shall death withdraw and dearth be justice,
And Daw the dyker die for hunger,
But if God of his goodness grant us a truce."

He proposes to feed the lazy wasters on beans:

"And gif the groomes grudge, bid them go swynk,
And he shall sup the sweeter when he hath deserved."

The ploughman asks Hunger the reason why both himself
and his servants are unable to work:

"I wot well, quod Hunger, what sickness you aileth.
Ye have maunged over much, and that maketh you groan....
Let not sir Surfeit sitten at thy board....
And gif thy diet be thus, I dare lay mine ears
That Physic shall his furred hoods for his food sell,
And his cloak of calabre with all the knaps of gold,
And be fain, by my faith, his physic to let,
And learn to labour with land, for lyflode is swect:
For murtherers are many leeches, Lord them amend!
They do men kill through their drinks, or destiny it would.
By Saint Poul, quod Piers, these aren profitable words."

In another place, Hawkin the minstrel confesses to gluttony:

"And more meat ate and drank than nature might digest,
And caught sickness some time for my surfeits oft."

A liking for the best of food, and plenty of it, when it was to
be had, has clearly been an English trait from the earliest times.
Conversely thrift does not appear to have been a virtue or a
grace of the labouring class in England. Thus a bad harvest
brought wide-spread scarcity, and two bad harvests brought
famine and famine-pestilences. The contrasts were sharp because the standard of living was high. And although three, at

least, of the English famines were disgraceful to so rich a country, and were probably the occasion of the foreign reproach of "Anglorum fames;" yet the significant fact remains that the disease of the European peasantry, which is the truest index of an inferior diet, namely ergotism, has little or no place in our annals of sickness.

CHAPTER II.

THE history of leprosy in Britain can hardly be the history of leprosy alone, but of that disease along with others which were either mistaken for it or conveniently and euphemistically included under it. That there was leprosy in the country is undoubted; but it is just as certain that there was *lues venerea*; that the latter as a primary lesion led an anonymous existence or was called *lepra* or *morphaea* if it were called anything; that the remote effects of the lues were not known as such, being taken for detached or original outcomes of the disordered humours and therefore in the same general class as leprous manifestations; and that the popular and clerical notions of leprosy were too superstitious and inexact, even if the diagnostic intention had been more resolute than it was, to permit of any clear separation of the leprous from the syphilitic, to say nothing of their separation from the poor victims of lupus and cancer of the face, of scrofulous running sores, or of neglected skin-eruptions more repulsive to the eye than serious in their nature. I shall give some proof of each of those assertions—as an essential preliminary to any correct handling of the historical records of British leprosy.

Leprosy in Medieval Medical Treatises.

The picture given of true leprosy in the medieval treatises on medicine is unmistakeable. There are two systematic writers about the year 1300 who have left a better account of it than the Arabian authors from whom they mostly copied. While the writers in question have transferred whole chapters unaltered from Avicenna, Rhazes and Theodoric, they have improved upon their models in the stock chapter 'De Lepra.' It so happens that those two writers, Bernard Gordonio and Gilbertus Anglicus, bear names which have been taken to indicate British nationality, and the picture of leprosy by the latter has actually been adduced as a contemporary account of the disease observed in England[1]. Gordonio was a professor at Montpellier, and his experience and scholarship are purely foreign. The circumstances of Gilbert the Englishman are not so well known; but it is tolerably certain that he was not, as often assumed, the Gilbert Langley, Gilbert de l'Aigle, or Gilbertus de Aquila, who was physician to Hubert, archbishop of Canterbury (✝ 13 July, 1205)[2], having been a pupil at Salerno in the time of Aegidius of Corbeil (about 1180). The treatise of Gilbertus Anglicus bears internal evidence of a later century and school; it is distinguished by method and comprehensiveness, and is almost exactly on the lines of the *Lilium Medicinae* by Gordonio, whose date at Montpellier is known with some exactness to have been from 1285 to about 1307. Future research may perhaps discover where Gilbert taught or was taught; meanwhile we may safely assume that his scholarship and system were of a foreign colour. The medical writer of that time in England was John of Gaddesden, mentioned in the end of the foregoing chapter; he is the merest plagiary, and the one or two original remarks in his chapter 'De Lepra' would almost justify the epithet of "fatuous" which Guy de Chauliac applied to him.

Although we cannot appeal to Gilbertus Anglicus for native English experience any more than we can to his *alter ego*, Gordonio, yet we may assume that the picture of leprosy which they give might have been sketched in England as well as in Italy or in Provence. The conditions were practically

---

[1] Simpson, *Edin. Med. and Surg. Journ.* 1842, vol. LVII. p. 136.

[2] Ralph of Coggeshall (Rolls ed. p. 156) describes the death of Hubert on 13 July, 1205, but does not mention the name of his physician.

uniform throughout Christendom; the true leprosy of any one part of medieval Europe is the true leprosy of the whole.

Gilbert's picture[1], as we have said, is unmistakeable, and the same might be said of Bernard's[2]—the eyebrows falling bare and getting knotted with uneven tuberosities, the nose and other features becoming thick, coarse and lumpy, the face losing its mobility or play of expression, the raucous voice, the loss of sensibility in the hands, and the ultimate break-up or *naufragium* of the leprous growths into foul running sores. The enumeration of nervous symptoms, which are now recognised to be fundamental in the pathology of leprosy, shows that Gilbert went below the surface. Among the "signa leprae generalia" he mentions such forms of hyperaesthesia as *formicatio* (the creeping of ants), and the feeling of "needles and pins;" and, in the way of anaesthesia, he speaks of the loss of sensibility from the little finger to the elbow, as well as in the exposed parts where the blanched spots or thickenings come—the forehead, cheeks, eyebrows, to which he adds the tongue. Gilbert's whole chapter 'De Lepra' is an obvious improvement upon the corresponding one in Avicenna, who says that *lepra* is a cancer of the whole body, cancer being the *lepra* of a single member, and is probably confusing lupus with leprosy when he describes the cartilages of the nose as corroded in the latter, and the nostrils destroyed by the same kind of *naufragium* as the fingers and toes. All students of the history or clinical characters of leprosy, from Guy de Chauliac, who wrote about 1350, down to Hensler and Sprengel, have recognised in Gilbert's and Bernard's account of it the marks of first-hand observation; so that we may take it, without farther debate, that leprosy, as correctly diagnosed, was a disease of Europe and of Britain in the Middle Ages.

Having got so far, we come next to a region of almost inextricable confusion, a region of secrecy and mystification, as well as of real contemporary ignorance. We may best approach it by one or two passages from Gilbert and Gordonio themselves.

[1] Gilberti Anglici *Compendium Medicinae*, ed. Michael de Capella. Lugduni, 1512, Lib. VII. cap. "De Lepra," pp. 337–345.

[2] Bernardi Gordonii *Lilium Medicinae*. Lugd. 1551, p. 88.

The systematic handling of *lepra* in their writings is one thing, and their more concrete remarks on its conditions of origin, its occasions, or circumstances are another. What are we to make of this kind of leprosy ?—" In hoc genere, causa est accessus ad mulierem ad quam accessit prius leprosus ; et corrumpit velocius vir sanus quam mulier a leproso....Et penetrant [venena] in nervos calidos et arterias et venas viriles, et inficiunt spiritus et bubones, et hoc velocius si mulier," etc. Or to quote Gilbert again : " Ex accessu ad mulieres, diximus superius, lepram in plerisque generari post coitûs leprosos[1]." Or in Gordonio : " Et provenit [lepra] etiam ex nimia confibulatione cum leprosis, et ex coitu cum leprosa, et qui jacuit cum muliere cum qua jacuit leprosus[2]." That these circumstances of contracting *lepra* were not mere verbal theorizings inspired by the pathology of the day and capable of being now set aside, is obvious from a *historia* or case which Gordonio introduces into his text. " I shall tell what happened," he says ; and then proceeds to the following relation :[3]

" Quaedam comtissa venit leprosa ad Montem Pessulanum [Montpellier], et erat in fine in cura mea ; et quidam Baccalarius in medicina ministrabat ei, et jacuit cum ea, et impregnavit eam, et perfectissime leprosus factus est." Happy is he therefore, he adds, who learns caution from the risks of others.

Here we have sufficient evidence, from the beginning of the fourteenth century, of a disease being called *lepra* which does not conform to the conditions of leprosy as we now understand them. The same confusion between leprosy and the *lues venerea* prevailed through the whole medieval period. Thus, in the single known instance of a severe edict against lepers in England, the order of Edward III. to the mayor and sheriffs of London in 1346[4], the reasons for driving lepers out of the City are given,—among others, because they communicate their disease " by carnal intercourse with women in stews and other secret places," and by their polluted breath. It was pointed

---

[1] *Compend. Med.   Ed. cit.* p. 344.
[2] *Lilium Medicinae.*   Lugd. 1551, p. 89.
[3] *Ibid.* p. 89.
[4] For fuller reference, see p. 103.

out long ago by Beckett in his paper on the antiquity of the *lues venerea*[1], that the polluted breath was characteristic of the latter, but not of leprosy. Of course the pollution of their breath might have meant no more than the theoretical reasoning of the books (as in Gilbert, where the breath of lepers, as well as the mere sight of them, is said to give the disease, p. 337), but the breath was probably obnoxious in a more real way, just as we know, from Gordonio's case at Montpellier, that the other alleged source of "leprous" contagion was no mere theoretical deduction. As the medieval period came to an end the leper-houses (in France) were found to contain a miscellaneous gathering of cases generically called leprous; and about the same time, the year 1488, an edict of the same purport as Edward III.'s London one of 1346, was issued by the provost of Paris against *les lépreux* of that city. The year 1488 is so near the epidemic outburst of the *morbus Gallicus* during the French campaigns on Italian soil in 1494–95, that the historian has not hesitated to set down that sudden reappearance of leprous contagion, in a proclamation of the State, to a real prevalence already in Paris of the contagious malady which was to be heard of to the farthest corners of Europe a few years after[2].

There is no difficulty in producing evidence from medieval English records of the prevalence of *lues venerea*, which was not

---

[1] *Philos. Trans. of Royal Society*, XXXI. 58: "Now in a true leprosy we never meet with the mention of any disorder in those parts, which, if there be not, must absolutely secure the person from having that disease communicated to him by coition with leprous women; but it proves there was a disease among them which was not the leprosy, although it went by that name; and that this could be no other than venereal because it was infectious."

He then quotes from Trevisa's translation of Bartholomew Glanvile, *De proprietatibus rerum*, passages which he thinks relate to syphilis, although they are obviously the distinctive signs of lepra taken almost verbatim from Gilbertus Anglicus. He implies that the later so-called leper-houses of London were really founded for syphilis when it became epidemic. In the will of Ralph Holland, merchant taylor, mention is made of three leper-houses, the Loke, Hackenay and St Giles beyond Holborn Bars, as if these were all that existed in the year 1452. But in the reign of Henry VIII. there were six of them besides St Giles's,—Knightsbridge, Hammersmith, Highgate, Kingsland, the Lock, and Mile End; and these, says Beckett, were used for the treatment of the French pox, which became exceedingly common after 1494–6.

[2] Martin, *Histoire de France*, VII. 283.

concealed under the euphemistic or mistaken diagnosis of leprosy. Instances of a very bad kind, authenticated with the names of the individuals, are given in Gascoigne's *Liber Veritatum*, under the date of 1433[1].

In the medieval text-books of Avicenna, Gilbert and others, there are invariably paragraphs on *pustulae et apostemata virgae*. In the only original English medical work of those times, by John Ardern, who was practising at Newark from 1349 to 1370, and came afterwards to London, appearances are described which can mean nothing else than condylomata[2]. From a manuscript prescription-book of the medieval period, in the British Museum, I have collected some receipts (or their headings) which relate, as an index of later date prefixed to the MS. says, to "the pox of old[3]."

[1] One of Gascoigne's references was copied by Beckett (*Phil. Trans.* XXXI. 47), beginning : " Novi enim ego, Magister Thomas Gascoigne, licet indignus, sacrae theologiae doctor, qui haec scripsi et collegi, diversos viros, qui mortui fuerunt ex putrefactione membrorum suorum et corporis sui, quae corruptio et putrefactio causata fuit, ut ipsi dixerunt, per exercitium copulae carnalis cum mulieribus. Magnus enim dux in Anglia, scil. J. de Gaunt, mortuus est ex tali putrefactione membrorum genitalium et corporis sui, causata per frequentationem mulierum. Magnus enim fornicator fuit, ut in toto regno Angliae divulgabatur," etc. In the *Loci e Libro Veritatum*, printed by Thorold Rogers (Oxford, 1881), the following consequences are mentioned : " Plures viri per actum libidinosum luxuriae habuerunt membra sua corrupta et penitus destructa, non solum virgam sed genitalia : et alii habuerunt membra sua per luxuriam corrupta ita quod cogebantur, propter poenam, caput virgae abscindere. Item homo Oxoniae scholaris, Morland nomine, mortuus fuit Oxoniae ex corruptione causata per actum luxuriae." p. 136.

[2] *A most excellent and compendious method of curing woundes in the head and in other partes of the body; translated into English by John Read, Chirurgeon; with the exact cure of the Caruncle, treatise of the Fistulae in the fundament, out of Joh. Ardern, etc.* London, 1588.

[3] MS. Harl. 2378 :—No 86 is : "Take lynsed or lynyn clothe and brēne it & do ye pouder in a clout, and bynd it to ye sore pintel." Also. "Take linsed and stamp it and a lytel oyle of olyf and a lytl milk of a cow of a color, and fry them togeder in a panne, and ley it about ye pyntel in a clout." No. 87 is "for bolnyng of pyntel." No. 88 is " For ye kank' on a mānys pyntel." On p. 103 is another "For ye bolnyng of a mānys yerde....Bind it alle abouten ye yerde, and it salle suage." On folio 19: "For ye nebbe yt semeth leprous...iii dayes it shall be hole." "For ye kanker" might have meant cancer or chancre. The prescriptions in Moulton's *This is the Myrour or Glasse of Helth* (? 1540) correspond closely with these in the above Harleian MS. The printed book gives one (cap. 63), "For a man that is Lepre, and it take in his legges and go upwarde." There is also a prescription for "morphewe."

Some have refused to see in such cases any real correspondence with the modern forms of syphilis because only local effects are described and no constitutional consequences traced. But no one in those times thought of a primary focus of infection with its remoter effects at large, in the case of any disease whatsoever. Even in the great epidemic of syphilis at the end of the fifteenth century, the sequence of primary and secondary (tertiaries were unheard of until long after), was not at first understood ; the eruption of the skin, which was compared to a bad kind of variola, the imposthumes of the head and of the bones elsewhere, together with all other constitutional or general symptoms, were traced, in good faith, to a disordered liver, an organ which was chosen on theoretical grounds as the *minera morbi* or laboratory of the disease[1]. The circumstances of the great epidemic were, of course, special, but they were not altogether new. No medieval miracle could have been more of a suspension of the order of nature than that *luxuria, immunditia*, and *foeditas*, with their attendant *corruptio membrorum*, should have been free from those consequences, in the individual and in the community, which are more familiar in our own not less clean-living days merely because the sequence of events is better understood. That such vices abounded in the medieval world we have sufficient evidence. They were notorious among the Norman conquerors of England, especially notorious in the reign of William Rufus[2]; hence, perhaps, the significance of the phrase *lepra Normannorum*. That particular vice which amounts to a felony was the subject of the sixth charge (unproved) in the indictment of the order of the Templars before the Pope Clement V. in 1307. Effects on the public health traceable to such causes, for the most part *sub rosa*, have been often felt in the history of nations, from the Biblical episode of Baal-peor down to modern times. The evidence is written at large in the works of Astruc, Hensler and Rosenbaum. We are here concerned with a much smaller matter, namely, any evidence from England which may throw light upon the classes of cases that were called leprous if they were called by a name at all.

[1] Nicolas Massa, in Luisini.
[2] Freeman, *The Reign of William Rufus.* App. vol. II. p. 499.

Under the year 1258, Matthew Paris introduces a singular paragraph, which is headed, "The Bishop of Hereford smitten with polypus." The bishop, a Provençal, had made himself obnoxious by his treacherous conduct as the agent of Henry III. at the Holy See in the matter of the English subsidies to the pope. Accordingly it was by the justice of God that he was deformed by a most disgraceful disease, to wit, *morphea*, or again, "morphea polipo, vel quadam specie leprae[1]." According to the medical teaching of the time, as we find it in Gilbertus Anglicus, *morphaea* was an infection producing a change in the natural colour of the skin; it was confined to the skin, whereas *lepra* was in the flesh also; the former was curable, the latter incurable; *morphaea* might be white, red, or black[2]. The account of *morphaea* by Gordonio is somewhat fuller. All things, he says, that are causes of *lepra* are causes of *morphaea*; so that what is in the flesh *lepra* is *morphaea* in the skin. It was a patchy discoloration of the skin, reddish, yellowish, whitish, dusky, or black, producing *terribilis aspectus*; curable if recent, incurable if of long standing; curable also if of moderate extent, but difficult to cure if of great extent[3]. In this description by Gordonio a modern French writer on leprosy[4] discovers the classical characters of the syphilis of our own day: "not one sign is wanting."

No doubt the medical writers drew a distinction between *morphaea* and *lepra*, as we have seen in quoting Gilbert and Gordonio. Gaddesden, also, who mostly copies them, interpolates here an original remark. No one should be adjudged leprous, he says, and separated from his fellows, merely because the "figure and form" (the stock phrase) of the face are corrupted: the disease might be "scabies foeda," or if in the feet, it might be "cancer." Nodosities or tubercles should not be taken to mean leprosy, unless they are confirmed (inveterate) in the

[1] *L.c.* v. 679, "Episcopus Herefordensis polipo percutitur.—Episcopus Herefordensis turpissimo morbo videlicet morphea, Deo percutiente, merito deformatur, qui totum regnum Angliae proditiose dampnificavit;" and again v. 622.

[2] *Compend. Med. Ed. cit.* p. 170.

[3] *Lilium Med. Ed. cit.* p. 108.

[4] Brassac, Art. "Elephantiasis" (p. 465) in *Dict. Encycl. des Sciences Médicales.*

face[1]. But how uncertain are these diagnostic indications, as between *lepra* and *morphaea*, *lepra* and " scabies foeda," *lepra* and " cancer in pedibus!" If there were any object in calling the disease by one name rather than another, it is clear that the same disease might be called by a euphemism in one case and by a term meant to be opprobrious in another. Although leprosy was not in general a disease that anyone might wish to be credited with, yet there were circumstances when the diagnosis of leprosy had its advantages. It was of use to a beggar or tramp to be called a leper : he would excite more pity, he might get admission to a hospital, and he might solicit alms, under royal privilege, although begging in ordinary was punishable. It is conceivable also that the diagnosis of leprosy was a convenient one for men in conspicuous positions in Church and State. It is most improbable that the " lepra Normannorum" was all leprosy; it is absurd to suppose that leprosy became common in Europe because returning Crusaders introduced it from the East, as if leprosy could be " introduced" in any such way ; and it is not easy to arrive at certitude, that all the cases of leprosy in princes and other high-placed personages (Baldwin IV. of Jerusalem who died at the age of twenty-five,[2] Robert the Bruce of Scotland,[3] and Henry IV. of England[4]) were cases that would now be diagnosed leprous.

Instances may be quoted to show that the name of leper was flung about somewhat at random. Thus, in an edict issued by Henry II., during the absence of Becket abroad for the settlement of his quarrel with the king, it was decreed that anyone who brought into the country documents relating to the threatened papal interdict should have his feet cut off if he were a regular cleric, his eyes put out if a secular clerk, should be hanged if a layman, and be burned if a *leprosus*—that is to

---

[1] *Rosa Anglica.* Papiae, 1492.

[2] That Baldwin IV.'s disease excited interest in him is clear from the reference of William of Newburgh, who calls him (p. 242) "princeps Christianus lepram corporis animi virtute exornans."

[3] Chronicon de Lanercost (Bannatyne Club, p. 259): "Dominus autem Robertus de Brus, quia factus fuerat leprosus, illa vice [anno 1327] cum eis Angliam non intravit." The rubric on folio 228 of the MS. has "leprosus moritur."

[4] The original account is by Gascoigne, *Loci etc.* ed. Rogers, Oxon. p. 228.

say, a beggar or common tramp. Again, in the charges brought for Henry III. against the powerful minister Hubert de Burg in 1239, one item is that he had prevented the marriage of our lord the king with a certain noble lady by representing to the latter and to her guardian that the king was "a squinter, and a fool, and a good-for-nothing, and that he had a kind of leprosy, and was a deceiver, and a perjurer, and more of a craven than any woman[1]" etc.

There is also a curious instance of the term leprous being applied to the Scots, evidently in the sense in which William of Malmesbury, and many more after him, twitted that nation with their cutaneous infirmities. When the Black Death of 1348–9 had reached the northern counties of England, the Scots took advantage of their prostrate state to gather in the forest of Selkirk for an invasion, exulting in the "foul death of England." Knighton says that the plague reached them there, that five thousand of them died, and that their rout was completed by the English falling upon them[2]. But the other contemporary chronicler of the Black Death, Geoffrey le Baker[3], tells the story with a curious difference. The Scots, he says, swearing by the foul death of the English, passed from the extreme of exultation to that of grief; the sword of God's wrath was lifted from the English and fell in its fury upon the Scots, "et [Scotos] per lepram, nec minus quam Anglicos per apostemata et pustulos, mactavit." The *apostemata* and *pustuli* were indeed the buboes, boils and carbuncles of the plague, correctly named; but what was the *lepra* of the Scots? It was probably a vague term of abuse; but, if the clerk of Osney attached any meaning to it, it is clear that he saw nothing improbable in a disease called *lepra* springing up suddenly and spreading among a body of men.

---

[1] "Item matrimonium inter dominum regem et quandam nobilem mulierem nequiter impedivit, dum clanculo significavit eidem mulieri et suo generi, quod rex strabo et fatuus nequamque fuerat, et speciem leprae habere, fallaxque fuerat et perjurus, imbellis plusquam mulier, in suos tantum saevientem, et prorsus inutilem complexibus alicujus ingenuae mulieris asserendo." Matthew Paris, *Chron. Maj.*, Rolls ed., III. 618–19.

[2] *Chronicon Angliae* in Twysden, col. 2600.

[3] *Chronicle of Geoffrey le Baker*, edited by E. Maunde Thompson. Oxford, 1889, p. 100.

We conclude, then, that *lepra* was a term used in a generic sense because of a real uncertainty of diagnosis, or because there was some advantage to be got from being called *leprosus*, or because it was flung about at random.   But there is still another reason for the inexact use of the terms *lepra* and *leprosus* in the medieval period, namely, the dominant influence of religious tradition.   The heritage or accretion of religious sentiment not only perverted the correct use of the name, but led to regulations and proscriptions which were out of place even for the real disease.

The Biblical Associations of Leprosy.

Among the synonyms for *leprosi* we find the terms "pauperes Christi, videlicet Lazares," the name of "Christ's poor" being given to lepers by Aelred in the twelfth century and by Matthew Paris in the thirteenth.   The association of ideas with Lazarus is a good sample of the want of discrimination in all that pertains to medieval leprosy.   The Lazarus of St Luke's Gospel, who was laid at the rich man's gate full of sores, is a representative person, existing only in parable.   On the other hand, the Lazarus of St John's Gospel, Lazarus of Bethany, the brother of Martha and Mary, the man of many friends, is both a historical personage and a saint in the calendar.   But there is nothing to show that he was a leper.   He had a remarkable experience of restoration to the light of day, and it was probably on account of an episode in his life that made so much talk that he received posthumously the name of Lazarus, or "helped of God[1]."   The name of the man in the parable is also generic, just

[1] Professor Robertson Smith has kindly written for me the following note : "The later Jews were given to shorten proper names ; and in the Talmud we find the shortening *La'zar* (with a guttural, which the Greeks could not pronounce, between the *a* and the *z*), for Eliezer or Eleazar. Λάζαρος is simply *La'zar* with a Greek ending, and occurs, as a man's name, not only in the New Testament but in Josephus (*B. Jud.* v. 13, 7).   This was quite understood by early readers of the Gospels ; the Syriac New Testament, translated from the Greek, restores the lost guttural, and uses the Syriac form, as employed in 1 *Macc.* viii. 17 to render the Greek 'Ελεάζαρος.   Moreover the Latin and Greek *onomastica* explain Lazarus as meaning 'adjutus,' which shows that they took it from (Hebrew) 'to help'—the second element in the compound Eliezer.   The etymology 'adjutus' (or the like)

as generic as that of his contrast Dives is; but specifically there was nothing in common between the one Lazarus and the other. Yet St Lazarus specially named as the brother of Martha and Mary (as in the charter of the leper-house at Sherburn) became the patron of lepers. The ascription to Lazarus of Bethany of the malady of Lazarus in the parable has done much for the prestige of the latter's disease; in the medieval world it brought all persons full of sores within a nimbus of sanctity, as being in a special sense " pauperes Christi," the successors at once of him whom Jesus loved and of "Lazarus ulcerosus." Doubtless the lepers deserved all the charity that they got; but we shall not easily understand the interest exceptionally taken in them, amidst abounding suffering and wretchedness in other forms, unless we keep in mind that they somehow came to be regarded as Christ's poor.

Next to the image of Lazarus, or rather the composite image of the two Lazaruses, the picture of leprosy that filled the imagination was that of the thirteenth and fourteenth chapters of Leviticus. That picture is even more composite than the other, and for leprosy in the strict sense it is absolutely misleading. The word translated "leprosy" is a generic term for various communicable maladies, most of which were curable within a definite period, sometimes no longer than a week. It rested with the skill of the priesthood to discriminate between the forms of communicable disease, and to prescribe the appropriate ceremonial treatment for each; the people had one common name for them all, and beyond that they were in the hands of their priests, who knew quite well what they were about. The Christian Church dealt with all those archaic institutions of an Eastern people in a child-like spirit of verbal or literal interpre-

'helped by God,' would no doubt powerfully assist in the choice of the designation lazars (for lepers). Suicer, in his *Thesaurus*, quotes a sermon of Theophanes, where it is suggested that every poor man who needs help from those who have means might be called a Lazarus."

Hirsch (*Geog. and Hist. Path.* II. 3) says that the Arabic word for the falling sickness comes from the same root (meaning "thrown to the ground") as the Hebrew word "sâraat," which is the term translated "leprosy" in Leviticus xiii. and xiv. In Isaiah liii. 4, the Vulgate has "et nos putavimus eum quasi leprosum," where the English Bible has "yet we did esteem him stricken."

tation, doubtless finding the greater part of them a meaningless jargon. But some verses would touch the imagination and call up a real and vivid picture, such verses, for example, as the following :

"And the leper in whom the plague is, his clothes shall be rent, and his head bare, and he shall put a covering upon his upper lip, and shall cry, Unclean, unclean. All the days wherein the plague shall be in him he shall be defiled ; he is unclean ; he shall dwell alone ; without the camp shall his habitation be."

Even in that comparatively plain direction, the obvious suggestion that the unclean person would not always be unclean, and that there was a term to his stay outside the camp, would go for little in reading the scripture. The medieval religious world took those parts of the Jewish teaching that appealed to their apprehension, and applied them to the circumstances of their own time with as much of zeal as the common sense of the community would permit. We have clear evidence of the effect of the Levitical teaching about "leprosy" upon English practice in the ordinances of the St Albans leper hospital of St Julian, which will be given in the sequel.

The Medieval Religious Sentiment towards Lepers.

Several incidents told of lepers by the chroniclers bring out that exaggerated religious view of the disease. Roger of Howden has preserved the following mythical story of Edward the Confessor. Proceeding one day from his palace to the Abbey Church in pomp and state, he passed with his train of nobles and ecclesiastics through a street in which sat a leper full of sores. The courtiers were about to drive the wretched man out from the royal presence, when the king ordered them to let him sit where he was. The leper, waxing bold after this concession, addressed the king, " I adjure thee by the living God to take me on thy shoulders and bring me into the church ;" whereupon the king bowed his head and took the leper upon his shoulders. And as the king went, he prayed that God would give health to the leper ; and his prayer was heard, and the leper was made whole from that very hour, praising and glorifying God[1].

It is not the miraculous ending of this incident that need surprise us most; for the Royal touch by which the Confessor wrought his numerous cures of the blind and the halt and the scrofulous, continued to be exercised, with unabated virtue, down to the eighteenth century, and came at length to be supervised by Court surgeons who were fellows of the Royal Society. It is the humility of a crowned head in the presence of a leper that marks an old-world kind of religious sentiment. The nearest approach to it in our time is the feet-washing of the poor by the empress at Vienna on Corpus Christi day.

A similar story, with a truer touch of nature in it, is told of Matilda, queen of Henry I.; and it happens to be related on so good authority that we may believe every word of it. Matilda was a Saxon princess, daughter of Margaret the Atheling, the queen of Malcolm Canmore. The other actor in the story was her brother David, afterwards king of Scots and, like his mother, honoured as a saint of the Church. The narrator is Aelred, abbot of Rievaulx, in the North Riding of Yorkshire, celebrated for his Latin style and his care for Saxon history. The abbot was a friend of St David, whose virtues he celebrates at length; the incident of queen Matilda and the lepers was one that he often heard from David's own lips (quod ex ore saepe Davidis regis audivi). The princess Matilda, taking more after her mother than her father, had been brought up in an English convent under her aunt, the abbess of it. When it came to a marriage between her and Henry I., an alliance which was meant to reconcile the Saxons to Norman rule, the question arose in the mind of Anselm whether the princess Matilda had not actually taken the veil, and whether he could legally marry her to the king. Questioned as to the fact, the princess made answer that she had indeed worn the veil in public, but only as a protection from the licentious insolence of the Norman nobles. She had no liking for the great match arranged for her, and

---

[1] Roger of Howden. Edited by Stubbs. Rolls series, No. 51, vol. I. p. 110. Aelred, the chief collector of the miraculous cures by Edward the Confessor, appears to have omitted this one.

consented unwillingly although the king was enamoured of her. Such was her humility that Aelred designates her "the Esther of our times." The marriage was on the 15th of November, 1100; and in the next year, according to the usual date given, the young queen sought relief and effusion for her religious instincts by founding the leper hospital of St Giles in the Fields, "with a chapel and a sufficient edifice." Matthew Paris, a century and a half after, saw it standing as queen Matilda had built it, and made a sketch of it in colours on the margin of his page, still remaining to us in a library at Cambridge, with the description, "Memoriale Matild. Regine."

The story which her brother David told to the abbot of Rievaulx is as follows:

When he was serving as a youth at the English Court, one evening he was with his companions in his lodging, when the queen called him into her chamber. He found the place full of lepers, and the queen standing in the midst, with her robe laid aside and a towel girt round her. Having filled a basin with water, she proceeded to wash the feet of the lepers and to wipe them with the towel, and then taking them in both her hands, she kissed them with devotion. To whom her brother: "What dost thou, my lady? Certes if the king were to know this, never would he deign to kiss with his lips that mouth of thine polluted with the soil of leprous feet." But she answered with a smile: "Who does not know that the feet of an Eternal King are to be preferred to the lips of a mortal king? See, then, dearest brother, wherefore I have called thee, that thou mayest learn by my example to do so also. Take the basin, and do what thou hast seen me do." "At this," said David, narrating to the abbot, "I was sore afraid, and answered that I could on no account endure it. For as yet I did not know the Lord, nor had His Spirit been revealed to me. And as she proceeded with her task, I laughed—*mea culpa*—and returned to my comrades[1]."

---

[1] Ailredi Abbatis Rievallensis *Genealogia Regum Anglorum.* In Twysden's *Decem Scriptores*, col. 368. "Cum, inquit [David], adolescens in curia regia [Anglica] servirem, nocte quadam in hospicio meo cum sociis meis nescio quid agens, ad thalamum reginae ab ipsa vocatus accessi. Et ecce domus plena leprosis, et regina in medio stans, deposito pallio, lintheo se precinxit, et posita in pelvi aqua, coepit lavare pedes eorum, et extergere, extersosque utrisque constringere manibus et devotissime osculari. Cui ego: 'Quid agis,' inquam, 'O domina mea? Certe si rex sciret ista, nunquam dignaretur os tuum, leprosorum pedum tabe pollutum, suis labiis osculari.' Et illa surridens ait: 'Pedes,' inquit, 'Regis aeterni quis nescit labiis regis morituri esse praeferendos? Ecce, ego idcirco vocavi te, frater carissime, ut exemplo mei talia discas operari. Sumpta proinde pelvi, fac quod me facere intueris.' Ad

The example of his sister, however, was not lost upon him ; for when he acquired the earldom and manor of Huntingdon, and so became an opulent English noble, he founded a leper-hospital there.   Aelred sees him in Abraham's bosom with Lazarus.

The meaning of all this devotion to lepers is shown in the name which Aelred applies to them—*pauperes Christi.*   In washing their feet the pious Matilda was in effect washing the feet of an Eternal King; and that, in her estimation, was better than kissing the lips of a mortal king.

Again, in the Life of St Hugh of Lincoln we see the good bishop moved to treat the leprous poor with a sort of attention which they can hardly have needed or expected, merely because they were, as his biographer says, the successors of *Lazarus ulcerosus,* and the special *protégés* of Jesus.   Not a few, says the biographer, were kept in seclusion owing to that disease, both men and women.   Bishop Hugh would take up his abode among them and speak to them words of good cheer, promising them the flowers of Paradise and an immortal crown.   Having sent the women lepers out of the way, he would go round among the men to kiss them, and when he came to one who was more atrociously marked by the disease than another, he would hold him in a longer and more gracious embrace.   It was too much for the bishop's biographer : " Spare, good Jesus, the unhappy soul of him who relates these things"—horrified, as he says he was, at seeing the "swollen and livid faces, deformed and sanious, with the eyelids everted, the eyeballs dug out, and the lips wasted away, faces which it were impossible to touch close or even to behold afar off[1]".   But these horrible disfigurements of the face are by no means the distinctive marks of leprosy.   The dragging down of the eyelids is an effect of leprosy but as likely to happen in lupus or rodent ulcer.   The loss of the eyeball may be a leprous sign, or perhaps from tumour. The wasting of the lips is a characteristic feature of lupus, after it has scarred, or if there be an actual loss of substance, of epithelial

hanc vocem vehementer expavi, et nullo modo id me pati posse respondi.   Necdum enim sciebam Dominum, nec revelatus fuerat mihi Spiritus ejus.   Illa igitur coeptis insistente, ego—mea culpa—ridens ad socios remeavi."
[1] *Vita S. Hugonis Lincolnensis.*   Rolls series, 39, p. 163-4.

cancer; in leprosy, on the other hand, the lips, as well as other prominent folds of the face, undergo thickening, and will probably remain thickened to the end. The sufferers who excited the compassion of St Hugh must have merited it; only they were not all lepers, nor probably the majority of them[1].

Two leper-stories are told to the honour of St Francis of Assisi. Seeing one day a friar of his order named James the Simple, consorting on the way to church with a leper from the hospital under his care, St Francis rebuked the friar for allowing the leper to be at large. While he thus admonished the friar, he thought that he observed the leper to blush, and was stricken with a sudden remorse that he should have said anything to hurt the wretched man's feelings. Having confessed and taken counsel, he resolved, by way of penance, to sit beside the leper at table and to eat with him out of the same dish, a penance all the greater, says the biographer, that the leper was covered all over with offensive sores and that the blood and sanies trickled down his fingers as he dipped them in the dish. The other story is a more pleasing one. There was a certain leper among those cared for by the friars, who would appear from the description of him to have been one of the class of truculent impostors, made all the worse by the morbid consideration with which his disease, or supposed disease, was regarded. One of his complaints was that no one would wash him; whereupon St Francis, having ordered a friar to bring a basin of perfumed water, proceeded to wash the leper with his own hands[2].

These four tales, all of them told of saints except that of Matilda—she somehow missed being canonised along with her mother St Margaret and her brother St David—will serve to show what a halo of morbid exaggeration surrounded the idea of leprosy in the medieval religious mind. We live in a time of saner and better-proportioned sentiment; but the critical spirit,

<hr>

[1] The bishop left by his will 100 marks to be distributed "per domos leprosorum" in his diocese and a like sum "per domos hospitales," and three marks each to the leper-houses at Selwood and outside Bath and Ilchester. *Hist. MSS. Commiss.* x. pt. 3, p. 186.

[2] *Monumenta Franciscana.* Rolls series, No. 4. Introd. by Brewer, p. xxiv.

which has set so much else in a sober light, has spared the medieval tradition of leprosy. Not only so, but our more graphic writers have put that disease into the medieval foreground as if it had been the commonest affliction of the time. We are taught to see the figures of lepers in their grey or russet gowns flitting everywhere through the scene; the air of those remote times is as if filled with the dull creaking of St Lazarus's rattle. Our business here is to apply to the question of leprosy in medieval Britain the same kind of scrutiny which has been applied to the question of famines and famine-fevers, and remains to be applied next in order to the great question of plague—the kind of scrutiny which no historian would be excused from if his business were with politics, or campaigns, or economics, or manners and customs. The best available evidence for our purpose is the history of the leper-houses, to which we shall now proceed.

The English Leper-houses.

The English charitable foundations, or hospitals of all kinds previous to the dissolution of the monasteries, including alms-houses, infirmaries, Maisons Dieu and lazar-houses, amount to five hundred and nine in the index of Bishop Tanner's *Notitia Monastica*. In the 1830 edition of the *Monasticon Anglicanum*, the latest recension of those immense volumes of antiquarian research, there are one hundred and four such foundations given, for which the original charters, or confirming charters, or reports of inquisitions, are known; and, besides these, there are about three hundred and sixty given in the section on "Additional Hospitals," the existence and circumstances of which rest upon such evidence as casual mention in old documents, or entries in monastery annals, or surviving names and traditions of the locality. Our task is to discover, if we can, what share of this charitable provision in medieval England, embracing at least four hundred and sixty houses, was intended for the class of *leprosi*; what indications there are of the sort of patients reckoned *leprosi*; how many sick inmates the leper-houses had, absolutely as well as in proportion to their clerical staff; and how far those refuges were in request among the people, either from a natural desire to find a refuge or from the social pressure upon them to keep themselves out of the way.

It is clear that the endowed hospitals of medieval England were in no exclusive sense leper-hospitals, but a general provision, under religious discipline, for the infirm and sick poor, for infirm and ailing monks and clergy, and here or there for decayed gentlefolk. The earliest of them that is known, St Peter's and St Leonard's hospital at York, founded in 936 by king Athelstane, and enlarged more especially on its religious side by king Stephen, was a great establishment for the relief of the poor, with no reference to leprosy; it provided for no fewer than two hundred and six bedesmen, and was served by a master, thirteen brethren, four seculars, eight sisters, thirty choristers and six servitors. When Lanfranc, the first Norman archbishop of Canterbury, set about organising the charitable relief of his see in 1084, he endowed two hospitals, one for the sick and infirm poor in general, and the other for *leprosi*[1]. The former, St John Baptist's hospital, was at the north gate, a commodious house of stone, for poor, infirm, lame or blind men and women. The latter was the hospital of Herbaldown, an erection of timber, in the woods of Blean about a mile from the west gate, for persons *regia valetudine fluentibus* (?), who are styled *leprosi* in a confirming charter of Henry II.[2] The charge of both these houses was given to the new priory of St Gregory, over against St John Baptist's hospital, endowed with tithes for secular clergy. The leper-house at Herbaldown was divided between men and women; but in a later reign (Henry II.) a hospital entirely for women (twenty-five leprous sisters) was founded at Tannington, outside Canterbury, with a master, prioress and three priests. There was still a third hospital at Canterbury, St Lawrence's, founded about 1137, for the relief of leprous monks or for the poor parents and relations of the monks of St Augustine's.

[1] William of Malmesbury, *Gesta pontificum*, Rolls ed., p. 72.

[2] In 1574 it was found providing indoor relief for fifteen brethren and fifteen sisters, and outdoor relief for as many more.

London had two endowed leper-hospitals under ecclesiastical government, as well as certain spitals or refuges of comparatively late date. The hospital and chapel of St Giles in the Fields was founded, as we have seen, by Matilda, queen of Henry I., in 1101, and was commonly known for long after as Matilda's hospital. It was built for forty *leprosi*, who may or may not all have lived in it; and it was supported in part by the voluntary contributions of the citizens collected by a proctor. Its staff was at first exceptionally small for the number of patients,—a chaplain, a clerk and a messenger; but as its endowments increased several other clerics and some matrons were added. By a king's charter of 1208 (10th John), it was to receive sixty shillings annually. It is next heard of, in the Rolls of Parliament, in connexion with a petition of 1314–15 (8 Ed. II.), by the terms of which, and of the reply to it, we can see that there were then some lepers in the hospital but also patients of another kind. It is mentioned by Wendover, under the year 1222, as the scene of a trial of strength between the citizens and the *comprovinciales extra urbem positos*[1]: at that date it stood well in the country, probably near to where the church of St Giles now stands at the end of old High Holborn. The drawing of the hospital on the margin of Matthew Paris's manuscript shows it as a house of stone, with a tower at the east end and a smaller one over the west porch, and with a chapel and a hall, but probably no dormitories for forty lepers[2].

The other endowed leper-house of the metropolis was the hospital of St James, in the fields beyond Westminster. It was of ancient date, and provided for fourteen female patients, who came somehow to be called the *leprosae puellae*[3], although youth is by no means specially associated with leprosy. This

[1] Roger of Wendover. Rolls ed. II. 265.

[2] In the MS. of Matthew Paris's *Chronica Majora* in the library of Corpus Christi College, Cambridge, No. 26 in the Parker Collection, p. 220. The late Rev. S. S. Lewis, fellow and librarian of the College, who most liberally had a fac-simile of the drawing made for me, would date it a little before 1250. (Rolls edition, by Luard, II. 144.)

[3] *Rotuli Chartarum*, 1199–1216. Charter of confirmation, 1204 (5 Joh.) p. 117 b.

house grew rich, and supported eight brethren for the religious services of the sixteen patients[1].

It is usual to enumerate five, and sometimes six, other leper-hospitals, in the outskirts of London—at Kingsland or Hackney, in Kent Street, Southwark (the Lock), at Highgate, at Mile End, at Knightsbridge and at Hammersmith. But the earliest of these were founded in the reign of Edward III. (about 1346) at a time when the old ecclesiastical leper-houses were nearly empty of lepers. It would be misleading to include them among the medieval leper-houses proper, and I shall refer to them in a later part of this chapter.

The example of archbishop Lanfranc at Canterbury and of queen Matilda in London was soon followed by other founders and benefactors. The movement in favour of lepers—there was probably too real an occasion for it to call it a craze—gained much from the appearance on the scene of the Knights of the Order of St Lazarus of Jerusalem. Those knights were the most sentimental of the orders of chivalry, and probably not more reputable than the Templars or the main body of the Hospitallers from which they branched off. If we may judge of them by modern instances, they wanted to do some great thing, and to do it in the most theatrical way, with everybody looking on. What real services they may have rendered to the sick poor, leprous or other, there is little to show. The head-quarters of the order were at Jerusalem, the Grand Master and the Knights there being all *leprosi*—doubtless in a liberal sense of the term. We should be doing them no injustice if we take them to have been Crusaders so badly hit by their vices or their misfortunes as to be marked off into a separate order by a natural line. However, many others enlisted under the banner of St Lazarus who were not *leprosi*; these established themselves in various countries of Europe, acquired many manors and built fine houses[2]. In England their chief house was at Burton in Leicestershire; it

---

[1] In the *Valor Ecclesiasticus* of Henry VIII. its revenue is put at £100.

[2] The commanderies of the Knights of St Lazarus were numerous in every province of France. For an enumeration of them see *Les Lepreux et les Chevaliers de Saint Lazare de Jérusalem et de Notre Dame et de Mont Carmel.* Par Eugene Vignat, Orleans, 1884, pp. 315–364.

was not by any means a great leper-hospital, but a Commandery or Preceptory for eight whole knights, with some provision for an uncertain number of poor brethren—the real Lazaruses who, like their prototype, would receive the crumbs from the high table. The house of Burton Lazars gradually swallowed up the lands of leper-hospitals elsewhere, as these passed into desuetude, and at the valuation of Henry VIII. it headed the list with an annual rental of £250. Their establishment in England dates from the early part of the twelfth century, and although the house at Burton appears to have been their only considerable possession, they are said, on vague evidence, to have enlisted many knights from England, and, curiously enough, still more from Scotland. A letter is extant by the celebrated schoolman, John of Salisbury, afterwards bishop of Chartres, written in the reign of Henry II. to a bishop of Salisbury, from which it would appear that the "Fratres Hospitales" were regarded with jealousy and dislike by the clerical profession; "rapiunt ut distribuant," says the writer, as if there were something at once forced and forcible in their charities[1].

Coincidently with the appearance in England of the Knights of St Lazarus, we find the monasteries, and sometimes private benefactors among the nobility, beginning to make provision for lepers, either along with other deserving poor or in houses apart. After the hospitals at Canterbury and London (as well as an eleventh-century foundation at Northampton, which may or may not have been originally destined for *leprosi*), come the two leper-houses founded by the great abbey of St Albans. As these were probably as good instances as can be found, their history is worth following.

In the time of abbot Gregory (1119 to 1146), the hospital and church of St Julian was built on the London road, for six poor brethren (*Lazares* or *pauperes Christi*) governed by a master and four chaplains. The mastership of St Julian's is twice mentioned in the abbey chronicles as a valuable piece of preferment. In 1254 the lands of the hospital were so heavily taxed, for the king and the pope, that the *miselli*, according to Matthew

[1] *Joannis Sarisburiensis Opera omnia*, ed. Giles 1, 141 (letter to Josselin, bishop of Salisbury).

Paris, had barely the necessaries of life. But a century after, in 1350, the revenues were too large for its needs, and new statutes were made; the accommodation of its six beds was by no means in request, the number of inmates being never more than three, sometimes only two, and occasionally only one[1]. The fate of the other leper-house of St Albans abbey, that of St Mary de Pratis for women, is not less instructive. The date of its foundation is not known, but in 1254 it had a church and a hospital occupied by *misellae*[2]. A century later we hear of the house being shared between illiterate sisters and nuns. The former are not called lepers, but simply poor sisters; whatever they were, the nuns and they did not get on comfortably together, and the abbot restored harmony by turning the hospital into a nunnery pure and simple[3]. Similar was the history of one of the richest foundations of the kind, that of Mayden Bradley in Wiltshire. It was originally endowed shortly before or shortly after the accession of Henry II. (1135) by a noble family for an unstated number of poor women, generally assumed to have been *leprosae*, and for an unstated number of regular and secular clerics to perform the religious offices and manage the property. It had not existed long, however, when the bishop of Salisbury, in 1190, got the charter altered so as to assign the revenues to eight canons and — poor sisters, and so it continued until the valuation of Henry VIII., when it was found to be of considerable wealth. In like manner the hospital of St James, at Tannington near Canterbury, founded in the reign of Henry II. for twenty-five "leprous sisters," was found, in the reign of Edward III. (1344), to contain no lepers, its "corrodies" being much sought after by needy gentlewomen[4].

Another foundation of Henry II.'s reign was the leper-hospital

[1] "Vix seu raro inveniuntur tot leprosi volentes vitam ducere observantiis obligatam ad dictum hospitale concurrentes." Walsingham, *Gesta Abbatum*, Rolls ed. II. 484.

[2] Matthew Paris, *Chron. Maj.* V. 452.

[3] Walsingham, *Gesta Abbatum*, II. 401.

[4] "The sisters of St James's were bound by no vows, and at this period [1344] were not all, or even any of them, lepers; and in consequence a place in the hospital was much sought after by needy dependents of the Court." Report on MSS. of the Dean and Chapter of Canterbury, in *Hist. MSS. Commission Reports*, IX. p. 87.

of St Mary Magdalen at Sponne, outside the walls of Coventry. It was founded by an Earl of Chester, who, having a certain leprous knight in his household, gave in pure alms for the health of his soul and the souls of his ancestors his chapel at Sponne with the site thereof, and half a carucate of land for the maintenance of such lepers as should happen to be in the town of Coventry. There was one priest to celebrate, and with him were wont to be also certain brethren or sisters together with the lepers, praying to God for the good estate of all their benefactors. "But clear it is," says Dugdale, "that the monks shortly after appropriated it to their own use." However, they were in time dispossessed by the Crown, to which the hospital belonged until the 14th of Edward IV[1].

One of the most typical as well as earliest foundations was the hospital of the Holy Innocents at Lincoln, endowed by Henry I. We owe our knowledge of its charter to an inquisition of Edward III. It was intended for ten *leprosi*, who were to be of the outcasts (*de ejectibus*) of the city of Lincoln, the presentation to be in the king's gift or in that of the mayor or other good men of the city, and the administration of it by a master or warden, two chaplains and one clerk. In the space of two centuries from its foundation the character of its inmates had gradually changed. Edward III.'s commissioners found nine poor brethren or sisters in it; only one of them was *leprosus*, and he had obtained admission by a golden key; also the seven poor women had got in *per viam pecuniam*. In Henry VI.'s time provision was made for the possibility of lepers still requiring its shelter—*quod absit*, as the new charter said.

In the same reign (end of Henry I.) the hospital of St Peter was founded at Bury St Edmunds by abbot Anselm, for priests and others when they grew old and infirm, leprous or diseased. The other hospital at Bury, St Saviour's, had no explicit reference to leprosy at all. It was founded by the famous abbot Samson about 1184, for a warden, twelve chaplain-priests, six clerks, twelve poor gentlemen, and twelve poor women. About a hundred years later the poor sisters had to go, in order to make room for old and infirm priests.

---

[1] Dugdale's *History of Warwickshire*, p. 197.

Sometime before his death in 1139, Thurstan, archbishop of York, founded a hospital at Ripon for the relief of "all the lepers in Richmondshire;" the provision was for eighteen patients, a chaplain and sisters. At an uncertain date afterwards the house was found to contain a master, two or three chaplains and some brethren, who are not styled *leprosi;* and from the inquisition of Edward III. we learn that its original destination had been for the relief as much of the poor as the leprous (*tam pauperum quam leprosorum*), and that there was no leprous person in it at the date of the inquisition.

The mixed character of hospitals commonly reckoned leper-hospitals is shown by several other instances. St Mary Magdalene's at Lynn (1145) provided for a prior and twelve brethren or sisters, nine of whom were to be whole and three leprous. St Leonard's at Lancaster (time of king John) was endowed for a master, a chaplain, and nine poor persons, three of them to be leprous. St Bartholomew's at Oxford provided for a master, a clerk, two whole brethren and six infirm or leprous brethren; but the infirm or leprous brethren had all been changed into whole brethren by the time of Edward III[1]. So again the Normans' spital at Norwich was found to be sheltering "seven whole sisters and seven half-sisters."

The leper-hospital at Stourbridge, near Cambridge, was founded for lepers by king John, the one king in English history who cared greatly about his leprous subjects. It was committed to the charge of the burgesses of Cambridge, but it was shortly after seized by Hugo de Norwold, bishop of Ely, and within little more than fifty years from its foundation (7 Ed. I.) it was found that the bishop of Ely of that day was using it for some purposes of his own, but "was keeping no lepers in it, as he ought, and as the custom had been[2]."

The ostentatious patronage of lepers by king John, of which something more might be said, was preceded by a more important interposition on their behalf by the third Council of the

[1] On Nov. 24, 1200, king John signed at Lincoln letters of simple protection to the *leprosi* of St Bartholomew's, Oxford (*Rot. Chart.* 1199–1216, p. 99).

[2] *Rotuli Hundredorum*, II. 359–60. The famous Stourbridge Fair originally grew out of a right of market-toll granted in aid of the leper-hospital.

Lateran in 1179 (Alexander III.). The position of *leprosi* in the community had clearly become anomalous, and one of the decrees of the Council was directed to setting it right. Lepers, who were "unable to live with sound persons, or to attend church with them, or to get buried in the same churchyard, or to have the ministrations of the proper priest," were enjoined to have their own presbytery, church, and churchyard, and their lands were to be exempt from tithe[1]. Within two or three years of that decree, in or near 1181, we find a bishop of Durham, Hugh de Puiset, endowing the greatest of all the English leper-hospitals, at Sherburn, a mile or more outside the city of Durham. The bishop was a noted instance of the worldly ecclesiastic of his time. He was accused by the king of misappropriating money left by the archbishop of York, and his defence was that he had spent it on the blind, the deaf, the dumb, the leprous, and such like deserving objects[2]. William of Newburgh has left us his opinion of the bishop's charity: it was a noble hospital lavishly provided for, "but with largess not quite honestly come by" (*sed tamen ex parte minus honesta largitione*[3]). The hospital of bishop Hugh, dedicated to the Saviour, the Blessed Virgin, St Lazarus, and his sisters Mary and Martha, still exists as Christ's Hospital, a quadrangular building enclosing about an acre in a sunny valley to the south of the city, with a fine chapel, a great hall (of which the ancient raftered roof existed into the present century), a master's lodge, and a low range of buildings on the west side of the square for the poor brethren, with their own modest hall in the middle of it. The original foundation was certainly on a princely scale, as things then went: it was for five "convents" of lepers, including in all sixty-five persons of both sexes, with a steward or guardian to be their own proper representative or protector, three priests, four attendant clerks, and a prior and prioress. We hear nothing more of the hospital for a century and a half, during which time it had doubtless been filled by a succession of poor brethren, or sick

[1] The decrees of the Third Lateran Council are given by several historians of the time, among others by William of Newburgh, pp. 206-223.
[2] Roger of Howden, Rolls edition, II. 265.
[3] William of Newburgh, Rolls edition, p. 437.

poor brethren, but whether leprous brethren, or even mainly leprous, may well be doubted after the recorded experiences of Ripon, Lincoln and Stourbridge. Its charter was confirmed by bishop Kellaw about 1311–1316; and in an ordinance of 1349 we still read, but not without a feeling of something forced and unreal, of the hospital ministering to the hunger, the thirst, the nakedness of the leprous, and to the other wants and miseries by which they are incessantly afflicted. But within ninety years of that time (1434) the real state of the case becomes apparent; the poor brethren had been neglected, and the estates so mismanaged or alienated to other uses, that new statutes were made reducing the number of inmates to thirteen poor brethren and two lepers, the latter being thrown in, "if they can be found in these parts," in order to preserve the memory of the original foundation[1].

To these samples, which are also the chief instances of English leper-hospitals, may be added two or three more to bring out another side of the matter. In the cases already given, it has been seen that the provision for the clerical staff was either a very liberal one at first or became so in course of time. The hospitals, whether leprous or other, were for the most part dependencies of the abbeys, affording occupation and residence to so many more monks, just as if they had been "cells" of the abbey. The enormous disproportion of the clerical staff to the inmates of hospitals (not, however, leprous) is seen in the instances of St Giles's at Norwich, St Saviour's at Bury and St Cross at Winchester. The provision was about six for the poor and half-a-dozen for the monks. But even the purely nosocomial part of these charities was in not a few instances for the immediate relief of the monasteries themselves. St Bartholomew's at Chatham, one of the earliest foundations usually counted among the leper-hospitals, was for sick or infirm monks. The hospital at Basingstoke, endowed by Merton College, Oxford, was for incurably sick fellows and scholars of Merton itself. The leper-hospital at Ilford in Essex was founded about 1180 by the rich abbey of Barking, for the leprous tenants and servants of the abbey, the provision being

---

[1] See the various charters and memorials in Surtees' *History of Durham.*

for a secular master, a leprous master, thirteen leprous brethren, two chaplains and a clerk. St Lawrence's at Canterbury (1137) was for leprous monks or for the poor parents and relations of monks. St Peter's at Bury St Edmunds, founded by abbot Anselm in the reign of Henry I., was for priests and others when they grew old, infirm, leprous, or diseased.

The instances which have been detailed in the last few pages, perhaps not without risk of tediousness, have not been chosen to give a colour to the view of medieval leprosy; they are a fair sample of the whole, and they include nearly all those leper-hospitals of which the charters or other authentic records are known[1]. It is possible by using every verbal reference to leprosy that may be found in connexion with all the five hundred or more medieval English hospitals in Bishop Tanner's *Notitia Monastica* or in Dugdale's *Monasticon*, to make out a list of over a hundred leper-hospitals of one kind or another. But there are probably not thirty of them for which the special destination of the charity is known from charters or inquisitions ; and even these, as we have seen, were not all purely for lepers or even mainly for lepers. As to the rest of the list of one hundred, the connexion with leprosy is of the vaguest kind. Thus, four out of the five hospitals in Cornwall are called lazar-houses or leper-hospitals, but they were so called merely on the authority of antiquaries subsequent to the sixteenth century. The same criticism applies almost equally to the eight so-called leper-hospitals, out of a total of fourteen medieval hospitals of all kinds, in Devonshire. It is clear that "lazar-house" became an even more widely generic term than the terms *lepra* and *leprosus* themselves[2].

[1] Two of the larger houses for lepers not mentioned in the text were St Nicholas's at Carlisle and the hospital at Bolton in Northumberland, each with thirteen beds.

[2] By collecting every reference to lepers or lazar-houses in Tanner's *Notitia Monastica* or in Dugdale's *Monasticon* Sir J. Y. Simpson has made out a table of some hundred leper-houses in Britain (*Edin. Med. and Surg. Journ.* 1841 and 1842). Simpson's table has been added to by Miss Lambert in the *Nineteenth Century*, Aug.—Sept. 1884, by the Rev. H. P. Wright (*Leprosy* etc. 1885), who says at the end of his long list: "There were hundreds more," and by Mr R. C. Hope (*The Leper in England*, Scarborough, 1891), whose list runs to 172.

Perhaps the most remarkable development of that verbalist handling of the

Thus our doubts as to the amount of true leprosy that once existed in England, and was provided for in the access of chivalrous sentiment that came upon Christendom in the twelfth and thirteenth centuries, tend to multiply in a compound ratio. We doubt whether many of the so-called leper-houses or lazar-houses in the list of one hundred, more or less, that may be compiled from the *Monasticon*, were not ordinary refuges for the sick and infirm poor, like the three or four hundred other religious charities of the country. We know that, in some instances of leper-hospitals with authentic charters, the provision for the leprous was in the proportion of one to three or four of non-leprous inmates. We know that as early as the end of the thirteenth century the *leprosi* were disappearing or getting displaced even from hospitals where the intentions of the founder were explicit. And lastly we doubt the homogeneity of the disease called *lepra* and of the class called *leprosi*.

As to the foundations of a later age they were no longer under ecclesiastical management, and they seem to have been mostly rude shelters on the outskirts of the larger towns. In 1316 a burgess of Rochester, who had sat in Parliament, left a house in Eastgate to be called St Katharine's Spital, "for poor men of the city, leprous or otherwise diseased, impotent and poor"—or, in other words, a common almshouse. The remarkable ordinance of Edward III. in 1346, for the expulsion of lepers from London, seems to have been the occasion of the founding of two so-called lazar-houses, one in Kent Street, Southwark, called "the Loke[1]," and the other at Hackney or Kingsland. These are the only two mentioned in the subsequent orders to the porters of the City Gates in 1375; and as late as the reign of Henry VI. they are the only two, besides the ancient Matilda's Hospital in St Giles's Fields, to which bequests

matter has been reserved for a recent medical writer, who has constructed, from the conventional list of leper-hospitals, a map of the *geographical distribution of leprosy* in medieval Britain. (*British Medical Journal*, March 1, 1890, p. 466.)

[1] The Lock was doubtless the house of the "Leprosi apud Bermondsey" who are designated in the Royal Charter of 1 Hen. IV. (1399) as recipients, along with the *leprosi* of Westminster (St James's), of "five or six thousand pounds." (*Rotuli Chartarum*, 1 Hen. IV.)

were made in the will of Ralph Holland, merchant taylor[1]. Another of the suburban leper-spitals was founded at Highgate by a citizen in 1468[2], and it is not until the reign of Henry VIII. that we hear of the spitals at Mile End, Knightsbridge and Hammersmith[3]. By that time leprosy had ceased to be heard of in England ; but another disease, syphilis, had become exceedingly common ; and it is known that those spitals, together with the older leper-hospitals, were used for the poorer victims of that disease. Stow is unable to give the exact date of any of these foundations except that at Highgate. He assumes that the others were all built on the occasion of the ordinance of 20 Edward III. ; but it is probable that only two of them, the Lock and the Kingsland or Hackney spital were built at that time[4].

An early instance of a leper-spital or refuge apparently without ecclesiastical discipline is mentioned in a charter roll of 1207–8, in which king John grants to the leprosi of Bristol a croft outside the Laffard gate, whereon to reside under the king's protection and to beg with impunity. On the roads leading to Norwich there were four such shelters, outside the gates of St Mary Magdalene, St Bennet, St Giles and St Stephen respectively ; these houses were each under a keeper, and were supported by the alms of the townsfolk or of travellers ; only one of the four is alleged to have had a chapel attached. The date of these is unknown, but they were probably late. On the roads leading from Lynn, there were three such erections, at Cowgate, Letchhythe and West Lynn, which are first mentioned in a will of 1432. These non-religious and unendowed leper-

---

[1] Beckett, *Phil. Trans.*, vol. 31, p. 60.

[2] Stow, *Survey of London*, ed. of 1890, p. 437.

[3] Beckett, *l.c.* The Knightsbridge house was earlier. See next note.

[4] *Survey of London*, pop. ed. p. 436. Bequests to lepers occur in various wills of London citizens, in Dr Sharpe's *Calendar of Wills*, vol. II. Lond. 1890. In a will dated 21 April, 1349, the bequest is to "the poor lazars without Southwerkebarre and at Hakeney" (p. 3). On 1 July, 1371, another bequeaths money to "the three colleges of lepers near London, viz. at *le loke*, at St Giles de Holbourne, and at Hakeney" (p. 147). On 7 April, 1396, bequests are made to "the lepers at le loke near Seynt Georges barre, of St Giles without Holbournebarre, and le meselcotes de Haconey" (p. 341). The "lazar house at Knyghtbrigge" appears, for the first time, in a will dated 21 Feb. 1485, along with "the sick people in the lazercotes next about London" (p. 589).

spitals were probably rude erections on the outskirts of the town, at the door of which, or on the roadside near, one or more lepers would sit and beg. The liberty of soliciting alms was one of their privileges, only they were not allowed to carry their importunity too far; hence the ordinance of most countries that the lepers were not to enter mills and bake-houses; and hence some ordinances of the Scots parliament limiting the excursions of the leper folk. One of the most considerable privileges to lepers was granted to the lepers of Shrewsbury in 1204 by king John, who did not lose the chance of earning a cheap reputation for Christian charity by his ostentatious patronage of the *pauperes Christi :* they were entitled to take a handful of corn or flour from all sacks exposed in Shrewsbury market.

Leper-houses in Scotland and Ireland.

Most of the leper-spitals of Scotland would appear to have been of the poorest kind, unendowed and unprovided with priests. The richest foundation for lepers in Scotland was at Kingcase, near Prestwick in Ayrshire, endowed with lands and consisting of a hospital of eight beds. One or more leper-hospitals were built by the rich abbeys on the Tweed (at Aldcambus in Berwickshire and probably at another place). Another great ecclesiastical centre in Scotland, Elgin, had a leper-house at Rothfan, with accommodation for seven lepers, a chaplain, and a servant. After these, the Scots leper-houses may be taken to have been mere refuges, in which the lepers supported themselves by begging. One such secular hospital was in the Gorbals of Glasgow, founded in 1350. Liberton, near Edinburgh, is supposed to mean Leper-town, and to have been a resort of the sick on account of its medicinal spring. The hospital at Greenside, then outside Edinburgh, was built in 1589. There was a leper-spital outside the Gallow-gate of Aberdeen, on a road which still bears the name of the Spital. Similar shelters may be inferred to have existed at Perth, Stirling, Linlithgow and other places. James IV., in his journeys, used to distribute small sums to the sick folk in

7—2

the "grandgore" (syphilis), to the poor folk, and to the lipper-folk, "at the town end[1]."

There were some leper-hospitals in Ireland, but it is not easy to distinguish them in every case from general hospitals for the sick poor. Thus the hospital built by the monks of Innisfallen in 869 is merely called *nosocomium*, although it is usually reckoned an early foundation for lepers in Ireland. A hospital at Waterford was "confirmed to the poor" by the Benedictines in 1185. St Stephen's in Dublin (1344) is specially named as the residence of the "poor lepers of the city" in a deed of gift about 1360–70; a locality of the city called Leper-hill was perhaps the site of another refuge. Lepers also may have been the occupants of the hospitals at Kilbrixy in Westmeath (St Bridget's), of St Mary Magdalene's at Wexford (previous to 1408), of the house at "Hospital," Lismore (1467), at Downpatrick, at Kilclief in county Down, at Cloyne, and of one or more of four old hospitals in or near Cork. The hospital at Galway, built "for the poor of the town" about 1543, was not a leper-house, nor is there reason to take the old hospital at Dungarvan as a foundation specially for lepers[2].

The Prejudice against Lepers.

It will have been inferred, from many particulars given, that the segregation of lepers in the Middle Ages was far from complete, and that many ministered to them without fear and without risk. The same hospital received both *leprosi* and others, the hospitals were served by staffs of chaplains, clerks and sometimes women attendants ; and yet nothing is anywhere said of contagion being feared or of the disease spreading by contagion. The experience of these medieval hospitals was doubtless the same as in the West Indies and other parts

---

[1] *Accounts of the Lord High-Treasurer of Scotland.* Rolls series I. 1473–1498, pp. 337, 356, 361, 378, 386.

[2] These are all the so-called "medieval leper-hospitals" collected by Belcher (*Dubl. Quart. Journ. of Med. Sc.* 1868, August, p. 36) chiefly from Archdall's *Monasticon Hibernicum.* He points out that the very early references to leprosy in the *Annals of the Four Masters* included various kinds of cutaneous maladies.

of the world in our own day. It is true that the medical writers pronounce the disease to be contagious, *ut docet Avicenna;* but the public would seem to have been unaware of that, and they certainly lost nothing by their ignorance of the medical dogma, which, in the text-books, is merely the result of a concatenation of verbalist arguments. At the same time it is clear that there was a certain amount of segregation of the leprous. The inmates of the hospital at Lincoln are significantly described as "de ejectibus" of the city. The third Lateran Council based one of its decrees upon what must have been a common experience, namely, that lepers were unable to mix freely with others, and that they were objected to in the same church, and even as corpses in the same churchyard. There are some particular indications of that feeling to be gathered from the chroniclers.

One of the most remarkable histories is that of a high ecclesiastic in the pre-Norman period. In the year 1044, Aelfward, bishop of London, being stricken with leprosy (*lepra perfusus*) sought an asylum in the monastery of Evesham, of which he was the prior. The monks may have had more than one reason for not welcoming back their prior; at all events they declined to let him stay, so that he repaired to the abbey of Ramsey, where he had passed his noviciate and been shorn a monk. He carried off with him from Evesham certain valuables and relics; and his old comrades at Ramsey, undeterred by his leprosy or counter-attracted by his treasures, took him in and kept him until his death. The incident can hardly be legendary for it is related in the annals of Ramsey Abbey by one who wrote within a hundred years of the event[1].

Another case, which may also be accepted as authentic, is given by Eadmer in his *Life of Anselm*. Among the penitents who sought counsel and consolation of Anselm while he was still abbot of Bec in Normandy, with a great name for sanctity,

---

[1] *Chronicon Abbatiae Rameseiensis.* Rolls series, 1886, p. 157. The chronicler has nothing farther to say as to the cause of the leprosy, than the opinion of "a certain philosopher," that whatever turns us from health to the vices of disease acts by the weight of too much blood, by superfluous heat, by humours exuding in excess, or by the spirits flowing with unwonted laxity through silent passages.

was a certain powerful noble from the marches of Flanders. He had been stricken with leprosy in his body, and his grief was all the greater that he saw himself despised beneath his hereditary rank, and shunned by his peers *pro obscenitate tanti mali*[1].

Besides such notable cases, we find more evidence in the ordinances of the hospital of St Julian at St Albans, which have been preserved more completely than those of any other leper-house. Forasmuch as the disease of leprosy is of all infirmities held the most in contempt, the unfortunate person who is about to be received into the St Albans house is directed to work himself up into a state of the most factitious melancholy; he is reminded, not only of the passage in Leviticus about "Unclean, unclean!", but also of the blessed Job, who was himself a leper (in the 14th century his boils became identified with the plague, and in the end of the 15th century the patriarch was claimed as an early victim of the *lues venerea*); and further of the verse in the 53rd of Isaiah: "Et nos putavimus eum leprosum, percussum a Deo, et humiliatum[2]." The St Albans house, with its six beds, appears to have been carefully managed, and its inmates well provided for; but the unreal atmosphere of the place had been too much for the leprous or other patients of the district; for we find it on record that they could hardly be persuaded to don its russet uniform, and submit themselves for the rest of their lives to its discipline.

There can be no question, then, that persons adjudged leprous were shunned, driven out or ostracised by public opinion, and even legislated against. The reality of these practices should not be confounded with a real need for them. Least of all should they be ascribed to a general belief in the contagiousness of the disease. In practice no one heeded the medical dogma of leprous contagion, because no one attached any concrete meaning to it or had any real experience of it. There was prejudice against lepers, partly on account of Biblical tradition, and partly because the "terribilis aspectus" of a leper was repulsive or uncanny. Further, in genuine leprosy, the most wretched part of the victim's condition was not his appear-

---

[1] Eadmer, *Vita S. Anselmi*, Rolls edit., p. 355.

[2] Walsingham, *Gesta Abbatum*, Rolls edit. II. Appendix C. p. 503.

ance (which in a large proportion of cases may present little that is noticeable to passing observation), but his unfitness for exertion, his listlessness, and depression of spirits, owing to the profound disorganisation of his nerves. A leprous member of a family would be a real burden to his relatives; and in a hard and cruel age he would be little better off than the stricken deer of the herd or the winged bird of the flock. To become a beggar was his natural fate; and as a beggar he became privileged, by royal patent or by prescription, while beggars in ordinary were under a ban.

It is undoubted that the privilege of begging accorded to lepers was abused, and was claimed by numbers who feigned to be lepers[1]. The one severe edict against lepers in England was the ordinance of Edward III. for the exclusion of lepers from London in 1346; it is clear, however, from the text of the ordinance that the occasion of it was not any fixed persuasion of the need for isolating leprous subjects, but some intolerable behaviour of lepers or of those who passed as such. The mayor and sheriffs are ordered to procure that all lepers should avoid the city within fifteen days, for the reason that persons of that class, as well by the pollution of their breath, etc. "as by carnal intercourse with women in stews and other secret places, detestably frequenting the same, do so taint persons who are sound, both male and female, to the great injury etc.[2]" That is the

---

[1] Brassac, Art. "Éléphantiasis," in *Dict. Encycl. des Sc. Méd.* p. 475, says: "Il y avait aussi des vagabonds et des paresseux qui, sans nulle crainte de la contagion, et désireux de vivre sans rien faire, simulaient la lèpre pour être admis aux léproseries. On y trouvait encore des personnes qui s'imposaient une réclusion perpétuelle pour vivre avec les lépreux et faire leur salut par une vie de soumission aux règles de l'Église."

[2] The ordinance is translated in full from the City archives by H. T. Riley, *London in the Thirteenth, Fourteenth and Fifteenth Centuries*, pp. 230–231. The following is the preamble of it :—

"Edward, by the grace of God, etc. Forasmuch as we have been given to understand that many persons, as well of the city aforesaid as others coming to the said city, being smitten with the blemish of leprosy, do publicly dwell among the other citizens and sound persons, and there continually abide and do not hesitate to communicate with them, as well in public places as in private; and that some of them, endeavouring to contaminate others with that abominable blemish (that so, to their own wretched solace, they may have the more fellows in suffering,) as well in

old confusion which we have already noticed in Bernard Gordonio and Gilbert; it is an edict against *lepra* in its generic
sense, and against the same class that William Clowes charac-
terizes so forcibly in his book on the *morbus Gallicus* in 1579.
At a date intermediate between those two, in 1488, an order was
made by the provost of Paris, that "lepers" should leave the
city; but that is too late a date for leprosy, although not too early
for syphilis.   On the 24th August, 1375, the porters of the City
Gates were sworn to prevent lepers from entering the city, or from
staying in the same, or in the suburbs thereof; and on the same
date, the foreman at 'Le Loke' (the Lock Hospital in Southwark)
and the foreman at the leper-spital of Hackney took oath that
they will not bring lepers, or know of their being brought, into
the city, but that they will inform the said porters and prevent
the said lepers from entering, so far as they may[1].

When all word of leprosy had long ceased in England the
porters of the City Gates had the same duties towards beggars in
general.   Thus in Bullein's *Dialogue* of 1564, the action begins
with a whining beggar from Northumberland saying the Lord's
Prayer at the door of a citizen.   The citizen asks him, "How
got you in at the gates?" whereupon it appears that the
Northumbrian had a friend at Court: "I have many countrymen
in the city," among the rest an influential personage, the Beadle
of the Beggars[2].

While it cannot be maintained that lepers were tolerated or
looked upon with indifference, yet it was for other reasons than
fear of contagion that they were objectionable.   The prejudices
against them have been already illustrated from periods as early
as the eleventh century.   They were, to say the least, undesirable
companions, and in certain occupations they must have been
peculiarly objectionable.   Thus, on the 11th June, 1372, in the

---

the way of mutual communications, and by the contagion of their polluted breath, as
by carnal intercourse with women in stews and other secret places, detestably
frequenting the same, do so taint persons who are sound, both male and female, to
the great injury of the people dwelling in the city aforesaid, and the manifest peril of
other persons to the same city resorting:—We" etc.

[1] Riley, p. 384.

[2] *Dialogue of the Fever Pestilence.*   Early Eng. Text Soc.

city of London, John Mayn, baker, who had often times before
been commanded by the mayor and aldermen to depart from
the city, and provide for himself some dwelling without the
same, and avoid the common conversation of mankind, seeing
that he the same John was smitten with the blemish of leprosy
—was again ordered to depart[1]. It does not appear whether
the baker departed that time, nor is there any good diagnosis of
his leprosy; there was certainly a prejudice against him, but the
occasion of it may have been nothing more than the eczematous
crusts on the hands and arms, sometimes very inveterate, which
men of his trade are subject to.

It is clear also from a singular case in the *Foedera*, that a
false accusation of leprosy was sometimes brought against an
individual, perhaps out of enmity, like an accusation of witch-
craft.   In 1468 a woman accused of leprosy appealed to Edward
IV., who issued a chancery warrant for her examination.

The writ of 3rd July, 1468, is to the king's physicians, "sworn to the
safe-keeping of our person," William Hatteclyff, Roger Marschall, and
Dominic de Serego, doctors of Arts and Medicine; and the subject of
the inquisition is Johanna Nightyngale of Brentwood in Essex, who was
presumed by certain of her neighbours to be infected by the foul contagion
of *lepra*, and for whose removal from the common intercourse of men a
petition had been laid in Chancery. She had refused to remove herself
to a solitary place, *prout moris est;* the physicians are accordingly ordered
to associate with themselves certain legal persons, to inquire whether the
woman was leprous, and, if so, to have her removed to a solitary place
honestiori modo quo poteris. On the 1st of November, 1468, the court
of inquiry reported that they found the woman to be in no way leprous,
nor to have been. The woman had been brought before them : they had
passed in review twenty-five or more of the commonly reputed signs of *lepra*,
but they had not found that she could be convicted of leprosy from them, or
from a sufficient number of them; again, passing in review each of the four
species of lepra (*alopecia, tinia, leonina,* and *elephantia*) and the forty or
more distinctive signs of the species of *lepra*, they found not that the woman
was marked by any of the species of *lepra*, but that she was altogether free
and immune from every species of *lepra*[2].

[1] Riley, p. 365.
[2] Rymer's *Foedera*, v. pt. 2, p. 166.

Laws against Lepers.

The ordinance of 21 Edward III. (1346) against the harbouring of lepers in London is the only one of the kind (so far as I know) in English history; the Statutes of the realm contain no reference to lepers or leprosy from first to last; the references in the Rolls of Parliament are to the taxing of their houses and lands. The laws which deprived lepers of marital rights and of heirship appear to have been wholly foreign; in England, leprosy as a bar to succession was made a plea in the law courts. It appears, however, that a law against lepers was made by a Welsh king in the tenth century [1]. It is not easy to realize the state of Welsh society in the tenth century; but we know enough of it in the twelfth century, from the description of Giraldus Cambrensis, to assert with some confidence that "leprosy" might have meant anything—perhaps the "lepra Normannorum [2]."

In Scotland the laws and ordinances, civil and ecclesiastical, against lepers have been more numerous. In 1242 and 1269, canons of the Scots Church were made, ordering that lepers should be separated from society in accordance with general custom. In 1283–84, the statutes of the Society of Merchants, or the Guildry, of Berwick provided that lepers should not enter the borough, and that "some gude man sall gather alms for them." In 1427 the Parliament of Perth authorised ministers and others to search the parishes for lepers [3].

We conclude, then, that little was made of leprosy by English legislators (rather more by the Scots), just as we have found that in the endowment of charities, the leprous had only

---

[1] Wharton's *Anglia Sacra*, II. Praef. p. 32.

[2] The expression "leprosa Sodomorum" occurs in a Latin poem from a medieval MS. found in Switzerland. The verses are printed in full by Hensler, *Geschichte der Lustseuche*, p. 307.

[3] These and other particulars relating to lepers in Scotland are given in Simpson's *Antiquarian Notices of Leprosy in Scotland and England* (*Edin. Med. and Surg. Journ.* Oct. 1841, Jan. and April 1842), a series of excellent papers which have been for many years the source of most that has been written of medieval leprosy in this country.

a small share, and that share a somewhat exaggerated one owing to the morbid sentimentality of the chivalrous period. The most liberal estimate of the amount of true leprosy at any time in England would hardly place it so high as in the worst provinces of India at the present day. In the province of Burdwan, with a population of over two millions, which may be taken to have been nearly the population of England in the thirteenth century, there are enumerated 4604 lepers, or 2·26 in every thousand inhabitants. But even with that excessive prevalence of leprosy, and with no seclusion of the lepers, a traveller may visit the province of Burdwan, and not be aware that leprosy is "frightfully common" in it. In medieval England the village leper may have been about as common as the village fool; while in the larger towns or cities, such as London, Norwich, York, Bristol, and Lincoln, true lepers can hardly have been so numerous as the friars themselves, who are supposed to have found a large part of their occupation in ministering to their wants. A rigorous scepticism might be justified, by the absence of any good diagnostic evidence, in going farther than this. But the convergence of probabilities does point to a real prevalence of leprosy in medieval England; and those probabilities will be greatly strengthened by discovering in the then habits of English living a *vera causa* for the disease.

Causes of Medieval Leprosy.

What was there in the medieval manner of life to give rise to a certain number of cases of leprosy in all the countries of Europe? Granting that not all who were called *leprosi* and *leprosae*, were actually the subjects of *lepra* as correctly diagnosed, and that the misnomer was not unlikely to have been applied in the case of princes, nobles and great ecclesiastics, we have still to reckon with the apparition of leprosy among the people in medieval Europe and with its gradual extinction, an extinction that became absolute in most parts of Europe before the Modern period had begun.

Of the "importation" of leprosy into Britain from some

source outside there can be no serious thought; the words are a meaningless phrase, which no one with a real knowledge of the conditions, nature and affinities of leprosy would care to resort to. The varying types of diseases, or their existence at one time and absence at another, are a reflex of the variations in the life of the people—in food and drink, wages, domestic comfort, town life or country life, and the like. No one doubts that the birth-rate and the death-rate have had great variations from time to time, depending on the greater or less abundance of the means of subsistence, on overcrowding, or other things; and the variation in the birth-rate and death-rate is only the most obvious and numerically precise of a whole series of variations in vital phenomena, of which the successions, alternations, and novelties in the types of disease are the least simple, and least within the reach of mere notional apprehension or mere statistical management. The apparition and vanishing of leprosy in medieval Europe was one of those vital phenomena. It may be more easily apprehended by placing beside it a simple example from our own times.

The pellagra of the North Italian peasantry (and of Roumania, Gascony and some other limited areas) is the nearest affinity to leprosy among the species of disease. Strip leprosy of all its superficial and sentimental characters, analyse its essential phenomena, reduce its pathology to the most correct outlines, and we shall find it a chronic constitutional malady not far removed in type from pellagra. In both diseases there are the early warnings in the excessive sensibility, excessive redness and changes of colour, at certain spots of skin on or about the face or on the hands and feet. In both diseases, permanent loss of sensibility follows the previous exaggeration, blanching of the skin will remain for good at the spots where redness and discoloration were apt to come and go, and these affections of the end-regions of nerves will settle, in less definite way, upon the nervous system at large,—the cerebro-spinal nervous system, or the organic nervous system, or both together. What makes leprosy seem a disease in a different class from that, is the formation of nodules, or lumps, in the regions of affected skin in a certain proportion of the cases. If leprosy were all anaesthetic leprosy, its affinities to pellagra would be more quickly perceived ; it is because about one-half of it has more or less of the tuberculated character that a diversion is created towards another kind of pathology. But the fact that some cases of leprosy develop nodules along the disordered nerves does not remove the disease as a whole from the class to which pellagra belongs. In both diseases we are dealing essentially with a profound disorder of the nerves and nerve-centres, commencing in local skin-affections which come and go and at length settle, proceeding to implicate the nervous functions generally, impairing the efficiency of the individual, and bringing him to a miserable end. The two diseases diverge each along its own path, leprosy becoming more a hopeless disorder of the nerves of tissue-nutrition, and so taking on a structural character mainly but not exclusively, and pellagra becoming more a hopeless disorder of the organic nervous system (digestion, circulation, etc.) with implication of the higher nervous functions, such as the senses, the intellect, and the emotions, and so taking on a functional character mainly but not exclusively. The correlation of structure and function is one that goes all through pathology as well as biology ; and here we find it giving character to each of two chronic disorders of the nervous system, according as the structural side or the functional side comes uppermost.

What, then, are the circumstances of pellagra, and do these throw light upon the medieval prevalence of leprosy ? Pellagra has been proved with the highest attainable scientific certainty to be due to a staple diet of bread or porridge made from damaged or spoilt maize. It followed the introduction of maize into Lombardy at an interval of two or three generations, and its distribution corresponds closely to the poorer kinds of maize on colder soils, and to the class of the peasantry who get the worst kind of corn or meal for their food. The cases of the disease among the peasantry of Lombardy and some other maize-growing provinces of Northern Italy, were about one hundred thousand when last estimated ; the endowed charitable houses and lunatic asylums are full of them. The connexion of the disease with its causes is perfectly well understood ; but the economic questions of starvation wages, of truck, of large farms with

bailiffs, and of agricultural usage, have proved too much for the
chambers of commerce and the Government; so that there is as yet
little or no sign of the decline of pellagra in the richest provinces
of Italy.   This disease is not mentioned in the Bible, therefore it
has no traditional vogue; it is not well suited to knight-errantry,
because it is a common evil of whole provinces; its causes are
economic and social, therefore there is no ready favour to be
earned by systematic attempts to deal with them ; and there is
absolutely no opening for heroism and self-sacrifice of the more
ostentatious kind.   These are among the reasons why this
great object-lesson of a chronic disorder of nutrition, proceeding
steadily before our eyes, has been so little perceived.   It is in
pellagra, however, that we find the key to the ancient problem
of leprosy.   The two diseases are closely allied in the insidious
approach of their symptoms, in their implicating the tissue-
nutrition through the nerves, or the nervous functions through the
nutrition, in their cumulating and incurable character, and in
their transmissibility by inheritance.   Thus nosologically allied,
they may be reasonably suspected of having analogous causes;
and as we know the cause of modern pellagra to be something
noxious in the habitual diet of the people, we may look for the
cause of medieval leprosy in something of the same kind.

The dietetic cause is not far to seek, and it cannot be stated
better than in the following well-known passage by the philosophical Gilbert White in his *Natural History of Selborne*[1]:—

" It must, therefore, in these days be, to a humane and thinking person,
a matter of equal wonder and satisfaction, when he contemplates how nearly
this pest is eradicated, and observes that a leper is now [1778] a rare sight.
He will, moreover, when engaged in such a train of thought, naturally
inquire for the reason.   This happy change perhaps may have originated
and been continued from the much smaller quantity of salted meat and
fish now eaten in these kingdoms ; from the use of linen next the skin ;
from the plenty of bread ; and from the profusion of fruits, roots, legumes,
and greens, so common in every family.   Three or four centuries ago, before
there were any enclosures, sown-grasses, field-turnips, or field-carrots, or
hay, all the cattle which had grown fat in summer, and were not killed for
winter use, were turned out soon after Michaelmas to shift as they could
through the dead months ; so that no fresh meat could be had in winter

---

[1] Letter to Barrington, 8 January, 1778.

or spring. Hence the marvellous account of vast stores of salted flesh found in the larder of the eldest Spencer even so late in the spring as the 3rd of May (600 bacons, 80 carcases of beef, and 600 muttons)[1]. It was from magazines like these that the turbulent barons supported in idleness their riotous swarms of retainers, ready for any disorder or mischief. But agriculture is now arrived at such pitch of perfection, that our best and fattest meats are killed in the winter; and no man needs eat salted flesh, unless he prefers it, that has money to buy fresh.

"One cause of this distemper might be no doubt the quantity of wretched fresh and salt fish consumed by the commonalty at all seasons as well as in Lent, which our poor now would hardly be persuaded to touch...The plenty of good wheaten bread that now is found among all ranks of people in the south, instead of that miserable sort which used, in old days, to be made of barley or beans, may contribute not a little to the sweetening their blood and correcting their juices."

Let us add to this, that the meat diet of the poorer class, whether serfs or freemen, would be apt to consist of the more worthless portions, the semi-putrid pieces in the salted sides of bacon, mutton or beef, and that badly-cured pork was in many parts the usual kind of flesh-food; and we shall have no difficulty in finding the noxious element in the diet of the Middle Ages, which the dietetic hypothesis of leprosy requires. Some who have advocated that hypothesis for modern leprosy, have laid themselves open, notwithstanding the ability and industry of their research, to plausible objections which have no bearing if the hypothesis be sufficiently safe-guarded. Leprosy, like every other *morbus miseriae*, needs a number of things working together to produce it, its more or less uniform specific character or distinctive mark being determined by the presence of one factor in particular. The special factor should be generalised as much as possible, so as to cover the whole circumstances of leprosy: it is not only half-cured or semi-putrid fish[2], but half-cured or

---

[1] These numbers seem to stand for the contents of the larders in all the various manors of De Spenser.

[2] Mr Jonathan Hutchinson has been adding, year after year, to the evidence that semi-putrid fish, eaten in that state by preference or of necessity, is the chief cause of modern leprosy, and he has successfully met many of the apparent exceptions. Norway has had leprosy in some provinces for centuries; and it is significant that William of Malmesbury, referring to those who went on the first Crusade, says: "Scotus familiaritatem pulicum reliquit, Noricus cruditatem piscium." (*Gesta Regum*, Eng. Hist. Soc. II. 533.)

semi-putrid flesh of any kind. The most general expression for leprosy is a semi-putrid or toxic character of animal food, just as for the allied pellagra, it is a semi-putrid or toxic character of the bread or porridge. Moreover it is that noxious or unnatural thing in the food, not once and again, or as a *bonne bouche*, but somewhat steadily from day to day as a chief part of the sustenance, and from year to year. As the rain-drops wear the stones, so the poison in the daily diet tells upon the constitution. Once more, such special causes may be present in a country generally, among the poor of all the towns, villages and hamlets, and yet only one person here and there may show specific effects that are recognisable as a disease to which we give a name. Unless there be present the aiding and abetting things, the special factor will hardly make itself felt; and if there be not the special factor, there may be some other *morbus miseriae* but there will not be that one. These aiding things are for the most part the usual concomitants of poverty and hardships, wearing out the nerves far more than is commonly supposed and producing in ordinary an excessive amount of nervous affections among the poor. But among the poor themselves, as well as among the well-to-do, there are special susceptibilities in individuals and in families. One person may have the same unwholesome surroundings as another and the same poisonous element in his diet, but he may fall into no such train of symptoms as his leprous neighbour because he is not formed in quite the same way, because he has "no nerves," or is of a hardier stock, or because his unwholesome manner of life comes out in some other form of disease (scrofula perhaps, less probably gout), or for some other reason deeply hidden in his ancestry and his personal peculiarities. The chances would be always largely against that particular combination of factors needed to make leprosy. It was a *morbus miseriae* of the Middle Ages, but on the whole not a very common one; and it was easily shaken off by the national life when the conditions changed ever so little. It was all the more easily shaken off by reason of the facilities for divorce, the prohibition of marriage, and the monastic discipline.

The staple diet as a cause of leprosy was suspected in the Middle Ages, and by writers as ancient as Galen. It is not with-

out significance that the minute directions for the dieting of
the lepers in the rich hospital of Sherburn, near Durham, urge
special caution as to the freshness of the fish : when fresh fish
was not to be had, red herrings might be substituted, but only
if they were well cured, not putrid nor corrupt.   Those directions
were in accordance with the best medical teaching of the time
on the dietetics of leprosy, or on how to prevent leprosy, as it is
given with considerable minuteness in Gordonio and Gilbert[1].

On the other hand we find a singular ordinance of the Scots
Parliament at Scone in 1386, or some forty years after the date
of the Durham regulations : " Gif any man brings to the market
corrupt swine or salmond to be sauld, they sall be taken by the
Bailie and incontinent without ony question sall be sent to the
lepper-folke ; and gif there be na lepper-folke, they sall be
destroyed alluterlie[2]."   Nothing could be more significant for
the prevalence and persistence of leprosy in Scotland[3].   Putrid
fish and pork did actually come to market; the dangers of them
as regarded the production of leprosy were unsuspected; and the
lepers (genuine or mistaken) were actually directed to be fed
with them.   Such food for "lepers" could only have fed the
disease; and if it be the case that genuine leprosy was met with
in Edinburgh and Glasgow more than two centuries after it ceased
to be heard of in England, we need be at no loss to assign the
reason why the disease was more inveterate in the one country
than in the other.

[1] In his section *De preservatione a lepra* (p. 345) Gilbert advises to avoid, among
other things, all salted fish and meat, and dried bacon.

[2] Acts of Robert III. in the *Regiam Majestatem*, p. 414 (quoted by Simpson, *Ed.
Med. and Surg. Journ.* vol. 57, p. 416).

[3] Dr Gilbert Skene, of Aberdeen, and afterwards of Edinburgh, in his book on
the plague (1568), has an incidental remark about "evil and corrupt meats" which
may be taken in a literal sense: "As we see dailie the pure man subject to sic
calamitie nor the potent, quha are constrynit be povertie to eit evill and corrupte
meittis, and diseis is contractit, heir of us callit pandemiall." (Bannatyne Club
edition, p. 6.)

CHAPTER III.

THE BLACK DEATH.

THE most likely of the fourteenth-century English annalists to have given us a good account of the Black Death was the historian Ranulphus Higden, author of the *Polychronicon*, who became a monk of St Werburgh's abbey at Chester about the beginning of the century, and lived to see the disastrous year of 1349[1]. That part of his history which relates to his own period he brings down year by year to 1348, with less fulness of detail in the later years, as if old age were making him brief. Under the year 1348 he begins the subject of the great mortality, speaks of the incessant rains of the second half of the year from Midsummer to Christmas, refers to the ravages of the plague at Avignon, the then ecclesiastical capital of Christendom, just mentions England and Ireland, and then lets the pen fall from his hand. Higden is believed to have resumed his annals after 1352; but he was then a very old man, and the last entries are unimportant. But the period from 1348 to 1352 is an absolute blank. He comes to the edge of the great subject of that time, as if he had intended to deal with it comprehensively, beginning with a notice of the previous weather, which is by no means irrelevant, and after two or three lines more he breaks off. Most of the monastic chronicles are interrupted at the same point; if there is an entry at all under the year 1349 it is for the most part

---

[1] Higden's *Polychronicon.* Edited for the Rolls series by Babington and Lumby, vol. VIII.

merely the words *magna mortalitas.* The prevailing sense of desolation and despair comes out in the record made by a friar of Kilkenny, who kept a chronicle of passing events, and escaped the fate of his brethren in the convent only long enough to record a few particulars of the great mortality[1] :

"And I, friar John Clyn, of the Order of Friars Minor, and of the convent of Kilkenny, wrote in this book those notable things which happened in my time, which I saw with my eyes, or which I learned from persons worthy of credit. And lest things worthy of remembrance should perish with time, and fall away from the memory of those who are to come after us, I, seeing these many evils, and the whole world lying, as it were, in the wicked one, among the dead waiting for death till it come—as I have truly heard and examined, so have I reduced these things to writing ; and lest the writing should perish with the writer, and the work fail together with the workman, I leave parchment for continuing the work, if haply any man survive, and any of the race of Adam escape this pestilence and continue the work which I have commenced."

There is nothing in the English chronicles so directly personal as that, but there are some facts recorded of the mortality in four of them which have contemporary value, or almost contemporary. The best of these accounts, as a piece of history, is that of Henry Knighton, canon of Leicester[2], who acknowledges his indebtedness to Higden's *Polychronicon* for the events down to 1326, but after that date either writes from his own observation or takes his facts from some unknown contemporary source. The next in importance is Geoffrey le Baker[3], a clerk of the abbey of Osney, near Oxford, whose account of the arrival of the Black Death in England has obtained wide currency as copied literally in the 1605 edition of

---

[1] *The Annals of Ireland.* By Friar John Clyn, of the Convent of Friars Minor, Kilkenny, and Thady Dowling, Chancellor of Leighlin. Edited from the MSS. etc. by R. Butler, Dean of Clonmacnois. Dublin, 1849 (Irish Archæological Society). The last entry by Clyn himself appears to be the words "magna karistia" etc., under 1349. There is added "Videtur quod author hic obiit;" and then two entries of pestilence made in 1375 in another hand.

[2] Henricus de Knighton, *Chronicon Angliae,* in Twysden's *Decem Script. Angl.* col. 2598 *et seq.* An edition of Knighton's *Chronicle,* by Lumby, is in progress for the Rolls series.

[3] *Chronicle of Geoffrey le Baker.* Edited by E. Maunde Thompson, Oxford, 1889.

8—2

Stow's *Annals.* The third is Robert de Avesbury[1], whose *History of Edward III.* serves as a chronicle for the city of London more particularly. The fourth is the Malmesbury monk who wrote, about 1367, the chronicle known as the *Eulogium*[2].

From the systematic paragraphs of those writers, and from various other incidental notices, an outline of the progress of the pestilence in England, Scotland and Ireland, may be traced. It entered English soil at a port of Dorsetshire—said in the *Eulogium* to have been Melcombe (Weymouth)—in the beginning of August, 1348. It is said to have spread rapidly through Dorset, Devon and Somerset, almost stripping those counties of their inhabitants, and to have reached Bristol by the 15th of August. The people of Gloucester in vain tried to keep out the infection by cutting off all intercourse with Bristol; from Gloucester it came to Oxford, and from Oxford to London, reaching the capital at Michaelmas, according to one account, or at All Saints (1st November) according to another. Although the 15th of August is definitely given as the date of its arrival at Bristol from the Dorset coast, it must not be assumed that the infection covered the ground so quickly as that in the rest of its progresses. We have a measure of the rate of its advance south-westward through Devonshire to Cornwall, in a contemporary entry in the register of the Church of Friars Minor at Bodmin[3]: confirming the independent statements that the pestilence entered England at the beginning of August, the register goes on to record that it reached the town of Bodmin shortly before Christmas, and that there died in that town about fifteen hundred persons, as estimated.

The corporation records of Bridport, a town near to the place in Dorset where the infection landed, show that four bailiffs held

---

[1] Robertus de Avesbury, *Historia de Mirabilibus Gestis Regis Ed. III.*, Oxon. 1720. Also in the Rolls series. Edited by E. Maunde Thompson.

[2] *Eulogium Historiarum.* Rolls series, No. 9. Edited by Haydon, III. 213.

[3] *Itineraria Symonis Simeonis et Willelmi de Worcestre.* Edited by Nasmith from the MSS. in the library of Corpus Christi College, Cambridge. Cantab. 1778, p. 113: "parum ante nativitatem Domini intravit villam Bodminiae, ubi mortui fuerunt circa mille quingentos per estimacionem."

office, instead of two, in the 23rd of Edward III., *in tempore pestilentiae;* the 23rd of Edward III. would begin 25 Jan. 1349, but the municipal year would probably have extended from September 1348, so that Bridport may have had the infection before the end of that year[1]. It seems probable that the smaller towns, and the villages, all over the South-west, had been infected in the end of 1348, but somewhat later than Bristol and Gloucester. The mandate of Ralph, bishop of Bath and Wells, "On confessions in the time of the pestilence," is dated Wynchelcomb, 4. id. Jan. M.CCC.XLVIII. (10 January, 1349) and it speaks of the contagion spreading everywhere, and of many parish churches and other cures in his diocese being left without curate and priest to visit the sick and administer the sacraments[2].

The autumn of 1348 may be taken, then, as correct for the South-west; and there is no doubt that the infection had been severe enough in London before the end of that year to move the authorities to action.

"Owing to the increasing severity of the sudden plague day by day at Westminster and places adjoining," Parliament was prorogued on the 1st of January, 1349[3]. There was a further prorogation on the 10th of March, for the reason given that "the pestilence was continuing at Westminster, in the city of London, and in other places, more severely than before" (*gravius solito*)[4]. This agrees with Avesbury's statement that the epidemic in London reached a height (*in tantum excrevit*) after Candlemas, 1349, and that it was over about Pentecost. One of the best proofs of the season and duration of the Black Death in London is got from the number of wills enrolled in the Husting Court

---

[1] Histor. MSS. Commission, VI. 475.

[2] Wilkins, *Concilia* II. 745 : "Contagium pestilentiae moderni temporis undique se dilatans etc."

[3] Rymer's *Foedera*, v. 655 :—"Quia tamen subita plaga Pestilentiae Mortalis in loco praedicto et aliis partibus circumvicinis adeo indies invalescit, quod de securo accessu Hominum ad locum illum formidatur admodum hiis diebus."

[4] *Ibid.*—"Et quia dicta Pestilentia Mortalis in dicto loco Westmonasteriensi ac in civitate Londoniae, ac alis locis circumvicinis, gravius solito invalescit (quod dolenter referimus) per quod accessus Magnatum et aliorum nostrorum Fidelium ad dictum locum nimis periculosus foret," &c. This second prorogation was *sine die.*

of the city in the successive months. Those who died of the plague leaving wills were, of course, but a small fraction of the whole mortality; but the wills during some eight months of 1349 are ten or fifteen times more numerous than in any other year before or after, excepting perhaps the year of the *pestis secunda*, 1361. Starting from 3 in November, 1348 (none in December), the probates rise to 18 in January, 1349, 42 in February, 41 in March, none in April (owing to paralysis of business, doubtless), but 121 in May, 31 in June, 51 in July, none in August and September, 18 in October, 27 in November, and then an ordinary average[1]. Thus it would have had a duration of some seven or eight months in the capital, with a curve of increase, maximum intensity, and decrease, just as the great London epidemics of the same disease in the 16th and 17th centuries are known from the weekly bills to have had.

It does not appear to have been felt at all in Norwich and other places in the Eastern Counties until the end of March, 1349, its enormous ravages in that part of England falling mostly in the summer. There is a definite statement that it began at York about the feast of the Ascension, by which time it had almost ceased in London, and that it lasted in the capital of the northern province until the end of July. The infection almost emptied the abbey of Meaux, in Holdernesse, of its monks, and the abbey lands of their tenants; and the date given in the abbey chronicle is the month of August, 1349. The spring and summer of that year appear to have been the seasons of the great mortality all over England, excepting perhaps in the southern counties where the outbreak began; even at Oxford, which is one of the towns mentioned as on the route of the pestilence from Dorsetshire to London, the mortality is entered under the year 1349, which was also the year of its enormous prevalence among the farmers and peasants on the manor of Winslow, in the county of Bucks.

Its invasion of the mountainous country of Wales (by no means exempt from plague in the 17th century) may have been a season later—*anno sequenti*, says Le Baker, which may mean either 1349 or 1350. In the Irish annals, the first mention of

---

[1] *Calendar of Wills* (Husting Court, London), ed. Sharpe, Lond. 1889, i. 506-624.

the pestilence is under the year 1348; but it was probably only the rumour of the mortality at Avignon and elsewhere abroad that caused the alarm in Ireland among ecclesiastics and in gatherings of the people. It was first seen on the shores of Dublin Bay, at Howth and Dalkey, and a little farther north on the coast at Drogheda; it raged in Dublin "from the beginning of August until the Nativity[1]," which may mean the year 1348, although the year 1349 is the date given for the great mortality in Ireland in later chronicles.

The experience of Scotland illustrates still farther the slow progression of the plague, and its dependence to some extent upon the season of the year. Two English chroniclers (Le Baker and Knighton) mention that it got among the Scots assembled in the forest of Selkirk for an invasion at the time when the mortality was greatest in the northern counties, the autumn of 1349. But the winter cold must have held it in check as regards the rest of Scotland; for it is clear from Fordoun that its great season in that country generally was the year 1350. Thus the Black Death may be said to have extended over three seasons in the British Islands—a partial season in the south of England in 1348, a great season all over England, in Ireland and in the south of Scotland in 1349, and a late extension to Scotland generally in 1350. The experience of all Europe was similar, the Mediterranean provinces receiving the infection as early as 1347, and the northern countries, on the Baltic and North Seas, as late as 1350.

Symptoms and Type of the Black Death.

This sweeping pestilence was part of a great wave of infection which passed over Europe from the remote East, and of which we shall trace the antecedents in the latter part of this chapter.

---

[1] Clyn. But his account for Kilkenny, where he lived, makes the epidemic either earlier or later there than at Dublin: "Ista pestilencia apud Kilkenniam in XL⁴ invaluit; nam vito die Marcii viii fratres predicatores infra diem Natalem obierunt," the Lent referred to being either that of 1349 or of 1350. The difficulty about assigning the landing of the infection near Dublin in the beginning of August to the year 1348 is that the English importation had only then taken place. But of course Ireland may have got it direct from abroad.

The type and symptoms of the disease are sufficiently well-known from foreign descriptions—by Guy de Chauliac and Raymond de Chalin, both of Avignon, by Boccaccio, and by the Villani of Florence. It was the bubo-plague, a disease which is known to have existed in Egypt in the time of the Ptolemies, and made its first great incursion from that country into Europe in the reign of Justinian in the year 543 (see Chapter I.). Its second great invasion, but from a new direction, was the Black Death of 1347–9; and from that time it remained domesticated in the soil of Europe for more than three hundred years as "the plague." The first medical descriptions of it by native British writers are comparatively late. Manuscript treatises or "ordinances" on the plague circulated in England from the reign of Richard II., most of them being copies of a short work of no great value by one John of Burgoyne or John of Bordeaux. There is also extant an English translation in manuscript, assigned to the 14th century (but belonging to the end of it, if not to the 15th), of a really good work on the plague by the bishop of Aarhus, in Denmark, of which I shall have more to say in the next chapter. But none of these give English experience ; and the earliest of our 16th century plague-books, by Phaer, is a compilation mostly, if not entirely, from the Danish bishop's treatise, the latter having been printed in its English form in or near 1480. It is not until we come to the work of Dr Gilbert Skene of Edinburgh, printed in 1568, that we find a treatise on plague showing traces of first-hand observation and reflection. Then follow the essay of Simon Kellwaye on the London plague of 1593, and that of the well-known Elizabethan poet and physician Thomas Lodge, on the plague of 1603. Thus the reign of the plague in Britain was approaching an end before the native medical profession began to write upon it. Its eventful history from its arrival in 1348 down to a comparatively late period has to be constructed from other materials than the records or systematic writings of the faculty.

The type of the Black Death in England is sufficiently indicated by Le Baker, who was probably living at Osney, near Oxford, when the infection began, and indubitably by friar Clyn of Kilkenny. Le Baker mentions the *apostemata* or swellings in diverse parts, their sudden eruption, and their extreme hardness and dryness, so that hardly any fluid escaped when they were lanced according to the usual method of treating them[1]. He speaks also of a peculiarly fatal form, from which few or none recovered ; it was characterised by " small black pustules " on the skin, probably the livid spots or "tokens" which came to be considered the peculiar mark of the plague, and were certainly the index of a malignant type of it, just as the corresponding haemorrhages are in pestilential fever (or typhus) and in yellow fever. The disease, he adds, was swift in doing its work : one day people were in high health and the next day dead and buried. Knighton also says, with special reference to Bristol, that the attack was fatal sometimes within twelve hours, and usually within three days at the most. The treatment, which would have been, according to all subsequent experience, the privilege only of those who could pay for it, would appear to have consisted in lancing the risings or botches in the armpits, neck, or groins ; these were the lymph-glands enlarged to the size of a walnut or of a hen's egg, and of a livid colour,—the most striking and certain of all the plague-signs.

Clyn's account of the disease, as he saw it at Kilkenny in 1349, is important for including one remarkable symptom on which great importance has been laid as distinctive of the Black Death among the epidemics of bubo-plague, namely haemorrhage from the lungs : " For many died from carbuncles, and boils, and botches which grew on the legs and under the arms ; others from passion of the head, as if thrown into a frenzy ; others by vomiting blood[2]." It was so contagious, he says, that those who touched the dead, or even the sick, were incontinently infected that they died, and both penitent and confessor were borne together to the same grave. Such was the fear and horror of it

[1] *Op. cit.* p. 98: "Torserunt illos apostemata e diversis partibus corporis subito irrumpencia, tam dura et sicca quod ab illis decisis vix liquor emanavit ; a quibus multi per incisionem aut per longam pacienciam evaserunt. Alii habuerunt pustulos parvos nigros per totam corporis cutem conspersos, a quibus paucissimi, immo vix aliquis, vitæ et sanitati resilierunt."

[2] "Nam multi ex anthrace et ex apostematibus, et pustulis quae creverunt in tibiis et sub asellis, alii ex passione capitis, et quasi in frenesim versi, alii spuendo san-guinem, moriebantur," p. 36.

that men scarce dared exercise the offices of pity, namely, to visit the sick and bury the dead. Clyn's list of symptoms includes all the most prominent features of the plague as we shall find them described for the great epidemics of the Stuart period—the botches in the armpits or groins, the carbuncles, the boils (or blains), and the frenzy or delirium, as well as the special symptom of the great mortality—vomiting of blood.

Of the botch, which was the most striking sign of the plague, the following description, by Woodall (1639), may be introduced here, to supplement the more meagre accounts of the bubo-plague on its first appearance. Woodall had himself suffered from the bubo or botch on two occasions, in its comparatively safe suppurating form ; his description relates to the hard, tense, and dry botch, especially mentioned by Le Baker for 1349, and always the index of great malignity :

"But the pestilential bubo or boyle commeth ever furiously on, and as in a rage of a Feaver, and as being in haste ; sometimes it lighteth on or near the inguen thwart, but more often lower upon the thigh, pointing downward with one end, the upper end towards the belly being commonly the biggest or the fullest part of the bubo, the whole thigh being also inflamed [1]."

Of this disease, says Le Baker, few of the first rank died, but of the common people an incalculable number, and of the clergy and the cleric class a multitude known to God only. It was mostly the young and strong who were cut off, the aged and weakly being commonly spared. No one dared come near the sick, and the bodies of the dead were shunned. Both Le Baker and Knighton speak of whole villages and hamlets left desolate, and of numbers of houses, both great and small, left empty and falling to ruin. It was not merely one in a house that died, says friar Clyn of Kilkenny, but commonly husband, wife, children and domestics all went the same way of death ; the friar himself wrote as one *inter mortuos mortem expectans*. Without naming the locality, Avesbury says that in a single day, twenty, forty,

---

[1] *A Treatise faithfully and plainely declaring the way of preventing, preserving from and curing that most fearfull and contagious disease called the Plague. With the Pestilential Feaver and other the fearful symptomes and accidents incident thereto.* By John Woodall, surgeon to St Bartholomew's Hospital, &c. London, 1639.

sixty or more corpses were buried in the same trench[1]. The stereotyped phrase in the monastic chronicles is that not more than a tenth part of the people were left alive. However, the author of the *Eulogium*, a monk of Malmesbury who brought his history down to 1366, gives a numerical estimate at the other extreme. He says that the plague entered England at Melcumbe, destroyed innumerable people in Dorset, Devon and Somerset, and, having left few alive in Bristol, proceeded northwards, leaving no city, nor town, nor hamlet, nor scarcely a house, in which it did not cut off the greater part of the people, or the whole of them; but he adds, somewhat inconsequently, "so that a fifth part of the men, women and children in all England were consigned to the grave[2]." These are the vague contemporary estimates of the mortality—ranging from nine-tenths to one-fifth of the whole population. It is possible, however, to come much nearer to precision by the systematic use of documents; and in that exercise we shall now proceed, in an order from the more general to the more particular.

Estimates of the Mortality.

There are two State documents the language of which favours the more moderate kind of estimate. In a letter of the king[3], dated 1 December, 1349, or after the epidemic was over, to the mayor and bailiffs of Sandwich, ordering them to watch all who took ship for foreign parts so as to arrest the exit of men and money, the preamble or motive is: "Quia non modica pars populi regni nostri Angliae praesenti Pestilentia est defuncta." (Forasmuch as no mean part of the people of our kingdom of England is dead of the present pestilence.) The Statute of Labourers, 18 November, 1350, begins: "Quia magna pars populi, et maximé operariorum et servientium jam in ultima pestilentia est defuncta." (Forasmuch as a great part of the people, principally of artisans and labourers, is dead in the late

---

[1] Robertus de Avesbury, Rolls ed., p. 177.
[2] *Eulogium Historiarum.* Rolls ser. No. 9, III. 213.
[3] Rymer's *Foedera*, v. 668.

pestilence.) The statute would have emphasized the loss of artizans and labourers as these were its special subjects, but the *maximé operariorum et servientium* may be fairly taken in a literal sense to mean that the adult and able-bodied of the working class suffered most. One of the contemporary chronicles says that the women and children were sent to take the places of the men in field labour[1]. It is also significant that the "second plague" of 1361 is named by two independent chroniclers the *pestis puerorum*, or plague of the juveniles, as if it were now their turn. The *pestis secunda* was also notable, both in England and on the Continent, for the numbers of the nobility which it carried off, and in that respect it was contrasted with the Black Death.

Next we come to certain numerical statements as to the mortality of 1349, which have an air of precision. They relate to Leicester, Oxford, Bodmin, Norwich, Yarmouth and London. In Leicester, according to Knighton, who was a canon there at the time or shortly after, the burials from the Black Death were more than 700 in St Margaret's churchyard, more than 400 in Holy Cross parish (afterwards St Martin's), more than 380 in St Leonard's parish, which was a small one, and in the same proportion in the other parishes, which were three or four in number, and none of them so large as the two first named. Knighton's round numbers for three parishes are not improbable, considering that Leicester was a comparatively populous town at the time of the poll-tax of 1377: the numbers who paid the tax were 2101, which would give, by the usual way of reckoning, a population of 3939. The population of the same three parishes in 1558, or shortly after the period when English towns were described in the statute of 32 Henry VIII. as being much decayed, would have been about 820 in St Margaret's, 800 in St Martin's (Holy Cross), and 160 in St Leonard's[2]. In 1712, when the hosiery industry had been flourishing for thirty years, the population of St Margaret's was about 1900 and of St Martin's about 1750, the estimated population of the whole

---

[1] "Pro quorum defectu [referring to the fugitive villeins] mulieres et parvuli invise missi sunt ad carucas et ad plaustra fuganda." *Eulogium.* Rolls ed. III. 214.

[2] Nichols, *History of Leicestershire,* I. 534.

town having been 6450, or about one-half more than we may assume it to have been in 1349.

In order to realise what the pestilence of 1349 meant to these parishes of Leicester, let us take the actual burials from the parish register of one of them, St Martin's, in the comparatively mild plague years of 1610 and 1611, a period when the population, as calculated from the annual averages of births and deaths, would have been from 3000 to 3500, probably less, therefore, by some hundreds than it was in the years before the Black Death. In 1610 there were 82 burials in St Martin's parish, or about twice the average of non-plague years; in 1611 there were 128 burials, or three to four times the annual average[1]. Knighton's 400 deaths for the same parish in 1349 would mean that the ordinary burials were multiplied about ten times; while his figures for two other parishes would mean a still greater ratio of increase[2].

For Oxford the estimate is not less precise or more moderate. "'Tis reported," says Anthony Wood, under the year 1349, "that no less than sixteen bodies in one day were carried to one churchyard[3]."

The information for Bodmin, in Cornwall, comes from William of Worcester[4] who read it, about a century after the event, in the register of the Franciscan church in that town. The entry in the register was doubtless made at the time, and as made by Franciscans familiar with burials it deserves some credit for approximate accuracy. The deaths are put down in round numbers at fifteen hundred, which may seem large for Bodmin at that date. But the truth is that the Cornish borough

---

[1] Nichols, *l. c.*

[2] For a series of years the burials in the St Martin's register are as follow :

1610	82	1611	128	1612	39	1613	25	1614	34
1615	60	1616	41	1617	31	1618	37	1619	28
1620	25	1621	43	1622	27	1623	37	1624	24.

[3] *History and Antiquities of the University of Oxford.* Ed. Gutch I. 449. He says also : "The school doors were shut, colleges and halls relinquished, and none scarce left to keep possession or make up a competent number to bury the dead." The rest of his account of the Black Death is copied from Le Baker's Chronicle of Osney.

[4] *Itinerarium, l. c.*

was a place of relatively greater importance then than afterwards. In the king's writ of 1351, for men-at-arms, in which each town was rated on the old basis before the Black Death, Bodmin comes fourteenth in order, being rated at eight men, while such towns as Gloucester, Hereford and Shrewsbury are rated at ten each. It may well have had a population of three or four thousand, of which the numbers said to have died in the great mortality would be less than one-half.

Perhaps the most satisfactory reckoning of the dead from contemporary statements is that which can be made for London. The disease, as we know, reached the capital at Michaelmas or All Souls (1st November), and its prevalence led to a prorogation of Parliament on the 1st of January, and again on the 10th of March, the reason assigned for the farther prorogation being that the pestilence was raging *gravius solito*—more severely than usual. The winter mortality must have been considerable, although doubtless the season of the year kept it in check, as in all subsequent experience. But there is evidence that three more burying-places became necessary early in the year 1349. One of these, of no great extent, was on the east side of the City, in the part that is now the Minories[1]; and two were on the north side, not far apart. Of the latter, one formerly called Nomansland, in West Smithfield, was also of small extent[2]; but the other was a field of thirteen acres and a rood, which became in the course of years the property of the Carthusians and the site of the Charterhouse (partly covered now by Merchant Taylors School). The larger burial-ground, called Manny's cemetery after its donor sir Walter Manny, the king's minister and high admiral, was consecrated by the bishop of London and opened for use at Candlemas, 1349. Now comes in the testimony of Avesbury, the only chronicler of good authority for London in those years. The mortality increased so much, he says (*in tantum excrevit*), that there were buried in Manny's cemetery from the feast of the

---

[1] Stow's *Survey*. "Portsoken Ward."

[2] "Lying without the walls on the north part of the city between the land of the abbot of Westminster and the prior of St John of Jerusalem." French Chronicle of London (p. 56), as quoted by Stubbs, in preface (p. lxxxi) to *Annales Londonienses.* Rolls series, No. 76.

Purification (when it was opened) until Easter more than 200 in a single day (*quasi diebus singulis*), besides the burials in other cemeteries[1]. The language of the chronicler implies that the burials in the new cemetery rose to a maximum of 200 in a day. The Black Death must have been like the great London plagues of later times in this respect, at least, that it rose to a height, remained at its highest level for some two, three or four weeks, and gradually declined. A maximum of 200 in a day, in the cemetery which would have at that stage received nearly all the dead, would mean a plague-mortality from first to last, or an epidemic curve, not unlike that of the London plague of 1563, for which we have the exact weekly totals[2]: the five successive weeks at the height of that plague (Sept. 3 to Oct. 8) produced mortalities of 1454, 1626, 1372, 1828 and 1262; and the epidemic throughout its whole curve of intensity from June to December caused a mortality of 17,404. If Avesbury's figures had been at all near the mark, the Black Death in London would have been a twenty-thousand plague, or to make a most liberal allowance for burials in other cemeteries than Manny's when the epidemic was at its worst, it might have been a thirty-thousand plague. Even at the smaller of those estimates it would have been a much more severe visitation upon the London of Edward III. than the plague with 17,404 deaths was upon the London of the 5th of Elizabeth.

The mortality of London in the Black Death has been usually estimated at a far higher figure than 20,000 or 30,000. There was a brass fixed to a stone monument in the Charter-house churchyard (Manny's cemetery), bearing an inscription which was read there both by Stow and Camden. Stow gives the Latin words, of which the following is a translation: "Anno Domini 1349, while the great pestilence was reigning, this cemetery was consecrated, wherein, and within the walls of the

---

[1] Robertus de Avesbury, *Historia Edwardi III.* Rolls ed. p. 407. "Quotidie multos vita privavit, et in tantum excrevit quod a festo Purificationis usque post Pascha, in novo tunc facto cimiterio juxta Smithfeld plus quam cc corpora defunctorum, praeter corpora quae in aliis cimiteriis civitatis ejusdem sepeliebantur, quasi diebus singulis sepulta fuerunt......In festo Pentecostes cessavit Londoniis."

[2] Stow's *Memoranda.* Camden Soc., 1880.

present monastery, were buried more than fifty thousand bodies of the dead, besides many more from that time to the present, on whose souls may God have mercy. Amen." Camden says the number on the brass was forty thousand, but his memory had probably misled him[1]. This has been accepted as if trustworthy, apparently because it was inscribed upon a monument in the cemetery; and it has been argued that if one cemetery received 50,000 corpses in the plague, the other cemeteries and parish churchyards of London would have together received as many more, so that the whole mortality of London would have been 100,000[2].

But that mode of reckoning disregards alike the scrutiny of documents and the probabilities of the case. The inscription bears upon it that it was written subsequent to the erection of the Carthusian monastery, which was not begun until 1371[3]. The round estimate of 50,000 is at least twenty-two years later than the mortality to which it relates, and may easily have been magnified by rumour in the course of transmission. Even if it had contemporary value we should have to take it as the roughest of guesses. The latter objection applies in a measure to Avesbury's estimate of 200 burials in a day at the height of the epidemic; but clearly it is easier to count correctly up to 200 in a day than to 50,000 in the space of three or four months. On the ground of probability, also, the number of 50,000 in one cemetery (or 100,000 for all London) is wholly incredible. The evidence to be given in the sequel shows that the mortality was about one-half the population. Assuming one-half as the death-rate, that would have brought the whole population of London in the 23rd of Edward III. up to about 200,000—a number hardly exceeded at the accession of James I., after a great expansion which had proceeded visibly in the Elizabethan period under the eyes of citizens like John Stow, had crowded the half-occupied space between the City gates and the bars of the Liberties, and had overflowed into the out-parishes to

---

[1] Camden's *Britannia*, ed. Gough, II. 9.

[2] Rickman, *Abstract of the Population Returns of* 1831. London, 1832. Introduction, p. 11.

[3] Stow's *Survey*, p. 392.

such an extent that proclamations from the year 1580 onwards were thought necessary for its restraint[1].

Hardly any details of the Black Death in London are known, but the few personal facts that we have are significant. Thus, in the charter of incorporation of the Company of Cutlers, granted in 1344, eight persons are named as wardens, and these are stated in a note to have been all dead five years after, that is to say, in the year of the Black Death, 1349, although their deaths are not set down to the plague[2]. Again, in the articles of the Hatters' Company, which were drawn up only a year before the plague began (Dec. 13, 1347), six persons are named as wardens, and these according to a note of the time were all dead before the 7th of July, 1350[3], the cause of mortality being again unmentioned probably because it was familiar knowledge to those then living. It is known also that four wardens of the Goldsmiths' Company died in the year of the Black Death. These instances show that the plague, on its first arrival, carried off many more of the richer class of citizens than it did in the disastrous epidemics of the sixteenth and seventeenth centuries. The same is shown by the number of wills, already given. Perhaps the greatest of the victims of plague in London was Bradwardine, "doctor profundus," the newly-appointed archbishop of Canterbury, who died at Lambeth, with the fatal botch in the armpits, on 26 Aug. 1349, just a week after landing at Dover from Avignon.

The often-quoted figures for Norwich, 57,374 deaths in the city from the pestilence of 1349, are wholly incredible. They are derived from an entry in the borough records in the Gildhall[4]: "In yis yere was swiche a Dethe in Norwic that there

---

[1] The population of London is stated on good authority, that of its archdeacon, in a letter to Pope Innocent III. (*Petri Blessensis Opera omnia,* ed. Giles, vol. II. p. 85), to have been 40,000 about the years 1190–1200, a period of great expansion or activity. By the usual reckoning of the poll-tax in 1377 the population would have been 44,770; and in the year 1349 it was probably not far from those numbers. This matter comes up again in the next chapter.

[2] *Memorials of London in the 13th, 14th and 15th centuries,* edited from the Archives of the City, A.D. 1246–1419, by H. T. Riley. Lond. 1868, p. 219.

[3] *Ibid,* pp. 239–40.

[4] Blomefield, *History of Norfolk,* III. 93.

died of ye Pestilence LVII Mil III C LXXIIII besyd Relygius and Beggars." We should probably come much nearer the truth by reading "XVII Mil." for "LVII Mil." It does not appear at what time the entry was made, nor by what computation the numbers were got. Norwich was certainly smaller than London; in the king's writ of 1351 for men-at-arms, London's quota is 100, and that of Norwich 60; the next in order being Bristol's, 20, and Lynn's, 20. These were probably the old proportions, fixed before the Black Death, and re-issued in 1351 without regard to what had happened meanwhile, and they correspond on the whole to the number of parishes in each city (about 120 in London and 60 in Norwich[1]). Norwich may have had from 25,000 to 30,000 people before the pestilence, but almost certainly not more. The city must have suffered terribly in 1349, for we find, by the returns in the Subsidy Roll showing the amount raised by the poll-tax of 1377 and the numbers in each county and town on whom it was levied, that only 3952 paid the tax in Norwich, whereas 23,314 paid it in London[2]. That is a very different proportion from the 60 to 100, as in the writ for men-at-arms; and the difference is the index of the decline of Norwich down to the year 1377. In that year, the population, by the usual reckoning from the poll-tax, would have been about 7410; and it is conceivable that at least twice that number had died of the plague within the city during the spring and summer of 1349.

The figures given of the mortality at Yarmouth, 7052, are those inscribed upon a document or a brass that once stood in the parish church; it was seen there in the fifteenth century by William of Worcester, a squire of the Fastolf family connected with Yarmouth, who gives the numbers as 7000, giving also the exact dimensions of the great church itself[3]. They are adduced by the burgesses of Yarmouth in a petition of 17 Henry VII.

---

[1] Peter of Blois, who as archdeacon of London was in a position to know, gives in his letter to the pope the number of parish churches in the City at 120.

[2] Popham, "Subsidy Roll of 51 Edward III.," in *Archæologia*, VII. (1785) p. 337.

[3] *Itineraria, et cet.* ed. Nasmith, Cantab. 1778, p. 344. See also Weever, *Funeral Monuments*, p. 862, according to whom the record of the great mortality was on a chronological table hanging up in the church.

(1502), as follows: "Buried in the parish church and churchyard of the said town 7052 men." Yarmouth, like Norwich, suffered unusually from the Black Death; in 1377, by the poll-tax reckoning, its population was about 3639. It may be assumed to have lost more than half its people; but it recovered quickly, was made a seat of the wool-staple, and threatened to rival Norwich.

Clyn's statement that 14,000 died in Dublin from the beginning of August until Christmas may also be taken merely as illustrating the inability of early writers to count correctly up to large numbers.

The most trustworthy figures of mortality in the Black Death which were recorded at the time are those given for the inmates of particular monasteries; and these are such as to give colour to the remark interpolated in Higden's *Polychronicon* that "in some houses of religion, of twenty there were left but twain."

At St Albans, the abbot Michael died of the common plague at Easter, 1349, one of the first victims in the monastery. The mortality in the house increased daily, until forty-seven monks, "eminent for religion," and including the prior and sub-prior, were dead, besides those who died in large numbers in the various cells or dependencies of the great religious house[1]. At the Yorkshire abbey of Meaux, in Holdernesse, the visitation was in August, although the epidemic in the city of York was already over by the end of July[2]. The abbot Hugh died at Meaux on the 12th of August, and five other monks were lying unburied the same day. Before the end of August twenty-two monks and six lay-brethren had died, and when the epidemic was over there were only ten monks and lay-brethren left alive out of a total of forty-three monks (including the abbot) and seven lay-brethren. The chronicler adds that the greater part of the tenants on the abbey lands died also[3]. In the Lincolnshire monastery of Croxton, all

[1] Walsingham, *Gesta Abbatum.* Rolls ed. II. 370. Abbot Michael, he says, "tactus est communi incommodo inter primos de suis monachis qui illo letali morbo percussi sunt."
[2] Th. Stubbs' *Chronicle of York* in Twysden, col. 1732.
[3] *Chronicon Monasterii de Melsa*, Rolls ed. III. 36.

the monks died save the abbot and prior[1]. In the hospital of Sandon, Surrey, the master and brethren all died[2].

At Ely 28 monks survived out of 43[3]. In the Irish monasteries the mortality had been equally severe: in the Franciscan convent at Drogheda, 25 friars died; in the corresponding fraternity at Dublin, 23; and in that of Kilkenny 8 down to the 6th of March[4], with probably others (Clyn himself) afterwards.

The following mortalities have been collected for East Anglian religious houses: At Hickling, a religious house in Norfolk, with a prior and nine or ten canons ('Monasticon'), only one canon survived. At Heveringham in the same county the prior and canons died to a man. At the College of St Mary in the Fields, near Norwich, five of the seven prebendaries died. Of seven nunneries in Norfolk and Suffolk, five lost their prioress as well as an unknown number of nuns[5]. At the nunnery of Great Winthorp on the Hill, near Stamford, all the nuns save one either died of the plague or fled from it, so that the house fell to ruin and the lands were annexed by a convent near it[6].

The experience of Canterbury appears to have been altogether different, and was perhaps exceptional. In a community of some eighty monks only four died of the plague in 1349[7]. It is known, however, that when the new abbot of St Albans halted at Canterbury on his way to Avignon after his election at Easter, one of the two monks who accompanied him was there seized with plague and died[8].

---

[1] Rymer's *Foedera.*

[2] Lowth, *Life of William of Wykeham*, p. 93, with a ref. to Regist. Edyngdon, pt. 1. fol. 49.

[3] Bentham, *Hist. of Ely.*

[4] Clyn.

[5] Jessopp, "The Black Death in East Anglia" in *Nineteenth Century*, April 1885, p. 602. The sources of these interesting particulars are not given.

[6] Peck's *Antiquarian Annals of Stamford*, Bk. XI. p. 47.

[7] *Hist. MSS. Commission's Reports*, IX. p. 127: "Hi quatuor tantum moriebantur de pestilencia." The reporter on the MSS. of the Dean and Chapter conjectures that the monastery may have owed its comparative immunity to the fact that it was supplied with water brought by closed pipes from the hills on the north-east of the city.

[8] Walsingham, *Gesta Abbatum.*

These monastic experiences in England were the same as in other parts of Europe. At Avignon, in 1348, sixty-six Carmelite monks were found lying dead in one monastery, no one outside the walls having heard that the plague was amongst them. In the English College at Avignon the whole of the monks are said to have died[1].

What remains to be said of the death-rate in the great mortality of 1349 is constructive or inferential, and that part of the evidence, not the least valuable of the whole, has been worked out only within a recent period. The enormous thinning of the ranks of the clergy was recorded at the time, in general terms, by Knighton, and the difficulty of supplying the parishes with educated priests is brought to light by various things, including the founding of colleges for their education at Cambridge (Corpus Christi) and at Oxford (Durham College). The first to examine closely the number of vacancies in cures after the great mortality was Blomefield in the third volume of the *History of Norfolk* published in 1741. The Institution Book of the diocese of Norwich, he says (with a reference to No. IV. of the *Lib. Instit.*), shows 863 institutions to benefices in 1349, " the clergy dying so fast that they were obliged to admit numbers of youths, that had only devoted themselves for clerks by being shaven, to be rectors of parishes[2]." A more precise use of Institution Books, but more to show how zealous the clergy had been in exposing themselves to infection than to ascertain the death-rate, was made (1825) for the archdeaconry of Salop. It was found that twenty-nine new presentations, after death-vacancies, had been made in the single year of 1349, the average number of death vacancies at the time having been three in two years[3]. The first systematic attempt to deduce the mortality of 1349 from the number of benefices vacant through death was

---

[1] Knighton.

[2] *History of Norfolk*, III. 94.

[3] Owen and Blakeway, *History of Shrewsbury*, I. 166:—" The average number of institutions to benefices on vacancies by death in the archdeaconry of Salop, for ten years before 1349, and ten years after, is one and a half per annum, or fifteen in the whole ; in that year alone the number of institutions on vacancies by death is twenty-nine, besides other institutions the cause of whose vacancies is not specified and therefore may also have been the same."

made in 1865 by Mr Seebohm, by original researches for the diocese of York and by using Blomefield's collections for the diocese of Norwich[1]. In the archdeaconry of the West Riding there were 96 death vacancies in 1349, leaving only 45 parishes in which the incumbent had survived. In the East Riding 60 incumbents died out of 95 parishes. In the archdeaconry of Nottingham there were deaths of priests in 65 parishes, and 61 survivals. In the diocese of Norwich there were 527 vacancies by death or transfer, while in 272 benefices there was no change. Thus the statement made to the pope by the bishop of Norwich, that two-thirds of the clergy had died in the great mortality is almost exact for his own diocese as well as for the diocese of York. These figures of mortality among the Norfolk clergy were confirmed, with fuller details, by a later writer[2]: the 527 new institutions in the diocese of Norwich fall between the months of March and October—23 before the end of April; 74 in May; 39 from 30th May to 10th June; 100 from 10th June to 4th July; 209 in July; and 82 more to October. According to another enumeration of the same author for East Anglia, upwards of 800 parishes lost their parsons from March 1349 to March 1350, 83 parishes having been twice vacant, and 10 three times.

There is no mistaking the significance of these facts as regards the clergy: some two-thirds of a class composed of adult males in moderate circumstances, and living mostly in country villages, were cut off by the plague in Norfolk and Suffolk, in Yorkshire and Shropshire, and probably all over England. That alone would suffice to show that the virus of the Black Death permeated the soil everywhere, country and town

---

[1] F. Seebohm, "The Black Death and its Place in English History," *Fortnightly Review*, Sept. 1 and 15, 1865:—"In the library of the Dean and Chapter, at York Minster, are voluminous MSS., known by the name of *Torr's MSS.*, which contain the clergy list of every parish in the diocese of York, and which, in by far the greater number of instances, state not only the date of each vacancy, but whether it was caused by death, resignation or otherwise of the incumbent." *L.c.* p. 150.

[2] Jessopp, "The Black Death in East Anglia," *Nineteenth Century*, April 1885, pp. 600–602. This author remarks that the evidence from manor court rolls and from the Institution Books of the clergy "has hardly received any attention hitherto, its very existence being entirely overlooked, nay, not even suspected."

alike. It is this universality of incidence that chiefly distinguishes the Black Death from the later outbreaks of plague, which were more often in towns than in villages or scattered houses, and were seldom in many places in the same year. But there remains to be mentioned, lastly, evidence inferential from another source, which shows that the incidence in the country districts was upon the people at large. That evidence is derived from the rolls of the manor courts.

It was remarked in one of the earliest works (1852) upon the history of an English manor and of its courts, that "the real life or history of a nation is to be gathered from the humble and seemingly trivial records of these petty local courts[1]," and so the researches of the generation following have abundantly proved. Much of this curious learning lies outside the present subject and is unfamiliar to the writer, but some of it intimately concerns us, and a few general remarks appear to be called for.

The manor was the unit of local government as the Normans found it. The lord of the manor and the cultivators of the soil had respectively their rights and duties, with a court to exact them. There are no written records of manor courts extant from a period before the reign of Edward I., when justice began to be administered according to regular forms. But in the year 1279 we find written rolls of a manor court[2]. From the reign of Edward III. these rolls begin to be fairly numerous ; for example, there is extant a complete series of them for the manor of Chedzey in Somerset from 1329–30 to 1413–14. The court met twice, thrice, or four times in the year, and the business transacted at each sitting was engrossed by the clerk upon a long roll of parchment. The business related to fines and heriots payable to the lord by the various orders of tenants on various occasions, including changes in tenancy, successions by heirship, death-duties, the marriages of daughters, the births of illegitimate children, the commission of nuisances, poaching, and

---

[1] G. Poulett Scrope, M.P., F.R.S., *The Manor and Barony of Castle Combe.* London, 1852, p. 168.

[2] The court rolls of the Manor of Snitterton, Norfolk, in the British Museum. Professor Maitland has lately edited some of the earliest rolls of manor courts for the Selden Society.

all matters of petty local government. The first court of the year has usually the longest roll, the parchment being written on one side, perhaps to the length of twenty or twenty-four inches; the margin bears the amount of fines opposite each entry; there are occasionally jury lists where causes had to be tried. Of the community whose business was thus managed a notion may be formed from the instance of the Castle Combe manor[1]: in 1340 it had two open fields, each of about 500 acres, on its hill-slopes, cultivated by 10 freemen tenants, 15 villeins, 11 other bondsmen cultivating a half-acre each; 8 tenants of cottages with crofts, 12 tenants of cottages without crofts, as well as 3 tenants of cottages in Malmesbury.

It will be readily understood that an unusual event such as the great mortality of 1348–49 would leave its mark upon the rolls of the manor courts; the death-vacancies, with their fines and heriots, and all entries relating to changes in tenancy, would be unusually numerous. Accordingly we find in the rolls for that year that there was much to record; at the first glance the parchments are seen to be written within and without, like the roll in the prophet's vision; and that is perhaps all that the inspection will show unless the student be expert in one of the most difficult of all kinds of ancient handwriting,—most difficult because most full of contractions and conventional forms. But by a few those palaeographic difficulties have been surmounted (doubtless at some cost of expert labour), and the results as regards the great mortality of 1349 have been disclosed.

The manor of Winslow, in Buckinghamshire, belonging to the great abbey of St Albans, was a large and typical one[2]. Besides the principal village it had six hamlets. At the manor courts held in 1348–9 no fewer than 153 holdings are entered as changing hands from the deaths of previous holders, the tenancies being either re-granted to the single heir of the deceased or to reversioners, or, in default of such, retained by the lord. Of the 153 deceased tenants, 28 were holders of

---

[1] G. Poulett Scrope, *op. cit.* pp. 151–2.

[2] F. Seebohm, *The English Village Community*, London, 1882. The Manor Court Rolls of Winslow, upon which Mr Seebohm bases his work, are in the library of the University of Cambridge.

virgates and 14 of half-virgates ; or, in other words, there died 42 small farmers, cultivating from forty to fifteen acres each, in half-acre strips scattered all over the common fields of the manor. These 42 held twice as much land as all the remaining 111 together ; the latter more numerous class were the crofters, who cultivated one or more half-acre strips : they would include the various small traders, artisans and labourers of the village and its hamlets; while the former class represented "the highest grades of tenants in villenage."

Of both classes together 153 had died in the great mortality. What proportion that number bore to the whole body of tenants on the manor may be inferred from the following : out of 43 jurymen belonging almost exclusively to the class of larger holders, who had served upon the petty jury in 1346, 1347 and 1348, as many as 27 had died in 1349; so that we may reckon three out of every five adult males to have died in the Winslow district, although it would be erroneous to conclude that the same proportion of adult women had died, or of aged persons, or of infants and young children.

Another more varied body of evidence has been obtained from researches in the rolls of manor courts in East Anglia[1].

In the parish of Hunstanton, in the extreme north of Norfolk, with an area of about 2000 to 2500 acres, 63 men and 15 women had been carried off in two months : in 31 of these instances there were only women and children to succeed, and in 9 of the cases there were no heirs at all ; the whole number of tenants of the manor dead in eight months was 172, of whom 74 left no heirs male, and 19 others had no blood relations left to claim the inheritance. The following is the record of the manor court of Cornard Parva, a small parish in Suffolk : on 31st March, 1349, 6 women and 3 men reported dead; on 1st May, 13 men and 2 women, of whom 7 had no heirs ; at the next meeting on 3 November, 36 more deaths of tenants, of whom 13 left no heirs. At Hadeston, a hamlet of Bunwell, twelve miles from Norwich, which could not possibly have had 400 inhabitants, 54 men and 14 women were carried off in six

---

[1] Rev. Augustus Jessopp, D.D. "The Black Death in East Anglia," *Nineteenth Century*, Dec. 1884.

months, 24 of them without anyone to inherit. At the manor
court of Croxton, near Thetford, on 24th July, 17 deaths are
reported since last court, 8 of these without heirs. At the
Raynham court, on the same day, 18 tenements had fallen into
the lord's hands, 8 of them absolutely escheated, and the rest
retained until the heir should appear. At other courts, the suits
set down for hearing could not be proceeded with owing to the
deaths of witnesses (e.g. 11 deaths among 16 witnesses) or
of principals. The manor court rolls of Lessingham have an
entry, 15th January, 1350, that only thirty shillings of tallage
was demanded, "because the greater part of those tenants who
were wont to render tallage had died in the previous year by
reason of the deadly pestilence[1]."

[1] Under the heading "The Black Death in Lancashire," Mr A. G. Little has
printed, with remarks, in the *English Historical Review*, July, 1890, p. 524, the data
submitted to a jury of eighteen who had been empannelled to settle a dispute between
the archdeacon of Richmond and Adam de Kirkham, dean of Amounderness, touching
the account rendered by the dean, as proctor for the archdeacon, of fees received for
instituting to vacant livings, for probates of wills, and for administration of the goods
of intestates. The dean's account to the archdeacon is said to run "from the Feast
of the Nativity of our Lady [8 September] in the year of our Lord 1349 unto the
eleventh day of January next following;" but it may not imply, and almost certainly
does not, that the vacancies in benefices, the probates and the letters of administration,
or the corresponding deaths of individuals, fell between those dates. The archdeacon
alleges what fees Adam de Kirkham had received, but had not accounted for, and the
jury find what Adam did actually receive. Nine benefices of one kind or another are
mentioned as vacant, three of them twice. The numbers said to have died in the
several parishes, with the number of wills and of intestate estates, I have extracted
from the data and tabulated as follows:

Parish	Men & Women dead	With wills (above 100 sh.)	Intestate (above 100 sh.)
Preston	3000	300	200
Kirkham	3000	—··	100
Pulton	800	—	40
Lancaster	3000	400	80
Garestang	2000	400	140
Cokram	1000	300	60
Ribchestre	[illegible]	70	40
Lytham	140	80	80
St Michel	80	50	40
Pulton	60	40	20

Of the alleged 300 who died in Preston parish, leaving wills, five married couples are

Further research upon the records of the manor courts will doubtless show that the experience of Buckinghamshire, Norfolk, Suffolk and Lancashire was not singular. From the Castle Combe rolls nothing has been extracted as to the mortality in 1348–9, except one entry (Nov. 13, 1357) that a certain tenement was ruinous, having remained in the lord's hands since the time of the pestilence for want of a purchaser; but it would be unsafe to conclude that this sequestered manor of Wiltshire had not shared the common fate. The accounts of certain manors in Hertfordshire were headed, for thirty years after the Black Death, with a list of those who had vacated tenancies by death in that pestilence[1]. A decayed inscription cut in the stone of the parish church of Ashwell, in the same county, records the great mortality of 1349 and the great tempest in January, 1362[2]. The tenants of the abbey of Meaux, in the Holdernesse division of Yorkshire, were nearly all dead, as well as the monks within the monastery walls. On the manor of Ensham, near Oxford, "there remained hardly two tenants[3]."

The immediate effects of the great mortality were not so striking as might have been supposed. Although it fell upon town and country in one terrific blow, yet some places had recovered from it before others felt it; it was over in Bristol (so far as we know) before it came to a height in London, and nearly over in London before it began in York. The dead were expe-

named, the probate fees being respectively ½ marc, 6 sh., 40 d., 4 sh., and 40 d. The archdeacon's whole claim for the 300 was 20 marcs, which the jury reduced to 10 pounds. Of the alleged 200 intestates in the same parish, two married couples, one woman, and "Jakke o þe hil" are named. In the parish of Garstang, the executors of 6 deceased are named, whose probate fees in all amounted to 16 sh. 10 d., the whole claim of the archdeacon for 400 deceased leaving wills being £10, and the award of the jury 40 sh. In the parish of Kirkham, on a claim of 20 marcs for probate fees not accounted for, "the jury say that he received £4;" on a claim of £10 for quittance, the jury say 20 sh. This was a parish in which 3000 are said to have died, the number of wills being not stated. The numbers had obviously been put in for a forensic purpose, and are, of course, not even approximately correct for the actual mortality, or the actual number of wills proved, or of letters of administration granted. The awards of the jury amounted in all to £48. 10s. See also *Eng. Hist. Review*, Jan. 1891.

[1] Thorold Rogers, *History of Agriculture and Prices*, I. 296–7.
[2] Cussan's *Hertfordshire*, vol. I. Hundred of Odsey, p. 37.
[3] *Sat. Rev.* 16 Jan. 1886, p. 82.

ditiously buried in trenches; vacancies among the clergy were promptly filled; the manor courts met and transacted business, and had their records engrossed for the most part in the usual clerkly style. So great a dislocation of society naturally gave rise to some irregularities: stripping the dead is reported from one district in Norfolk, fights and quarrels came into court more often than ever in 1349 and 1350, and we read of two women who each had three husbands in as many months[1]. Knighton says that sheep and cattle were left to wander about untended, and that they often perished in ditches by the wayside. A murrain occurred the same year; at one place five thousand sheep died in the pasture and were left to putrefy[2]. The price of a horse fell from forty shillings to half a marc; a fat ox could be bought for four shillings, a cow for twelve pence, a heifer for sixpence, a fat sheep for four pence, a stone of wool for nine pence[3]. On the other hand, when the harvest of 1349 had to be gathered, the price of labour rose enormously. According to Knighton, a reaper got eightpence a day, with his food, and a mower twelvepence. The extant accounts tabulated by Thorold Rogers confirm the contemporary statement: the rates for threshing the harvest of 1349 were those of panic and compulsion, being unparalleled, whether before or after, in the Eastern, Midland and Southern counties; the immediate effect of the scarcity of hands was to nearly double the wages of labour for the time being. Many villeins or bondsmen took the opportunity of escaping to the towns or to distant manors, where they could make their own terms. Of the last kind of incident, probably a very common one, we have an instance recorded[4]:

[1] Jessopp, *l.c.* April 1885, p. 611–12.

[2] The priory of Christ Church, Canterbury, lost the following live stock in the murrain of 1349: oxen, 757, cows and calves, 511, sheep, 4585. (*Hist. MSS. Commission*, v. 444.)

[3] The author of the *Eulogium*, who wrote not later than 1367, and is for his own period an authority like Knighton, gives the following prices: wheat, 12 pence a quarter, barley 9 pence, beans 8 pence; a good horse 16 shillings (used to be 40 sh.), a large ox 40 pence, a good cow 2 sh. or 18 pence. Of the scarcity of servants he says: "Pro quorum defectu mulieres et parvuli invise missi sunt ad carucas et ad plaustra fuganda."

[4] "The English Manor;" two articles in the *Saturday Review*, 9th and 16th

At an inquest, some years after the Black Death, upon sundry manors near Oxford belonging to Christ Church, it was ascertained that, "in the time of the mortality or pestilence, which was in the year 1349, there remained hardly two tenants in the said manor [Ensham], and these had wished to leave, had not brother Nicholas de Upton, then abbot of the said manor, compounded anew with them, as well as with other tenants who came in."

So far as regards the immediate effects of the great mortality. Its after-effects, felt within a year or two, upon the economics and morals of the country, upon the power of the old governing class, upon the dispersion of industries and the new life of towns, upon the system of farming, upon the development of the legal profession in London, and upon various other things, are a much more intricate and disputable subject, some part of which will be dealt with in the next chapter in connexion with the subsequent history of plague or its domestication upon the soil of England. Many things in England were noted as having happened "sithen the Pestilence," to quote the stock phrase of the 'Vision of Piers the Ploughman,' and not the least of them was the frequent recurrence of plague, or a prevalence of sickness so steady that the poet compares it to the rain coming in through a leaky roof.

Some historians have doubted whether after all the Black Death made so very much difference to the course of affairs[1]. It is perhaps inevitable that scholars, accustomed to deal only with obvious human causation, should look with some distrust

Jan. 1886, p. 82 [by Professor Sir Frederick Pollock], the sources of information being as yet unpublished. He says: "The prospect of better terms brought in new tenants."

[1] Stubbs, *Constitutional History of England*, 1875, II. 434. Höniger, dealing with the German evidence of the Black Death, concludes that the great mortality was almost without significance for the political course of affairs; that the great loss of life was unable to check the revival of trade and industry which had already begun or to retard the splendid development of the German free towns; that the low state of morals belonged to the period and was no worse after the epidemic than before; that no new impulse was given or point of view brought out, unless, perhaps, the idea of sanitary regulation; and that the scarcity of labour was merely an incident to be taken advantage of in the struggle against the existing order which was already going on. (*Der schwarze Tod in Deutschland.* Berlin, 1882, p. 133.)

upon the large claims made, in the way of moral and social consequences, for a phenomenon which has been apt to be classed with comets and earthquakes. The sudden thinning of the population may indeed become a subject for economists without any regard to the causation, and irrespectively of the means by which the numbers were reduced; and that has been the only historic interest of the great mortality hitherto. But the operation of pestilence is peculiar; the thinning of the population is not effected as if in the due course of nature; the analogy is closer with a decimating or exterminating war. The invasion of the Black Death was part of the great human drama, just as if a swarming people or a barbarous conqueror had been visibly present in it. If things were moving in the fourteenth century towards a particular issue, as historians find in their retrospect that they were, then the coming of a great plague was part of that movement, organically bound up with the other forces of it, and no more arbitrary than they. Thus it becomes of interest to trace the antecedents of the Black Death before we attempt to follow out its consequences; and it is not the less of interest to do so, that the train of events leads us as far eastwards as the soil of China, and to the incidents that attended the collapse of the greatest government of the Middle Ages, the empire of the Great Khan.

The Antecedents of the Black Death.

When the Black Death in its progress westwards came to Constantinople in 1347, the emperor-historian, John Cantacuzenes, was present in his capital to witness the arrival of the pestilence; in his history he wrote that it came among them from the country of the hyperborean Scythians, that is to say, the Tartars of the Crimea. The other contemporary Byzantine historian, Nicephorus Gregoras, says that the pestilence began among the Scythians in the Crimea and at the mouths of the Don. The Russian annals, which are an independent source, and likely enough to have a correct tradition, also say that the plague was God's punishment on the people of the Don territory and of several other localities with obsolete names, including the famous city of Sarai on the Volga[1]. The Chersonese, and the country from the Don to the Volga, or from the Euxine to the Caspian, are the regions thus clearly indicated as the scene of the first outburst of the Black Death; but there was no clue to its unaccountable appearance there, or to the connexion between its outburst on the confines of Europe and the distant home in the East which the rumour of the day vaguely assigned to it. The more definite association of the Black Death with China dates from 1757, when the abbé Des Guignes, in his *Histoire des Huns*[2], took up the old tradition of the Arab historian, Aboel Mahasin, that the plague began in Tartary, that the smell of corpses spread on every side, that the infection passed from Cathay or Tartary to the Tartars of the Kaptchac (Crimea), and from them to Constantinople and Europe on the one hand, and to Asia Minor, Syria, Egypt and North Africa on the other. He pointed out also that the overland caravan trade was a ready means of transport for the infection. That which specially attracted his attention as the historian of the Mongol power was the other statement of the Arab historian in the same context, that China had been visited by floods so disastrous that men, beasts, and even birds perished, and that the country was almost depopulated. Upon that hint Des Guignes collected from the Chinese annals of the first half of the fourteenth century a considerable list[3] of calamities, which had actually happened— floods causing the loss of millions of lives, earthquakes, and the like, appending the catalogue without comment as a note to the text where he has occasion to mention the Black Death. Des Guignes' note was reproduced verbatim by Hecker in his essay on the Black Death in 1832, and the unwonted series of phenomena in China was made the basis of certain mystical speculations as to the effect of earthquakes in causing a "progressive infection of the zones," a perturbation of "the earth's organism," a "baneful commotion of the atmosphere," or the like. In that nebulous and unsatisfactory state the old tradition of the Black Death originating in China has remained to the present hour;

[1] Richter, *Geschichte der Medicin in Russland*, I. 215.
[2] *Histoire des Huns*, V. 223–4.
[3] *Ib.* p. 226, note.

the intuition of the Peking Jesuit had merely been appropriated and set forth in his own way by the German "Naturphilosoph[1]."

Meanwhile, in 1842 a clue to Des Guignes' conjecture of a connexion between the importation of the Black Death and the China land-route was found (but not followed up) in the discovery by Henschel of a Latin manuscript in the Rhediger Library at Breslau[2]. This was a narrative compiled by one Gabriel de Mussis, a jurist of Piacenza, who had been practising as a notary or advocate among the Genoese and Venetians trading around the shores of the Euxine and Caspian, and had been an eyewitness of the outbreak of the plague in that region. De Mussis has no theory of the origin of the plague; he merely narrates the events as they unfolded themselves before his own eyes; so much was he in the midst of them that he was a passenger on board the very ship which brought the first seeds of the Black Death direct from the Crimea to Genoa as early as the spring of 1347.

The substance of this story is that the Italian merchants, who were then settled in considerable numbers at the various termini or entrepôts of the overland trade from China and Central Asia by the more northern route, were harassed by the Tartar hordes; that they had stood a siege in Tana, on the Don, but had been driven out of it, and had sought refuge for themselves and their merchandise within the walls of Caffa, a small fortified post on the Crimean Straits (of Kertch), built by Genoese not long before; that Caffa was besieged in due course by the Tartar barbarians; that the investment lasted nearly three years; that the merchants and others, crowded into the narrow space within the walls, were put to great straits and could hardly breathe, being only partially relieved by the arrival of a ship with supplies; that the plague broke out among the besieging Tartar host and daily destroyed thousands; that the Tartars threw the pestilent dead bodies inside the walls by their engines of siege, so that the infection took hold of those within the fort; that the Tartars dispersed in panic and spread the infection all over the shores of the Euxine, Caspian

---

[1] *Der schwarze Tod im vierzehnten Jahrhundert*, Berlin, 1832. Engl. Transl. by Babington, Lond. 1833. This well-known work presents the more picturesque aspects of the Black Death in various countries, without thoroughness for any. England has a large space in the book; but the author has not gone for his information farther than the chapter on the Black Death in Barnes's *Life of Edward III*.

[2] Printed in Häser's *Archiv für die gesammte Medicin*, 1842, II. pp. 26–59; and reprinted in his *Geschichte der Med. u. epid. Krankheiten*, III. 157, 3d ed., Jena, 1882.

and Levant; that such of the Italian traders as were able, De Mussis himself with them, escaped from Caffa in a ship; and that the infection appeared in Genoa in its most deadly form a day or two after the arrival of the ship, although none of those on board were suffering from the plague.

These are all the circumstances related by De Mussis of the beginning of the outbreak as known to himself at first hand: the rest of his narrative is occupied with various incidents of the plague in Europe, with pious reflections, and accounts of portents. His single reference to China is as follows: "In the Orient, about Cathay, where is the head of the world and the beginning of the earth, horrible and fearful signs appeared; for serpents and frogs, descending in dense rains, entered the dwellings and consumed countless numbers, wounding them by their venom and corroding them with their teeth. In the meridian parts, about the Indies, regions were overturned by earthquakes, and cities wasted in ruin, tongues of flame being shot forth. Fiery vapours burnt up many, and in places there were copious rains of blood and murderous showers of stones." De Mussis has certainly no scientific intention; nor can it be said that any scientific use has been made of his manuscript since its discovery. For Häser, its editor, merely reproduces in his history the passage from Hecker on the three overland routes between Europe and the East, without remarking on the fact that De Mussis definitely places the outbreak of the plague at the European terminus of one of them: its remote origin is involved in "impenetrable obscurity;" all we can say is that it came from the East, "the cradle of the human race[1]."

But the entirely credible narrative by De Mussis of the outbreak of plague at the siege of Caffa is just the clue that was wanting to unravel the meaning of the widespread rumour of the time, that the plague came from China. Let us first examine somewhat closely the source of that rumour. It finds its most definite expression in an Arabic account of the Black Death at Granada, by the famous Moorish statesman of that

---

[1] *Geschichte der Medicin*, Bd. III. "Epidemische Krankheiten." Jena, 1882, p. 139. He gives point to this phrase by an account of the local plagues of recent times in Gujerat and Kumaon.

city, Ibn-ul-Khatib[1].   Besides giving the local circumstances for Granada, he makes various remarks on the nature of the plague, and on its mode of spreading, which are not exceeded in shrewdness and insight by the more scientific doctrines of later times.   Its origin in China he repeats on the authority of several trustworthy and far-travelled men, more particularly of his celebrated countryman Ibn-Batuta, or "the Traveller," whose story was that the plague arose in China from the corruption of many corpses after a war, a famine, and a conflagration.

The mention of Ibn-Batuta, as the authority more particularly, has a special interest.   That traveller was actually in China from 1342 to 1346.   In his book of travels[2] he tells us how on his way back (he took the East-Indian sea-route to the Persian Gulf) he came at length to Damascus, Aleppo and Cairo in the summer of 1348, and was a witness of the Black Death at each of those places, and of the mixed religious processions at Damascus of Jews with their Hebrew Scriptures and Christians with their Gospels.   But he says not one word anywhere as to the origin of the plague in China, whence he was journeying homewards.   He continued his journey to Tangier, his birthplace, and crossed thence to Spain about the beginning of 1350.   At Granada he spent some days among his countrymen, of whom he mentions in his journal four by name; but the most famous of them, Ibn-ul-Khatib, he does not mention. However, here was Ibn-Batuta at Granada, a year or two after the Black Death, discoursing on all manner of topics with the most eminent Moors of the place; and here is one of them, Ibn-ul-Khatib, in an account of the Black Death at Granada, quoting the report of Ibn-Batuta that the pestilence arose in China from the corruption of unburied corpses.   None of the other statements of an Eastern origin can compare with this in precision or in credibility; they all indeed confuse the backward extension of the plague from the Euxine eastwards to Khiva,

[1] His essay is one of the Escurial MSS., and has been printed, with a German translation, by M. H. Müller, in the *Sitzungsberichte der Münchener Akad. der Wissensch.* 1863.
[2] *Voyages d'Ibn Batoutah* in 4 vols., for the Société Asiatique, Paris, 1853, I. 227–9, and IV. 309.

Bokhara and the like, with its original progress towards Europe from a source still farther east. The authority of Ibn-Batuta himself is not, of course, that of historian or observer; although he was in China during part, at least, of the national calamities which the Chinese Annals record, he says nothing of them, and probably witnessed nothing of them. But the traveller was a likely person to have heard correctly the gossip of the East and to have judged of its credibility; so that there is a satisfaction in tracing it through him.

The siege of Caffa, and the general circumstances of it, we may take as historical on the authority of the Italian notary who was there; but it may be doubted whether the plague began, as he says, among the nomade hordes outside the fort. In sieges it has been not unusual for both sides to suffer from infective disease; and although it is not always easy to say where the disease may have begun, the presumption is that it arose among those who were most crowded, most pressed by want, and most desponding in spirit. It is, of course, not altogether inconceivable that the Tartar besiegers of Caffa had bred a pestilential disease in their camp; the nomades of the Cyrenaic plateau have bred bubo-plague itself more than once in recent years in their wretched summer tents, and plague has appeared from time to time in isolated or remote Bedouin villages on the basaltic plateaus of Arabia. There is nothing in the nomade manner of life adverse to pestilential products, least of all in the life of nomades encamped for a season. But such outbreaks of bubo-plague or of typhus fever have been local, sporadic, or non-diffusive. On the other hand the plague which arose at the siege of Caffa was the Black Death, one of the two greatest pestilences in the history of the world. Let us then see whether there is any greater likelihood of finding inside the walls of Caffa the lurking germs of so great a pestilence. Within the walls of the Genoese trading fort were the Italian merchants driven in from all around that region, with their merchandise—as De Mussis says, *fugientes pro suarum tutione personarum et rerum*. Previous to their three years' siege in Caffa they, or some of them, had stood a siege in Tana, and had retreated to the next post on the homeward route. Tana was at the eastward bend of the Don, whence the road across the steppe is shortest to the westward bend of the Volga; a little above the bend of the Volga was the great city of Sarai—whence the caravans started on their overland journey along northern parallels, across mountain ranges and the desert of Gobi, to enter China at its north-western angle, just within the end of the Great Wall[1]. The merchandise of Sarai and Tana was the return merchandise of China—the bales of silks and fine cloths, spices and drugs, which had become the articles of a great commerce between China and Europe since Marco Polo first showed the way, and which continued to reach Europe by the caravan routes until about 1360: then the route was closed owing to the final overthrow of the authority of the Great Khan, which had once secured a peaceful transit from the Yellow Sea to the Black Sea—so completely closed that men forgot, two hundred years after, that it had ever existed.

Did these bales of Chinese stuffs, carried into Caffa for protection, contain the seeds of the Black Death? There is, at least, nothing improbable in the seeds of plague lurking in bales of goods; that mode of transmission was afterwards recognized as highly characteristic of the plague during its Levantine days. Nor is there anything improbable in the seeds of an infection being carried thousands of miles across the deserts of Central Asia; cholera came in that way from India in 1827–8 by the caravan-route to Cabul, Balkh, Bokhara, Khiva and the Kirghiz Steppe to Orenburg, and again in 1847 to Astrakhan; and the slow land-borne viruses of those two great epidemics exceeded in virulence the later importations of cholera by the sea route from the East. Still farther, there is nothing improbable in the germs of plague lying latent for a long time, or in the disease existing as a potency although not manifested in a succession of cases. The next stage of its progress, from Caffa to Genoa, illustrates that very point; for we know that there were no cases of plague on board ship, although the very atmosphere or smell of the new arrival seemed sufficient to taint the whole air of

---

[1] See Sir Henry Yule's *Cathay and the Way Thither* (2 vols. Hakluyt Society) and his edition of *The Book of Marco Polo*, for numerous particulars of the overland trade to China by the northern parallels, in the 14th century.

Genoa, and to carry death to every part of the city within a couple of days. And lastly the long imprisonment of a virus in bales of goods, the crowding of merchants and merchandise into the narrow space of a walled seaport, amidst the almost inevitable squalor and fœtor of a three years' siege, were the very circumstances needed to raise the potency of the assumed virus to an unusual height, to give it a degree of virulence that would make it effective, and a power of diffusion that would spread and continue the liberated infection after the manner of the greatest of pestilences.

Thus, if we have to choose between the origin of the plague-virus among the Tartar hordes besieging the China merchants within the walls of Caffa, and the pre-existence of that virus, for a long time latent, among the goods or effects of the besieged, the latter hypothesis must be accorded the advantage in pro-bability. Accepting it, we follow the virus back to Tana on the Don, from Tana to Sarai on the Volga, from Sarai by a well-trodden route which need not be particularized[1], for many weeks' journey until we come to the soil of China. According to a dominant school of epidemiologists it is always enough to have traced a virus to a remote source, to the "roof of the world" or to the back of the east wind, and there to leave it, in the full assurance that there must have been circumstances to account for its engendering there, perhaps in an equally remote past, if only we knew them. If, however, we follow the trail back definitely to China, it is our duty to connect it there with an actual history or tradition, immemorial if need be, of Chinese plague. But there is no such history or tradition to be found. We know something of the China of Kublai Khan, fifty years before, from the book of Marco Polo; and the only possible reference to plague there is an ambiguous statement about "carbuncles" in a remote province, which was probably Yun-nan. Not only so, but if we scrutinize the Chinese Annals closely, we shall find that the thirty years preceding the Black Death were indeed marked by many great calamities and loss of

[1] The stages, distances, expenses, &c. from Tana to Peking are given in Pegolotti's mercantile handbook (written about 1340), in Yule's *Cathay and the Way Thither*, vol. II.

life on a vast scale, by floods, droughts, earthquakes, famines and famine-fevers, but not by pestilence unconnected with these; on the other hand, the thirty or forty years after the Black Death had overrun Europe, beginning with the year 1352, are marked in the Chinese Annals (as summarized in the *Imperial Encyclopædia* of Peking, 1726) by a succession of "great plagues" in various provinces of the Empire, which are not associated with calamitous seasons, but stand alone as disease-calamities pure and simple[1]. If the Black Death connects at all with events in China, these events were natural calamities and their attendant loss of life, and not outbreaks of plague itself; for the latter, assuming them to have been bubo-plague, were subsequent in China to the devastation of Europe by the plague.

We are left, then, to make what we can of the antecedent calamities of China; and we may now revert to the curious rumour of the time that the relevant thing in China was the corruption of many corpses left unburied after inundation, war and conflagration. So far as war and conflagration are concerned they are quite subordinate; there was no war except an occasional ineffective revolt in some remote western province, and the conflagrations were minor affairs, noticed, indeed, in the Annals, but lost among the greater calamities. The floods, droughts and famines were events of almost annual recurrence for many years before, so that no period in the Annals of China presents such a continuous picture of national calamity, full as Chinese history has at all times been of disasters of the same kind. It was the decadence of the great Mongol empire, founded by Genghiz and carried by Kublai to that marvellous height of splendour and prosperity which we read of in the book of Marco Polo. The warlike virtues of the earlier Mongol rulers had degenerated in their successors into sensual vices during the times of peace; and the history of the country, priest-ridden, tax-burdened, and ruled by women and eunuchs, neglected in its thousand water-ways and in all the safeguards against floods and famine which wiser rulers had set up, became from year to year an illustration of the ancient Chinese maxim,

---

[1] C. A. Gordon, M.D. in *Reports of Med. Officers to the Imperial Maritime Customs of China*, London, 1884.

that misgovernment in the palace is visited by the anger of the sky.

The following epitome of the calamities in China is taken from De Mailla's *Histoire générale de la Chine.* Paris, 1777, 9 vols. 4to., a translation of the abridged official annals.

The year 1308 marks the beginning of the series of bad seasons. Droughts in some places, floods in others, locusts and failure of the crops, brought famine and pestilence. The people in Kiang-Hoaï were reduced to live on wild roots and the bark of trees. In Ho-nan and Chan-tong the fathers ate the flesh of the children. The imperial granaries were still able to supply grain, but not nearly enough for the people's wants. The provinces of Kiang-si and Che-kiang were depopulated by the plague or malignant fever which followed the famine. The ministers sent in their resignations, which were not accepted.

In 1313 the same events recur, including the resignations of ministers. An epidemic carried off many in the capital, and the whole empire was desolated by drought. At a council of ministers to devise remedies and avert further calamities it was proposed by some to copy the institutions of ancient empires celebrated for their virtue, and by others to abolish the Bhuddist priesthood of Foh as the cause of all misfortunes. The throne is now occupied by Gin-tsong, an emperor of a serious and ascetic disposition. In 1314 he revived the old Chinese system of competitive examinations and the distinctive dress among the grades of mandarins, which the earlier Mongol rulers had been able to dispense with. Next year there is a public distribution of grain, and a check to the exactions of tax-gatherers in the distressed districts. In 1317, it appears that the provincial mandarins, in defiance of express orders, had neglected the laws of Kublai with reference to the distribution of grain, although it was dangerous to defer such public aid longer; they had failed also to relax their rigour in collecting the taxes. One day the emperor found at Peking a soldier in rags from a distant garrison, and discovered that a system of embezzlement in the army clothing department had been going on for five years. Gin-tsong is reported to have said to his ministers, "My august predecessors have left wise laws, which I have always had at heart to follow closely; but I see with pain that they are neglected, and that my people are unhappy."

In 1318 we read of a great flood in one province, of multitudes drowned, and of a public distribution of grain. In 1320, forty of the Censors of the Empire remonstrated against the cruel exactions of "public leeches," and against a practice of calumniating honest men so as to get them out of the way. The emperor Gin-tsong died in that year, aged thirty-three, and with his death the last serious attempt to check the flood of corruption came to an end. In 1321 there is drought in Ho-nan, followed by famine. In 1324 we read of droughts, locusts, inundations and earthquakes. The emperor demanded advice of the nobles, ministers and wise men, and received the following answer: "While the palace of the prince is full of eunuchs, astrologers, physicians, women, and other idle people, whose maintenance costs the State an enormous sum, the people are plunged in extreme misery. The empire is a family, and the emperor its father: let him listen to the cries of the miserable." In 1325 famine follows the disasters of the year before; and we learn that the people were supplied from the full granaries of the rich, who were paid, not out of the State treasury, but by places in the mandarinate! In 1326 the tyranny and licentiousness of the Bhuddist lamas reaches a climax, and an edict is issued against them. The year 1327 is marked by a series of calamities and portents—drought, locusts, ruined crops, earthquakes, inundations. In 1330, again floods and the harvest destroyed, a cruel famine in Hou-Kouang, millions of acres of land ruined, and 400,000 families reduced to beggary. In 1331 the harvest is worse than in the year before—in Che-kiang there were more than 800,000 families who did not gather a single grain of corn or rice,—and all the while enormous taxes were ground out of universal poverty.

In 1333 begins the long and calamitous reign of Shun-ti, who came to the throne a weak youth of thirteen. Next year the misfortunes of China touch their highest point. Inundations ruined the crops in Chan-tong; a drought in Che-kiang brought famine and pestilence; in the southern provinces generally, famine and floods caused the deaths of 2,270,000 families, or of 13,000,000 individuals. In 1336 inundations in Chan-tong ruined the harvest; in Kiang-nan and Che-kiang the first harvest was a failure from drought, multitudes perished of hunger, and a plague broke out. The emperor, insensible to the misfortunes of his people, abandons himself to his pleasures. Next year sees the first of those provincial revolts, led by obscure Chinese peasants, which eventually overthrew the dynasty in 1368. Floods occurred in more than one river basin, by which multitudes of men and beasts were drowned; in the valley of the Kiang (a tributary of the Hoang-ho) four millions perished. For several years we read of numerous and repeated shocks of earthquakes, in 1341 of a great famine, in 1342 of a famine so severe that human flesh was eaten, in 1343 of seven towns submerged, in 1344 of a great tract of country inundated by the sea in consequence of an earthquake, in 1345 of earthquakes in Pe-chili, in 1346 of earthquakes for seven days in Chan-tong, and of a great famine in Chan-si. In 1347 earthquakes in various provinces, and drought in Ho-tong, followed by many deaths. The record of disasters in De Mailla's abridged annals, and in Des Guignes, who had clearly access to fuller narrations, comes to an end for a time at the year 1347.

It will be observed that in these records there is comparatively little said of epidemic sickness. The references to pestilence would in no case suggest more than the typhus fever which has been the usual attendant upon Chinese famines, and has never shown the independent vitality and diffusive properties of plague.   But the minor place occupied by actual pestilence in China, in the years before the Black Death in Europe, is brought out even more clearly on comparing that period with the section of the Chinese annals for the generation following.   In the chronology of Chinese epidemics drawn up by Gordon (London, 1884) from the Peking *Encyclopædia* of 1726, there are, from 1308–1347, just the same entries of pestilence as are given above from De Mailla's and Des Guignes' French adaptation of the Annals.   (Gordon makes the obvious mistake of attributing to pestilence the enormous loss of life which the Annals clearly assigned to floods and famines, with their attendant sickness.) But with the year 1352 we enter upon a great pestilential period, as clearly marked in the history of China by the annual recurrence of vast epidemics as the decades before it were marked by the unusual frequency of floods, famines and earthquakes. Every year from 1352 to 1363, except 1355, has an entry of "great pestilence" or "great plague" (yi-li), in one province or another, although the old tale of floods and famines has come to an end in the Annals.   The last of the nearly continuous series of great pestilences is in 1369, when there was a great pest in Fukien, and "the dead lay in heaps on the ground."   There is then a break until 1380, and after that a longer break until 1403. It would thus appear as if the great pestilential period of China in the fourteenth century had not coincided with the succession of disastrous seasons, but had followed the latter at a distinct interval.   Conversely the years of plague from 1352 to 1369 do not appear to have been years of inundations and bad harvests ; they stand out in the chronology, by comparison, as years of plague-sickness pure and simple; and although nothing is said to indicate the type of bubo-plague, yet the disease can hardly be assumed to have been the old famine fevers or other sickness directly due to floods and scarcity, so long as not a word is said of floods and famines in that context or in the Annals generally. The suggestion is that the soil of China may not have felt the full effects of the plague virus, originally engendered thereon, until some few years after the same had been carried to Europe, having produced there within a short space of time the stupendous phenomenon of the Black Death. If there be something of a paradox in that view, it is the facts themselves that refuse to fall into what might be thought the natural sequence.

The historian Gaubil thinks that the national Annals make the most of these recurring calamities, having been written by the official scribes of the next dynasty, who sought to discredit the Mongol rule as much as possible[1]; but it is not suggested that the compilers had invented the series of disasters,—now in one province or river basin, now in another, at one time with thirteen millions of lives lost, at another with four hundred thousand families reduced to beggary, this time a drought, and next time a flood, and in another series of years a succession of destructive earthquakes.

We are here concerned with discovering any possible relation that these disasters, coming one upon another almost without time for recovery, can have had to the engendering of the plague-virus. According to the rumours of the time, it was the corruption of unburied corpses in China which caused the Black Death; and certainly the unburied corpses were there, a *vera causa*, if that were all. Recent experiences in China make it easy for us to construct in imagination the state of the shores of rivers after those fatal inundations of the fourteenth century, or of the roadsides after the recurring famines. Thus, of the famine of 1878 it is said[2]: "Coffins are not to be got for the corpses, nor can graves be prepared for them. Their blood is a dispersed mass on the ground, their bones lie all about...Pestilence [it is otherwise known to have been typhus fever] comes with the famine, and who can think of medicine for the plague or coffins for the multitude of the dead?" Or, again, according to a memorial in the official Peking Gazette of 16 January, 1878, "the roads are lined with corpses in such numbers as to distance all efforts for their interment[3]."

There is much of sameness in the history of China from century to century; what happened in 1878, and again on a

[1] Gaubil, *Histoire de Gentchiscan*, Paris, 1739.

[2] *The Famine in China*, London, 1878—a translation of a Chinese appeal for charity, with illustrations.

[3] Parliamentary Papers, 1878, China, No. 4.

lesser scale two or three years ago, must have happened on an unparalleled scale year after year during the ill-starred period which ended about 1342; there must have been no ordinary break-down in the decencies and sanitary safeguards of interment in such years as 1334, when thirteen millions (two million, two hundred and seventy thousand families) were swept away by the floods of the Yang-tsi, or destroyed by hunger and disease. But we are not left altogether to the exercise of the imagination. A strangely vivid picture remains to us of a scene in China in those years, which a returning missionary saw as in a vision. The friar Odoric, of Pordenone, had spent six years in Northern China previous to 1327 or 1328, when he returned to Italy by one of the overland routes. The story of his travels[1] was afterwards taken down from his lips, and it is made to end with one gruesome scene, which is brought in without naming the time or the place. It is a vision of a valley of death, invested with the same air of generality as in Bunyan's allegory of the common lot.

"Another great and terrible thing I saw. For, as I went through a certain valley which lieth by the River of Delights (*flumen deliciarum*) I saw therein many dead corpses lying. And I heard also therein sundry kinds of music, but chiefly nakers, which were marvellously played upon. And so great was the noise thereof that very great fear came upon me. Now, this valley is seven or eight miles long; and if any unbeliever enter therein, he quitteth it never again, but perisheth incontinently. Yet I hesitated not to go in that I might see once for all what the matter was. And when I had gone in I saw there, as I have said, such numbers of corpses as no one without seeing it could deem credible. And at one side of the valley, in the very rock, I beheld as it were the face of a man very great and terrible, so very terrible indeed that for my exceeding great fear my spirit seemed to die in me. Wherefore I made the sign of the Cross, and began continually to repeat *Verbum caro factum*, but I dared not at all come nigh that face, but kept at seven or eight paces from it. And so I came at length to the other end of the valley, and there I ascended a hill of sand and looked around me."

Narrated as it is of no specified place and of no one year of his journey, it may stand, and perhaps it was meant to stand, for a common experience of China in the period of Mongol decadence. Whether he left the country by the gorges of the

[1] In Yule's *Cathay and the Way Thither* (Hakluyt Society), 1. 156.

Yang-tsi and the Yun-nan route, or along the upper basin of the Hoang-ho by the more usual northern route to the desert of Gobi, his vision of a Valley of Corpses is equally significant.

The Theory of the Plague-Virus.

The question that remains is the connexion, in pathological theory, between the bubo-plague and the corruption of the un- buried dead or of the imperfectly buried dead. Some such connexion was the rumour of the time, before any scientific theory can well have existed. Also the factor in question was undoubtedly there among the antecedents, if it were not even the most conspicuous of the antecedents. But we might still be following a wandering light if we were to trust the theory of the Black Death to those empirical suggestions, striking and plaus- ible though they be. It is not for the Black Death only, but for the great plagues of the Mohammedan conquests, which preceded the Black Death by many centuries and also followed that great intercurrent wave until long after in their own strict succession, for the circumscribed spots of plague in various parts of Asia and Africa in our own day, and above all for the great plague of Justinian's reign,—it is for them all that a theory of bubo-plague is needed. A survey of the circumstances of all these . plagues will either weaken or strengthen, destroy or establish, the theory that the virus of the Black Death had arisen on the soil of China from the cadaveric poison present in some peculiar potency, and had been carried to Europe in the course of that overland trade at whose terminus we first hear of its virulence being manifested.

The theory of the origin of the plague-virus from the corrup- tion of the dead was a common one in the sixteenth century. It was held by Ambroise Paré among others, and it was elabo- rately worked out for the Egypt of his day by Prosper Alpinus, physician to the Venetian Consulate at Cairo towards the end of the same century. But the most brilliant exposition of it, one of the finest exercises of diction and of reasoning that has ever issued from the profession of medicine, was that given for the origin in Egypt of the great plague of Justinian's reign by Etienne Pariset, secretary to the Académie de Médecine and commissioner from France to study the plague in Syria and Egypt in 1829[1].

In the plague-stricken Egypt of that time, overburdened with population and still awaiting the beneficent rule of Mehemet Ali, Dr Pariset had his attention forcibly directed to the same contrast between the modern and ancient manner of disposing of the dead, and to the insuitability of the former to the Delta, which had been remarked by Prosper Alpinus in 1591, and by De Maillet, French consul at Cairo, in 1735, and had been specially dwelt upon by *philosophes* of the eighteenth century, such as Montesquieu, Volney and De Pauw. On the one hand he saw under his eyes various revolting things in the Delta,—brick tombs invaded by water, an occasional corpse floating at large, canals choked with the putrefying bodies of bullocks dead of a murrain, the courtyards of Coptic and Jewish houses, and the floors of mosques, churches and monasteries filled with generations of the dead in their flooded vaults and catacombs. On the other hand he saw, on the slopes of the Libyan range and on the edge of the desert beyond the reach of the inundation, the occasional openings of a vast and uncounted series of rock-grottoes in which the Egyptians of the pre-Christian era had carefully put away every dead body, whether of bird, or of beast, or of human kind. He was persuaded of the truth of Volney's remark, "In a crowded population, under a hot sun, and in a soil filled deep with water during several months of every year, the *rapid* putrefaction of bodies becomes a leaven of plague and of other disease[2]." The remark of De Pauw, although it is not adduced, was equally to the point: "Neither men nor beasts are any longer embalmed in Egypt; but the ancient Egyptians seem to have done well in following that mode, and in keeping the mummies in the deepest recesses of excavated rocks....Were we to note here all that those two nations [Arabs and Turks] have left undone, and everything that they ought not to have done, it would be easy to understand how a country formerly not altogether unhealthy, is now become a hotbed of the

---

[1] Etienne Pariset, *Causes de la Peste.* Paris, 1837.
[2] Volney, *Voyages en Syrie et en Egypte.* Paris, 1792.

plague[1]." These eighteenth-century reflections, casual and dis-
cursive after the manner of the time, were amplified by Pariset
to scientific fulness and order, and set in permanent classical
form. Like De Pauw and Volney, he extolled the ancient
sanitary wisdom of Egypt, and excused the priestly mask of
superstition for the implicit obedience that it secured. De
Pauw had pointed out that the towns most remarkable for the
worship of crocodiles,—Coptos, Arsinoë (Crocodilopolis), and
Athribis,—were all situated on canals at some distance from the
Nile; the crocodiles could never have got to them unless the
canals were kept clear; according to Aelian and Eusebius the
crocodile was the symbol of water fit to drink; so that the superstitious worship of the animal was in effect the motive for
keeping the canals of the Nile in repair. The priests of Egypt,
says Pariset, with their apparatus of fictions and emblems,
sought to veil from the profane eyes of the vulgar and of
strangers the secrets of a sublime philosophy[2]. They made
things sacred so as to make them binding, so as to constrain by
the force of religion, as Moses did, their disciple. They had to
reckon with the annual overflow of the Nile, with a hot sun,
and a crowded population. Suppose that all the dead animal
matter, human or other, were to be incorporated with the soil
under these rapid changes of saturation and drying, of diffusion
and emanation, what a mass of poison, what danger to the
living! What foresight they showed in avoiding it, what
labour and effort, but what results! Can anyone pretend that a
system so vast, so beautiful, so coherent in all its parts, had been
engendered and conserved merely by an ignorant fanaticism, or
that a people who had so much of wisdom in their actions had
none in their thoughts? Looking around him at the Egypt of
the Christian and Mohammedan eras, he asks, What has become
of that hygiene, attentive, scrupulous and enlightened, of that

[1] Cornelius de Pauw, *Philosophical Reflections on the Egyptians and Chinese*,
Engl. Transl. Lond. 1795, 2 vols.

[2] It is noteworthy that Herodotus represents the question of disposal of the dead
as having been raised by the Egyptians: they decided in favour of embalming and
rock entombment, as against cremation or burial, the reason given for the preference
being that fire was "a savage beast," in the one case, while in the other case, the
devouring beast was the worm. Bk. III. § 16.

marvellous police of sepulture, of that prodigious care to preserve the soil from all admixture of putrescible matters? The ancient learning of Egypt, the wisdom taught by hard experience in remote ages and perfected in prosperous times, had gradually been overthrown, first by the Persian and Greek conquests which weakened the national spirit, then by the Roman conquest which broke it, then by the prevalence of the Christian doctrines, and lastly by the Mohammedan domination, more hostile than all the others to sanitary precaution.

Pariset's remaining argument was that ancient Egypt, by its systematic care in providing for a slow mouldering of human and animal bodies beyond the reach of the inundation, had been saved from the plague; in the historic period there had been epidemics, but these had been of typhus or other sickness of prisons, slavery, and famines. According to Herodotus, Egypt and Libya were the two healthiest countries under the sun. But when St Paul's vehement argument as to the natural and the spiritual body began to make way, when men began to ask the question, " How are the dead raised up, and with what body do they come?" the ancient practice of Egypt was judged to be out of harmony with Christian doctrine. Embalming was denounced as sinful by St Anthony, the founder of Egyptian monachism, in the third century; and by the time that the church of North Africa had reached its point of highest influence under St Augustine, bishop of Hippo, the ancient religious rites of Egypt had everywhere given place to Christian burial[1]. Bubo-plague had already been prevalent in at least one disastrous epidemic in Lower Egypt at the time of the great massacres of Christians in the episcopate of Cyprian; and in the year 542 it broke out at Pelusium, one of the uncleannest spots in the Delta, spread thence on the one hand along the North African coast, and on the other hand by the corn ships to Byzantium, and grew into the disastrous world-wide pestilence which has ever since been associated with the reign of Justinian.

After the Mohammedan conquest things went from bad to

---

[1] Curiously enough it was among the Christians of Egypt that the controversy as to the *corruptibles* and the *incorruptibles* raged most furiously. See Gibbon.

worse; and from the tenth century until the year 1846, plague had been domesticated on the soil of Egypt.

The theory of Pariset was communicated by him to the Académie de Médecine on 12 July, 1831, and finally published in a carefully designed and highly finished essay in 1837. It was received with much disfavour; according to his colleague Daremberg, the learned librarian of the Academy, nothing but its brilliant style could have saved it from being forgotten in a week. It was vigorously opposed by Clot Bey, on behalf of Egyptian officialdom, because it fixed upon Egypt the stigma of holding in the soil an inherent and abiding cause of the plague[1]. Besides the general objection that it was the theorizing of a *philosophe*, exception was taken to particular parts of the argument. Thus Labat demonstrated by arithmetic that the mummied carcases of all the generations of men and animals in Egypt for three thousand years would have required a space as large as the whole of Egypt, which should thus have become one vast ossuary. And as to the fact, he added, embalming was the privilege of the rich, and of some sacred species of animals. Clot Bey asserted that the whole class of slaves were not thought worthy of embalming. He found also, in the language used by Herodotus, evidence that the people of Egypt felt themselves to be under "the continual menace" of some great epidemic scourge and took precautions accordingly—the very ground on which Pariset based his theory. The objection which weighed most with Daremberg was the fact that, just about the time when Pariset had asserted the immunity of Egypt from plague in her prosperous days, evidence had been found, in the newly-discovered collections of Oribasius, that a bubonic disease was recorded for Egypt and Libya by a Greek physician two centuries before the Christian era, and by another Greek medical writer about the beginning of our era.

It does not appear to have occurred to the opponents of Pariset's theory that the two chief objections, first that embalming was far from general, and second that cases of plague did occur in ancient Egypt, answered each other. But, as matter of fact, it can be shown that there were cheaper forms of embalming

[1] Clot Bey, *Peste en Egypte.* Paris, 1840.

practised for the great mass of the people. Again, it was found by De Maillet that bodies not embalmed at all, but laid in coarse cloths upon beds of charcoal under six or eight feet of sand at an elevation on the edge of the great plain of mummies at Memphis, and beyond the reach of the water, were as perfectly preserved from putrid decay as if they had been embalmed, the dry air and the nitrous soil contributing to their slow and inoffensive decomposition[1]. These facts tended to support the notion that it was not ceremony which really determined the national practice, but utility, into which neither art nor religion necessarily entered. The existence also of bubonic disease in the period of the Ptolemies proved that the risk assumed in Pariset's theory was a real risk, the precautions having been not always sufficient to meet it.

The plague which overran the known world in Justinian's reign (542) was, according to this theory, the effect on a grand scale of an equally grand cause, namely, the final overthrow of a most ancient religion and national life, which had not been built up for nothing and had a true principle concealed beneath its superstitions. The parallelism between China and ancient Egypt has been a favourite subject. In China whatever of religion there is runs upon the Egyptian lines—reverence for the dead or worship of ancestors. The Chinese do not indeed embalm their dead, but they practise an equivalent art of preservation which may be read in almost identical terms in the book of Marco Polo and in modern works on the social life of China[2]. To prevent the products of cadaveric decay from passing into the soil may be said to be the object of their practices. The pains taken to secure dry burial-places are especially obvious in those parts of the country, such as the " reed lands " of the Yang-tsi, which are subject to inundations, annual or occasional[3]. Much of the national art of Feng-shui is concerned, under the mask of divination, with these common-sense aims.

[1] Benoit de Maillet, *Description de l'Egypte.* Paris, 1735, p. 281. See also Wilkinson, *Ancient Egyptians,* III. 456, 465.

[2] Justus Doolittle, *Social Life of the Chinese,* 2 vols. New York, 1867, I. 33, 198, 213.

[3] T. T. Cooper, *Travels of a Pioneer of Commerce,* Lond. 1871, p. 23, 33.

C.

Both Egypt and China are liable to have their river-basins flooded at one time and parched to dust at another. These extreme fluctuations of the ground water are now known to scientific research to be the cause of peculiar and unwholesome products of putrefaction in the soil: given a soil charged with animal matters, the risk to those living upon it is in proportion to the range of fluctuation of the ground water. If it happen as an annual thing that the pores of the ground are now full of water, now full of air, or if these extreme alternations be a common liability, then a soil with the products of animal decomposition dispersed through it will be always unwholesome, and unwholesome on a national scale. It is often held that even vegetables rotting on the ground are pestiferous; Ambroise Paré believed that the rotting carcase of a stranded whale caused an outbreak of bubo-plague at Genoa; but human decomposition is something special—at least for the living of the same species[1]. Most special of all is it when its gross and crude matters pass rapidly into the ground, getting carried hither and thither by the movements of the ground water, and giving off those half-products of oxidation which the extreme alternations from air to water, or from water to air, in the pores of the ground are known to favour. There may be nothing offensive to the sense, but the emanations from such a soil will in all probability be poisonous or pestilent. In particular circumstances of locality the permeation or leavening of the soil with the products of organic decomposition produces Asiatic cholera; in still more special circumstances the result is yellow fever; in circumstances familiar enough to ourselves the result is typhoid fever, and probably also summer diarrhœa or British cholera. These are all soil poisons. Bubo-plague also is a soil poison; and it is claimed as specially related to the products of *cadaveric* decomposition, diffused at large in such a soil as soil-poisons are ordinarily engendered in.

---

[1] This is one of the remarks in Dr Gilbert Skene's treatise on the Plague, Edinburgh, 1568 (reprinted for the Bannatyne Club, 1840):—Among the causes are "deid cariounis unbureit, in speciale of mankynd, quhilkis be similitude of nature is maist nocent to man, as everie brutall is maist infectand and pestilentiall to thair awin kynd," p. 6.

It is possible to subject that theory of the plague to the test of facts still further. Thus bubo-plague dogged the steps of Mohammedan conquest from the first century after the Hegira, now in Syria when Damascus was the capital, now in Irak when Bagdad was the centre of Mohammedan rule, now in Egypt when the seat of empire shifted to Grand Cairo; and, over a great part of the period, simultaneously in all the regions of Islam. That long series of plague-epidemics has been recorded in Arabic annals, and has lately been published in an abstract accessible to all, with a summary of conclusions[1].

What are the conclusions of the learned commentator on the Arabic annals, as to the general causes of the thousand years of Mohammedan plague?—" War, with the wasting of whole nations, in disregard of all established rights, with plundering of towns and concentration of great masses of men ill provided for and unregulated, who developed the seeds of communicable and malignant diseases. Add to these things the negligent or wholly neglected burial of those who had fallen in battle, the straits and privations of the wounded, and the effects of a hot climate, especially in flooded and swampy tracts of country... The kind of burial, in very shallow and often badly covered graves, which used to be practised in most Eastern towns, and in part is still practised, may also have had disastrous consequences not unfrequently."

The Theory tested by Modern Instances.

With that general statement for the long succession of plague-epidemics in Islam during nine centuries from the Hegira, beginning with a Syrian epidemic in A.D. 628 and ending with a close succession of twelve epidemics in Egypt from 1410 to 1492, we may pass to the more detailed accounts of the conditions under which bubo-plague has been found in various localities, often circumscribed spots far apart and out of the way, during recent years. These spots are so varied, have so little apparently in common, and are so capriciously chosen in the midst of their

---

[1] A. von Kremer, "Ueber die grossen Seuchen des Orients nach arabischen Quellen." *Sitzungsber. der Wien. Akad.*, Philos.-histor. Classe, Bd. 96 (1880), p. 69.

several regions of the globe, that they do not readily fall into any order or classification. What are we to make of a few spots of plague among nomade Arabs of the Cyrenaic plateau; of plague in some stricken villages high up in the highlands of Kurdistan, or in low-lying towns such as Resht, near the shore of the Caspian, or amidst the black ooze of amphibious habitations in the lower valley of Tigris and Euphrates; of true bubonic disease in some few Bedouin villages or small towns on the summits of the basaltic plateaus that rise like gigantic warts from the Arabian desert; of bubo-plague in Yun-nan, at or near the capital Talifoo, where the Mohammedan and Chinese influences have been struggling for mastery, as well as among the cabins in the rocky valleys of the Salwen; of some forty or fifty Himalayan hamlets picked out as plague-spots among the six thousand villages of Kumaon; and of the now extinct but comparatively recent centres of the same disease in the walled towns and walled villages of Kutch, Kattiwar, and Marwar? And lastly what are we to make of those cases of typhus fever with buboes which have been observed in villages of the Yusufzai valley, near Peshawur, in 1852; in the Chinese town of Pakhoi, on the gulf of Tonking, in 1886; occasionally among the fever-cases in Burdwan since the health of that province underwent so disastrous a change about the year 1870; and, on credible report, among the troops in the Russo-Turkish war of 1879? It is surely unnecessary, at least, to refute the sterile dogmatism that these are all the effects of one pre-existing virus, carried, we know not how, from point to point of the globe in an unbroken succession. It is a far cry even on a small-scale map from Kumaon to Kutch, from Yun-nan to the Gulf of Tonking, from Resht to the Armenian highlands, from the centre of Arabia to Tripoli, and from Mesopotamia to North Yemen. And what is the use of assuming that there has always been bubo-plague in the "cradle of the human race," and concluding that the Black Death was one of its excursions westwards, so long as the plagues of Islam were going on from decade to decade, all through the Middle Ages, at no great distance from Byzantium and from Western Europe? Are not Damascus, Bagdad and Grand Cairo of more account as plague-foci than a few villages in the Himalaya or in Kattiwar, even granting that the plague may have been in the latter at an earlier date than we know? It is not communication that connects the several seats of plague, scattered widely in time and place; but it is community of conditions, or of the causes and associated circumstances which breed the plague in each separately. Let us take them in some sort of order.

Among the most remarkable habitats of modern bubo-plague are the villages on the basalt plateaus of the Arabian desert. We have information of these plague-spots from Doughty[1], who did not indeed visit Assir, the most notorious of them, but several others more to the north and east. He describes the ruined villages of Mogug, Gofar, Hâyil and others, where the people had died of plague some years before. A year of dearth preceded the plague in some, if not in all of them. The author is struck by the carelessness of burial, or the difficulties of it in the baked soil, although he does not directly connect that with the epidemics. Thus, in passing the graveyard of Hâyil, one of the plague-towns, he remarks: "Aheyd was a man of much might and glory in his day; he lies a yard under the squalid gravel in his shirt." Of Kheybar, with vague traditions of plague, he says: "We passed through a burial-ground of black volcanic mould and salt-warp; the squalid grave heaps are marked with headstones of wild basalt. That funeral earth is chapped and ghastly, bulging over her enwombed corses, like a garden soil in spring-time which is pushed by the new spring plants. All is horror at Kheybar!" He is led to the following general remarks: "The care of sepulture was beyond measure in the religions of antiquity, which were without humility. Under the new religion [of Arabia] the deceased is wound in a shirt-cloth of calico, and his corse is laid in the shallow pit of droughty earth." Again, of Bedouin burials in general: "The deceased is buried the same day or on the morrow. They scrape out painfully with a stick and their hands in the hard-burned soil a shallow grave. I have seen their graves in the desert ruined by foul hyenas, and their winding-sheets lay half above ground."

[1] Ch. M. Doughty, *Travels in Arabia Deserta*, 2 vols. Cambridge, 1888.

Of the best known of these Arabian plague-spots the plateau of Assir, to the south-east of Mecca, we have the following information relating to the years 1874–79[1]; the chief plague-locality is Namasse, the principal town of Beny Sheir, with five other villages.

The site is on a mountain ridge too high for camels, the climate is cold and moist, the soil fruitful, springs abundant, and no standing water. The houses are built of stone, and stand close together. The ground-floor of each house is used as the stable; and as the winter in these mountains is very severe, so that water freezes, the inhabitants live with their cattle in a horrible state of filth. According to information from the district super-intendent, there had been plague in a few villages every two or three years for the previous thirty-five or forty years. It has seldom extended further than five or six leagues. The region is a mountain canton, with no trade; it is cut off from the rest of the world. The disease is mostly attended with buboes in the groins, armpits, and neck, but not always; sometimes petechial spots were spoken of; in the sheikh Faïk's own household the disease began with rigors, and developed buboes, petechiæ, headache and burning thirst. Dr Nury counted up in six villages, with a population of eight hundred, cases of plague to the number of 184 (68 men, 45 women, 50 boys and 21 girls), with 155 deaths and 29 recoveries.

Let us now place beside this the accounts of the plague in the mountains village of Kumaon[2].

Of the plague-villages of Danpore and Munsharee, near the snow, we read:

"Their houses are generally built of stone, one storey high. On the ground-floor herd the cattle; in this compartment the dung is allowed to accumulate till such time as there is no room left for the cattle to stand erect; it is then removed and carefully packed close around all sides, so that the house literally stands in the centre of a hot-bed....In many instances we have seen it accumulated above the level of the floor of the upper story in which the family lives." In that compartment, four feet high, with no window and a door of some three feet by eighteen inches, ten or fifteen people live, lying huddled together with the door shut. Their food is as poor as their lodging. When plague breaks out, the family ties are rudely loosened: those who can, flee to the jungle, leaving the stricken to their fate.

---

[1] Communicated to Herr von Kremer (*l.c.*) by Nury Effendi, who visited Assir, and wrote a report preserved in MS. in the Archives at Constantinople.

[2] "Report regarding Mahamurree in Kumaon and Garhwal in 1851–52." By F. Pearson and Mookerjee. Agra, 1852 (Extracts in *Ind. Annals of Med. Sc.*, I. 358). Also extracts (*Ib.*) from Renny's Report, 1851.

The following is by Renny: " Fourteen died at a place in the forest half a mile or more from Duddoli, respecting which I had the best description yet given to me of the career of the sickness. Here were only two houses, or long low huts, occupied by two separate families, the heads being two brothers, sixteen souls in all. These two huts had to contain also thirty head of cattle, large and small, at the worst season of the year. In these two huts the Mahamurree [bubo-plague] commenced about ten or eleven months ago, corresponding to the time it appeared in Duddoli. At this place the sixteen residents kept together till fourteen died, and one adult only, a man of about thirty years of age, with his female child of six years old, survived. There was no particular disorder among the cattle, but the outbreak of the plague was preceded and accompanied by a great mortality among the rats in their houses."

Let us now take the accounts, twenty-five years later, of the plague in the same district in 1876–77[1].

Confirming the earlier statements as to the extraordinary filth of the houses—the cattle under the same roof and the baskets of damp and unripe grain—he directs attention specially to the disposal of the dead. The custom of the country is to burn the body beside the most convenient mountain stream terminating in the Ganges. But from that good practice the people have deviated in regard to bodies dead of any pestilence (small-pox, cholera, plague), which are buried. Of all countries the Himalaya is least suited to the burial of the dead. For, by reason of the rocky subsoil, it is seldom possible to dig a grave more than two feet deep; and, as a rule, the pestilent dead are laid in shallow trenches in the surface soil of the field nearest to the place of death, or of the terrace facing the house, or even of the floor of the house itself. This bad practice is begotten of fear to handle the body, and has been long established. Such mismanagement of the dead is sufficient to account for the continuous existence of the active principle of plague-disease, sometimes dormant for want of opportunity, but ever ready to affect persons suitably prepared by any cause producing a low or bad state of health. In the houses of families about to suffer from an outbreak of plague, rats are sometimes found dead on the floor. Planck had seen them himself; all that he had seen appeared to have died suddenly, as by suffocation, their bodies being in good condition, a piece of rag some-times clenched in the teeth. He mentions nine villages, all of them endemic seats of plague, in which the premonitory death of rats in the infected houses was testified. The affected villages were not one in a hundred of all the villages of Kumaon, and were widely scattered throughout

[1] Planck, *Ninth Report of the Sanitary Commissioner, N. W. Prov.* Allahabad, 1877, pp. 40–95. (Extracts, p. 39, of *Papers relating to the Plague, Parl. Papers*, 1879.)

the northern half of the province. Even in each of those few villages, the plague is confined to one house, or one terrace, or one portion of the village.

Let us turn next to the small spots of bubo-plague in the remote province of Yun-nan. Our information comes from members of the British and French Consular services[1].

The plague occurs in towns and villages and is the cause of much mortality. After ravaging villages scattered about the plains, it frequently ascends the mountains, and takes off many of the aborigines inhabiting the high lands. What, in M. Rocher's opinion, aggravates the evil is the practice of not burying the bodies of those who die of this disease. Instead of being buried, the body is placed on a bier and exposed to the sun. As a consequence of this practice the traveller passing the outskirts of a village where the plague is raging is nearly choked with the nauseous smell emanating from the exposed and rotting corpses. Burial is the usual mode of disposal, although many of the villages are on rocky mountain sides, as in Kumaon. The rats are first affected; as soon as they sicken, they leave their holes in troops, and after staggering about and falling over each other, drop down dead. Mr Baber had the same information from a French missionary in the upper valley of the Salwen, a long, low valley about two miles broad, walled in by immense precipices, so hot in summer that the inhabitants go up the hill sides to live. The approach of bubo-plague (the buboes may be as large as a hen's or goose's egg) may often be known from the extraordinary behaviour of the rats, who leave their holes and crevices and issue on to the floors without a trace of their accustomed timidity, springing continually upwards from their hind legs as if they were trying to jump out of something. The rats fall dead, and then comes the turn of the poultry, pigs, goats, etc. The good father had a theory of his own that the plague is really a pestilential emanation slowly rising in an equable stratum from the ground, the smallest creatures being first engulfed. The larger plague-centre at or near the capital, Talifoo, appears to be related to Mohammedan warfare, and possibly to the neglect to bury the dead, which is an admitted fact, although not connected by the narrator with the prevalence of plague.

The other Chinese plague-spot is hundreds of miles away, on the shores of the Gulf of Tonking. The best known centre of plague is the port of Pakhoi, the native quarter of which is described as peculiarly filthy. The houses are little cleaner than

---

[1] Baber, in *Parliamentary Papers*, 1878, "China." No. 6. Rocher (*Province Chinoise de Yun-nan*) quoted, without the reference, in *Med. Reports of Chinese Imperial Maritime Customs*, No. 15, 1878, Shanghai, p. 25.

the streets, the floors being saturated with excrement, and the drains being either close to the surface or open altogether. An outbreak of plague there in 1882 is minutely described by Dr Lowry[1].

It occurred in the hot weather of June (85° Fahr. day, 76° Fahr. night) ; for fear of thieves the houses are carefully shut up even on the hottest night. The epidemic caused about 400 to 500 deaths in a population of 25,000. The disease does not spread. In nearly every house where the disease broke out, the rats had been coming out of their holes and dying on the floors : Dr Lowry dissected several of them, and found the lungs congested. In the human subject, except for the buboes, the disease resembled typhus : "anyone going to the bedside of a patient would certainly at first think it was that disease he had to deal with." The same disease occurred at Lien-chow, a city twelve miles off. Another English physician in the service of the China Maritime Customs heard of a malady with the symptoms of plague in certain districts of Southern Kiangsi in the autumn of 1886 ; but no particulars were to be had. Typhus was prevalent, and very fatal, every year in the towns, villages and hamlets of Northern Kiangsi.

One curious piece of evidence as to the death of rats, not associated with plague in men, comes from a more northern province of China. In the autumn of 1881, on the opposite side of the Yang-tsi from Nanking and in the western suburbs of the ancient capital, the rats emerged from holes in dwellings, jumped up, turned round, and fell dead. Baskets and boxes filled with their bodies were cast into the canal. "Here," says Dr Macgowan, "was evidently a subsoil poison which affected the animals precisely in the same way as the malaria of the Yun-nan pest. Happily the subterranean miasm at Nanking did not affect animals that live above ground[2]."

The evidence from Kutch, Kattiwar, and Marwar relates to the years 1815–20, and 1838. In circumstances peculiar in some respects, namely, of walled towns and stockaded villages, but the same as those already given in the matter of filth from cattle crowded into the human dwellings, we find bubo-plague breaking out so long as the unwholesome state of things lasted under Mahratta rule and until British rule had been fairly at work. The causes of the bubo-plague, says Whyte, were the same as of typhus—walled and crowded towns, cattle housed with human beings, slow wasting diseases among the cattle, which were not

---

[1] J. H. Lowry, *Med. Rep. Chinese Mar. Customs*, No. 24, 1882, p. 27.
[2] D. J. Macgowan, *Ib.* 1882.   Report for Wenchow.

killed for food but kept for milk and ghee. He questions whether, in shutting out their enemies, they had not shut in one far more powerful[1]. Here also we have various independent witnesses[2] testifying to the premonitory death of the rats; they lay dead in all places and directions—in the streets, houses, and hiding-places of the walls. This happened in every town that was affected in Marwar, so that the inhabitants of any house instantly quitted it on seeing a dead rat.

Relation of Typhus to Bubo-plague.

The smallest and the most easily surveyed of all the recent foci of bubo-plague, is that among the Bedouin of the Cyrenaic plateau in North Africa (port of Benghazi), a desert region corresponding to one of the most famous corn-lands of antiquity.

There was no difference of opinion that the small outbreak of plague in 1874 began simultaneously in the tents of Orphas and the tents of Ferig-el-Hanan, containing together about a hundred souls[3]. These Arabs keep cows, sheep and goats; some of them also cultivate small patches of corn. They are subject to periodic famines, and there had been much want among them in 1869, 1870, 1871, 1872 and 1873, attended by epidemics of typhus, cholera and smallpox. In the winter they found employment among the traders of Merdjé, and at the end of March, 1873, had quitted that village to place their animals in the neighbouring hill-pastures. The ground had been saturated, after long drought, by the rains of the winter. Their tents are pitched in hollows which may be filled by water in a few minutes. The encampments, like those of the Bedouin in Arabia, are excessively filthy and are often the scene of typhus fever. In April, 1874, the plague began, the first case being in a child; the buboes were in the groin, armpit or neck. The other symptoms were bilious vomiting, black vomit, haematemesis, petechiae, anthraceous boils, pains in the head, collapse, and delirium. A few cases were mild, but the majority grave and fatal; in several cases there was a relapse with new buboes. The disease was brought from the tents to the village of Merdjé, in which 270 were attacked in a population of

---

[1] Thomas Whyte, "Report on the Disease which prevailed in Kattywar, etc. in 1819–20." *Trans. Med. Phys. Soc. Bombay*, I. 155. Bombay, 1838.

[2] I have curtailed the evidence from Gujerat; it will be found at large in the following writers: Gilder, *Bombay Med. Trans.* I. 193; McAdam, *ib.* 183; F. Forbes, *ib.* II. |1, and Thesis on Plague, Edin. 1840; Glen, *Quart. Journ. Cal. Med. Soc.* I. 433; Ranken, *Report on Pali Plague*, Calcutta, 1838; and Whyte, as above.

[3] L. Arnaud, *Peste de Benghazi*, Constantinople, 1875; *Essai sur la Peste*, Paris, 1888; *Une Mission pour la Peste*, Paris, 1888.

310, with 100 deaths. The total known attacks from 5 April to 24 July were 533 in a population of 734, with 208 deaths and 325 recoveries, 201 resisting the infection. The sanitary state of the village was as bad as that of the tents : the houses, entered by a low door, had windows not to the sun, but to the courtyard, which is a stable choked with filth ; the floors of the houses are covered with filth. The graveyard is in the centre of the village, beside a pool of standing water : the graves are shallow, and the corpses are sometimes unearthed by jackals. Both in the village and in the encampments a fall of rain was followed by a new series of attacks. The advice of the sanitary commisioner was to make graves at least six feet deep, and to cover them with lime.

These events in 1874 were an exact repetition of those of 1858. In both years heavy rains followed long drought, giving promise of an abundant harvest after a period of famine. The dry years, in both instances, were attended with sickness, typhus and other; the first wet season turned the sickness to plague, that is to say, it added the complication of buboes and haemorrhagic symptoms to the characters of typhus. The meaning of that seems to be that the saturation of the ground generated a soil-poison where there had previously been the milder aerial poison of typhus. This view of plague, as a typhus of the soil, or a disease made so much more malignant than typhus just because of underground fermentation of the putrescible animal matters, is borne out by the facts already given for China and for India. The latter country furnishes other illustrations of typhus fever becoming complicated with buboes, and so becoming something like plague. Perhaps the best instance is the fever observed in the Yusufzai valley, near Peshawur, in 1852[1].

It arose mostly in the filthy Mohammedan houses, shared by cattle and human beings ; but it invaded some of the cleaner Hindoo houses also. The disease began in low, marshy situations, which were covered with water after rain and heavy night dews. It was of the type of typhus, or relapsing fever, with yellowness of the skin, bleeding from the gums, and from the bowels, and often from the nose. One of the observers says: "The only other concomitant affection worthy of note is swelling of the lymphatic glands over various parts of the body; this, however, is only met with in a very few instances." The other authority says : "Inflammati n

---

[1] T. Farquhar, M.D., "Typhus Fever in the Eusofzai," *Ind. Annals of Med. Sc.* II. 504 ; R. Lyell, M.D., "Fever of the Yusufzai Valley," *Ib.* II. p. 16.

and suppuration of the glands in the groin, axilla, and neck occurred in some that survived the first or second relapse." To this outbreak, which is removed only in degree from the Benghazi plague, the Pakhoi plague, and the Pali plague (Gujerat), may be added some others, about which the information is more general. Thus, the fevers which have become notorious in Burdwan since the health of that province changed so disastrously owing to the damming of the ground-water, are said to have been attended now and then with buboes. The typhus fever at Saugor in 1859 was occasionally complicated with suppuration of the lymphatic glands: "In the Doab, as in the subsequent gaol attack, the glands in the groin were very rarely affected; those in the neck were more frequently affected, but this was not a prominent feature in the disease[1]." Again, General Loris Melikoff told the correspondent of the *Golos* that twenty men died in a day in the Russo-Turkish war in the winter of 1878, with glandular swellings; everywhere there was Schmutz, Schmutz! And lastly, in the epidemic of 1878 at Vetlianka, on the Volga, which is reckoned among the historic occurrences of bubo-plague in Europe, the first ten cases in November, 1878, had suppurating glands in the axilla, did not take to bed, and recovered; there had been ordinary typhus in the filthy fisher cottages in 1877, and there was typhus concurrent with the disease which at length became, and was at length recognized as, true bubo-plague in the winter of 1878—79[2].

One thing which distinguishes these recent outbreaks of plague from the great plague of Justinian's reign, in part from the series of Mohammedan plagues, and from the Black Death, is that they have for the most part shown no independent vitality and no diffusive power. As in typhus fever itself (except on great occasions), they have been almost confined to those who lived in the filthy houses, and to those who came within the influence of the pestilential emanations. The great plagues of the 6th and 14th centuries had, on the other hand, a diffusive power which carried them over the whole known world. The buboes of Egypt and of China became familiar as far as Norway and Greenland.

But, apart from diffusiveness, the conditions of recent local plagues are not unlike those of the great historical epidemics. The very same observation of the rats leaving their holes, which is so abundantly confirmed from the recent plague-spots of Southern China, of Yun-nan, of Kumaon, and of Gujerat, was

[1] Surgeon-General J. Murray, M.D., at Epidemiological Society, 11 May, 1878. *Med. Times and Gaz.* I. 1878, p. 597.
[2] Alex. Rittmann, *Chronik der Pest*. Brünn, 1879.

familiar in the plague-books of London and of Edinburgh in the Elizabethan period. Of the great outbreak in 1603, Thomas Lodge writes : " And when as rats, moules, and other creatures (accustomed to live underground) forsake their holes and habitations, it is a token of corruption in the same, by reason that such sorts of creatures forsake their wonted places of aboade[1]." That is only one of many proofs that the virus of plague has its habitat in the soil, although it may be carried long distances clinging to other things. In its most diffusive potency it is a soil-poison generated, we may now say with some confidence, out of the products of cadaveric decay[2]; in its less diffusive but hardly less malignant potency, it is a soil-poison generated out of the filth of cattle housed with human beings, or out of domestic filth generally, and in nearly all the known instances of such generation, associated with, but perhaps not absolutely dependent upon, carelessness in the disposal of the dead after famine or fever; in the least malignant form, when plague is only a small part of an epidemic of typhus and with the buboes inclined to suppurate, it appears to be still a soil-poison, and to differ from typhus itself, just because the pestilential product of decomposing filth has been engendered in the pores of the ground, rather than in the atmosphere of living-rooms.

The Black Death, which here concerns us immediately, is one of the two great instances of a plague-virus with vast diffusive power, enormous momentum, and centuries of endurance. So great effects may be said to postulate adequate causes; and one must assume that the virus had been bred from cadaveric decomposition in circumstances of peculiar

[1] Thomas Lodge, *Treatise of the Plague*, Lond. 1603, chap. III. Skene, in his Edinburgh essay on plague in 1568, gives as a sign of impending plague the moles and "serpents" leaving their holes: "As when the moudewart and serpent leavis the eird, beand molestit be the vapore contenit within the bowells of the samin." He adds what agrees still farther with modern experience in Yun-nan : "If the domesticall fowls become pestilential, it is ane signe of maist dangerous pest to follow." (Bannatyne Club ed. p. 9).

[2] The writer of the article "Peste" in the *Dict. Encycl. des Sc. Med.*, Dr Mahé, inclines on the whole to the view that the poison of plague is somehow related to cadaveric products : " Parmi ces accusations d'insalubrité publique, il en est une qui repose sur un objectif plus positif en apparance" viz. the "miasme des cadavres."

aggravation and on some vast or national scale. The sequence
of events carries us to China; and the annals of China do
furnish evidence that the assumed cause was there on a vast
scale through a long period of national disaster, while the
national customs of China for the disposal of the dead, like
those of ancient Egypt, point to the existence of a real risk
from allowing the soil to be permeated at large by the crude or
hasty products of cadaveric decomposition.

It is our duty to construct the best hypothesis we can,
sparing no labour. No one really dispenses with theory, whatever his protestations to the contrary; those who are the loudest
professors of suspended judgment are the most likely to fall
victims to some empty verbalism which hangs loose at both
ends, some ill-considered piece of argument which ignores the
historical antecedents and stops short of the concrete conclusions.
It has been so in the case of infective diseases, and of bubo-
plague in particular. The virus of the plague, we are told, is
specific; it has existed from an unknown antiquity, and has
come down in an unbroken succession; we can no more discover
how it arose, than we can tell how the first man arose, or the
first mollusc, or the first moss or lichen; its species is, indeed, of
the nature of the lowest vegetable organisms.

The objection to that hypothesis of plague is that it involves
a total disregard of facts. It is a mere formula, which saves all
trouble, dispenses with all historical inquiry, and appears to be
adapted equally to popular apprehension and to academic ease.
The bubo-plagues of history have not, in fact, been all of the
same descent; notably the Black Death was a wave of pestilence
which Mohammedan countries, accustomed as they had been to
native bubo-plagues for centuries before, recognized as an
invasion from a foreign source, as an interruption of the sequence
of their own plagues. Again, the attempt to link in one series
the various scattered and circumscribed spots of plague now or
lately existing must fail disastrously the moment it is seriously
attempted. The hypothesis of one single source of the plague,
of a species of disease arising we know not how, beginning we
know not when or where, but at all events reproduced by
ordinary generation in an unbroken series of cases, *ab aevo, ab*

ovo, is the merest verbalism, wanting in reality or concreteness, and dictated by the curious illusion that a species of disease, because it reproduces itself after its kind, must resemble in other respects a species of living things.

The diffusive power of the virus of the Black Death, which has been equalled only by that of the plague in Justinian's reign, may seem to have depended upon the favouring conditions that it met with. But although favouring conditions count for much, they are not all. The Black Death raged as furiously as anywhere among the nomade Tartars who were its first victims ; the virus, as soon as it was let loose, put forth a degree of virulence which must have been native to it, or brought with it from its place of engendering. None the less the incidence of the Black Death in Europe had depended in part upon the preparedness of the soil. It came to Europe in the age of feudalism and of walled towns, with a cramped and unwholesome manner of life, and inhabited spots of ground choked with the waste matters of generations. But even amidst these generally fostering conditions, there would have been more special things that determined its election. It is a principle exemplified in all importations of disease from remote sources, in smallpox among the aerial contagions and in Asiatic cholera among the soil-poisons, that the conditions which favour diffusion abroad are approximately the same amidst which the infection had been originally engendered. A soil-poison of foreign origin makes straight for the most likely spots in the line of its travels; it may not, and often does not confine itself to these, but it gives them a preference. Thus, if we conclude on the evidence that the bubo-plague is a soil-poison having a special affinity to the products of cadaveric decomposition, we shall understand why the Black Death, when it came to England, found so congenial a soil in the monasteries, and in the homes of the clergy. Within the monastery walls, under the floor of the chapel or cloisters, were buried not only generations of monks, but often the bodies of princes, of notables of the surrounding country, and of great ecclesiastics. In every parish the house of the priest would have stood close to the church and the churchyard. One has to figure the virus of the Black Death not so much as carried by individuals from place to place in their persons, or in their clothes and effects, but rather as a leaven which had passed into the ground, spreading hither and thither therein as if by polarizing the adjacent particles of the soil, and that not instantaneously like a physical force, but so gradually as to occupy a whole twelvemonth between Dorset and Yorkshire. Sooner or later it reached to every corner of the land, manifesting its presence wherever there were people resident. Such universality in the soil of England, we have reason to think, it had. But it appears to have put forth its greatest power in the walled town, in the monastery, and in the neighbourhood of the village churchyard.

CHAPTER IV.

ENGLAND AFTER THE BLACK DEATH, WITH THE EPIDEMICS TO THE TUDOR PERIOD.

THE great mortality came to an end everywhere in England by Michaelmas, 1349. The pestilence had lasted some fourteen months, from its first appearance on the Dorset coast at the beginning of August, 1348, until its subsidence in the northern counties in the autumn of 1349. It came to an end, as all devastating epidemics do, through having spent its force, exhausted its pabulum, run through all the susceptible subjects. A letter-writer of Charles I.'s reign has put into colloquial language the corresponding reason for a pause in the ravages of the plague towards the end of its stay in London : " And I think the only reason why the plague is somewhat slackened is because the place is dead already, and no bodie left in it worth the killing[1]." The exhausted state of the country, and of all Europe, is not easy for us to realize. Petrarch, a witness of the Black Death in Italy, foresaw the incredulity of after ages, or their inability to image the state of things—the empty houses, the abandoned towns, the squalid country, the fields crowded with the dead, the vast and dreadful solitude over the whole world. If you inquire of historians, he continues, they are silent; if you consult the physicians, they are at their wits' end ; if you question the philosophers, they shrug their shoulders, wrinkle their brows, and lay the finger on the lip. Is it possible that posterity can

---

[1] Sir Tobie Matthews' *Letters*. Lond. 1660, p. 110.

believe these things? For we who have seen them can hardly believe them[1].

The blow fell upon every country of Europe within a period of two or three years; and it must have paralysed all trade and industry, war and politics, for the time being. Edward III.'s wars in France, which had resulted in the victory of Crecy in 1346 and the conquest of Calais in 1347, had been suspended by a truce, which was renewed from time to time. Thus, in the very midst of the pestilence, on the 2nd of May, 1349, the envoys of the English and French kings, "in their tents between Calais and Guines," agreed upon a form of treaty continuing the truce until Pentecost, 1350[2]. In the last days of 1349, Edward III. in person, with a small force, was able to repel an attack upon his new possession of Calais[3]. It was in the year after the Black Death (1350) according to both Stow and Selden, that Edward III. held a great feast at Windsor, to which his heralds invited knights from abroad, to celebrate the institution of the Order of the Garter, the statutes of the Order having been drawn up the year before. What is styled "the necessary defence of the realm," was a chief subject of concern throughout the year 1350. On the 12th February an order was made to the sheriffs of counties for a supply of so many arrows from each[4]. On the 20th March the mayors and bailiffs of 110 towns are ordered to provide their respective quotas of men-at-arms—London 100, Norwich 60, Bristol 20, and so on—and to send them to Sandwich "for the necessary defence of our realm[5]." On the 1st of May a commission was issued to engage mariners for certain ships, and on the 20th May, an order for ships, pinnaces and barges.

On the 22nd July and 10th August there are proclamations relating to the piratical fleet of Spanish ships, intercepting the English traders to Gascony, and threatening an invasion of England[6]; the Spaniards were routed, their ships taken, and

---

[1] *Epist. de rebus familiar.* Lib. viii. epist. 7. The citation of these contemporary illustrations of the Black Death was begun in the last century by Sprengel (*Beiträge*, &c., p. 37).

[2] *Foedera*, III. 184; it was renewed on 30th June for a year longer.

[3] Avesbury.   [4] *Foedera*, III. 192.   [5] *Ib.* 193.   [6] *Ib.* 200, 201.

the Channel cleared, in a famous engagement off Winchelsea, on 29th August, 1350, which the king directed in person[1]. On 15th June, three days before the first of the ordinances against the Labourers, the king issued two orders to counties, to raise men "for our passage against the parts over sea"—one to the Welsh lords, and the other to the sheriffs of English counties, the demands being in all for 4170 bowmen from England, and for 1350 men from Wales[2]. Whatever these edicts may have resulted in, it was not until four years after that the king really resumed his wars with France. On the 8th September, 1355, the Black Prince sailed from Plymouth with a fleet of some three hundred ships carrying an army of knights, men-at-arms, English bowmen and Welshmen, to the Garonne, for his famous raid across the south of France[3]. Later in the autumn the king collected at Portsmouth[4] and Sandwich, and at Calais, a force of three thousand men-at-arms, two thousand mounted bowmen, and an immense number of bowmen on foot, with which he took the field on the 2nd November[5]. The same summer, a fleet of forty great ships was fitted out at Rotherhithe, for a force of foot under Henry, duke of Lancaster, to aid the king of Navarre; it sailed on the 10th of July, but was unable to clear the Channel, and for various reasons did not proceed[6]; next year, however, the duke of Lancaster crossed from Southampton to Normandy with a force in forty-eight ships[7].

Thus was the war with France resumed six years after the great mortality. The means for equipping these expeditions had been provided by loans raised on the security of the enormous subsidy which the Parliament of 1353–54 was induced to vote, in the form of an export duty of fifty shillings on every sack of wool shipped to foreign countries during the next six years. According to Avesbury's calculation, Edward had a revenue, from that source, of a thousand marks a day; it was the common opinion, he says, that more than 100,000 sacks of

[1] Le Baker's *Chronicle of Osney*. Avesbury.   [2] *Foedera*, III. 221.
[3] Avesbury, Rolls ed. 425.
[4] Blomefield (*Hist. of Norfolk*, III.) says that the writ to Norwich in 1355 was for 120 men-at-arms to be sent to Portsmouth by Sunday in mid-Lent.
[5] Avesbury, pp. 427–8.   [6] *Ib.* p. 425.   [7] *Ib.* p. 461.

wool were exported in a year[1].   But another and perhaps better authority gives the annual export of wool in the middle of the fourteenth century at nearly 32,000 sacks[2].

Direct effects of the Black Death.

Meanwhile internal affairs were demanding the king's attention, although they occupy less space in the extant State papers than the warlike preparations.   On the 23rd August, while the mortality was raging in the north, a proclamation was issued to the sheriff of Northumberland against the migration of people to Scotland, with arms, victuals, goods and merchandise, the pestilence not being mentioned[3].   The first State paper which relates to the recent great mortality is the king's proclamation of 1st December, 1349, to the mayor and bailiffs of Sandwich, and of forty-eight other English ports, including London[4].   The proclamation begins:

" Forasmuch as no mean part of the people of our realm of England is dead in the present pestilence, and the treasure of the said realm is mostly exhausted, and (as we have learned) numbers of this our kingdom are daily passing, or proposing to pass, to parts over sea with money which they were able to have kept within the realm, Now we, taking heed that if passage after this manner be tolerated, the kingdom will in a short time be stripped both of men and of treasure, and so therefrom grave danger may easily arise to us and to the said realm, unless a fitting remedy be speedily appointed

---

[1] Avesbury, p. 431.

[2] Thorold Rogers, *Hist. of Agric. and Prices,* I. 367, ''according to an account quoted by Misselden in his *Circle of Commerce.*''   The sack of wool contained 52 cloves of 7 lbs. each, or 364 lbs.   It appears from a statute of 5 Ric. II. that 240 wool-fells were equivalent, for duty, to one sack of wool.   In Rogers' tables, the wool-fell is usually priced at about the value of 1½ lbs. of wool, which was at the same time about the average clip of a sheep.   The present average clip would be at least four times as much.   The colonial bale of wool is of the same weight as the medieval sack, but would represent 40 to 60 fleeces, instead of about 240.   At the smallest of the estimates in the text, the wool of 7,680,000 sheep would have been exported in a year.   Avesbury's estimate would mean an annual export to foreign countries of the clip of about 24,000,000 sheep.   The average price of a sack of wool just before the Black Death was about £4 in money of the time; the period immediately following the plague was one of low prices; but from 1364 to 1380, the price was uniformly high.

[3] *Foedera,* III. 186.   [4] *Ib.* III. 191.

—do command the mayor and bailiffs of Sandwich (and of forty-eight other ports) to stop the passage beyond sea of them that have no mandate, especially if they be Englishmen, excepting merchants, notaries, or the king's envoys."

The edict was probably directed more against the drain of treasure than against the emigration of people; but this not uninteresting question really belongs to other historians, who do not appear to have dealt with it[1].

On the 18th of June, 1350, the first summer after the mortality, there was issued the first proclamation, to the sheriffs of counties, on the demands of the labourers and artificers for higher wages, entitled "De magna parte populi in ultima pestilentia defuncta, et de servientium salariis proinde moderandis[2]." The preamble or motive is one that cannot but seem strange to modern ideas, although it must have been correct and conventional according to feudal notions : "Forasmuch as some, having regard to the necessities of lords and to the scarcity of servants, are unwilling to serve unless they receive excessive wages, while others prefer to beg in idleness, rather than to seek their living by labour—be it therefore enacted that any man or woman, bond or free, under the age of sixty, and not living by a trade or handicraft, nor possessing private means, nor having land to cultivate, shall be obliged, when required, to serve any master who is willing to hire him or her at such wages as were usually paid in the locality in the year 1346, or on the average of five or six years preceding ; provided that the lords of villeins or tenants shall have the preference of their labour, so that they retain no more than shall be necessary for them." It was strictly forbidden either to offer or to demand wages above the old rate. Another clause forbids the giving of alms to beggars. Handicraftsmen of various kinds are also ordered to be paid at the old rate. Lastly, victuallers and other traders are directed to sell

---

[1] Jessopp (*l.c.*) giving a general reference to the *Foedera*, and probably having the Sandwich letter in view, says there was "mad, unreasoning, insensate panic among well-to-do classes—the trader and the moneyed man, the *bourgeoisie* of the towns," and "a stampede," (presumably to foreign parts). But the mortality was all over by 1st December, 1349 ; and the exodus, whatever motive it may have had, was almost certainly deliberate.

[2] *Foedera*, III. 198.

their wares at reasonable prices[1]. The same ordinance, with
some added paragraphs, was reissued on the 18th November,
1350, to the county of Suffolk and to the district of Lindsey
(Lincolnshire), the latter being one of the chief sheep-grazing
parts of England ; in those two localities, it is stated in so many
words, the labourers had set at nought the ordinance of 18th
June[2]. When Parliament met—for the first time since the
mortality—on the 9th of February, 1351, it was acknowledged
that the commissions to sheriffs issued by the king and his
council had been ineffective, and that wages had been at twice
or thrice the old rate[3]. The Parliament, having legislated for a
number of technical matters in connexion with the enormous
number of wills and successions, proceeded next to the labour
question, and passed the famous Statute of Labourers, by which
the generalities of the ordinance of 18th June, 1350, are replaced
by an elaborate schedule of wages for harvest-time and other
times[4]. One clause of the Act is specially directed against the
migration of labourers to other counties. It was the ancient
manorial system that was threatened most of all by the depopulation. The surviving labourers sought work where they
could command the best wages, and at the same time could
escape from the few degrading bonds of servitude which still

---

[1] The last clause of the ordinance implies that not only the labourers but also the
employers of labour were taking the natural advantage of the situation. There appears
to be some particular evidence of this for Bristol (Rev. W. Hunt, *Bristol*, p. 77):
the masters in various crafts and trades were so reduced in numbers that the survivors
could charge what they pleased. Thus, the attempt to coerce labourers and skilled
workmen was a one-sided affair; although, in practice, it related mostly to farm-
labour, where the one-sidedness did not appear.

[2] *Foedera*, III. 210.   [3] *Rot. Parl.* II. 225.

[4] This was the first parliamentary Statute of Labourers (25 Ed. III. cap 2). The
king's ordinance of 18th June, 1350 (re-issued for Suffolk and Lindsey on 18th Nov.),
is usually reckoned the first Statute of Labourers, and is invariably assigned to the
23rd year of Edward III., being so entered in the *Statutes of the Realm*. It is clear,
however, from the text of the ordinance in the *Foedera* that it belongs to the 24th of
Edward III., its exact date being 18th June, 1350. Longman, in his *History of the
Life and Times of Edward III.*, correctly states in one place (I. 309) that the ordinance
of 18th June, 1350, was "the first step," but on the very next page, after stating that
the ordinance failed, he proceeds, according to the usual chronology of 23 Ed. III. and
25 Ed. III., to say that "therefore, two years afterwards," the statute of 25 Ed. III.
was made in Parliament. The interval was only some eight months.

clung to the *nativi* or serfs of a manor. But the Manor Court was still the unit of government, and the Act would have been inoperative except on that basis. That fundamental intention of the statute of the 9th February, 1351, comes out, not only in the explicit clause against migrations, but also by contrast, in the special permission given to the labourers of the counties of Stafford, Derby and Lancaster, to the people of Craven, and to the dwellers in the Marches of Wales and Scotland, to go about in search of work in harvest "as they were wont to do before this time[1]."

The immediate effect of the depopulation had been to mobilise, as it were, the labouring class. Many of them must have taken the road at once; for, in the first ordinance of 18th June, 1350, before the harvest of that year had begun, it is stated that certain of the labourers preferred to live by begging instead of by labour, and it is therefore forbidden to give alms to beggars. According to Knighton, the effect of the ordinance itself was to swell the ranks of the wandering poor; when some were arrested, imprisoned, or fined in terms of the commission to the sheriffs, others fled to the woods and wastes (*ad silvas et boscos*)[2]. These escapes continued for years after; the rolls of the Manor Court of Winslow have entries of many such cases long after the pestilence[3]. Many of these fugitive villeins formed the class of "wasters," often referred to in the *Vision of Piers the Ploughman*: "waster would not work, but wander about," or he would work only in harvest, squander his earnings, and for the rest of the year feel the pinch of hunger "until both his eyen watered." But it is clear that others went to distant manors, and settled down again to steady employment, freed from their bonds as *nativi*; and it cannot be doubted that some went to the towns[4].

---

[1] *Rot. Parl.* II. 234.

[2] Knighton, in Twysden's *Decem Scriptores*, *l.c.*

[3] Seebohm, *The English Village Community.* Chapter I.

[4] The Statute of Labourers was re-enacted with increased stringency six years after (31 Ed. III.), and again in 1360 and 1368. All the labour statutes were confirmed in the 12th year of Richard II. (cap. 34). Legislative attempts of the same kind continued to be made as late as the 5th of Elizabeth (1562–3), with particular reference to sturdy beggars. See copious extracts from the Statutes in Sir George

In order to realize the causes and circumstances of the labour difficulty after the enormous thinning of the population, it may be well to recall the composition of the village communities. In each manor the arable land was in two portions—on the one hand the immense open fields (two or perhaps three) in which the villagers had each so many half-acre strips, and on the other hand the lord's demesne, or home-farm. Part of the latter would often be let to free tenants, or even to villeins, who would count for the occasion as free tenants. For the cultivation of his demesne the lord was dependent on his tenants in villenage, who owed him, in form, so many days' work in the year, but in reality were often able to commute their personal services for a money payment and are said to have done so very generally[1]. Thus the lord of the manor was no longer able to call upon his serfs to plough or to sow or to reap; he had to hire them for his occasions. The free tenants would also be dependent to some extent upon hired labour; and as some even of the villeins cultivated up to forty acres or more, in the open fields of the manor, these would also have to hire unless their families were old enough to help. All that labour for hire would naturally be supplied by the poorer villagers, the cottars and bordars, who would seldom cultivate more than a few half-acres, and in some cases perhaps none[2]. The lower order of tenants in villenage formed accordingly the class of labourers; and it was their demands which gave occasion for the ordinances of 1350 and the statute of 1351. In each manor the lord would have been affected more than all the rest by the scarcity of labour, in respect of the extensive demesne or home-farm managed by his bailiff. It is conjectured that he tried, in some cases, to go back to his rights of customary service from his

Nicholls's *History of the English Poor Law*, vol. i. Lond. 1854. "An Act for regulating Journeymen Tailors" was made in 7 Geo. I. (cap. 13).

[1] "There is no trace of the villenage described in Glanville and Bracton, among the tenants of a manor 500 years ago. All customary services were commutable for money payments; all villein tenants were secure in the possession of their lands; and the only distinction between socage and villein occupation lay in the liberation of the former from certain degrading incidents which affected the latter." Thorold Rogers, "Effects of the Black Death, &c." *Fort. Rev.* III. (1865) p. 196.

[2] Seebohm, *The English Village Community.* Lond. 1882. Chapter I.

villeins, which had gradually become commutable for rents paid in money, and that the attempts to do so led to insubordination[1]. He had to pay wages, notwithstanding all his rights of lordship. The wages paid in the harvest of 1349 were, says Rogers, those of panic. In the form of petition which brought the labour-question before Parliament in February 1351, it is stated that the wages demanded were at double or treble the old rate ; of the year preceding (1350) it is recorded that the wages paid to labourers for gathering the harvest on the manor of Ham, belonging to the lord Berkeley, amounted to 1144 days' work, on the old scale of commutation[2].

The labourers, although the lowest order on the manors, were accordingly masters of the situation. Personal service to the lord, measurable merely by days, and having no reference to fluctuations in the rate of wages, had become obsolete ; nor do the ordinance of 1350 and the statute of 1351 give any hint of trying to revive it. If the men refused to be hired at the old rate, they were to be arrested and imprisoned.

There were, of course, many things besides the statute, tending to keep the majority of peasants on the manors where they had been born ; so that the formal abolition of villenage remained to be carried by rebellion in 1381, while many traces of it in practice remained for long after. Those who stayed on their old manors, or removed to another county or hundred to become tenants under new lords, were able to get permanently better wages ; the price of labour remained about forty per cent. higher than it had been before the mortality; so that the statute was on the whole ineffective. But another large proportion of the labouring class appears to have been driven to a wandering life. It is not easy to explain on economical principles why the class of "wasters," of whom we hear so much, should have been called into existence. Hands were scarce, and wages were high;

---

[1] Seebohm, p. 31. Such attempts by landowners, to go back to personal service from their villein tenants, appear to have become more systematic in the generation following, and to have been a cause of the Peasants' Rebellion in 1381. See v. Oschenkowski, *England's wirthschaftliche Entwickelung*, Jena, 1879, confirming the opinion of Thorold Rogers.

[2] Smith, *Lives of the Berkeleys*, p. 128: "in 24 Edward III." (Cited by Denton, *England in the 15th Century.*)

the conditions look on the surface to be entirely adverse to the creation of a class of sturdy beggars and idle tramps. But the economic conditions were really complex; and when all has been said on the head of economics, there will remain something to be explained on the side of ethics.

Not only the labourers but also the employers of labour were cut off in the mortality. A great part of the capital of the country passed suddenly into new hands. Before the Parliament of 1351 legislated upon wages, it was occupied with a number of technical difficulties about wills. Of the proving of wills and the granting of letters of administration on a great scale we have had an instance from an archdeaconry in Lancashire. In Colchester, a town with some four hundred burgesses, one hundred and eleven wills were proved[1]. In the Husting Court of London, three hundred and sixty wills were enrolled and proved from 13th January, 1349, to 13th January, 1350. An immense number of persons came into money who could not all have had the inclination, even if they had the skill and aptitude, for employing it as capital. If there were wasters among the labourers, there were wasters also among the moneyed class. The mortality produced, indeed, that demoralisation of the whole national life which has been usually observed to follow in the like circumstances. " Almost all great epochs of moral degradation are connected with great epidemics," says Niebuhr, generalizing the evidence which Thucydides gives specially for the plague of Athens[2]. The fourteenth century was by no means a period of high morality before the Black Death; but it was undoubtedly worse after it. Langland's poem of the vision of Piers the Ploughman is one long diatribe against the vices of the age, and some of the worst of them he expressly dates " sith the pestilence time." It will be convenient to take these ethical illustrations, before we proceed with the effects of the mortality upon material prosperity and population, and with the domestication of plague on the soil.

So far from the labouring class being the chief sinners, it is in the humbler ranks that the root of goodness remains. Langland's hero, the Ploughman, is obviously chosen to represent

---

[1] Morant, *Hist. of Essex.*

[2] Niebuhr, *Lectures on Ancient History.* Engl. transl. London, 1852, II., p. 53.

"that ingenuous simplicity and native candour and integrity," which, as Burke says, "formerly characterized the English nation," and, one may add, have been at all times its saving grace. It was in that class that the reforming movement, led by Wyclif twenty years after, had its strength. Lollardy and the Peasants' Rebellion were closely allied. The grievance of the latter was that the gulf between the gentleman and the workman had become wider than in nature it should be. An ultimate and very indirect effect of the great mortality was to strengthen the middle class by recruits from beneath; it created the circumstances which produced the English yeoman of the fifteenth century. But we are here engaged with the immediate effect; and that was to broaden the contrast between the rich and the poor.

Luxury had already touched so high a point as to call for a statute against extravagant living, the curious sumptuary law of 1336 which prohibited many courses at table. Nothing could be more significant of its later developments in London than the sarcastic description, which fills an unusual space in one of the chroniclers, of the fantastic excesses of dress and ornament among the male sex about the year 1362[1]. Some of the names of the men's ornaments occur also in Langland's verses:

> "Sir John and Sir Goffray hath a gerdel of silver,
> A basellarde or a ballok-knyf with botones overgilt."

These effeminate fashions actually led to a Statute of Dress in 1363, in which also the lower class are forbidden to ape their betters. It is perhaps to these hangers-on of wealth that Langland refers in his bitter lines:

> "Right so! ye rich, ye robeth that be rich | and helpeth them that helpeth you, and giveth where no need is. | As who so filled a tun of a fresh river | and went forth with that water to woke with Thames. | Right so! ye rich, ye robe and feed | them that have as ye have, them ye make at ease."

But, as for the poor, Avarice considers them fair game:

> "I have as moche pite of pore men as pedlere hath of cattes, | that wolde kill them if he cacche hem myghte, for covetise of their skynnes."

---

[1] *Eulogium Historiarum.* Rolls ed. III. 230.

In London the preaching clergy are accused of pandering to the avarice of the rich:

"And were mercy in mean men no more than in rich | mendicants meatless might go to bed. | God is much in the gorge of these great masters, | but among mean men his mercy and his works. | Friars and faitours have found such questions, | to plese with proud men sithen the pestilence tyme, | and prechers at Saint Poules, for pure envye of clerkis, | that folke is nought firmed in the feith ne fill of their goodes. | ...Ne be plentyous to the pore as pure charitye wolde, | but in gayness and in glotonye forglotten her goode hem selve, | and breken noughte to the beggar as the Boke techeth."

The friars had lost altogether the enthusiasm of their early days:

"And how that friars followed folk that was rich, | and folk that was poor at little price they set; | and no corpse in their kirk-yard nor in their kirk was buried, | but quick he bequeath them aughte or should help quit their debts."

As for the monks, the same might have been said of them before; but now more land had been thrown into their possession by the mortality:

"Ac now is Religion a ryder, a rowmer bi streetes,
A leader of love-days, and a lond-buyer,
A pricker on a palfrey fro manere to manere,
An heap of houndes at his ers, as he a lord were.
And but if his knave kneel, that shall his cup bringe,
He lowreth on hym, and axeth hym who taught hym curtesye."

According to Langland's poem, the country clergy left their livings and came up to London:—

"Parsons and parish priests plained them to the bishop | that their parishes were poor sith the pestilence time; | to have licence and leave at London to dwell | and syngen there for simony, for silver is sweet. | Bishops and bachelors, both masters and doctours, | that have cures under Christ and crowning in token and sign, | that they should shrive their parishours, preach and pray for them and the poor feed, | live in London in Lent and all"—

some of them serving the king in the offices of Exchequer and Chancery, and some acting as the stewards of lords.

It is undoubted that the business of the courts in London received a great impetus after the mortality, as one can readily understand from the number of inheritances, successions, and feudal claims that had to be settled. Several of the Inns of Chancery date from about that time. Gascoigne, who was "cancellarius" at Oxford about 1430, and had access to the rolls of former "cancellarii," was struck by the increase of legists after the commotion of 1349: "Before the great pestilence there were few disputes among the people, and few pleas; and, accordingly, there were few legists in the realm of England, and few legists in Oxford, at a time when there were thirty thousand scholars in Oxford, as I have seen in the rolls," etc.[1]

The country clergy, such of them as remained in their cures were a notoriously illiterate class; according to Knighton, they could read the Latin services without understanding what they read. Langland makes a parson confess his poor qualifications to be the spiritual guide of his flock; on the other hand he was not without skill in the sports of the field: "But I can fynde in a felde or in a furlonge an hare." At one of the manor courts in Wiltshire in 1361, a gang of the district clergy were convicted of night poaching[2].

Such being the state of matters among the upper and middle classes, it is not surprising to find a lax morality among the lower orders. The ploughman is as severe a satirist of his own class as he is of the rich. In London we have a picture of the interior of a tavern crowded with loafers of all sorts "early in the morning." In the country also the contrast is drawn between the industrious and the idle class:

"And whoso helpeth me to erie [plough] or sowen here ere I wende | shall have leve, bi oure Lorde to lese here in harvest, | and make him merry there-mydde, maugre whoso begruccheth it: | save Jakke the jogeloure and Jonet of the stewes, | and Danget the dys-playere, and Denot the bawd, | and Frere the faytoure and folk of his order, | and Robyn the rybaudoure for his rusty wordes."

To live out of wedlock was nothing unusual:

"Many of you ne wedde nought the wimmen that ye with delen, | but as

---

[1] *Loci e Libro Veritatum*, ed. Rogers. Oxon. 1880, p. 202; and, from Gascoigne's MS., in Anthony Wood, *Hist. and Antiq. Univ. Oxford*, Ed. Gutch, I. 451: "What I shall farther observe is that before it began there were but few complaints among the people, and few pleas; as also few Legists in England, and very few at Oxford."

[2] *Manor and Barony of Castle Combe*, sub anno 1361.

wilde bestis with wehe worthen up and worchen, | and bryngeth forth barnes that bastardes men calleth."

Ill-assorted marriages also appear to have been common :

" It is an oncomely couple, bi Cryst, as me-thinketh, | to gyven a yonge wenche to an olde feble, | or wedden any widwe for welth of hir goodis, | that never shall bairne bere but if it be in armes. | Many a paire sithen the pestilence have plight hem togiders : | the fruit that thei brynge forth aren foule wordes : | in jalousye joyeles and jangling in bedde | have thei no children but cheste and choppyng hem betweene."

Chapmen did not chastise their children. Old traditions of weather-lore, and of reckoning the yield of harvest, were forgotten.

As a set-off to the uniformly bad picture of the times given by Langland, we may turn to the gay and good-humoured scenes of the 'Canterbury Tales.' But Chaucer was emphatically the poet of the cultured class, and it is proper to his muse to keep within the limits of a well-bred cynicism. Again, Langland's strictures on the avarice and other vices of the rich may seem to be a mere echo of a very old cry, which finds equally strong expression in Roger of Wendover, about the year 1235, and in Robert of Brunne's 'Handlyng Synne' in the year 1303. But the Vision of the Ploughman is too consistent, and too concrete, to be considered as a mere homily on the wickedness of the times, such as might have been written of almost any age or of any country in which the Seven Mortal Sins were still called by their plain names. The words "sithen the pestilence" recur so often, that this contemporary author must be held as sharing the belief that the Black Death made a marked difference to the morals of the nation throughout all classes.

More lasting effects on Farming, Industries, and Population.

Turning from things moral to things material, we shall find that the Great Mortality left its mark on the cultivated area of the country, on rents of land, on the kind of tenure and the system of farming, on industry, trade and municipal government, on the population, and, on what chiefly concerns us, the subsequent health of the country.

Corn-growing would appear to have met with at least a temporary check. Three water-mills near Shrewsbury fell in annual value by one half, owing to the scarcity of corn to grind[1]. Richmond, one of the chief corn-markets in Yorkshire, is said, on rather uncertain evidence, to have been permanently reduced for the same reason; besides losing an enormous number by the plague itself (vaguely stated at 2000), the town lost its corn-trade through the land around falling out of cultivation, so that some of the burgesses, being unable to pay rent, had to wander abroad as mendicants[2].

The general statements of Knighton, Le Baker and others for England (not to mention numerous rhetorical passages of foreign writers), to the effect that whole villages were left desolate, are borne out by the petitions recurring in the Rolls of Parliament for many years after. There are also some references to the continuing desolateness of particular places, which are probably fair samples of a larger number.

Thus a rich clergyman in Hertfordshire had given, just before the Black Death, all his lands and tenements in Brag-hinge, Herts, to the prior and convent of Anglesey, Cambridge-shire, in consideration that they should find at their proper expense a chantry of two priests for ever in the church of Anglesey, to say masses for the souls of the benefactor and his family. But on the 10th of May, 1351, he remitted the charge and support of one of the two said priests, on the ground that, "on account of the vast mortality, lands lie uncultivated in many and innumerable places, not a few tenements daily and suddenly decay and are pulled down, rents and services cannot be levied, but a much smaller profit is obliged to be taken than usual[3]." An instance of a long-abiding effect is that of the manor of Hockham belonging to the earl of Arundel, which was not tenanted for thirty years[4].

[1] Owen and Blakeway, *op. cit.* I. 165.

[2] Clarkson's *History of Richmond.* Richmond, 1821 (authority not quoted).

[3] Hailstone, *History of Bottisham and the Priory of Anglesey.* Camb. 1873. (Transact. Camb. Antiq. Soc. 8vo. series, vol. XIV.)

[4] Cited by Jessopp, *l.c.*

The history of rents is peculiar. The immediate effect, as we learn from Knighton, as well as from the rolls of particular manor courts, was a remission of them by the lords, lest their tenants in villenage should quit the lands. There was, indeed, a competition among landlords for tenants to occupy their manors, so that the cultivators could make their own terms. Of that we have had an instance from the manor of Ensham, belonging to Christ Church, Oxford[1]. But, after a few years, rents appear to have come back to near their old level. The following figures have been compiled from the Tower records of assizes made for the purpose of taxation[2]:

1268	9d.	1271	12d.	1336	11½d.	1338	11½d.
1348–9	—	1359	9¼d.	1368	10½d.	1381	9¾d.
1417	6d.	1422	4d.	1429	4d.	1432	6d.
1446	8d.						

The great fall, it will be seen, was in the next century.

Perhaps the most striking effect upon agriculture of the upheaval produced by the great mortality was, as Thorold Rogers has shown, in changing the system of farming and in creating the type of the English yeoman. The system of farming the lord's demesne or home-farm by a bailiff, never very profitable, became, says that historian, quite unproductive, owing especially to the permanent rise in wages. The small men who took the lord's land to farm—they had been doing so to some extent before[3]—had not sufficient of their own for stock and seed; but they got advances from the lord, which were repaid in due course. It was a kind of *métairie* farming. It prevailed for about fifty years, by which time the ordinary system of farming on lease was becoming general. Finally, and especially in the Civil Wars of the fifteenth century, much of the land which had belonged in fee to the feudal lords, passed away by purchase to the tenant farmers[4]. Thus arose the

---

[1] See p. 141.   [2] Clutterbuck, *History of Hertfordshire.*

[3] Seebohm, for the Manor of Winslow, *op. cit.*, p. 34.

[4] Thorold Rogers, *Fort. Rev.* III. (1865), p. 196. In his *History of Agriculture and Prices*, IV., the same learned and sagacious student of English developments thus sums up the agrarian consequences of the Black Death:—"The indirect effects of this great event were even more remarkable. The great landowner ceases to carry on

famous breed of English yeomen—the "good yeomen whose limbs were made in England."

The effect of the mortality upon trade and industry was, momentarily, to paralyse them. Of the great wool-trade, Rogers, the historian of English prices, says : " Nothing, I think, in the whole history of these prices is more significant of the terror and prostration induced by the plague than the sudden fall in the price of wool at this time. It is a long time before a recovery takes place[1]." But from 1364 to 1380, the price of wool was uniformly above the average ; and, if there be any accuracy in Avesbury's figures already given for the years following 1355, the export of bales of wool to the Continent (100,000 sacks in a year, he says, each sack being a bale of the present colonial size, or weighing about three hundredweights) meant a very considerable amount of labour, tonnage and exchange. Among other articles of export, we hear specially of iron, in a petition to Parliament of 28 Ed. III. (1354); the price of iron had risen to four times what it was before the plague, and it was desired to stop the export of it and to fix the price[2].

The effect of the mortality upon the industries of the country was shown most in Norwich. That city was the centre of the Flemish cloth-weaving, which had been flourishing in Norfolk for some twenty years, under the direct encouragement of Edward III., and of a protective statute against foreign-made cloth. Before the pestilence, Norwich was the second city in the kingdom. In the king's warrant for men-at-arms, which was indeed issued in 1350, but may be taken as drawn up on the old lines and irrespective of the pestilence, the quota of

---

agriculture with his own capital, and farmers' rents of a fixed and almost invariable amount take the place of the lord's cultivation by bailiffs. Attempts were made for varying periods of time to continue the old system, especially by corporations. It is possible that the system of stock and land leasing, which became very general after the change commenced, may have been suggested by the hope that the old state of things might be restored....In the end all the great landowners conformed to the inevitable change, and let their land on short leases, and as a rule at low and almost fixed rents, to capitalist farmers."

[1] Thorold Rogers, *op. cit.*, I. 376.
[2] *Rot. Parl.*, II. 260. a.

Norwich is rated at 60, London's being 100, Bristol's and Lynn's 20 each, that of Coventry, Gloucester, Hereford, Shrewsbury, Winchester, Sarum, Oxford, Canterbury and Bury St Edmund's 10 each, and of other towns from 8 to 1 each, York not being mentioned. But in the Subsidy Roll of 1377, which shows how many persons, above the age of fourteen, paid the poll-tax of a groat in each county and in each principal town, Norwich comes sixth in the list instead of second, being far surpassed in numbers by York and Bristol, and surpassed considerably by Coventry and Plymouth. So far from being in a proportion to London of 60 to 100, it is now in a proportion of 3952 to 23,314, its whole population, as estimated, being 7410 against 44,770 in the capital which at one time it bade fair to rival. It had lost heavily in the Black Death, and so had the populous district around it, where the Flemish industries and trade were planted in numerous villages. By 1368, ten of the sixty very small parishes of Norwich had disappeared, and fourteen more disappeared by degrees, the ruins of twenty of them being still visible[1].

There is no mistaking the significance of these figures and facts for the second city of the kingdom. At least one generation passed before Norwich recovered something of its old prosperity. In the fifteenth century it was still the chief seat of the woollen manufactures; the county of Norfolk kept its old pre-eminence, although rival centres of industry had grown up. There were, however, causes at work which at length reduced the capital of East Anglia to a comparatively poor state. One of the intermediate glimpses that we get of it—they are not many, even in Blomefield's history—is the statute of 1455, to put down the enormous number of "pettifogging attorneys" in the city and county[2]. Its real decline was in the early Tudor reigns. When Henry VII. visited Norwich in 1497, the mayor in presenting the Queen's usual gold cup with a hundred pieces in it, took occasion to tell the monarch "howbeit that they are more poor, and not of such wealth as they have been afore

[1] Seebohm, *l. c. Fort. Rev.*, II. (1865), p. 157.
[2] Blomefield, III. *sub anno.*

these days[1]." When the town suffered much from fires about the year 1505, the city of London raised large sums in aid of its rebuilding. To the same period belongs a municipal order that no one should dig holes in the market-place to get sand, without the mayor's licence. In 1525, there was a general decay of work, the clothiers and farmers being unable to employ the artisans and labourers, who began to rise in revolt against the heavy taxes. An Act of 33 Hen. VIII. recites that the making and weaving of worsteds is wholly decayed and taken away from the city of Norwich and county of Norfolk—by the deceit and crafty practices of the great multitude of regrators and buyers of the said yarn. These evidences of decline in prosperity are in part long after the Black Death; but they seem to have been continuous from that event.

So far as concerns the other large towns of England, they did not all fare alike. The capital was more luxurious, and probably not less populous, after the mortality than before it. The chancery and exchequer business alone would have served to draw numbers to it; and we may be sure, from all subsequent experience, that the gaps left by the plague were filled up by influx from the provinces and from abroad in the course of two or three years. Nor does it appear from the poll-tax that York had suffered to anything like the same extent as Norwich; while Bristol and Coventry became towns of much greater consequence than before the plague. On the other hand, Lincoln is described, in a petition for relief in 1399 (1 Hen. IV.) as being "in the greater part empty and uninhabited." In the same year, Yarmouth has its houses "vacant and void," although, in 1369, it is said to have "gained so much upon Norwich" that it was made a seat of the wool-staple. Other towns which figure in petitions to Parliament as "impoverished and desolate of people," are Ilchester (1407) and Truro (1410). Camden instances the ancient borough of Wallingford, on the Thames, as having been permanently reduced by the Black Death, although the inhabitants, he says, traced the decay of the town to the diversion of traffic over the new bridges at Abingdon and Dorchester[2].

---

[1] Blomefield, III. *sub anno.*
[2] Camden's *Britannia.* Gough's ed. II. 9.

Some parts of Cambridge would appear to have borne the traces of the pestilence for a number of years after. A charter of the bishop of Ely, dated 12 September, 1365, mentions that the parishioners of All Saints (on the north-east side) are for the most part dead by pestilence, and those that are alive are gone to the parishes of other churches; that the parishioners of St Giles's (the adjoining parish, near the Castle) have died; and that the nave of All Saints is ruinous and the bones of dead bodies are exposed to beasts; therefore the bishop unites All Saints and St Giles's[1]. At that time the churches of those parishes would have been small, perhaps not much larger than the little church of St Peter still standing on the high ground opposite to the great modern church of St Giles.

These instances of the chequered history of English towns subsequent to the great mortality are not altogether favourable to the generality which has been put forward by an able historian[2], that the great social revolution produced by that event was to detach the people from the soil, to drive them into the towns, to increase the urban population disproportionately to the rural, to plant the germs of commerce and industry, and to determine that expansion of England which became manifest in the end of the Elizabethan period and under the Stuarts, the British nation being "doomed by its economic conditions to take the course which it has taken." Many things happened between the Black Death and the expansion of England. The fifteenth century intervened, which was in its middle period, at least, distinguished as much by the rise of the yeoman class as by the growth of trade guilds in the town. But that which mars the generality most of all was the decline of industries and the decay of towns (London and Bristol always excepted) in the reigns of Henry VII. and Henry VIII.; the country had to recover from that before the Elizabethan expansion,—before the nation began "to increase rapidly in population until at length it should overflow the limits of its island home."

---

[1] *Hist. MSS. Commission*, VI. 299. Register of Ely Priory, in Lord Leconfield's MSS.

[2] Seebohm, "The Black Death and its Place in English History." *Fort. Rev.* II. (1865), p. 278.

At the same time, one effect of the great mortality was to mobilise the class of agricultural labourers, and to drive a certain number of them into the towns. Proof of that migration comes from the statutes and the Rolls of Parliament.

An Act of 34 Edward III. (1360) imposes a fine of ten pounds to the king on the mayor and bailiffs of any town refusing "to deliver up a labourer, servant, or artificer" who had absented himself from his master's service, with a farther fine of five pounds to the lord. In 1376 the "Good Parliament" makes complaint that servants and labourers quitted service on the slightest cause, and then led an idle life in towns, or wandered in parties about the country, "many becoming beggars, others staff-strikers, but the greater number taking to robbing." More direct evidence of industries diverting hands from farm labour is found in the various statutes about apprentices. In the Act of 12 Ric. II. (1388) it is provided that "he or she which use to labour at the plough and cart or other labour or service of husbandry till they be of the age of twelve years, shall abide at that labour without being put to any mystery or handicraft; and if any covenant or bond of apprentice be from henceforth made to the contrary, the same shall be holden for none." A more definite provision of the same kind was made in 7 Hen. IV. (1405–6): "Notwithstanding the good statutes aforemade, infants whose fathers and mothers have no land, nor rent, nor other living, but only their service or mystery, be put to serve and bound apprentices to divers crafts within cities and boroughs, sometimes at the age of twelve years, sometimes within the said age, and that for the pride of clothing and other evil customs which servants do use in the same" etc.—the result being that farm labourers were scarce ; therefore no one, not having land or rent of twenty-shillings a year, to bind his son or daughter of whatsoever age to serve as apprentice within any city or borough. In the 8th of Henry VI. (1429) this statute was repealed so far as respected London, on account of the hindrance which the said statute might occasion to the inhabitants of that city[1].

It may be doubted if, after the Black Death, the towns underwent any marked industrial development, except in such cases as Coventry and Bristol. On the other hand, the cloth-weaving of East Anglia was dispersed over the country, more particularly to the western and south-western counties, so that the west of England gained an industrial character which it retained until the comparatively modern rise of the cloth-industries of Yorkshire and Lancashire. But it was in great part

[1] These and other labour-statutes are collected in *A History of the English Poor Law*, by Sir George Nicholls, 2 vols. London, 1854, I. 37–77.

a development of village industries upon the old manorial basis, as well as a migration of labour to the towns.

We have an authentic instance, and probably a typical instance, in the manor and barony of Castle Combe, of which the social history has been pieced together from the rolls of its manor court by one of the earliest students of that class of documents. Before the middle of the fifteenth century this village situated among the Wiltshire hills, difficult of access and almost secluded from the highways, had grown into a thriving community of weavers, fullers, dyers, glovers, and the like, with their attendant tradings and marketings, all upon its old manorial basis, and with its old agriculture going hand in hand with its new industries. There were free or copyhold tenants occupying their farms, while several clothiers and occupiers of fulling-mills held farms also, " driving a double and evidently a very thriving trade, accumulating considerable wealth and giving employment to a large number of artizans who had been attracted to the place for this purpose. Yet, strange to say, some of the wealthiest and most prosperous of these tradesmen were still subject to the odious bonds of serfship, adscript the soil[1]." It is clear, however, that the jury of the manor court took care that the lord should not have the best of it. The morals of this industrial village were, as might have been expected, somewhat lax[2]. At the same time the removal of nuisances was insisted upon by this self-governing community as effectively, perhaps, as if it had been under the Local Government Acts[3].

Another kind of effect than the industrial, upon the state of

---

[1] G. Poulett Scrope, *op. cit.*

[2] From 1416 to 1424, three different persons were fined at the manor court for keeping a common brothel in their houses. Forestalling of butter, cheese and eggs, on the way to market, came before the court in 1418.

[3] At the manor court in 1417, Thomas Selwin, a butcher, was convicted of throwing offal and other offensive matters into the common street and of making his dung-heap there, to the common hurt; also the said Thomas Selwin " tarde et de novo erexit unam latrinam foetidam in shopa sua ad commune nocumentum. Ideo ipse in misericordia." The next entry of nuisances, so far as extracts are given, is as late as 1590—various offences in the street and churchyard, and the glover washing his skins in the stream or otherwise befouling the water running by his house.

the towns, is exemplified in the case of Shrewsbury. The dislocation of the old social order had somehow touched the privileges and monopolies of municipal corporations and guilds, and given power to a hitherto unenfranchised class. The general question, besides being a somewhat new one, is foreign to this subject; but the reference to Shrewsbury is given, as the "late pestilence" is expressly connected with the municipal changes. A patent of the 35th of Edward III. (1361), relating to the town of Shrewsbury, recites the grievous debates and dissensions which had arisen therein, "through the strangers who had newly come to reside in the said town after the late pestilence, and were plotting to draw to themselves the government of the said town[1]."

It has been conjectured that population in the country at large speedily righted itself, according to the principle that population always tends to come close to the limit of subsistence. But there is reason to think that the means of subsistence were themselves reduced. We read of corn-land running to waste, although most of the references to desolation are perhaps to be taken as true for only one or two harvests following the plague. Again, it is undoubted that sheep-farming and the pasturing of cattle at length took the place of much of the old agriculture. It is not easy to make out when the change begins; but there are instances of rural depopulation as early as 1414[2], and the same had become a burning grievance in the time of cardinal Morton and the early years of sir Thomas More. It has been assumed, also, that the "positive checks" to population

---

[1] Cited in Owen and Blakeway's *History of Shrewsbury*, II. 524: "per advenas qui in dicta villa post ultimam pestilenciam de novo sunt inhabitati...at regimen dictae ville ad se attrahere...machinantes." By the "ultima pestilencia" could hardly have been meant the pestis secunda of 1361, the year of the patent, as the learned antiquaries suppose.

[2] *Rotul. Parl.* IV. 60. 7. The petition of Chesterton, near Cambridge: "And also they seiden that there was made gret waste in the same Manor of Chesterton of Housing, that is to say of Halles and of Chambers, and of other houses of office, that were necessary in the same Manor, and none housinge left standing therein, but gif it were a Shepcote or a Berne or a Swynsty and a few houses byside to putte in bestes."

had been taken off, when they ought in theory so to have been : that is to say, after the inhabitants had been enormously thinned. The statement of Hecker, that there was increased fecundity after the pestilence, appears to be an instance of that author's *a priori* habit of mind[1]. What we read in an English chronicle of the time is just the opposite, namely, that "the women who survived remained for the most part barren during several years[2]." The authority is not conclusive, but the statement is in keeping with what we may gather from Langland's poem as to ill-assorted and sterile marriages, and as to illicit unions, which, as Malthus teaches, are comparatively unfruitful. The alleged sterility is also in keeping with, although not strictly parallel to, the experience of crowded Indian provinces, such as Orissa, where a thinning of the population by famine and disease has been statistically proved to be followed by a marked decrease of fecundity. More direct evidence of a permanent loss of people occurs a generation after the Black Death, at a time when the circumstances of health were such as would explain it.

The poll-tax of 1377 was a means of estimating the population. The tax was levied on every person, male or female, above the age of fourteen. In estimating the population from the poll-tax returns, it is usual to add one-fifth for taxable subjects who had evaded it, and to reckon the taxable subjects above fourteen years as two-thirds of the whole population. On that basis of reckoning, the population of the whole of England, except Cheshire and Durham, in the year 1377 would have been 2,580,828 (or 1,376,442 who actually paid their groat each). The population of the principal towns is calculated, in the second column of the Table, from the numbers in the first column who actually paid the poll-tax, according to the Subsidy Roll of 51 Edward III.

[1] "After the cessation of the Black Plague a greater fecundity in women was everywhere remarkable—a grand phenomenon which, from its occurrence after every destructive pestilence, proves to conviction, if any occurrence can do so, the prevalence of a higher power in the direction of general organic life. Marriages were almost without exception prolific," etc.

[2] *Eulogium Historiarum,* III. 213.

Laity assessed for the Poll-tax of 1377 in each of the following Towns, being persons of either sex above the age of fourteen years.

	Taxed	Estimated Population		Taxed	Estimated Population
London	23,314	44,770	Ely	1722	3230
York	7248	13,590	Exeter	1560	2925
Bristol	6345	11,904	Hull	1557	2920
Plymouth	4837	9069	Worcester	1557	2920
Coventry	4817	9032	Ipswich	1507	2825
Norwich	3952	7410	Nottingham	1447	2713
Lincoln	3412	6399	Northampton	1447	2713
Sarum	3226	6048	Winchester	1440	2700
Lynn	3127	5863	Stamford	1218	2284
Colchester	2955	5540	Newark	1178	2209
Beverley	2663	4993	Wells	1172	2198
Newcastle-on-Tyne	2647	4963	Ludlow	1172	2198
Canterbury	2574	4826	Southampton	1152	2160
Bury St Edmunds	2442	4580	Derby	1046	1961
Oxford	2357	4420	Lichfield	1024	1920
Gloucester	2239	4198	Chichester	869	1630
Leicester	2101	3939	Boston	814	1526
Shrewsbury	2082	3904	Carlisle	678	1271
Yarmouth	1941	3640	Bath	570	1070
Hereford	1903	3568	Rochester	570	1070
Cambridge	1722	3230	Dartmouth	506	949

That this indirect census was taken on a declining population may be inferred from the language of contemporaries. In the year of the poll-tax (1377), Richard II. addressed certain questions to Wyclif concerning the papal exactions of tribute; the reformer's reply gives as the second objection to the tribute "that the people decreases by reason of (*praetextu*) the withdrawal of this treasure, which should be spent in England[1]."

In the political poems of the time there are numerous references to the pestilences and famines. One of these doggerel productions, "On the Council of London," 1382, contains a clear reference to a decrease of the people:

> "In nos pestilentia saeva jam crescit,
> Quod virorum fortium jam populus decrescit."

[1] *Fasciculi Zizan.* Rolls series, No. 5, ed. Shirley, p. 263: "Dimitto alias rationes palpabiles: quod exhinc regnum nostrum sensibiliter depauperetur pecunia; quod, praetextu subtractionis hujus thesauri, qui expenderetur in Anglia, decrescit populus;" etc.

[2] *Political Songs and Poems, Ed. II.—Ric. II.* Rolls series, No. 14, ed. T. Wright, I. 2. 53.

These general expressions in writings of the time will appear the more credible after we have carried the history of plague and other forms of epidemic sickness down through a whole generation from 1349.

The Epidemics following the Black Death.

Not the least of the effects of the Black Death upon England was the domestication of the foreign pestilence on the soil. For more than three centuries bubo-plague was never long absent from one part of Britain or another. The whole country was never again swamped by a vast wave of plague as in the fourteen months of 1348–49. Nor does it appear that the succeeding plagues of the fourteenth century, the *pestis secunda, tertia, quarta* and *quinta* were all of the same type as the first, or otherwise comparable to it. Disastrous as many subsequent English epidemics of bubo-plague were, they appear to have been localised in the North, perhaps, or in Norfolk, or confined to the young; and, above all, the bubo-plague became, in its later period, peculiarly a disease of the poor in the towns, although it did not cease altogether in the villages and country houses until it ceased absolutely in 1666. For three hundred years plague was the grand "zymotic" disease of England—the same type of plague that came from the East in 1347–49, continuously reproduced in a succession of epidemics at one place or another, which, by diligent search, can be made to fill the annals with few gaps, and, if the records were better, could probably be made to fill most years. Britain was not peculiar among the countries of Europe in that respect, although the chronology of plagues abroad has not been worked out minutely, except for an occasional province in which some zealous archaeologist had happened to take up the subject[1].

From 1349 to 1361 there is no record of pestilence in England. There was scarcity or famine in 1353, owing to an unfavourable harvest, but nothing is said of an unusual amount

---

[1] The only monograph that I know is Peinlich's *Pest in Steiermark*, 2 Bde. Graz, 1877–78. From 1349 to 1716, seventy years are marked in the annals of Styria as plague-years. Corradi gives the plague-years in Italy in his *Annali*.

of sickness. In 1361 came the *pestis secunda*, which would hardly have been so called had it not presented the same type as the great bubo-plague. There is little said of it in the chroniclers; but two of them mention that it was called the *pestis puerorum*, or plague of the juveniles; and a third gives the names of several great personages who died of it, including three bishops and Henry, duke of Lancaster, at his castle of Leicester, in Lent, 1362. This recrudescence, then, of the seeds of plague in English soil, may be taken as having cut off the nobles and the young: that is to say, the members of a class who had, by all accounts, escaped the first plague, and the rising generation who had either escaped the first plague as infants or had been born subsequent to it. The same selection of victims was observed, according to Guy de Chauliac, in the very same year at Avignon; in contrast to the Black Death, the second plague there cut off the upper and well-to-do classes, and an innumerable number of children[1]; among the former, it is said, were five cardinals and a hundred bishops. From Poland, also, it is reported that the return of the plague, which happened in 1360, affected mostly, although not exclusively, the upper classes and children. It is clear from the Continental evidence that the second pestilence was marked by the same buboes, carbuncles, and other signs as the first. In some places, at least, it must have been as destructive as the Black Death itself; thus, in Florence, says Petrarch (with obvious exaggeration) hardly ten in the thousand remained alive in the city after the epidemic of 1359, while Boccaccio estimates the mortality of the year at the equally incredible figure of a hundred thousand. In London many more wills than usual were enrolled in 1361, but not more than a third of the number enrolled in 1349: viz. 4 in February, 2 in March, 8 in April, 8 in May, 12 in June, 39 in July, 28 in October, 15 in November, 11 in December.

The *pestis secunda* is only one of a series of pestilences in the reigns of Edward III. and Richard II., which the chroniclers number in succession to the *pestis quinta* in 1391. The entries in the annals are for the most part so meagre and colourless that

[1] Guy de Chauliac for Avignon, in Häser, III. 176. Other foreign references in the same work.

they give us no help in realizing the share that a continuous infection in the soil, from the Black Death onwards, may have had in bringing about the disastrous state of the country in the latter half of the fourteenth century. Edward III. was ruined in reputation by his French wars, and ended his long reign in dishonour. His grandson Richard II. found the task of government too much for him, and was deposed. The history of this period is not complete without some account of the health of the country; a single line or sentence in a chronicle, to mark the date of a *pestis tertia* or *quarta* or *quinta*, hardly does justice to the place of national sickness among the events with which historians fill their pages. The graphic picture of the times is 'The Vision of Piers the Ploughman,' some passages of which may help us to realize what the bare enumeration of second, third, fourth and fifth pestilences meant. Some Latin poems of the time may be cited in support; and for more particular evidence of the type of pestilence which remained in England after the Black Death, we shall have to refer to certain extant manuscript treatises, from the latter part of the fourteenth century, which had been written in English to meet the wants of the people.

The Latin poems of the time of Edward III. and Richard II. need only be referred to so as to bring out by contrast the immense superiority of the 'Vision of Piers the Ploughman.' The poems of John of Bridlington, which are the most considerable of the Latin series of verses, contain numerous references to the epidemics of the time, both at home and abroad. Curiously, he dwells more upon the effects of famine—flux and fever—than upon the plague proper, which he nowhere distinguishes. Thus, of France about the time of the Black Death:

> "Destructis granis, deerit mox copia panis ;
> Poena fames panis, venter fluxu fit inanis."

Or again, with specific reference to the *pestis secunda* of 1361, which we know to have been bubo-plague :

> "...fluxus nocet, undique febris
> Extirpat fluxus pollutos crimine luxus."

Another reference, in the form of a prophecy, which from the context is clearly to the pestilence of 1368–69, again dwells exclusively upon famine:

> "In mensis justi pandetur copia crusti:
> Fundis falsorum premet arcta fames famulorum."

followed by a note in Latin: "from which it appears that the poor in those days were ill off for want of food[1]." One Latin poem of the end of the fourteenth century is expressly "On the Pestilence," in the following manner:

> "Ecce dolet Anglia luctibus imbuta,
> Gens tremit tristitia sordibus polluta,
> Necat pestilentia viros atque bruta.
> Cur? Quia flagitia regnant resoluta[2]."

Turning to the far more real or observant work of the same date by Langland, we find among his general references to sickness a most significant one in which he compares it to the continual dropping of rain through a leaky roof: "The rain that raineth where we rest should, be sicknesses and sorrows that we suffer oft." Again, in the allegory of Conscience and Nature, the former makes appeal to Nature to come forth as the scourge of evil-living:

"Nature Conscience heard, and came out of the planets, and sent forth his fore-goers, fevers and fluxes, coughs and cardiacles, cramps and tooth-aches, rheums and radegoundes and roynous scalls, boils and botches and burning agues, frenzies and foul evils—foragers of Nature had ypricked and preyed polls of people that largely a legion lose their life soon. Eld the hoary, he was in the vanguard, and bare the banner before Death, by right he it claimed. Nature came after, with many keen sores, as pokkes and pestilences, and much people shent. So Nature through corruptions killed many. Death came driving after, and all to dust dashed kings and knights, kaisers and popes, learned and lewd, he let no man stand that he hit even, that ever stirred after. Many a lovely lady, and lemans of knights, swooned and swelted for sorrow of Death's dints."

But "Conscience of his courtesy to Nature he besought, to cease and suffer and see whether they would leave pride privily and be perfect Christens. And Nature ceased then, to see the people amend. Fortune gan

---

[1] *Political Songs and Poems. Ed. II.–Ric. II.* Rolls series, No. 14, ed. T. Wright, I. 173, 190, &c.

[2] *Ibid.* I. 229, from a MS. in the library of Cambridge University.

flatter those few that were alive, and promised them long life; and Lechery he sent among all manner men, wedded and unwedded, and gathered a great host all against Conscience[1]."

Next came Avarice, Envy and other of the deadly sins, so that the respite which Nature had given was of no real avail.

A clear reference to pestilence continuing in the country comes in where the pope's exactions are mentioned. The pope did nothing in return for his English tribute:

> "Had I a clerk that could write, I would cast him a bill
> That he send me under his seal a salve for the pestilence,
> And that his blessing and his bulls botches might destroy.
> For, sith he hath the power that Peter himself had,
> He hath the pot with the salve, soothly as me thinketh."

Among the other consequences "sithen the pestilence," was this: "So is pride waxen, in religion and in all the realm among rich and poor, that prayers have no power the pestilence to let; ...ne for dread of the death withdraw not their pride."

The *pestis secunda* of 1361, or *pestis puerorum*, may perhaps be pointed to in the passage where chapmen are blamed for indulging their children, "ne for no pouste of pestilence correct them overmuch." The ill-assorted marriages had doubtless followed the great mortality itself; but the second pestilence, of 1361, which affected the upper classes especially, and is said by one chronicler to have cut off more men than women[2], may have been more specially pointed to in Langland's reference. Of that pestilence a chronicle of the next century has preserved a curious reminiscence: among its victims were men, doubtless of the upper class, "whose wives, as women out of gouvernance, took as well strangers to their husbands and other lewd and simple people, the which, forgetting their awe, worship and birth, coupled and married them with them that were of low degree and low reputation[3]."

Although Langland, when he speaks of changes "sith the

---

[1] The spelling has been modernized, a few old words changed, and the division into verses omitted.

[2] *Chronicon Angliae*, by a monk of St Albans. Rolls ed.

[3] Harleian MS. No. 1568, "Chronicle of England to A.D. 1419." (Printed with additions at the St Albans press about 1484.)

pestilence time," means the great mortality of 1349, he means in other places, the second, third, and perhaps also fourth pestilences[1]. The years of the pestilences down to the fifth are not the same in all the chronicles; there are indeed some nine outbreaks that might have been enumerated after the Black Death to the end of the century. Some of these are clearly associated with scarcity, and may have been of the old type of famine-sickness; dysentery is, indeed, mentioned in connexion with the sickness of 1391[2]. Again, an epidemic in London in 1382 is said by a chronicler to have affected children (boys and girls), while the same chronicler is explicit that the sickness in Norfolk the year after was confined to the young of both sexes under a certain age. Lastly, the epidemic of 1391 was so severe in the North as to recall the great mortality itself; but under the same year is the reference to sickness of the type of dysentery due to rotten fruit; and under the year before, 1390, two chroniclers agree that the epidemic was "mostly among children," or that it cut off "more young than old." It would be unsafe, therefore, to conclude that all the outbreaks of *pestis* in England subsequent to the Black Death, were of bubo-plague itself. The list of sicknesses in Langland's poem gives, indeed, as much space to fevers and fluxes, burning agues and frenzies, as to boils and botches, foul evils, pokkes and pestilences—by which latter group of synonyms the bubo-plague is meant. *Pestis*, it is well known, was a generic name in the medieval period, just as pest and pestilence are generic now. So generic was it that some may doubt whether bubo-plague, of the type of 1349, was included at all among the *pestes* of the generations following. Positive evidence of the continued existence of bubo-plague in England is, at least, not superfluous, and this will be the best place to bring it in.

---

[1] Skeat, whose great edition of 'The Vision of Piers the Ploughman,' has been brought out by the Early English Text Society, thinks that the ironical reference (Passus XIII. 248) to the pope sending a salve for the pestilence applies particularly to the "Fourth Pestilence" of 1375 and 1376, which was the *pestis tertia* of some chronicles.

[2] Flux and fever from famine are alone mentioned in the poems of John of Bridlington, which cover the period from the Black Death to the reign of Richard II.

Medical Evidence of the Continuance of Plague.

The plague was called "the botch" down to the Elizabethan and Stuart periods; and the "botches" in Langland's poem, or, as he writes it, "boches," were the familiar risings, under the arms and elsewhere, which had given the disease its popular name when it began to recur time after time. Apart from this verbal or philological evidence, there is a clear proof of the prevalence of true bubo-plague during the latter part of the fourteenth century, in the manuscript ordinances or rules of prevention and treatment which were in circulation. Most of the extant copies bear the name of one John of Burgoyne, or John of Bordeaux[1]. A fragment in comparatively late handwriting purports to be the ordinance of "a great Clark, Mr John Cordewe, at the prayer of King Richard and other the Lords, for pestilence[2]"; from which it may be concluded that this, the commonly used ordinance, dates from the time of Richard II. The names used in the text are "pestilence" and "pestilential sores," and the handling of the subject is the conventional one for the plague. The ordinance contains exceedingly little that is of practical interest, and it is difficult to believe that it can have been of real use to anyone. We are introduced to the subject with a few empty common-places; but whenever we come to business, we are plainly told to go and consult those who know—and this, be it observed, in a disease which was remarkably uniform in its type and circumstances:

"Wherefore they that have not dronken of that swete drynke of Astronomye may putte to these pestilentiall sores no fit remedies; for, because that they know not the cause and the quality of the sickness, they may not hele it, as sayeth the prince of physic Avicenna: 'How shouldest thou hele a sore and yknowe not the cause?' He that knoweth not the cause, it is impossible that he hele the sickness."

If there were any doubt about the date of John of Burgoyne,

---

[1] Egerton MS. No. 2572, Sloane MS. 443 ("xiv. cent."), as well as several copies of the 15th century.

[2] Lansdowne MS. 285, fol. 220.

or John of Bordeaux[1], it ought to be set at rest by the discovery that he corresponds in the closest way with the physician in the Prologue of the *Canterbury Tales.* Chaucer's doctor of physic stands for the well-grounded practitioner of the time—"grounded in astronomie," it is true, but at all events academically grounded, in contrast to the charlatans and pretenders who had not been to Paris or Bologna, probably knew no Latin, to say nothing of "astronomy," and therefore knew not how to let a patient die (or recover) *secundum artem.* The doctor of physic uses his astrological knowledge so much in the manner of John of Bordeaux, that one suspects Chaucer to have seen the passage quoted above, and to have condensed it into the two following lines :

> "The cause yknowne, and of his harm the rote,
> Anon he gave to the sick man his bote."

It was in the pestilence that this practitioner had made the money which he kept so tightly.   Richly clad he was ;

> "And yet he was but easy of dispense ;
> He kept that he wan in the pestilence.
> For gold in physic is a cordial :
> Therefore he loved gold in special."

This is John of Burgoyne all over ; it would have been an anachronism in England by more than two hundred years to have represented a physician as caring for any but paying patients, or as regarding an epidemic sickness from any other point of view than as a source of income.

Besides the "ordinance" of John of Burgoyne, which may be assigned to the reign of Richard II., there was another essay on the plague circulating in England in an English translation, of which the copy among the Sloane manuscripts is assigned to the fourteenth century[2]. The importance attached to this manuscript work is shown in the fact that it was chosen among the very first to be printed at an English press, probably in the year

---

[1] Mr Warner identifies him with the person who invented "Sir John Mandeville" and the travels of Sir John.   See an article in the *Quarterly Review*, April, 1891.

[2] Sloane MS. (British Museum) No. 2276, fol. 191–199.

1480[1]. It was reprinted in 1536, and the substance of it was copied into nearly all the English books on plague (from one to another) as late as the seventeenth century, much of its original matter passing under the name of one Phaer, or Phayre or Thayre, who was a compiler about the middle of the sixteenth century. Writers on early English printing have made much of the printed book of 1480; but they do not appear to have known of the manuscript which was used as the printer's "copy[2]." If one happens to use the latter first, and comes later to the printed book, he will observe the identity not merely in the words and spelling but even in the very form in which the type had been cut. The authorship of a manuscript which is thus invested with a various interest may deserve a few lines of inquiry.

The author of it describes himself in the (translated) introduction as " I the bisshop of Arusiens, Doctour of phisike," that is to say, bishop of Aarhus, in Denmark. In the text, he claims to have practised physic at Montpellier:

" In the Mount of Pessulane I might not eschewe the company of people, for I went from house to house, because of my poverty, to cure sick folk. Therefore bread or a sponge sopped in vinegar I took with me, holding it to my mouth and nose, because all aigre things stoppen the ways of humours and suffereth no venomous thing to enter into a man's body; and so I escaped the pestilence, my fellows supposing that I should not live. These foresaid things I have proved by myself[3]."

[1] 'A passing gode lityll boke necessarye and behouefull azenst the Pestilence.' British Museum, case 31, e. 13, 4to, twelve leaves. The MS. begins as follows : "Here begynneth a lytell boke necessary and behouefull azens the pestylence."

[2] Dibdin (*Antiq. Typogr.* II. 19) assigns the printing to Machlinia, and reproduces a page as a sample of his common type. Bliss (*Reliquiae Hearnianae*, II. 117) says that this sample page does not correspond with that of the British Museum copy. He adds that there is a fragment of the printed book in the library of St Peter's College, Cambridge, "pasted within the wooden covers of the binding of an edition (1499) of *Discipuli Sermones.*"

[3] In the earliest printed Latin texts of this work (Antwerp, 1485? Leipzig, 1495? and versified in Albertus Magnus, 'De Virtute Herbarum,' 1500?) he is named Kamitus, bishop of Arusia, a city in the realm of Denmark. In the copy of the English version in the British Museum, someone has called him Ramicius, having written on a leaf, "Ramicius Episcopus Arusiensis civitatis Daciae Regimen contra pestem," with the date 1698. The name of Kamitus, being judged improbable on the face of it, has been changed in the catalogue of the British Museum library into Canutus. But there was no Canutus among the bishops of Aarhus, nor a Kamitus,

The fact that this medieval treatise, whatever its exact date, was turned into English and circulated in manuscript, and that it was chosen for printing almost as soon as English printing began, in the reign of Edward IV., is sufficient evidence, if more were needed, that the English had to reckon with bubo-plague as one of their standing diseases throughout the latter part of the medieval period. Before we come to the chronology of English plagues in that period, from the Black Death to the accession of the Tudor dynasty in 1485, it will be convenient to consider here, with the help of the above treatise, how the endemic plague was viewed in those days,—what it was ascribed to in its origin, in its incidence upon houses and persons, and in its propagation, what was advised for its avoidance or prevention, and what was prescribed for its treatment. As the bishop's essay was the source of most that was taught on these matters in England for the next two or three hundred years, it will be an economy to give a brief account of it here once for all.

The remote causes, or warnings of the approach of pestilence, are given under seven heads, including the kind of weather, swarms of flies, shooting stars, comets, thunder and lightning out of the south, and winds out of the south; this list was reproduced, with little or no change, by the Elizabethan writers of popular health-manuals. The second section of the essay is on the "causes of pestilence." There are three causes :—

"Sometime it cometh from the root beneath ; other while from the root above, so that we may feel sensibly howwith change of the air appeareth

nor a Ramicius. The two bishops that appear to suit best are Olaus, or Olaf, who was bishop from 1371 to 1388, and Ulricus or Udalricus, or Olric Stycka, who succeeded in 1425 and held the see until 1449. Curiously enough, the latter, when he went to Rome in 1425 to represent Eric, king of Pomerania in a suit with the dukes of Sleswig, figures throughout the records of the suit as "Olaus, episcopus Arosiensis," although Olaus, bishop of Arusia, belonged to a former generation. It is, of course, the merest guessing; but I am inclined to think that the author of the essay on plague was either bishop Olaus, of 1371-1388, or bishop Udalricus, of 1425-1449, a man of character and ability, who also went by the name of Olaus; and that in any case the manuscript version of the essay in the English tongue is more likely to have been of the early part of the fifteenth century than of the fourteenth. The above facts are collected from various parts of Langbeck's *Script. Rer. Dan.:* the "Series Episcoporum Arhusiorum" is in vol. VII. p. 212. Nothing is there said of any bishop of Aarhus having written a book, or having been a physician at Montpellier.

14—2

unto us ; and sometime it cometh of both together, as well from the root above as from the root beneath, as we see a siege or privy next to a chamber, or of any other particular thing which corrupteth the air in his substance and quality, which is a thing may happen every day. And thereof cometh the ague of pestilence (and about the same many physicians be deceived, not supposing this ague to be a pestilence). Sometimes it cometh of dead carrion, or corruption of standing waters in ditches or sloughs and other corrupt places. These things sometime be universal, sometime particular." Then follow sentences on the "root above" which are somewhat transcendental. When both "roots" work together, when, by "th' ynp'ffyons[1]" above, the air is corrupt and by the putrefaction or rotten carrion of the vile places beneath,—an infirmity is caused in man. "And such infirmity sometimes is an ague, sometimes a posthume or a swelling, and that is in many things. Also the air inspired sometimes is venomous and corrupt, hurting the heart, that nature many ways is grieved, so that he perceiveth not his harm......

"These things written before are the causes of pestilence. But about these things, two questions be mooted. The first is, wherefore one dieth and another dieth not, in a town where men be dead in one house and in another house there dieth none. The second question is, whether pestilence sores be contagious.

"To the first question, I say it may hap to be of two causes : that is to say, of that thing that doth, and of that thing that suffereth. An ensample of that thing that doth : The influence of the bodies above beholdeth that place or that place, more than this place or this place. And one patient is more disposed to die than another. Therefore it is to be noted that bodies be more hot disposed, of open pores, than bodies infect having the pores stopped with many humours. Where bodies be of resolution or opening, as men which abusen them selfe with wymmen, or usen often times bathis ; or men that be hot with labour or great anger—they have their bodies more disposed to this great sickness.

"To the second question I say, that pestilence sores be contagious by cause of infect humoures bodies, and the reek or smoke of such sores is venomous and corrupteth the air. And therefore it is to flee from such persons as be infect. In pestilence time nobody should stand in great press of people, because some man of them may be infect. Therefore wise physicians, in visiting sick folk, stand far from the patient, holding their face toward the door or window. And so should the servants of sick folk stand. Also it is good to a patient every day for to change his chamber, and often times to have the windows open against the North and East, and to spar the windows against the South. For the south wind hath two causes of putrefaction. The first is, it maketh a man, being whole or sick, feeble in

[1] These words ("the impressions") are contracted in the printed book, exactly as in the manuscript. I have modernised the spelling for the most part.

their bodies. The second cause is, as it is written in the Third of Aphorisms, the south wind grieveth the hearing and hurteth the heart, because it
openeth the pores of man and entereth into the heart. Wherefore it is good
to an whole man in time of pestilence, when the wind is in the South, to
keep within the house all the day. And if it shall need a man to go out, yet
let him abide in his house till the sun be up in the East passing south-
ward."

These explanations of the incidence of plague are in part
repeated in the section of the essay where the author gives
directions for avoiding it. After enjoining penance, he proceeds:

"It is a good remedy to void and change the infect place. But some
may not profitably change their places. Therefore as much as to them is
possible, it is to be eschewed every cause of putrefaction and stinking, and
namely every fleshly lust with women is to be eschewed. Also the southern
wind, which wind is naturally infective : therefore spar the windows, etc.
Of the same cause, every foul stink is to be eschewed—of stable, stinking
fields, ways, or streets, and namely of stinking dead carrion ; and most of
stinking waters, where in many places water is kept two days or two nights,
or else there be gutters of water casten under the earth which caused great
stink and corruption. And of this cause some die in that house where such
things happen, and in another house die none, as it is said afore. Likewise
in that place where the worts and coles putrefied, it maketh noifull savour
and stinking. For in like wise as by the sweet odour of bawme the heart and
spirits have recreation, so of evil savours they be made feeble. Therefore
keep your house that an infect air enter not in. For an infect air most
causeth putrefaction in places and houses where folk sleep. Therefore let
your house be clean, and make clear fire of wood flaming : let your house be
made with fumigation of herbs, that is to say, with leaves of bay-tree,
juniper, yberiorgam—it is in the apothecary shops—wormwood etc....For a
little crust corrupteth all the body.
  "Also in the time of the pestilence it is better to abide within the house ;
for it is not wholesome to go into the city or town. Also let your house be
sprinkled, specially in summer, with vinegar and roses, and with the leaves
of vine tree. Also it is good to wash your hands ofttimes in the day with
water and vinegar, and wipe your face with your hands, and smell to them.
Also it is good always to savour aigre things."

Then follows his own Montpellier experience, already quoted.

The diagnostics come in casually along with the treatment :

"But some would understand how may a man feel when he is infect. I
say that a man which is infect, that day eateth not much meat for he is
replenished with evil humours ; and forthwith after dinner he hath lust to

sleep, and feeleth great heat under cold. Also he hath great pain in the forehead...He shall feel a swelling under the arm, or about the share, or about the ears...When a man feeleth himself infect, as soon as he may, let him be let blood plenteously till he swoon : then stop the vein. For a little letting of blood moveth or stirreth venom."

Then follow directions for bleeding, according to the position of the bubo—in the armpit, groin or neck, the direction " if on the back " probably having reference to the carbuncle[1]. The section on treatment, which is the last, ends with a prescription for a medicine " that the sooner a swelling be made ripe."

These are sufficiently clear indications of the bubonic nature of the disease called pestilence. At the same time the writer includes an ague as also pestilential, due to similar causes and arising on similar occasions. This is a use of the name ague which should not be mistaken for its common application to intermittent fever. Ague was simply (febris) acuta; and pestilential ague was a name for typhus fever in the sixteenth century (as in Jones' *Dyall of Agues*), as well as in Ireland until a much later period. This early association of acute pestilential fever with true bubo-plague means the same relationship of typhus to plague which was systematically taught by Sydenham, Willis, and Morton in the seventeenth century ; typhus in their time was the frequent attendant of plague,—a *pestis mitior ;* and it would appear to have been its attendant and congener in the fourteenth century also.

---

[1] "When a man feeleth himself infect, as soon as he may, let him be let blood plenteously till he swoon: then stop the vein. For a little letting of blood moveth or stirreth venom...Let him blood on the side of the body where the swelling appeareth. Therefore if a swelling appear under the right arm, let blood in the middle of the same arm, in the vein called *mediana.* If it appear under the left arm, let him blood in midst of the same, or in the vein of the liver which is about the little finger. And if it be about the share, let him blood about the heel upon the same side. If the swelling be in the neck, let him blood in the vein called *cephalica,* about the thumb in the hand of the same side; or in the vein the which is called *mediana* of the same arm, or in the hand of the same side about the little finger. And, overmore, if the swelling appear about the ear, let him blood in the vein called *cephalica* of the same side, or in the vein which is between the long finger and the thumb, lest many venomous things go into the brain." If the swelling is in the shoulders, bleed from the *mediana :* if on the back from *pedica magna,* and so on.

The Fourteenth Century Chronology continued.

Two epidemics contend in the chronicles for being the *pestis tertia*—that of 1368–69, and that of 1375. The former is described as a "great pestilence of men and the larger animals[1]," and it appears to have been associated with unfavourable seasons and with the beginning of that scarcity which Langland's poem refers to the month of April, 1370:

> Atte Londoun, I leve, liketh wel my wafres
> And louren whan thei lakken hem —It is nought longe passed,
> There was a careful comune whan no cart cam to towne
> With bred fro Strethforth, tho gan beggeres wepe
> And werkmen were agast a lite. This wole be thought longe
> In the date of our Drighte in a drye Aprille,
> A thousand and thre hondreth tweis thretty and ten
> My wafres there were gesen whan Chichestre was Maire[2].

The *pestis* of 1368 and 1369 may have been primarily a famine-sickness; but it does not follow that there was no bubo-plague mixed therewith. On the contrary, seasons of scarcity were often in after experience found to be the seasons of plague, the lowered vitality probably offering the opportunity to the plague-virus. Previous to the harvests of 1376 and 1377, which were abundant, there had been an unbroken period of high prices for many years, of which 1371 was remembered as "the grete dere yere[3]." But the *pestis tertia* appears to have been most severe in the summer of 1368; for, on 23 July of that year, Simon, archbishop of Canterbury, ordered public prayers for the

---

[1] Walsingham, *Hist. Angl.* I. 309. Adam of Murimuth, Engl. Hist. Soc.

[2] The Stratford bread-carts are explained in Stow's *Survey of London* ("Lime Street Ward"). In the famines of 1512 and 1527, they were besieged on the way by hungry citizens and had to be guarded. The same phrase of bread being "gesen" or scarce, occurs in a letter of 4 September, 1535, from Thomas Broke to Cromwell, secretary of State: "never knew good bread so geason in London at this time of the year; it is so musty, and of so evil wheat, that it is rather poisonous than nourishing; what was sold for a halfpenny, when you were here, is now a penny." (*Cal. State Papers*, Henry VIII. vol. IX. § 274.)

[3] Thorold Rogers. *A Short English Chronicle*, Camden Soc. 1880 :—"45 Edward III. This yere was called the grete dere yere, and that same yere was a quarter of whete at iiii nobles."

cessation of the pestilence[1], and it is under the same year that the wills of deceased London citizens are enrolled in unusual numbers, although not in such numbers as in the *pestis secunda* of 1361[2]. Public prayers for the cessation of pestilence (without reference to famine) and an unusual mortality of the richer citizens, point to the plague proper, which may or may not have been the type of sickness in the country districts in 1369, the second year of the epidemic[3].

There is, furthermore, some indirect evidence that pestilential disease, and probably bubo-plague, occurred in London subsequent to the scarcity of the dry April, 1370, to which Langland's verses relate. This evidence lies in the comparison of the wording of two ordinances of Edward III., one of 1369 and the other of 1371, both relating to nuisances in the city[4]. In an order of the king in Council (43 Edward III.) for stopping the carrying of slaughter-house offal from the shambles in St Nicholas parish, within Newgate, through the streets, lanes, and other places to the banks of the water of Thames near to Baynard's Castle, where there was a jetty for throwing the refuse from into the river, the motive assigned is that divers prelates, nobles, and other persons having houses in the line of traffic, had complained grievously of these offences to the sight and smell. But, in an amended order of 28th October, 1371, against the same nuisance and with a definite (but futile) relegation of all slaughtering to Stratford on the one side and Knightsbridge on the other, the motive is differently stated: "Whereas of late, from the putrefied blood of slaughtered beasts running in the streets, and the entrails thereof thrown into the water of Thames, the air in the same city has been greatly corrupted and infected, and whereby the worst of

---

[1] Wilkins, *Concilia*, III. 74: "De orando pro cessatione pestilentiae," dated Slyndon, 10 Cal. Aug. A.D. MCCCLXVIII.

[2] Sharpe, *Cal. of Wills*, vol. II.

[3] Otterbourne (ed. Hearne, p. 133) says that the *pestis tertia* was in 1368, and that it lasted two years. Nicolas (*Chronol. of History*, p. 389) gives from a Lansdowne MS. (no. 863, fol. 107) of the time of Charles I., the duration of the *pestis tertia* as 2 July—29 Sept., 1369, which should probably read "2 July, 1368—29 Sept. 1369."

[4] *Memorials of London*, etc. from the Council Records. Edited by H. T. Riley. Lond. 1867, p. 339 and p. 356.

abominations and stenches have been generated, and sicknesses and many other maladies have befallen persons dwelling in the same city and resorting thereto :—We, desiring to take precautions against such perils, and to provide for the decency of the said city, and the safety of the same our people " etc.

Up to this date, the Rolls of Parliament contain frequent references to the wasting and impoverishment of the country by pestilence. A petition of 1362 begs the king "to consider the divers mischiefs that have come to his commons by divers pestilences of wind and water, and mortality of men and beasts"—the destructive wind being the tornado-like storm, on the 16th January, 1362, "on Saturday at even," which was long remembered, and is commemorated, along with the Black Death itself, in an inscription in the church of Ashwell, Herts. Next year, another petition states that "pestilences and great winds have done divers mischiefs"—manors and tenements held direct from the king having become desolate and ruinous. In 1369 a petition states that "the king's ferms [rents] in every county of England are greatly abated by the great mortalities." The parliament of 1376, the "good Parliament" so-called, is able to point the moral of its petitions by frequent references to the pestilences "that have been in the kingdom one after another," the pestilences "of people and servants," the murrains of cattle, and "the failure of their corn and other fruits of the earth." The same language recurs in the second parliament of Richard II. in 1378 (the year after the poll-tax), and from that time until the end of his reign, it becomes stereotyped in the petitions deprecating heavy subsidies or excusing the smallness of the sums voted.

The pestilence of 1375 would appear to have been considered as one of the greater sort. The author of the *Eulogium* reckons it the *pestis tertia* (passing over that of 1368–69). The season was one of great heat, there was "grandis pestilentia" both in England and other countries, an infinity of both sexes died, the mortality being so swift that the pope, "at the instance of the cardinal of England" granted plenary remission to all dying contrite and confessing their sins[1]. That looks like an epidemic

---

[1] Walsingham, *Hist. Angl.* I. 319; Adam of Murimuth.

of true bubo-plague,—probably the *pestis quarta* correctly so-called[1].

In 1379 there was a great plague in the Northern parts, which were stripped of their best men ; the Scots made a raid, with the following prayer on their lips : "God and Sen Mungo, Sen Ninian and Seynt Andrew scheld us this day and ilka day fro Goddis grace, and the foule deth that Ynglessh men dyene upon"—foul death being the name given to plague also in 1349[2]. The northern counties send a petition to the parliament of 1379–80, that the king would "consider the very great hurt and damage which they have suffered, and are still suffering, both by pestilence and by the continual devastations of the Scots enemy[3]."

In the parliament of 1381–82 there is a petition from the convent of Salisbury as to want of money to repair the losses caused by the pestilence, of which the tenants are nearly all dead, and by the murrain of cattle. This is more than thirty years from the Black Death, and can hardly refer, as some earlier petitions may have done, to the enduring effects of that calamity. The sixth parliament of Richard II. (1382), has two of the stereotyped petitions deprecating a heavy subsidy on the ground of "the great poverty and disease" of the commons, through pestilence of people, murrain of cattle, failure of crops, great floods, etc.[4] This was the year after the Peasant Revolt, which had coincided with troubles of various kinds. A Norwich chronicle, perhaps of contemporary authority, enters, under the year 1382, a very pestilential fever in many places of the country, and very extraordinary inundations of the fens[5]. In

---

[1] The chroniclers are not agreed as to the chronology of the various 14th century plagues from the first (the Black Death) to the fifth. Some of the enumerations are clearly erroneous. Thus in *A Short English Chronicle* from the Lambeth MS. (ed. Gairdner for the Camden Society, 1880), the plague of 1361 is erroneously called "the threde pestilence," while the fourth is assigned to 1369 and the fifth to 1377 (for 1375). Otterbourne places the *quarta* in 1374 (for 1375), and the *quinta* (as others do) in 1391; but in the *Life of Richard II.*, by a monk of Evesham, the pestilence of 1382 is more correctly reckoned the fifth from the Black Death.

[2] Walsingham, *Hist. Angl.* I. 409. *Chronicon Angliae*, p. 239.

[3] *Rot. Parl.* IV. 806.

[4] *Ibid.* III. pp. 139 a, 147 a.

[5] Blomefield's *History of Norfolk*, III. p. 111.

London the epidemic of 1382 is said to have been "chiefly among boys and girls[1]." A primitive English poem of the time has for its subject the earthquake of 1382, and with that portent it associates not only the Peasant's Rebellion but also "the pestilens[2]."

The year 1383 was a bad one for the fruit, which was spoiled by "foetid fogs, exhalations and various corruptions of the air": from eating of the spoiled fruits many died, or incurred serious illness and infirmities[3]. By another account, a great pestilence in Kent and other parts of England destroyed many, sparing no age or sex. In Norfolk the sickness that year is said to have been confined to young persons[4]. This was only one of the occasions which might have been referred to in 'Piers Ploughman,' when the poor people thought to "poison Hunger" by bad food.

The next pestilence, that of 1390 and 1391, was so prolonged and so serious as to be compared with the Great Mortality itself. It is called the *pestis quinta* by two annalists[5], and is described not without some detail by several. It is clear that the seeds of disease were ready to burst forth at various parts of the country; for we read that in 1389, the king was in the south of England, and seeing some of his men prostrated by sudden death, he returned to Windsor[6]. Another outburst came the year after. Intense heat began in June and lasted until September; great mortality ensued, the epidemic continuing in diverse parts of England, but not everywhere, until Michaelmas; it cut off more young than old, as well as several famous soldiers[7]. The St Albans entry confirms this: "A great plague, especially of youths and children, who died everywhere in towns and villages, in incredible and excessive numbers[8]." After the epidemic

---

[1] Continuator of Higden, IX. 14.

[2] *Political Songs and Poems.* Rolls series, No. 14, I. p. 252:—
"The rysyng of the comuynes in londe,
The pestilens, and the eorthe-quake—
Theose three thinges I understonde."

[3] Walsingham, *Hist. Angl.* II. 109.

[4] Continuator of Higden, IX. 21, 27.

[5] *Eulogium Historiarum*, III. 369. Otterbourne, ed. Hearne: "From the nativity of St John Baptist to the feast of St Luke," 1391.

[6] Continuator of Higden, IX. 216.　　　　[7] *Ibid.* 237.

[8] Walsingham, *Hist. Angl.* II. 186.

there was scarcity, of which we have special accounts from Norfolk[1]. But the heaviest mortality fell in the year 1391. There was first of all scarcity, now in its second year, and aggravated by six weeks of continual gloom in July and August. At the time of the nuts, apples and other fruits of the kind, many poor people died of dysentery, and the sickness would have been worse but for the laudable care of the mayor of London who caused corn to be brought from over sea. In Norfolk and many other counties the sickness was compared even to the Great Mortality, and was probably a mixture of famine-pestilence with bubo-plague. At York "eleven thousand" were said to have been buried[2]. Another account says that the North suffered severely, and also the West, and that the sickness lasted all summer[3]. Under the year 1393 one annalist states that many died in Essex in September and October, "on the pestilence setting in[4]." The next evidence comes from the Rolls of Parliament; in the first parliament of Henry IV. (1399) a petition is presented "that the king would graciously consider the great pestilence which is in the northern parts," and send sufficient men to defend the Scots marches.

The first great outburst of plague in the fifteenth century falls somewhere between 1405 and 1407. "So great pestilence," says the St Albans annalist, under the year 1407, "had not been seen for many years." In London "thirty thousand men and women" are reported to have died in a short space; and "in

---

[1] Blomefield's *History of Norfolk*, III. 113 :—"1390. A great mortality increased in Norfolk and in many other counties in England, and it seemed not unlike the season of the great pestilence: it was occasioned by a great want of victuals, that forced many people to eat unwholesome food, and so brought distempers upon them. This dearth began under the sickle, and lasted to the following harvest [1391], but was not so much for want of corn, as money to purchase it, occasioned by the law made in relation to wool, by which wool became dog-cheap; for a stone of chosen and picked wool of the best sort was sold for 3 sh. and some for 22 pence or 2 sh., so that in these times the woollen manufacture was the great support of the nation." According to Thorold Rogers, these high prices of wool obtained from 1364 to 1380.

[2] Walsingham, II. 203. The Continuator of Higden (IX. 259) says 12,000. These estimates are, of course, the merest guesses, and extreme exaggerations. The whole population of York would have been under 15,000.

[3] Higden, *ibid.*

[4] Walsingham, II. 213; St Albans Annals of Ric. II. and Hen. IV.

country villages the sickness fell so heavily upon the wretched peasants that many homes that had before been gladdened by a numerous family were left almost empty[1]." But it is under the 7th of Henry IV. (1405) that Hall's chronicle narrates how the king, to avoid the city on account of the plague, sailed from Queenborough to a port in Essex, and so to Plashey, " there to pass his time till the plague were ceased" (p. 36). Another chronicle says that the plague of 1407 was mostly in the West country. In that year, the 9th of Henry IV., there is a petition from Ilchester in Somerset for a remission of dues "because the town is so impoverished and desolate of people that the burgesses are unable to pay the said ferme," and for the cancelling of all arrears due since the 43rd year of Edward III. (1369). In the 11th of Henry IV. (1410–11), the burgesses of Truro represent "that the said town is impoverished by pestilence and the death of men, and by invasions and loss by the enemy by sea, and by the surcharge of twelve lives, and by default of inhabitants in the said town "— a petition apparently similar in terms to one that had been submitted in the previous reign. In the 1st of Henry IV. (1399), petitions of the same kind had been presented from Lincoln and Yarmouth; the former was "in great part empty and uninhabited," while the latter had " its houses vacant and void, owing to pestilence and other things."

For the year 1413 there is a brief entry that "numbers of Englishmen were struck by plague and ceased to live[2]." A single chronicler mentions a pestilence in Norfolk in 1420[3]; but the Rolls of Parliament bear undoubted witness to a very severe prevalence of plague in the North about the same time: a petition from the Marches in 1421 speaks of "great numbers of persons dead by the great mortalities and pestilences which have raged for three years past and still reign ; where a hundred men used to be there are not ten, and these of small account ; where

---

[1] Walsingham, II. 276. The Chronicle of William Gregory (Camden Society, ed. Gairdner) enters under the year 1407, a great frost, for twenty-five weeks. It would be of real scientific interest to know the chronology exactly, whether the plague followed or preceded the long cold drought ; but the year of the plague is disputable, if any heed be paid to the date of 1406, given by later compilers.

[2] Walsingham, II. 297. Otterbourne, under 1411, says plague in Gascony.

[3] Annals of Bermondsey, in *Annales Monast.* Rolls ed. III. 485.

people of position kept twenty men at arms they now keep only themselves"; the enemy were making raids and food was scarce[1]. Another petition the same year (9 Henry V.) states that "both by pestilence within the realm and wars without there are not sufficient men of estate to hold the office of sheriff[2]." That was shortly after Agincourt and the conquest of France, when the fortunes of Henry V. were at their highest point. The horrors of the siege of Rouen (1419) were a favourite subject with poets of the time[3], but they were of a kind foreign to English experience in that age, and, indeed, in all periods of our history, save that of the Danish invasions. The Cromwellian Civil Wars, as we shall see, do indeed furnish many instances of plague, and some of typhus fever, in besieged or occupied towns; but, for the middle part of the fifteenth century, including the period of the wars of York and Lancaster, there is no good reason to suppose that fevers or other *morbi miseriae*, were rife among the common people, least of all among the peasantry.

The Public Health in the Fifteenth Century.

Our safest indications are got from the prices of commodities and the rates of wages, and these, according to the most competent authority, Thorold Rogers, were more favourable to the working class in the fifteenth century than at other periods: "As the agriculturist throve in the fifteenth century, so the mechanic and the artisan was also prosperous. This was the age in which the property of the guilds was generally acquired." On famines in particular, I shall quote one other passage, which entirely confirms the view that I had independently stated in the first chapter when speaking of Ergotism:

"Famine, in the strict sense of the word, has rarely occurred in England, owing to the practice which the inhabitants of this island have persistently

---

[1] *Rot. Parl.* IV. 143 a. It is probably under 1420 that the "great plague" at Newcastle, given in so many words in Brand's *History* under 1410, should be placed.

[2] *Ibid.* 148 b.

[3] *Histor. Collec. of a Citizen of London, 15th cent.* Camden Soc. ed. Gairdner, 1876 :

"They dyde faster every day
Thenn men myght them in erthe lay."

maintained of living mainly on the dearest kind of corn...The people lived abundantly, and, except when extraordinary scarcity occurred, regularly on the best provision which could be procured[1]."

One such period of extraordinary scarcity all over England fell in the years 1438–39. The chronicle of Croyland says that there were three wet harvests in succession, that famine had been almost constant for two years, and that the people were reduced to eating dried herbs and roots[2]. That would have been a famine of the old kind, like those of 1258 and 1315, wheat having touched 20s. But it should not lead us to suppose that the disastrous period of the end of Edward III.'s reign and of the reign of Richard II. was continued throughout the fifteenth century. It is true that the records of that century are scantier than for earlier periods ; the monastic chronicles have all ceased, except those of St Albans and Croyland, and the citizens' diaries, which took their place, have hardly begun. It is possible that a fuller record would have shown a greater prevalence of distress throughout the country. It is probably owing to the scantiness of the history that the views of the fifteenth century range from the extreme of optimism to the extreme of pessimism. Where little is known, much may be imagined. Thus, a recent writer on *England in the Fifteenth Century*[3], says that "all attempts to specify the years of scarcity would only mislead"; and again : "There is hardly any period of five years during that time [15th century] without these ghastly records." Another recent writer[4] remarks upon the fifteenth century being called a time of rude plenty, and sets against that "the famines, the plagues, the skin-diseases, the miserable quality of the food, the insecurity of life and property, the hovels in which the people lived, and the tyranny and oppression of a time of unsettled government." It is needless to controvert the merely subjective impression in an author's mind. But, in order to clear our ideas, let us take these things one by one. What were firstly the famines ? There is no

---

[1] *History of Agriculture and Prices in England*, IV. 105.
[2] Chronicle of Croyland, in Gale, I. 518 ; Rogers, IV. 233.
[3] Denton. London, 1886, p. 92.
[4] Mackay, *The English Poor*. London, 1890, p. 40.

great one but that of 1438–39, which was due to a succession of wet harvests, and was equally severe in Scotland and in France, having in them caused famine-sickness as well as plague. Of the plagues, which were certainly no worse than in the Elizabethan and Stuart times, I shall speak in detail almost at once. Of the skin-diseases, there is nowhere a word said: another writer[1] specifies leprosy as afflicting England "all over the country" in the fifteenth century, whereas it can be shown that the prevalence of that disease, such as it had ever been in England, had almost ceased, and its sentimental vogue passed, in the reign of Edward III. The miserable quality of the food and the wretched hovels have certainly no special relevancy to the period[2]; on the contrary, the picture that we get of the manor of Castle Combe in the fifteenth century is that of a prosperous community, although not a highly moral one. As to insecurity of life and property, and oppression of government, there seems to be some illusion because the time was that of the wars of York and Lancaster. But we have the significant observation of Philip de Comines, a contemporary French statesman who kept his eye on the state of other countries; writing of the effects of civil war, he says:—

"England has this peculiar grace that neither the country, nor the people, nor the houses are wasted or demolished; but the calamities and misfortunes of the war fall only upon the soldiers and especially the nobility, of whom they are more than ordinarily jealous: for nothing is perfect in this world."

The truth seems to be that the middle part of the fifteenth century was really the time "cre England's woes began, when

[1] W. Cunningham, *Growth of English Industry and Commerce.* 2nd ed. Camb. 1890, p. 105. He reproduces Denton's statement that "there was chronic typhoid in the towns." Denton professes to have found this in Hecker, who had certainly no knowledge of English towns in the 15th century, and is, in general, more entertaining as a *philosophe* than trustworthy for erudition.

[2] In 1741, during a prevalence of fever all over England, we hear of bread made of horse-beans, pease, and coarse unsound barley as the chief food of the poor. (*Gent. Magaz.* letters of 27 Nov. 1741 and 11 Jan. 1742). Thorold Rogers (*Agric. and Prices*, v. Preface) thinks that the staple food of the English labourer, wheaten bread, had first been changed, especially in the North, to rye, barley and oat bread, in the 17th century during the Civil Wars.

every rood of ground maintained its man," and that the Golden Age came to an end as soon as the dynastic and aristocratic quarrel was ended, and the nobles left free to turn their attention to their lapsing feudal rights. It is then that we begin to hear of enclosures, of adding house to house and field to field, of huge sheep-farms with no labourers on the soil, and of deserted villages. Goldsmith meant it of his own time; but Auburn flourishing belonged to the fifteenth century, and Auburn deserted was a common English experience in the time of Henry VIII. It is just because the fifteenth century is bounded on either side by periods of known distress among the commons, and is itself without a history, that one thinks of it as happy; and that view of it is borne out by the economic history which has been laboriously constructed for it.

So much being premised of the country's well-being at large, we may now return to the particular records of epidemics of plague.

Chronology of Plagues in the Fifteenth Century.

With the exception of an undoubted reference to influenza epidemic all over England in 1427 (a year of its prevalence in France also), which I shall postpone to a future chapter, the history down to the arrival of the sweating sickness in 1485, is concerned almost exclusively with notices of plague, and of plague mostly in the towns. It cannot be maintained that rural districts were exempt, or that some great epidemics of plague did not fall on town and country alike. Thus, the St Albans annalist, under the year 1431, has an entry of "pestilence at Codycote and divers places of this domain in this year." Again, in 1439, the Rolls of Parliament contain a petition to the king "how that a sickness called the Pestilence universally through this your realm more commonly reigneth than hath been usual before this time, the which is an infirmity most infective, and the presence of such so infect must be eschewed, as by noble Fisisseanes and wise Philosofors before this time plainly it hath been determined, and as experience daily showeth"—therefore to omit the ceremony of kissing the king in doing knightly

C.   15

service, "and the homage to be as though they kissed you."
That may have been a plague both of town and country during
famine, comparable to the epidemic of 1407, which, as "Walsingham" expressly says, was severely felt in the homes of the
peasantry as well as in London. But plague henceforth is
seldom universal; it becomes more and more a disease of the
towns, and when it does occur in the country, it is for the most
part at some few limited spots. A Paston letter of the years
between 1461 and 1466 gives us a glimpse of the sort of the
incidence of plague in country places, and of the avoidance of
such infected spots, which we shall find often mentioned in the
documents of the sixteenth and seventeenth centuries[1]. There
is, of course, no means of estimating the frequency of plague in
these almost sporadic circumstances. The disease must have
had its seats of election in the country, but we may safely
conclude that these, after the Black Death and the recurrences
thereof down, say, to 1407, were much fewer than in the towns.
One significant piece of evidence comes from the great monastery
of Canterbury. Among its records is an obituary, on twenty
sheets, of all the monks from 1286 to 1517. Out of a hundred
cases taken without selection from the record, there died, of
pestilence, 33; of phthisis, 10; of chronic diseases, 29. "Pestilence" appears to mean specifically bubo-plague; for we
find besides, among the sample hundred, two deaths from
flux, one of these corpses having been buried immediately
propter infexionem. The inference, under correction from
further inquiry, would be that one-third of the deaths in the
monastery of Canterbury during the first half of the reign of
plague in England were from that disease. And that was in a
monastery which, in the Black Death itself, is reported, in the
same record, to have lost "only four" out of a membership of
about eighty[2].

---

[1] *Paston Letters.* Ed. Gairdner, 1872, II. 254: John Wymondham of Fellbrigg
to John Paston, 10th Nov. "And forasmuch as there was a child dead at Asteleys,
and one other like to be dead in the same place, what time I rode out about my little
livelihood, my lady and I both thought pity on my mistress your wife to see her abide
there, and desired her to come to my poor house, unto such time as you should be
otherwise advised."

[2] *Histor. MSS. Commission*, IX. 127 b.

It remains to enumerate briefly the known instances of plague in London or other towns, from the last date given (1420) down to the beginning of the Tudor period (1485). Its prevalence "in England," but more probably in London only, in 1426, comes out in a letter from the Senate of Venice cautioning the captain of the Flanders galleys and the vice-captain of the London galleys[1]. We hear also of that plague in London owing to the fact that certain Scotsmen of rank, hostages for the ransom of the king of Scots, died of the plague in London. An envoy who proceeded to Scotland on 12th March, 1427, was instructed to ask that the dead hostages be replaced by others of equal rank; and if the king of Scots objected on the ground that they had died because they had been kept in places where the late pestilence raged, notwithstanding their request to be removed, the envoy was to say that the hostages had been kept in London, where the dukes of Bedford and Gloucester and all other lords of the Council remained during the time; and that the hostages were "neither pinned nor barred up" in any house, but went at large in the city, and might have taken any measures they pleased for their own preservation. It appears, however, that the council removed from the city, and that the courts were adjourned, at a stage of the epidemic subsequent to the deaths of the Scots. The last plea of the envoy was that, supposing the pestilence had prevailed throughout England, the king was not therefore bound to send the hostages out of England; from which hypothetical construction, we may conclude that the epidemic was special to London—one of a long series requiring the king's Court, the Parliament, and the Law Courts to be adjourned[2].

In 1433, the Parliament which met at Westminster on the 8th July, was prorogued on the 15th August, on account of the *gravis pestilentia* which began to arise in London and the suburbs[3]. A London chronicler enters, under the 12th of Henry VI. (1433) "a grete pestilence and a grete frost," a conjunction that would be interesting if the hard winter had pre-

---

[1] *Calendar of State Papers.* Venetian, vol. I. § 236.
[2] *Proceedings and Ordinances of the Privy Council.* Ed. Nicolas, III. p. xlv.
[3] *Rot. Parl.* IV. 420 b.

ceded¹. The plague revived in London in the following autumn ; for, on the 27th October, 1434, the Privy Council ordered all pleas then pending to be continued from the morrow of All Souls to the octaves of St Hilary on account of the epidemic². After three years, in 1437, the Chief Justice of the Common Pleas paid a visit to St Albans Abbey and remained there some time, "on account of the epidemic plague which was then reigning in the city of London³." Two years after, 1439, comes the entry in the Rolls of Parliament, already quoted, with reference to omitting the ceremony of kissing the king, because "a sickness called the Pestilence universally through this your realm more commonly reigneth than hath been usual before this time, the which is an infirmity most infective⁴." Thus we have in the decade from 1430 to 1440 no fewer than four distinct outbreaks of plague, three of them confined to the city of London, and one of them, that of 1439, general throughout the realm. The last was "a sickness called the pestilence," which should mean the bubo-plague. The year was one of great distress abroad, many thousands having died in Paris. It was a year of famine in Scotland, where the disease was undoubtedly dysentery in part ; but the information from Scotland (given in the sequel) points to the true plague supervening on the other. There was famine in England at the time when it was in France and in Scotland, so that the type of sickness may have been, in England also, fever and dysentery first and plague afterwards.

In 1444, on the 5th of June, the Rolls contain the entry that grave pestilence began to arise. A severe pestilence is reported at Oxford in 1448⁵. On the 30th May, 1449, Parliament is

---

¹ *Arnold's Chronicle*, p. xxxii.

² *Proc. and Ord. Privy Council*, IV. p. lxxx. Sir Harris Nicolas, in this con-nexion, remarks that Fabyan and all other chroniclers (he had overlooked Arnold) omit to mention pestilence, while they mention much less important things; but he is hardly warranted in his inference that plagues were so common-place as to be left unrecorded. A low level of plague would not be noticed, but a great epidemic certainly would.

³ Johannes Amundesham (of St Albans), *Annales*. Rolls ed. II. 127.

⁴ *Rot. Parl.* v. 31 b.

⁵ This is the only plague in the first half of the fifteenth century that Anthony Wood records; but he says, under the year 1500, that "no less than about thirty

adjourned to Winchester to avoid "the corrupt and infected airs" of Westminster. On the 6th November of the same year it adjourns to Ludgate, in the city of London, owing to the infection of the air in Westminster. The infected state of Westminster and other places around is again the subject of an entry on the 4th December, with this addition: "it has been sufficiently decreed as to avoiding and extinguishing the said corrupt and infectious air." About three months later, on 30th March, 1450, Parliament adjourns to Leicester on account of the insalubrity of the air at Westminster. In 1452 it adjourns on 20th November to Reading for the same reason, but is soon after adjourned to the 11th February, owing to plague in Reading itself:—"de magna mortalitate in dicta villa de Redyng jam regnante." These years must have been a really severe plague-period, for we find in 1454, a reference in the Paston Letters to the alarm caused by the plague in London. Wm. Paston writes to John Paston, 6 September: "Sergeant-at-law Billing came to London this week. He sent for me and asked me how I fared. I told him, here is pestilence, and said I fared the better he was in good hele, for it was noised that he was dead...Here is great pestilence. I purpose to flee into the country[1]."

From 1454 (and the year following in Scotland) there is a clear interval of ten years without mention of plague in the not very complete records of the time. With the year 1464 there began a series of outbreaks of plague which appear to have lasted in one part of the country or another with few intermissions until 1478. This plague-period is said to have been foretold in a remarkable prophecy. In the year 1462 a boy at Cambridge, while walking in a lane between King's College and the adjoining buildings of Clare and Trinity Halls, met an old man with a long beard, who addressed him thus: "Go now and tell to anyone that within these two years there will be such pestilence, and famine, and slaughter of men, as no one living has seen." Having said this he disappeared. Doubts

pests, both great and small, happened in this last century"—i.e. in the University of Oxford. I shall speak of their general effects in another chapter.

[1] *Paston Letters.* Ed. Gairdner, 1872, I. 302–3.

however, were at once thrown on the reality of these words; for the boy, on being questioned by Master Myleton, doctor of theology, and others, said that he neither saw the old man walking on the ground nor heard him speak[1].

The authentic intelligence of plague in England in 1464 is contained in a letter to the Seignory of Venice from Bruges, dated 5th October, 1464, to the effect that some Venetian merchants have arrived from London, which they had quitted on the 26th September. They say the plague is at work there at the rate of two hundred [deaths] per diem, "and thus writes [also] Carlo Ziglio." In April next year, 1465, we hear of it still in London, through a casual reference in a letter written by one of the Paston family[2]; and as prevailing all over England, through a formal entry in the chronicle of Croyland, the last of the monastic records which continued to be kept. There was an infection of the air, we read, in the whole of England, so that many thousands of people of every age came to their death suddenly, like sheep slaughtered[3].

The very next year, 1466, Parliament is adjourned from Westminster on account of the infection in London, to meet at Reading. Next summer, 1st July, 1467, there is another adjournment to Reading (6 November), because of the heat and because the plague was beginning to reign, by which certain members of the House of Commons had been cut off. After an interval of four years we hear of plague, in a Paston letter, and by a Southwell record. On 2 August, 1471, the residentiary canons of Southwell Minster vote themselves leave of absence for a month "quia regnat morbus pestiferus in villa Southwell, et furit excessivé morbus pestiferus[4]." On 13 September, 1471, Sir John Paston writes from near Winchester: "I cannot hear by

---

[1] *Three Fifteenth Century Chronicles.* Ed. Gairdner, for the Camden Society, 1880, from the Lambeth MSS., p. 163.

[2] Sir J. Paston to John Paston, 30 April, 1465. Another letter, of 18th August, has: "For the pestilence is so fervent in Norwych, that they dare no longer abyde there, so God help!" (*Paston Letters*, ed. Gairdner, II. 226), which probably refers to 1465 also. It is not mentioned by Blomefield.

[3] *Chronicle of Croyland*, in Gale, I. 541.

[4] Communicated to me by the Rev. W. Hunt, from a new volume of the Camden Society, edited by A. F. Leach, *Visitations and Memorials of Southwell Minster*, p. 11.

pilgrims that pass the country, nor none other man that rideth or goeth any country, that any borough town in England is free from that sickness. God cease it when it please him!" Apart from London the English town which has the most disastrous record for this period is Hull[1]. The plague was so severe there, in three epidemics close together, as almost to ruin the place. It broke out in 1472, and had swept off a great number of the inhabitants before the end of the year, including the mayor. In 1476 it broke out afresh, causing a great mortality. In 1478 it was more violent than ever, the number of its victims being given as 1580, including the mayor and all his family ; the people fled the town, the church was shut up, and the streets deserted and grass-grown. The epidemic appears to have been, as usual, an autumnal one, ceasing at the approach of winter. Meanwhile, in 1474, there is mention of a serious prevalence of plague in the Royal household, as well as elsewhere in London. The weather of the previous autumn, 1473, had been remarkable. Labourers are said to have died in the harvest-field from the excessive heat, and "fervues, axes, and the bloody flyx" (fevers, agues, and dysentery) to have been universal in divers parts of England ; but there was no dearth. The unusual character of that season, or of the season preceding, was indicated by the bursting forth of underground reservoirs of water[2].

The great plague of this period in London should most probably be placed under the years 1478–9. Merely to show the difficulties of the chronology it may be worth while citing the various accounts. The Greyfriars' Chronicle says, under the year 17 Edward IV., that the term was "deferred from Ester to Michaelmas because of the grete pestylens[3]." The 17th of Edward IV. was 1477. But Fabyan, who was now a citizen of London (afterwards sheriff and alderman), enters it under the civic year 1478–79, or the year which begins for him with the new lord mayor taking office on 30 October. His words are: "This year was great mortality and death in London and many other parts of this realm, the which began in the latter end of

---

[1] Tickell, *History of Kingston upon Hull*, 1798.

[2] *Warkworth's Chronicle.* Camden Society, p. 23 (under the year 13 Ed. IV.).

[3] *Chronicle of the Greyfriars.* Camden Society, No. 53, 1852, p. 22.

Senii [September] in the preceding year and continued in this year till the beginning of November, in the which passed time died innumerable people in the said city and many places elsewhere[1]." Grafton says, under the year 1478, that the chief mortality fell in four months of great heat, during which the pestilence was so fierce and quick that fifteen years' war had not consumed a third as many people[2]. To reconcile these dates we should have to take the year of the Greyfriars' Chronicle as 1478, so that the adjournment of the term from Easter to Michaelmas, might suit the four months in Grafton. At the same time, Fabyan's statement that the plague " continued in this year till November," is correct for 1479. Sir John Paston writes home from London, 29 Oct. 1479, of his danger from the sickness; he died there on 15th November; and his brother, who came up from Norfolk to bury him, writes to his mother, who wished him "to haste out of the air that he was in," that the sickness is " well ceased " in December.

The year 1478, the first of two plague-seasons in London, was also a year of plague at Hull, and at Newcastle and Southwell. The account for Newcastle, in its annals under 1478, is merely that great numbers died of the plague[3]. At Southwell, on 5 July, 1478, the canons residentiary again take leave of absence for the summer, " because it may be probably estimated that the dire pestilential affliction in the town of Southwell will continue, and because the venerable men, with their domestics, have a just fear of incurring the infection of the said pestiferous affliction[4]." Next year, 1479, an " incredible number " died of plague at Norwich[5], and at villages like Swainsthorp, where "they have died and been sick nigh in every house[6]."

Thus in two years, 1478–79, we hear of an epidemic of plague of the first rank in London, an epidemic most severe for the size of the place, at Hull, and epidemics at Southwell, Newcastle and Norwich. This is not unlike the plague-years that we often find in the centuries following. Whether it be that we

---

[1] Robert Fabyan's *Chronicle of England*, (editions in 1516 and 1533, and by Ellis, 1808), *sub anno.*   [2] *Grafton's Chronicle*, p. 742.
[3] Brand's *History of Newcastle.*   [4] *Visitations and Memorials*, p. 41.
[5] Blomefield.   [6] Paston, 6 Nov. 1479.

are merely coming to a time of better records, or that the disease itself was getting worse in English towns, these later years of Edward IV. are comparable to plague-periods under the Tudors and the Stuarts.

The period from the Black Death of 1349 to the reign of Edward IV. witnesses a considerable change in the habits, so to speak, of plague in England. In the earlier part of that period, the epidemics of "pestilence"—although they were not all of plague or wholly of plague—are general throughout England, like the great mortality itself but on a smaller scale. As late as 1407, or perhaps 1439, we still hear of "the disease called the pestilence" being universal and in the homes of the peasantry. The extent of the sickness in 1465, or even the type of it, is not sufficiently known. From that time onwards town and country are contrasted in the matter of plague ; it becomes usual to flee to the country so as to escape the pestilential air in town in the summer heats, and the unwholesomeness of the London air becomes on numerous occasions a real reason, or a pretext, for the adjournment of Parliament. All the while, the plague was the lineal descendant of the Black Death,—a virus so potent on its first entry into English soil as to overrun every parish of the land.

Plague and other pestilences in Scotland and Ireland, 1349–1475.

The materials for the history of plague in Scotland, including the Black Death and subsequent outbreaks down to the end of the medieval period, are much fewer than for England. From the English chroniclers (Knighton and Le Baker) we learn that the Black Death in the autumn of 1349 extended from the northern counties to the Scots army in the Forest of Selkirk. According to Fordoun, plague would have been general in Scotland in 1350; but as he includes in his reference "several years before and after" and "divers parts of the world," his statement that nearly a third part of the human race paid the debt of nature is perhaps a mere echo of the general estimate and without reference specially to Scotland[1]. His next general

---

[1] Fordoun, *Scotichronicon*, ed. Hearne, Oxon. 1722, p. 1039.

reference to pestilence is under the year 1362, when the same kind of disease and the same extent of mortality as in 1350 occurred throughout all Scotland[1]. But as he says elsewhere that the visit of David, king of Scots, to Aberdeenshire in 1361, when he took Kildrummy Castle from the earl of Mar, was determined in the first instance by the prevalence of plague in the southern part of his kingdom[2], it may be inferred that the epidemic had begun late in that year in the south, coincident with the *pestis secunda* of England, and had been interrupted by the coming on of winter, as in the first epidemic of 1349 and 1350. The next mortality recorded by Fordoun he names the fourth (*quarta mortalitas*) and assigns to 1401[3]. The question arises as to the third; and it appears that there were indeed two plague-years in Scotland between 1362 and 1401—namely, 1380 and 1392, both of them corresponding nearly to great plagues in the north of England. In the former year sir John Lyon, lord of Glamis, was unable to hold his court as auditor of the exchequer in certain places owing to the plague[4]. In 1392, also, the custumars of Haddington, Peebles, and Dumbarton did not attend the "chamberlain ayres" on account of the pestilence[5]. In 1402 (not in 1401, as Fordoun has it), the custumars of Stirling were absent from the audit by reason of the plague[6]; and in the same financial year (10 July, 1402, to 18 July, 1403), only one bailie from Dundee attended the audit at Perth, the others being dead in the pestilence[7].

For a whole generation there is no documentary evidence of plague in Scotland. But Fordoun has two entries of a disease which he calls *pestilentia volatilis*—it can hardly have been plague and may have been influenza—the one in 1430, having begun at Edinburgh in February, and the other in 1432 at Haddington[8].

Under the year 1439, an old chronicle, *Ane Addicioun of*

---

[1] *Scotichronicon*, p. 1056: "eadem...sicut prius jubileo...in toto regno Scotiae mirabiliter saeviebat."

[2] *Exchequer Rolls of Scotland.* Introduction to vol. II. p. xlviii.

[3] *Scotichronicon*, p. 1141.

[4] *Exchequer Rolls of Scotland*, III. 650.

[5] *Ibid.* III. 310. [6] *Ibid.* III. 553.

[7] *Ibid.* III. 579. [8] *Scotichronicon*, p. 1287 and p. 1298.

Scottis Cornicklis and Deidis records one of those seasons of famine and dysentery or lientery, with some more sudden sickness, which have been described for England in a former chapter. " The samen time there was in Scotland a great dearth, for the boll of wheat was at 40*s*., and the boll of ait meal 30*s*.; and verily the dearth was sae great that there died a passing [number of] people for hunger. And als the land-ill, the wame-ill, was so violent, that there died mae that year than ever there died, owther in pestilence, or yet in ony other sickness in Scotland. And that samen year the pestilence came in Scotland, and began at Dumfries, and it was callit the *Pestilence but Mercy*, for there took it nane that ever recoverit, but they died within twenty-four hours[1]." Here the " land-ill " or " wame-ill " (dysentery or lientery) is contrasted within " the pestilence," which latter is said to have supervened the same year, beginning at Dumfries and proving peculiarly deadly. This was a year of plague, said to be "universal," in England (where famine also was severe), and of an enormous mortality in France.

The continuator of Fordoun records under the year 1455 (James II.) a great pestilential mortality of men through the whole kingdom, an epidemic which would be again a year behind the corresponding plague in England[2]. We hear of it next definitely in the year 1475, which falls within the series of plague-years at Hull, and elsewhere in the southern part of the island. On account of an outbreak of pestilence the king of Scots adjourned the meeting of the estates from September 1475 to the Epiphany following[3], when the Parliament actually met. The same year there was a plague-hospital on Inchkeith, in the Firth of Forth, and not for the first time ; ten marts from the Orkneys were landed there for the quarantined patients[4].

---

[1] Cited by R. Chambers (*Domestic Annals of Scotland*, I. 57) from the Chronicle as printed by Thomas Thomson.

[2] *Scotichronicon*, p. 1565. Hearne's edition.

[3] Ferrerius, f. 393, cited in *Excheq. Rolls of Scot.* VIII. p. lx.

[4] *Excheq. Rolls of Scot.* VIII. 364. Accounts of William, bishop of Orkney, from 5 Aug. 1475 to 3 Aug. 1476: "et decem martis liberatis, de tempore pestis, egrotantibus in Incheskeith." Another item (£30. 13*s*. 4*d*.) is for forty-six marts destroyed "propter longam moram" in the lairs at Leith, "anno pestis, videlicet anno ultimo."

The references to plague in Scotland begin again about the year 1498; but these, according to the division of our subject, will come into another chapter.

The references to plagues in Ireland after the invasion of 1349 are extremely meagre; but they make it probable that outbursts of bubo-plague recurred at intervals, as well as occasional epidemics of flux and other diseases brought on by scarcity or bad corn. The continuators of Clyn's Kilkenny annals enumerate various *pestes—secunda, tertia, quarta* and *quinta*—just as the English annalists do. The *secunda* falls in 1362, its season in Scotland also[1]. The *tertia* is given under 1373; but also under 1370[2]. The *quarta* is in 1382 (or 1385), and the *quinta* in 1391. But there is little or no independent evidence that this chronology, originally made for England, is really good for Ireland also. The only other entry, until the Tudor period, is "fames magna in Hibernia" in 1410[3].

---

[1] But MS. annals are cited for the date 1361, in *The ancient and present State of the County and City of Cork.* By Charles Smith, M.D. 2 vols. Dublin, 1774. 2nd ed. II. p. 23.

[2] Thady Dowling [Elizabethan] "1370. Pestilentia magna in Hibernia, adeo quod propter immensitatem mortalitatis vocabatur ab antiquis tertia," p. 24.

[3] Dowling, p. 27.

CHAPTER V.

THE SWEATING SICKNESS.

THE strange disease which came to be known all over Europe as *sudor Anglicus*, or the English Sweat, was a new type or species of infection first seen in the autumn of 1485. Polydore Virgil, an Italian scholar and man of affairs, who arrived in England in 1501, became, in effect, the court historian of Henry VII.'s reign, and of the events which led up to the overthrow of Richard III. at Bosworth Field on the 22nd of August 1485; his account of the movements of Henry Tudor, from his landing at Milford Haven on Saturday the 6th of August until his triumphal entry into London on Saturday the 27th of the same month, is so minute that he must be assumed to have had access to journals written at the time. Polydore's account of the sweat begins with the statement that it showed itself on the first descent of Henry upon the island —*sub primum descensum in insulam*[1]. The last continuator of the ancient chronicle of Croyland abbey, who was still making his entries when Bosworth Field was fought, not far from Croyland, and who closed his annals the year after, records an incident which seems to show that the sweat had been prevalent before the battle. Thomas, lord Stanley, lay at Atherstone, not far from Bosworth, with five thousand men nominally in the service of Richard, and was summoned by the king to bring up his force before the battle. He excused himself, says the Croyland

---

[1] *Angl. Hist.* Basil. 1555, p. 567.

annalist, on the ground that he was suffering from the sweating
sickness[1]. I shall examine that evidence, and the general
statement of Polydore Virgil, in a later part of this chapter.
Meanwhile we may take it that the outbreak of the sweat was
somehow associated in popular rumour with the victorious
expedition of Henry Tudor. Writers on the English sweat
hitherto have had to depend on the somewhat meagre and not
always consistent statements of annalists for their knowledge
of its first authentic occurrence. I am now able to adduce
the testimony of a manuscript treatise on the new epidemic,
written by a physician while it was still prevalent in London,
and elaborately dedicated to Henry VII., if not composed by
his order[2]. The author is Thomas Forrestier, styled in the title
a Doctor of Medicine and a native of Normandy, tarrying in
London. Whatever his relation with the Tudor court may have
been, his name does not occur in the patents as one of the king's
physicians. It appears, indeed, that he had got into trouble in
London some two years after this date; for, on the 28th of
January, 1488, the king granted to him a general pardon, "with
pardon for all escapes and evasions out of the Tower of London
or elsewhere, and remissions of forfeiture of all lands and goods[3]."
Probably he went back after this to his native Normandy: at
all events, he is next heard of in practice at Rouen, where he
published, in 1490, a Latin treatise on the plague, one of the
first productions of the printing-press of that city.

It is in the opening sentences of his printed book on the
plague[4], and not in his manuscript on the sweat, that he fixes
the date when the latter began. The sweating sickness, he says,

---

[1] In Gale, *Script. Angl.* I. 573.

[2] British Museum Addit. MS., No. 27,582.

[3] *Materials illustrative of the Reign of Henry VII.* Rolls series, No. 60, s. d.

[4] *Tractatus contra pestilentiam thenasmonem et dissinteriam* [Rouen, 1490]:—
"Causae pestilentiae ut alias scripsimus: in quodam opusculo quod composuimus de
quadam rabiosa febre pestilentiali, quae in duodecim horis patientes cum calore et
sudore continuo interficiebat. Cujus febris adventus incepit sua vexilla extendere in
Anglia in civitate Londoniarum decima nova die mensis Septembris 1485, in qua die
[planetary signs] posuerunt. Ex qua febre pestilentiali plus quam quindecim millia
hominum ab hoc seculo morte repentina, tanquam ex pugnitione divina, recesserunt,
multique sine mora per vicos deambulantes absque confessione obierunt."

first unfurled its banners in England in the city of London, on the 19th of September, 1485; and then follow in the text certain astrological signs, representing the positions or conjunctions of heavenly bodies on that date. The London chronicles of the time assign dates for the beginning of the epidemic which differ somewhat from Dr Forrestier's. One of them, a manuscript of the Cotton collection, by an anonymous citizen of London, records the entry of Henry VII. into the capital on the 27th of August, and proceeds: "And the XXVII day of September began the sweating syknes in London, whereof died Thomas Hyll that yer mayor, for whom was chosen sir William Stokker, knyght, which died within V days after of the same disease. Then for him was chosen John Warde...And this yere died of that sickness, besides ii mayors above rehersed, John Stokker, Thomas Breten, Richard Pawson, Thomas Norland, aldermen, and many worshipful commoners[1]." In the better known but not always equally full chronicle of Fabyan, who was then a citizen, and afterwards sheriff and alderman, the date of Henry's reception by the mayor and citizens at Hornsey Park is given as the 28th of August, the reference to the sweat being as follows: "And upon the XI day of Octobre next following, than beynge the swetynge sykeness of newe begun, dyed the same Thomas Hylle, mayor, and for him was chosen sir William Stokker, knyght and draper, which dyed also of the sayd sickness shortly after." The only other particular date extant for the sweat of 1485 comes from the country: Lambert Fosse-dike, abbot of Croyland, died there of the sweating sickness, after an illness of eighteen hours, on the 14th of October[2].

Apart from the hitherto unknown manuscript of Forrestier, these are the only contemporary references. Stow, who must have had access to some journal of the time, says that the king

---

[1] MSS. Cotton. Vitellius A. XVI. *A Chronicle of England from 1st Henry III. to 1st Hen. VIII.*

[2] The Croyland Chronicle (in Gale's *Script. Angl.* I. 570 and 576) gives the 14th November in one place and the 14th October in another. But it is clear that the latter is the correct date, the letter from the prior of Croyland to Henry VII., announcing the death of the abbot and praying for a *congé d'élire*, being dated the 14th of October. (*Materials illustrative of the Reign of Henry VII.* vol. I. s.d. 21 Oct. 1485, Rolls series, No. 60.)

entered London on the 27th August and that "the sweating began the 21st September, and continued till the end of October, of the which a wonderful number died," including the two mayors and four other aldermen, as above. Hall's chronicle, which has been the principal source used by Hecker and others, reproduces the account of the sweat by Polydore Virgil almost word for word; and Polydore's account was certainly not begun until after 1504 and was not published until 1531. Bernard André, historiographer and poet laureate of Henry VII., was present at the entry into London on the 27th August; but he gives no particulars of the sweat of that autumn, in his 'Life of Henry VII.,' although it is probable that his 'Annals of Henry VII.' would have furnished some information had they not been lost for the year 1485, as it is to his extant annals for the year 1508 that we owe almost all that is known of the second epidemic of the sweat in that year. The state papers of the time do not contain a single reference to the epidemic, although it was so active in the city of London as to carry off two mayors and four aldermen within a few days, and was besides, as Polydore Virgil says, "a new kind of disease, from which no former age had suffered, as all agree." London was full of people, including some who had stood by Henry Tudor in France, others who had joined his standard in Wales, and still others who came to do homage to the new dynasty; and there is evidence remaining of hundreds of suitors, great and small, attending the court to receive the reward of their services in patents and grants, as well as evidence in the wardrobe accounts of the bustle of preparing for the Coronation on the 30th of October. But in all the extant state records of those busy weeks, there is not a scrap of writing to show that such a thing as a pestilence was raging within the narrow bounds of the city and under the walls of the royal palace in the Tower. It remains, therefore, to make what we can out of the medical essay which Dr Forrestier wrote for the occasion.

In his later reference of 1490, he says that more than fifteen thousand were cut off in sudden death, as if by the visitation of God, many dying while walking in the streets, without warning and without being confessed. That number of the dead need not be taken as at all exact: nor does it appear whether it is meant for London or for the whole country. But the dramatic suddenness of the attack is illustrated by particular cases in his original treatise of 1485, although deaths so sudden are unheard of in any infection :—

"We saw two prestys standing togeder and speaking togeder, and we saw both of them dye sodenly. Also in die — proximi we se the wyf of a taylour taken and sodenly dyed. Another yonge man walking by the street fell down sodenly. Also another gentylman ryding out of the cyte [date given] dyed. Also many others the which were long to rehearse we have known that have dyed sodenly." Gentlemen and gentlewomen, priests, righteous men, merchants, rich and poor, were among the victims of this sudden death. Of the symptoms he says : "And this sickness cometh with a grete swetyng and stynkyng, with rednesse of the face and of all the body, and a contynual thurst, with a grete hete and hedache because of the fumes and venoms." He mentions also "pricking the brains," and that "some appear red and yellow, as we have seen many, and in two grete ladies that we saw, the which were sick in all their bodies and they felt grete pricking in their bodies. And some had black spots, as it appeared in our frere (?) Alban, a noble leech on whose soul God have mercy !"

Both in his pathology and in his copious appendix of formulae he directs attention to the heart, as the organ that was suddenly overpowered by the pestilential venoms. Many died, he would have us believe, because they listened to the false leeches, who professed to know the disease and to have treated it before. A considerable part of his space is occupied with the denunciation of these irregular practitioners, their greed and their ignorance,—a theme which is a common one in the prefaces of Elizabethan medical works also. It appears that the false leeches wrote and put letters upon gates and church doors, or upon poles, promising to help the people in their sickness. They were also injudicious in the choice of their remedies—some ordaining powders and medicines that are hot until the thirtieth degree and over, others ale or wine, or hot spices, "and many other medicines they have, the which, the best of them, is nothing worth." These false leeches knew not the causes,— their complexions, their ages, the regions, the times of the year, the climate,—evidently the astrological lore which gave Chaucer's physician, a century earlier, his academical standing or his

C.   16

superiority to the vulgar quacks of his day. Those who fell into the hands of quacks, Forrestier implies, had an indifferent chance. Many died for want of help and good guiding; whereas many a one was healed that had received a medicine in due order, "and if he purge himself before." The clearly written and fully detailed formulae at the end of his essay are so far evidence that Forrestier did not traffic in secret remedies. The first part of the essay is occupied with the doctrine of causes— the nigh causes and the far. The far causes were astrological; but the nigh causes, although they are altogether inadequate to account for sweating sickness as a special type, and are indeed little else than the stock list of nuisances quoted in earlier treatises upon the plague, are suggestive enough of the condition of London streets and houses at the time, and will be referred to in a later part of the chapter.

The account of the treatment given by Polydore Virgil, and from him copied into Hall's chronicle, is probably the experience of later epidemics of the sweat, although it comes into the history under the year 1485. The evil effects of throwing off the bed-clothes, and of drinking great draughts of cold water, and, on the other hand, the benefits of lying still with the hands and feet well covered, are among the topics discussed in letters during the epidemic of 1517, one of those which came within the historian's own experience in England. But it is clear from Forrestier's essay of 1485 that there were great differences in the regimen of patients in the sweat during its very first season, some adopting the hot and cordial treatment, others, perhaps, the cooling, just as in the smallpox long after. Bernard André implies that there was a correct and an incorrect regimen also in the second epidemic of 1508, and there is evidence of conflicting advice in the letters on the sweats of 1517 and 1528. If there were any better regimen in the later epidemics than in the earlier, as Polydore Virgil says there was, it was merely the wisdom of avoiding extremes. Hence the misleading character of his remark that, after an immense loss of life, "a remedy was found, ready to hand for everyone." Bacon in his 'Reign of Henry VII.' took from Polydore almost word for word all that he says of the "remedy" of the sweat; and the unreal word-spinning thus begun was carried to its full development by bishop Sprat, the historian of the Royal Society (1667), who mistakes the "remedy" for some *arcanum* or potent drug, gives my lord Verulam the credit of preserving the prescription for the use of posterity, and adduces it as an encouragement to the Royal Society to seek among the secrets of nature for an equally efficacious "antidote" to the plague.

The language of historians is that the sweat of 1485 spread over the whole kingdom. We hear of it definitely at Oxford[1] where it "lasted but a month or six weeks" and is said to have cut off many of the scholars before they could disperse. It is heard of also with equal definiteness at Croyland abbey. There is also mention of it in a contemporary calendar of the mayor of Bristol, but without any special reference to that city[2]. Beyond these notices, there appears to be nothing to show that the sweat went all through England in the late autumn or early winter of 1485. But we may take the following passage by Forrestier, in the dedication of his tract to the king, as expressing the state of matters, with perhaps some exaggeration:

"When that thy highness and thy great power is vexed and troubled with divers sickness, and thy lordships and almost the middle part of thy realm with the venomous fever of pestilence, and, by the reason of that, young and old and of all manner of ages, with divers wailings and sadness they are stricken: therefore, excellent and noble prince, we are moved with every love and duty, and not for no lucre neither covetyse, to ordain a short governing against this foresaid fever[3]."

The Second Sweat in 1508.

After the first outburst of the sweat in 1485 had subsided, probably before winter was well begun, nothing more is heard of it for twenty-three years. It reappeared in 1508, a third time in 1517, a fourth time in 1528, and for the last time in 1551.

---

[1] Anthony Wood, I. 462.

[2] *The Maire of Bristowe is Kalendar* (by Robert Ricart, town-clerk of Bristol, 18 Ed. IV.). Camden Society, 1872, p. 46.

[3] The Bristol calendar says: "This yere Hary, Erle of Richmond landed at Milford Haven...And sone after there was a sodeyn sikenes in all places of Englond called the sweting syknes, whereof moche people dyed."

With each successive outbreak, our information becomes less meagre, while the epidemic of 1551 actually called forth an English printed book by Dr Caius, the epidemic of 1528 having called forth a whole crop of foreign writings on its spreading to the continent (for the first and only time) in the year following (1529). As the nature, causes, and favouring circumstances of the sweat cannot profitably be dealt with except on a review of its whole history, it will be necessary to take up at once and together the four subsequent epidemics of it in this country, leaving the intercurrent and probably much more disastrous epidemics of bubo-plague, during the same period, as well as the great invasion of syphilis in 1494–6, to be chronicled apart.

Our knowledge of the second outbreak of the sweat, in 1508[1], comes almost exclusively from Bernard André, whose *Annals of Henry VII.*[2] are fortunately preserved for that year (as they are also for 1504–5). Under the date of July, 1508, he says that some of the household of the Lord Treasurer were seized with the sweat, and died of it, "and everywhere in this city there die not a few." In August public prayers were made at St Paul's on account of the plague of sweat. In the same month the king's movements from place to place in the country round London are described as determined by the prevalence of the sweat. From Hatfield, whither he had gone to visit his mother on the 9th August, he went to Wanstead, where certain of his household "sweated;" on that account the king moved to Barking, and thence to other places about the 14th. He avoided Greenwich and Eltham, in both which places the chief personages of the royal palaces "had sweated," so much did the sickness then rage in all places (*per omnia loca*). Some of the king's personal attendants appear to have caught the infection; nor did it avail, says André, to run away or to follow the chase, *quoniam mors omnia vincit.* Other visits were paid down to the 17th August, and a strict edict was issued that no one from London

---

[1] The date of 1506 in Hecker is erroneous, having been taken from the very loose entry in Hall's chronicle (copied by Grafton), which might equally well belong to the year 1507. Bernard André's date of 1508 is unmistakeable; his annals go on continuously until the death of Henry VII. in April following.

[2] Bernard André's *Works.* Rolls series, No. 10, pp. 126–8.

was to come near the court, nor anyone to repair to the city, under penalties specified. The only one near the king's person who died of it was lord Graystock, a young Cumberland noble. The Lord Privy Seal and the Lord Chamberlain were both attacked but recovered; doctor Symeon, the dean of the Chapel Royal, died of it. There appears to have been a good deal of the sickness in various places, but many recovered, says André, with good tending. The king occupied himself with hunting the stag in the forests at Stratford, Eltham and other places round London.

From the provinces there is one item of information relating to Chester[1]: in the summer of 1507, it is said, the sweating sickness destroyed 91 in three days, of whom only four were women. At Oxford in 1508, or the year before Henry VII.'s death, there was a sore pestilence which caused the dispersion of divers students; but it is not called the sweat[2].

The Third Sweat in 1517.

Except for a single reference to the sweat in 1511, nothing is heard of it between the autumn of 1508 and the summer of 1517. The reference in 1511 occurs in a letter of Erasmus, from Queens' College, Cambridge, dated 25th August, in which he says that his health is still indifferent *a sudore illo*. This may possibly refer to the lingering effects of an attack in 1508, or to the influenza of 1510; and as all the other references in 1511 are to plague, and to alarms of plague, it may be doubted if the sweating sickness had really been prevalent in England in that year, or at any time between 1508 and 1517. We begin to hear of it definitely in the summer of the latter year. We have now reached a period from which numerous letters, despatches and other state papers have come down[3]. Among the most useful of

---

[1] Hemingway's *History of Chester*, I. 142.

[2] Anthony Wood's *History and Antiquities of the Univ. of Oxford.* I. 665.

[3] Calendared for the Rolls series by Brewer for the greater part of the reign of Henry VIII. (1509–1530), and after him by Gairdner, at present as far as 1538. The facts given in the next few pages may be taken as coming from the Calendar of State Papers, under their respective dates, unless it is otherwise stated in the notes

these for our purpose are the despatches of the Venetian ambassador and the apostolic nuncio from London, the letters of Pace to Wolsey when Henry VIII. was in the country and the cardinal not with him, the letters of Erasmus, sir Thomas More and others.

The first that we hear of sickness in London in 1517 is from a letter of the 24th June, written by a cardinal of Arragon to Wolsey, from Calais ; the cardinal, who was travelling like a noble, with a train of forty horses, had intended to visit London, but was waiting on the other side owing to a rumour that the sickness was prevalent in London. It is probable that this rumour had referred to the standing infection of English towns in summer and autumn, the bubo-plague ; for it is not until five weeks later that we hear of the sweating sickness under its proper name.

On the 1st of August the nuncio writes from London to the marquis of Mantua that a disease is broken out here causing sudden death within six hours ; it is called the sweating sickness; an immense number die of it.   On the 6th of August he occupies the greater part of a letter of three pages with an account of it. To some it proved fatal in twelve hours, to others in six, and to others in four ; it is an easy death.   Most patients are seized when lying down, but some when on foot, and even a very few when riding out.   The attack lasts about twenty-four hours, more or less.   It is fatal to take, during the fit, any cold drink, or to allow a draught of air to reach the drenching skin ; the covering should be rather more ample than usual, but there was danger in heaping too many bed-clothes on the patient.   A moderate fire should be kept up in the sick chamber ; the arms should be crossed on the patient's breast, and great care should be taken that no cold air reached the armpits[1].   The disease was on the increase, and was already spreading over England ;

---

[1] This appears to have been a common direction.   In a letter of 12 August, 1517, dated from the Fleet Prison by Thomas Leeke to his brother sir John Leeke (*Hist. MSS. Commission Reports*, X. pt. 4, p. 447), the writer says he has been sore vexed with the sweat and in danger of life : "If any of you have it, pray you to keep well and close about your breasts and your heart for twenty-four hours and then with God's grace there is no danger in it: there has been a marvellous great death for so short a time."

it was reported that more than four hundred students had died of it at Oxford, which was a small place but for the university there. Burials were occurring on every side; there had been many deaths in the king's household and in that of cardinal Wolsey, who was in the country "sweating." Such is the universal dread of the disease that there are very few who do not fear for their lives, while some are so terrified that they suffer more from fear than others do from the sweat itself.

On the same day (6th August), the Venetian ambassador, Sebastian Giustinian, who was on friendly terms with the nuncio and often indebted to him for information, writes to the Doge giving much the same account of "the new malady." He remarks upon the sudden onset, the rapidity of the issue when it was to be fatal, and the cessation of the sweat within twenty-four hours. His secretary had taken it, as well as many of his domestics. Few strangers are dead, but an immense number of Englishmen. On going to visit Wolsey, he found that he had the sweat; many of the cardinal's household had died of it, including some of his chief attendants; the bishop of Winchester also had taken it. On the 12th of August, the Venetian envoy writes that he himself and his son have had the sweat; Wolsey has had it three times in a few days, many of his people being dead of it, especially his gentlemen[1]. In London "omnes silent."

Wolsey's attack and relapses are confirmed by his own letter to the king; about the end of August he went on a pilgrimage to Walsingham, and remained there most of September, but even after his return he was "vexed with fever." The relapses of the sweat, which are mentioned by Forrestier in 1485, by André in 1508, and now again in 1517, may have been the origin of the saying in the form of a proverb, which occurs in

---

[1] In the letter of 12 August from the Fleet Prison, already quoted (*Hist. MSS. Reports, l.c.*), it is stated that fifteen are dead in the Cardinal's house, including Mr Cowper, the steward, Talboys, lord of Kyme, young Wastness, and one Grenell. In my lord of Durham's house, Dr Port and Dr Fysche are dead, with divers others. Of the Court, my lord Clinton, Mr Morgan, steward to the Queen, and one Mat. Jones, of the King's wardrobe, were buried at Richmond on Friday last, and divers more of the Court are dead.

an essay of the time by sir Thomas More,—that the relapse is worse than the original disease[1].

The death of a well-known personage, Ammonio, the Latin secretary of the king, is the subject of several letters, including one of the 19th August from More to Erasmus; he died at nine on the morning of the 17th August, after an illness of twenty hours: he had been congratulating himself on being safe by reason of his temperate life. More confirms the statement as to deaths in the university of Oxford, and he adds also at Cambridge. In London the sweat attacks whole families: "I assure you there is less danger in the ranks of war than in this city." His own family (? in Bucklersbury) are safe so far, and he has composed his mind for any eventuality. He hears that the sweat is now at Calais. On the 27th August, the Venetian envoy writes again that the disease is now making great progress; the king keeps out of the way at Windsor, with only three favourite gentlemen and Dionysius Memo, who is described as his physician, but in other letters as "the Reverend," and as a musician from Venice. On the 21st September the envoy has gone to the country to avoid "the plague *and* the sweating sickness." A few days later (26th Sept.) he writes that "the plague" is making some progress, and that the prolonged absence of the king, the cardinal and other lords from London owing to the sweat, had encouraged the citizens to a turbulent mood against .the foreign traders and residents; the state of matters was so threatening that three thousand citizens were under arms to preserve the peace. The references after September, 1517, are mostly to the "common infection" or plague, which was an almost annual autumnal event in London. There was probably some confusion, at the time, between that infection and the sweat, not, of course as regards symptoms, but in common report; thus it is not clear whether the fresh alarm in the king's court at or near Windsor on the 15th October, owing to the deaths of young lord Grey de Wilton and a German attendant of the king, refers to the sweat or to the plague. As late as the 2nd November, a letter from the

---

[1] *The Pitiful Life of King Edward the Fifth:* "Considering there is, as physicians say, and as we also find, double the peril in the relapse that was in the first sickness," p. 230. Camelot edition.

University of Oxford to Wolsey excuses delay in answering his two letters on the ground of the sweating sickness.

The prevalence of "sudor tabificus" at Oxford in 1517 is known from other sources as well: it is said to have caused "the dispersion and sweeping away of most, if not all, of the students[1];" and the nuncio, writing from London on the 6th of August, mentions the current but improbable statement that more than four hundred students had died in less than a week.

Besides these from Oxford, there are hardly any notices of the 1517 sweat in the country remote from London. A record at Chester mentions an outbreak of "plague," which is taken to mean sweating sickness; it is said also to have been "probably more serious than in 1507;" many died, others fled; and the grass grew a foot high at the Cross[2]. But these are the marks of true plague, which we know to have broken out in London, and in country districts as well, in the autumn and winter of 1517, or almost as soon as the short and sharp outburst of the sweat was past.

Among the references to prevailing diseases on the continent in 1517, besides sir Thomas More's rumour of the sweat in Calais, there is none which would lead us to suppose that the distinctive English malady had invaded Europe in that year. But there is a significant statement by Erasmus, hitherto overlooked, which almost certainly points to an epidemic of influenza on the other side of the North Sea the year after the sweat was prevalent in England. It is known that there was a suddenly fatal form of throat disease prevalent in the Netherlands that spring, which has been taken to be diphtheria; but the malady to which Erasmus refers can hardly have been the same as that. Writing from Louvain to Barbieri on the 1st June, 1518, he says that a new plague is raging in Germany, affecting people with a cough, and pain in the head and stomach, he himself having suffered from it. The significance of that epidemic, assuming it to have been influenza, will be dealt with in the sequel.

By means of the foregoing contemporary notices of the sweat

---

[1] Anthony Wood, *Hist. and Antiq.*, *sub anno* 1517.

[2] Hemingway's *History of Chester*, I. 142.

in 1517 we are able to judge of the general accuracy of the summary of it in Hall's chronicle, which has been hitherto almost the only source of information.   The sweat killed, he says, in three hours or two hours, which is something of an exaggeration of the shortest duration mentioned by the nuncio and the Venetian envoy in their letters of the 1st and 6th August.   Another general statement may be suspected of even greater exaggeration : " For in some one town half the people died, and in some other town the third part, the sweat was so fervent and the infection so great."   The sweat lasted, he says, to the middle of December.   Stow, in his *Annals*, more correctly states that the plague came in the end of the year, after the sweat.   The plague was much the more deadly infection of the two ; but even plague and sweat together, and at their worst, would hardly have destroyed one-half or one-third of the inhabitants of a town.

The Fourth Sweat in 1528.

As the despatches of the nuncio and the Venetian envoy in London give the best accounts of the sweat of 1517, it is in the despatches of the French ambassador, Du Bellay, that we find the most serviceable particulars of the sweat in 1528.   Du Bellay, bishop of Bayonne, and a witty diplomatist, was in London through the whole of it, and during that time sent letters to Paris, in three of which the sweat is a principal topic. From many other state letters of the time various particulars may be gathered, and in one letter by Brian Tuke, one of the king's ministers, we find some theorizings about the disease. The outbreak befell at the time when Henry VIII.'s passion for Mistress Anne Boleyn, sister to one of the ladies of the Court, was waxing strong ; it had the effect of parting the lovers for several weeks, the distance between them having been bridged over by an interchange of tender notes, of which those of the king remain open to the prying eyes of posterity.

The sweat is heard of as early as the 5th of June, 1528, when Brian Tuke writes to Tunstall, bishop of London, that he had fled to Stepney "for fear of the infection," a servant being ill at his house. The sickness must have made little talk for some ten days longer. On the 18th June, Du Bellay writes that it had made its appearance "within these four days[1]." On the 16th, the king at Greenwich was alarmed by the intelligence that a maid of Anne Boleyn's had been attacked by it[2]. He left in great haste for Waltham, and sent the young lady to her father's in Kent. " As yet," writes Du Bellay, "the love has not abated. I know not, if absence and the difficulties of Rome may effect anything." The king wrote to her at once: " There came to me in the night the most afflicting news possible...I fear to suffer yet longer that absence which has already given me so much pain." He sends his second physician (Dr Butts) to her. The alarm about her health seems to have been un-called for just then, although both she and her father caught the disease within a few days. By the 18th June, according to the French envoy, some 2000 had caught the sickness in London. It is, he says, a most perilous disease : " one has a little pain in the head and heart ; suddenly a sweat begins ; and a physician is useless, for whether you wrap yourself up much or little, in four hours, sometimes in two or three, you are despatched without languishing as in those troublesome fevers." The day before, on going to swear the truce, he saw the people "as thick as flies rushing from the streets or shops into their houses to take the sweat whenever they felt ill...In London, I assure you, the priests have a better time than the doctors, except that the latter do not help to bury. If this thing goes on, corn will soon be cheap. [The season was one of scarcity.] It is twelve [eleven] years since there was such a visitation, when there died 10,000 persons in ten or twelve days ; but it was not so bad as this has been." Writing again, twelve days after, on the 30th June, he says that some 40,000 had been attacked in London, only 2000

---

[1] The letter bears the date of 8 June, which would make the first of the sweat the same as in Tuke's letter ; but Brewer says the date should be the 18th June.

[2] Brewer (*Cal. State Papers*) reads the letter, " On Tuesday one of the ladies of the chamber, Mlle de Boulan, was infected with the sweat." But P. Friedmann (*Anne Boleyn*, Lond. 1884, I. 72) says the correct reading is a fille-de-chambre of Mlle de Boulan ; and it is known that Anne Boleyn did not take the sweat until some days after.

of whom had died ; "but if a man only put his hand out of bed during the twenty-four hours, it becomes as stiff as a pane of glass"—that is to say, by keeping themselves carefully covered, as we learn also from Polydore Virgil's history and letters on the sweat of 1517, they greatly increased the chance of recovery. In his third despatch, 21st July, he says the danger begins to diminish hereabout and to increase elsewhere ; in Kent it is very great. Anne Boleyn and her father have sweated, but have got over it. The notaries have had a fine time of it, nearly everyone having made his will, as those who took the disease in its fatal form "became quite foolish the moment they fell ill." His estimate of 100,000 wills is, of course, a humorous exaggeration. The sweat had been at its height in London, according to its wont, for only a few weeks, mostly in July. On the 21st of August one writes from London that "the plague at this day is well assuaged, and little or nothing heard thereof." From other parts of England there are few particulars of the sweat of 1528. We hear of it at Woburn on the 26th June, in a nunnery at Wilton on the 18th July, at Beverley on the 22nd July—it is reported as very serious in York-shire generally,—at Cambridge on the 27th July, and at several places in Kent about the same date. The "infection" at Dover as late as the 27th September may not have been the sweat, but the ordinary bubo-plague. But it is probably to the sweat that the deaths of four priests and two lay-brothers at Axholme, in Lincolnshire, are to be referred, as well as the heavy mortality in the Charterhouse, London[1].

As in the previous sweat of 1517, the letters of the time give us many glimpses of the invasion of great households in and around London, including the king's.

When the French ambassador was walking with Wolsey in his garden at York Place (Whitehall) on a day in June, word was brought to the cardinal that five or six of his household had

---

[1] In the *History of Cork* by C. Smith, M.D. (2nd ed., 1774) there is an entry under 1528: "a malignant disorder called the sweating sickness in Cork," with a reference to "MS. annals." It has been generally supposed that the sweat did not enter Ireland or Scotland in any of its five outbreaks.

taken the sweat, and the diplomatic interview was brought to an abrupt end. Du Bellay writes again in July that only four men in Wolsey's great house remained well. Among those in his household who died of it were a brother of lord Derby and a nephew of the duke of Norfolk. The cardinal, who had suffered from the sweat and its relapses in 1517, fled from it to Hampton Court on the 30th June, and shut himself up there with only a few attendants, having previously adjourned the law courts and stopped the assizes. On the 21st of July, Du Bellay writes that it was almost impossible to get access to Wolsey, and suggests that he might have to speak with him at Hampton Court through a trumpet. In the same letter the French ambassador refers to the circumstances of his own attack when he was visiting the archbishop of Canterbury (Warham), probably at Lambeth: "The day I sweated at my lord of Canterbury's, there died eighteen persons in four hours, and hardly anyone escaped but myself, who am not yet quite strong again." The bishop of London, Tunstall, writes to Wolsey from Fulham on the 10th July, that thirteen of his servants were sick of the sweat at once on St Thomas's day; he had caused the public processions and prayers to be made, which the king had wished for on the 5th July. The governor of Calais writes on the 10th July: "The sweat has arrived and has attacked many." Only two were dead, a Lancashire gentleman and a fisherman; but in a second letter of the same night, four more are dead, of whom two "were in good health yestereven when they went to their beds." Various other letters about the same date make mention of personal experiences of the sweat, or of domestics attacked, at country houses in the home counties. The most minute accounts are those for the king's household.

On the 16th June the king had left Greenwich hurriedly for Waltham. In a letter to Anne Boleyn, he writes that, when he was at Waltham, two ushers, two valets-de-chambre, George Boleyn and Mr Treasurer (Fitzwilliam) fell ill of the sweat, and are now quite well. "The doubt I had of your health troubled me extremely, and I should scarcely have had any quiet without knowing the certainty; but since you have felt nothing, I hope it is with you as with us." He had removed to Hunsdon (on 20th or 21st June) "where we are very well, without one sick person. I think if you would retire from Surrey, as we did, you would avoid all danger.   Another thing may comfort you: few women have this illness, and moreover none of our court, and few elsewhere, have died of it."   When Brian Tuke went to Hunsdon on the 21st June, the king spoke to him "of the advantages of this house, and its wholesomeness at this time of sickness." Two days after, Tuke having business with the king, found him "in secret communication with his physician, Mr Chambre, in a tower where he sometimes sups apart."   The king conversed with his minister about the latter's ill-health (seemingly stone), and showed him remedies, "as any most cunning physician in England could do."   As to the infection, the king spoke of how folk were taken, how little danger there was if good order be observed, how few were dead, how Mistress Anne and my lord Rochford (her father) both have had it, what jeopardy they have been in by the turning in of the sweat before the time, of the endeavours of Mr Butts who had been with them, and finally of their perfect recovery.   The king sends advice to Wolsey to use "the pills of Rhazes" once a week, and, if it come to it, to sweat moderately and to the full time, without suffering it to run in.   But the king's optimist views of the malady were quickly disturbed.   William Cary, married to Anne Boleyn's sister, died of the sweat suddenly at Hunsdon, having just arrived from Plashey, and two others of the Chamber, Poyntz and Compton, died about the same time either there or at Hertford, whither the king removed.   On the evening of the 26th June there fell sick at Hertford, the marquis and marchioness of Dorset, sir Thomas Cheyney, Croke, Norris and Wallop.   The king hastily left for Hatfield, on the 28th June, where still others appear to have taken the sickness.   Du Bellay, writing on the 30th, says all but one of the Chamber have been attacked.   From Hatfield the king went at once to Tittenhanger, a country house which belonged to Wolsey as abbot of St Albans, and there he elected to take his chance of the sweat, keeping up immense fires to destroy the infection. On the 7th July, Dr Bell writes from Tittenhanger to Wolsey that "none have had the sweat here these three days except

Mr Butts." Two days later, however, the marchioness of Exeter "sweated," and the king ordered all who were of the marquis's company to depart, he himself removing as far as Ampthill, whence he thought of removing on the 22nd July to Grafton, but was prevented by the prevalence of the infection there. Shortly after Anne Boleyn returned to the court. It is clearly to the period of her return that an undated letter of hers to Wolsey belongs ; after writing a few formal lines to make interest with the cardinal, she took her letter to the king for him to add a postscript, which was as follows: " Both of us desire to see you, and are glad to hear you have escaped the plague so well, trusting the fury of it is abated, especially with those that keep good diet as I trust you do."

Although the attacks mentioned in the correspondence of the time are many, the deaths are few. A letter of Brian Tuke's to Wolsey's secretary, on the 14th July, takes a somewhat sceptical line about the whole matter. His wife has " passed the sweat," but is very weak, and is broken out at the mouth and other places. He himself "puts away the sweat" from himself nightly (directly against the king's advice to him), though other people think they would kill themselves thereby. He had done that during the last sweat and this, feeling sure that, as long as he is not first sick, the sweat is rather provoked by disposition of the time, and by keeping men close, than by any infection, although the infection was a reality. Thousands have it from fear, who need not else sweat, especially if they observe good diet. He believes that it proceeds much of men's opinion. It has been brought from London to other parts by report ; for when a whole man comes from London and talks of the sweat, the same night all the town is full of it, and thus it spreads as the fame runs. Children, again, lacking this opinion, have it not, unless their mothers kill them by keeping them too hot if they sweat a little. It does not go to Gravelines when it is at Calais, although people go from the one place to the other.

The English Sweat on the Continent in 1529[1].

Whether the sweat went at length to Gravelines or other places in that direction does not appear; but there is abundant evidence that it showed itself in the course of the following year (1529) in many parts of the Continent, excepting France, and that its outbreak was often attended with a heavy mortality. It was observed in Calais, as we have seen, on the 10th of July, 1528. But it is not until the year after, on the 25th of July, 1529, that we hear of it again,—at Hamburg, where a thousand persons are said to have died of it within four or five weeks, most of them within nine days. On the 31st July it was at Lübeck, and about the same time at Bremen and the neighbouring ancient town of Verden; on 14th August in Mecklenburg; at Stettin on the 27th August, and at Wismar, Demmin, Rostock, Stralsund, and Greifswald about the same date; in Danzig on the 1st September; Königsberg, on the 8th; and so eastwards to Livonia in 1530, and to Lithuania, Poland and Russia, the information for which countries is vague. Copenhagen also suffered from it, and towns in the interior of East Prussia, such as Thorn and Kulm. Meanwhile the sweat had proceeded by way of Hanover and Göttingen, about the middle of August afflicting also Brunswick, Lüneburg, Waldeck, Hadeln, Einbeck, Westphalia, the valley of the Weser, and East Friesland. It reached Frankfurt on the 11th September, Worms shortly after, and Marburg at the end of the month, breaking up the conference there between Luther and Zwingli, and their respective adherents, on the doctrine of the Eucharist. Jülich, Liege and Cologne were reached about the middle of September, and

---

[1] The German writers have assumed that the sweat was prevalent abroad really in the same summer or autumn as in England, explaining the discrepant dates by the difference in the English calendar. But it was only the months of January and February, and March to the 24th, that were counted in the old year in England; the months of June, July, August, etc. in which the sweat occurred, are the same in the English and foreign calendar-years. In the English chronology of the sweat, those months belong quite clearly to the year 1528; and, in the German, Swiss, and Netherlands chronology of the sweat, just as clearly to the year 1529. The sweat on the Continent was a year later than in England.

Speyer about the 24th, Augsburg (where there was a most severe and protracted epidemic) on the 6th, Strasburg on the 24th. Freiburg in Breisgau, Mühlhausen and Gebweiler in Alsace, in October. In November, the sickness overran Wurtemberg, Baden, the Upper Rhine, the Palatinate, and the shores of the Lake of Constance. Among the other German provinces visited in due order were Franconia, Thuringia, Saxony, the Saxon Metal Mountains, Meissen, Mannsfeld, Halberstadt, Magdeburg, Wittenberg, Lusatia, the Mark of Brandenburg, and Silesia. In Vienna the sweat prevailed during the siege by Sultan Soliman from the 22nd September to the 14th October. At Berne it is heard of in December, and at Basle in January 1530. The Low Countries had not been affected so soon as their nearness to England might have led one to expect: the sickness is said to have approached them from the Rhine in the latter half of September. They suffered severely, one of the heaviest mortalities being reported for the town of Zierikzee, where three thousand are said to have died subsequent to the 3rd of October, 1529.

In this remarkable progress over the mainland of Europe, France was conspicuously avoided. The sweat does not appear to have entered Spain, nor to have crossed the Alps. But all the rest of the Continent, from the Rhine to the Oder (if not farther east) and from the Baltic to the Alps, was reached by the English sweat in much the same way as if it had been an influenza reversing the order of its usual direction. There need be no hesitation as to the correctness of the diagnosis; the disease was described by several foreign writers from their own observation, and their descriptions agree entirely with those of Forrestier, in 1485, of Polydore Virgil, perhaps for the epidemics of 1508 and 1517, and of the letter-writers who were describing the epidemic of the year before (1528), as they saw it in and around London. The striking thing in the accounts from the continent is the enormous range of its fatality; in some towns the proportion of deaths to cases was hardly more than in influenza, while in others it was the death-rate of a peculiarly pestilential or malignant typhus; and those differences cannot have depended wholly upon the method of treatment.

C.   17

These full accounts of the English sweat on the continent of Europe in 1529 are in striking contrast to the meagre records of it at home. They were compiled first in 1805 from the numerous contemporary chronicles, and printed pamphlets or fly-sheets on the sweat, by Gruner, professor at Jena, in his *Itinerary of the English Sweat*, and his *Extant writers on the English Sweat*, published in Latin[1]. In 1834 Hecker went over the ground again in his well-known essay, improving somewhat upon the positive erudition of Gruner, but at the same time hazarding a number of doubtful interpretative statements, especially as to the sweat in England, for which the meagreness of the English records then available may be his excuse. The erudition of Gruner, Hecker and Häser deserves every acknowledgement; but it is of value more especially for the extension of the sweat to the continent of Europe in 1529, where it had abundant materials at its service, in chronicles, printed essays, and "regiments." There are extant no fewer than twenty-one printed essays or sheets of directions on the English sweat, which were issued from the German, Netherlands, or Swiss presses between the month of October 1529 and the month of June 1531, two or three of them being in Latin and most of them brief summaries in the native tongue for popular use. The corresponding epidemic in England did not call forth a single piece by any medical man, so far as is known. Nor does the English treatment appear to have lost anything thereby; for it was based upon the profitable experience of previous epidemics as embodied in oral tradition. Down to the fifth epidemic in 1551, the only English writing on the sweat so far as is known was the manuscript of 1485, by Forrestier. Almost all that we know of the epidemics in England in 1508, 1517 and 1528 comes from Bernard André's annals and Polydore Virgil's history, and from the despatches of the apostolic nuncio, the Venetian ambassador and the French ambassador. The fifth and last out-

---

[1] Gruner's *Scriptores de sudore Anglico superstites* was reprinted by Häser, with additional citations and notes, in 1847. Hecker (*Der Englische Schweiss*, 1834) refers to the work by Gruner, *Itinerarium sudoris Anglici ex actis designatum*, Jena, 1805, which I have been unable to see. The account of the German invasion in the text is accordingly at second-hand.

break, in 1551, called forth two native writings, one for popular use in English in 1552, and another in Latin in 1555, both by Dr Caius, physician to Henry VIII. and Edward VI.; these are indeed better than nothing at all, but they are too much occupied with pedantry and lugubrious rhetoric to be of much service for historical purposes[1]. The information about the epidemic of 1551 is so scanty as to suggest that the sickness in that year can hardly have been so severe as in 1528; the state papers contain hardly anything relating to it, and we owe nearly all our knowledge of it to the diary of Machyn, a citizen of London, to Edward VI.'s diary, and to Dr Caius. Bills of mortality had been kept in London for two or three weeks when the epidemic was at its height, from which some totals of deaths are extant.

The Fifth Sweat in 1551.

It was not in London that the sweat of 1551 began, but at Shrewsbury—on the 22nd of March, according to the manuscript chronicle of that town[2], or on the 15th of April, according to Caius[3]. No record remains of its prevalence at Shrewsbury; the statement of Caius, that some 900 deaths had occurred in a single city corresponds to the facts for London, and has no more reference to Shrewsbury (where Caius never resided) than it has to Norwich (as in Blomefield's county history). The strange influence in the air or soil advanced from Salop, as we learn from Caius, by way of Ludlow, Presteign, Westchester, Coventry and Oxford, in only one of which places is anything known of it except Caius's remark that it proceeded "with great mortality." The best record of its prevalence on the way from Shrewsbury to London occurs in the parish register of Loughborough, in Leicestershire. Under the date of June, 1551, the register has an

---

[1] *A boke or counseill against the Sweate*, London, 1552. *De Ephemera Britannica*, London, 1555.

[2] "This yere the swetinge sycknes raignyd in England, and began first in this towne of Shrowsbery the xxii of Marche, and ran through the realme, and began in London the ixth of July." Quoted from MS. Chronicle, in Owen and Blakeway's *History of Shrewsbury*, p. 345.

[3] *Op. cit.* 1552, fol. 10. In the Latin work the date at "Salopia" is "17 Kal. May."

entry that "the swat called New Acquaintance, alias Stoupe! Knave and know thy Master, began on the 24th of this month." Then follow the names of 12 persons who were buried in four days, and, on the next page, under the heading of " The Sweat or New Acquaintance," the names of 7 more, all buried in three days—making a total of 19 in six days, presumably all dead of the sweat and presumably also the whole mortality from it in Loughborough, which had far heavier mortalities from the common plague in after years[1].

The date of its arrival at Oxford, on the way to London, is not known; but a physician then resident there, Dr Ethredge, has left it on record that it attacked sixty in Oxford in one night, and next day more than a hundred in the villages around ; very few died of it at Oxford, which showed that the air of that university was more salubrious than at Cambridge, where the two sons of the duchess of Suffolk died[2].

The sweat appeared suddenly in London about the beginning of July, and had a short but active career of some three weeks. Deaths from it began to be mentioned on the 7th, and are entered in the king's (Edward VI.'s) diary as having amounted on the 10th to the number of 120, in the London district, including "one of my nobles and one of my chamberlains," so that " I repaired to Hampton Court with only a small company." The royal diarist says that the victims fell into a delirium and died in that state[3]. On the 18th July, the king, in Council at Hampton Court, issued an order to the bishops, that they should " exhort the people to a diligent attendance at common prayer, and so avert the displeasure of Almighty God, having visited the realm with the extreme plague of sudden death[4]."

The diary of a London citizen says that "there died in London many merchants and great rich men and women, and young men and old, of the new sweat[5]." On the 12th died Sir

[1] Nichols, *Leicestershire*, III. 891.

[2] Edrichus, *In libros aliquot Pauli Æginetae*, &c.   London, 1588 (not paged).

[3] " Diary of Edward VI." in Burnet's *Hist. of Reformation*.   Stow (*Annales*) says it began on the 9th July and was most vehement on the 12th.

[4] *Calendar of State Papers*.   Domestic (under the date).

[5] *Machyn's Diary*.   Camden Society, No. 42, edited by J. Gough Nichols, p. 7. Machyn was an undertaker, and records deaths and funerals.

Thomas Speke, one of the king's council, at his house in Chancery Lane; next day died Sir John Wallop "an old knight and gentle[1]," the same who had survived an attack of the sweat in 1528 when at Hertford with Henry VIII. It is not clear whether some other deaths of notables in the same few days were due to the sweat. Three independent statements are extant of the mortality in London which had all been taken, doubtless, from the bills regularly compiled. One gives the deaths "from all diseases" in London from the 8th to the 19th July as 872, "no more in all, and so the Chancellor is certified[2];" another gives the deaths "by the sweating sickness" from the 7th to the 20th July as 938[3]; and Caius gives the deaths from the 9th to the 16th July as 761, "besides those that died on the 7th and 8th days, of whom no register was kept[4];" by the 30th of July, 142, more had died, by which time it had practically ceased in London[5]. Caius adds that it next prevailed in the eastern and northern parts of England until the end of August, and ceased everywhere before the end of September. The king, in a letter of the 22nd August, written during his progress, says that the most part of England at that time was clear of any dangerous or infectious sickness[6]. Records at York make mention of a great plague in 1551, but without describing it as the sweat[7]. The event which excited most attention was the death by the sweat of the two sons of the widowed duchess of Suffolk, the young duke Henry and his brother lord Charles Brandon on the 16th of July. They had been taken from Cambridge, for fear of the sweat, to the bishop of Lincoln's palace at Bugden, in Huntingdonshire, their mother accompanying them; they fell ill

---

[1] Machyn.   [2] *Ibid.* p. 8.

[3] Letter from London, in Harl. MS. No. 353, f. 107, cited by Nichols in notes to Machyn.

[4] Caius, *Boke or Counseill*, 1552, ff. 10–11.

[5] The Venetian ambassador (*Cal. S. P.* Venetian, v. 541) says that the sweat was at an end in London in twenty days. He says, also, that children under ten years were not subject "questo influsso." The excitement caused by the London epidemic is shown in an entry of money in the corporation records of Canterbury: "1551. To one of the King's servants that brought word how many were dede in the swett." (*Hist. MSS. Commiss.* IX. 154 b.)

[6] Edward VI. to Fitzpatrick.   [7] Drake's *Eboracum*, p. 128.

immediately upon their arrival, the elder dying after an illness of five hours and his brother half an hour after him[1].

Besides the cases of the two noble youths and others at Cambridge[2], there are no particulars of its prevalence in "the eastern and northern parts of England" (Caius). But we hear of it in the register of a country parish in Devonshire, under the same name of "Stup-gallant" as in the Loughborough register; and it is probable that those two casual notices indicate its diffusion all over England in the manner of influenza. That conclusion may find some support in the statement of one Hancocke, minister of Poole, Dorset, that "God had plagued this realm most justly with three notable plagues: (1) The Posting Sweat, that posted from town to town thorow England and was named 'Stop-gallant,' for it spared none. For there were some dancing in the Court at nine o'clock that were dead at eleven[3]." Its occurrence in Devonshire is proved by entries in the parish register of Uffculme: the whole burials in the year 1551 are 38; and of these no fewer than 27 occur in the first eleven days of August, and 16 of them in three days, the disease of which those persons died being named, in the register, "the hote sickness or stup-gallant[4]."

Comparing these records of the sweat of 1551 with those of the years 1517 and 1528, we may conclude that the latest of those three outbreaks was not more severe than the earlier, and that, in the Court circle, it was probably milder. The gloomy rhetoric of Caius had led Hecker to construct a picture of its disastrous progress along the valley of the Severn, in which there is not a single authentic detail. Caius says that he was a witness of it, but that must have been in London; and the figures for London, although they indicate a very sharp epidemic while it lasted, do not suggest a mortality greater at least than that of 1528. The Venetian ambassador in writing a general

---

[1] Nichols, notes to Machyn, giving a reference to *Gent. Magaz.* 1825, II. 206.

[2] Fuller (ed. Nichols, p. 183) says, under 1551: "Many in Cambridge died of this sweating sickness, patients mending or ending in twenty-four hours." The death of the two young noblemen was made an occasion for copies of verses by members of the University.

[3] Strype, *Memorials*, III. chap. 7 (cited in notes to Machyn).

[4] Lysons, *Magna Britannia*, VI. 539.

memoir on England four years after, says that all business was suspended in London, the shops closed and nothing attended to but the preservation of life ; but as he makes a gross exaggeration in stating the deaths in London at 5000 "during the three first days of its appearance," we may take it that his impressions were vague or his recollections grown dim[1].

Were it not for the isolated notices of the sweat in Leicestershire and Devonshire, we should hardly have been able to realize that country towns and villages had been visited by an epidemic which was appalling both by its suddenness and by its fatality while it lasted. The name of "Stop-gallant," by which it is called in these parish registers, shows the sort of impression which it ·made ; but so far as the mortality is concerned, that was often equalled, if not exceeded, in after years by forms of epidemic fever which had nothing of the sweating type, although they might also have been called "stop-gallant," and indeed were so-called in France (*trousse-galante*).

Apart from the notices in parish registers, we have the generalities of Dr Caius, which amount to no more than a funereal essay, in the scholastic manner, upon the theme of sudden death. It may be doubted whether Caius really knew the facts about the disease in the country. The 27 deaths within a few days in a small Devonshire village and the 19 in six days in a small Leicestershire town, are hardly to be reconciled with the statement in his Latin treatise of 1555, that "women and serving folk, the plebeian and humble classes, even the middle class," did not feel it, but the "proceres" or upper classes did : they fled from it, he says, to Belgium, France, Ireland and Scotland. It was for these that he was chiefly concerned ; and when he approaches his rhetorical task with the remark that "nothing is more difficult than to find suitable words for a great grief," we may take it that he was thinking rather of such moving cases as that of the widowed duchess of Suffolk, who had lost her two sons in one day, than of wide-spread sickness and death throughout the homes of the people.

Nothing more is heard of the sweat in England after the autumn of 1551, at least not under that name. Francis Keene,

[1] *Calendar of State Papers.* Venetian, v. 541, under the date of 18 Aug. 1554.

an "astronomer," prophesied in his almanack for 1575, that the sweat would return, "wherein he erred not much," says Cogan[1], "as there were many strange fevers and nervous sickness." Some years before that, in 1558 (a year after influenza abroad), there prevailed in summer "divers strange and new sicknesses," among which was a "sweating sickness," so described by Dr John Jones, who had it at Southampton. We are, indeed, approaching the period of frequent and widespread epidemics of fever and of influenza, in both which types of disease sweating was occasionally a notable symptom, as in the influenza of 1580 abroad, in the fatal typhus of 1644 at Tiverton, in the widespread English fevers of 1658, and in the London typhus as late as 1750. How those other types of fever, due as if to a "corruption of the air," are related generically to the English sweat is a question upon which something remains to be said before this chapter is concluded. But the history of the English sweat comes to a definite end with the epidemic of 1551. Sweating sickness of the original sort was never again the *signum pathognomicum* of a whole epidemic of fever. The English Sweat became an extinct species, after a comparatively brief existence on the earth of sixty-six years. Its successors among the forms of pestilential disease may have occasionally put forth the sweating character, as if in a sport of nature; but the most of the travelling, or posting, or universal fevers, and universal colds, are easily distinguished from the sweat—*nova febrium terris incubuit cohors*[2].

---

[1] Thomas Cogan, 'The Haven of Health: chiefly made for the comfort of students, and consequently for all those that have a care of their health, amplified uppon fiue wordes of Hippocrates, written Epid. 6. Labour, Meate, Drinke, Sleepe, Venus...Hereunto is added a Preseruation from the Pestilence: with a short Censure of the late sicknesse at Oxford.' London, 1589. New ed. 1596, p. 272.

[2] There is a single reference to a sweat on the Continent in 1551, which may really have been one of those epidemics of typhus (or influenza), with a sweating character, that were observed in 1557-8 and 1580. Brassavolus, writing *de morbo Gallico*, and illustrating the fact that epidemics were sometimes generated by drought (though mostly by humidity), says that the sweat in England, in former years, came with drought, and that at the time of his writing, the 15th September, 1551, that disease was vexing Flanders,—the season being extremely dry,—and had attacked many thousands. This was first noticed by Häser, *Op. cit.* III. (1882), p. 332. The reference to Brassavolus is Luisini's *Script. de lue venerea.* Lugd. Bat. 1728, f. p. 671.

Antecedents of the English Sweat.

The history of the English sweat presents to the student of epidemics much that is paradoxical although not without parallel, and much that his research can never rescue from uncertainty. Where did this hitherto unheard of disease come from? Where was it in the intervals from 1485 to 1508, from 1508 to 1517, from 1517 to 1528, and from 1528 to 1551? What became of it after 1551? Why did it fall mostly on the great houses,—on the king's court, on the luxurious establishments of prelates and nobles, on the richer citizens, on the lusty and well fed, for the most part sparing the poor? Why did it avoid France when it overran the Continent in 1529? No theory of the sweat can be held sufficient which does not afford some kind of answer to each of those questions, and some harmonizing of them all.

The history of Polydore Virgil is so well informed on all that relates to the arrival in England of Henry VII. that we may accept as the common belief of the time his two statements about the sweat, the first associating it in some vague way with the descent of Henry upon Wales, and the second pronouncing it a disease hitherto unheard of in England. Caius, who wrote in 1552 and 1555, and can have had no other knowledge of the events of 1485 than is open to a historical student of to-day, said that the sweat "arose, so far as can be known, in the army of Henry VII., part of which he had lately brought together in France, and part of which had joined him in Wales." Hecker, the modern reconstructer of the history (1834), has passed from the tradition of Polydore Virgil and of Caius, clean into the region of conjecture in assuming that the sweat had arisen among the French mercenaries on the voyage and on the march to Bosworth. On the other hand, the one contemporary medical writer in 1485, Forrestier, is explicit enough in his statement that the sweat "first unfurled its banners in England in the city of London, on the 19th of September," or some three weeks after Henry's entry into the city. There is nowhere a hint that it was prevalent among the troops, whether French, Welsh or English, who won the battle of Bosworth on the 22nd of August, the only pretext for asserting that it was prevalent in the neighbourhood before the battle being the gossip of the Croyland chronicle concerning lord Stanley's excuse to Richard III. for not bringing up his men, which gossip probably arose soon after when the sweat became notorious. Croyland was not very far from the camp of the Stanleys; and yet we know for certain (with the help of the state papers) that the death of the abbot Lambert Fossedike from the sweat happened there after an illness of eighteen hours on the 14th October, some seven or eight weeks from the date of Bosworth Field, and some three or four weeks after the outbreak of the disease in London. The probabilities of the case are all in favour of Forrestier's view that the first of the sweat in 1485 was its appearance in London; and we shall accordingly take that as our point of departure.

Henry covered the distance between Leicester and London in four days, having left the former, after a rest of two nights, on the Wednesday, slept at St Albans on the Friday, and entered London, very tired by his journey (says Bernard André), on Saturday evening, 27th August, three weeks to a day from his landing at Milford Haven. Whether his whole force travelled from Leicester at the same pace, and entered the city with him, does not appear; but it can hardly be doubted that Henry's following, French, Welsh and English, had found their way to London without loss of time, to make personal suit for the grants and patents that began to be issued under the royal seal in immense numbers after the first or second week in September. London must have been unusually full of people in the weeks before the Coronation on the 30th October. But the pestilence that broke out was not the " common infection " or plague, which might intelligibly have been fanned into a flame by a great concourse of people. It was the sweat,—a new disease, a stranger not only to England but to all the world. We shall understand the mysteriousness of the visitation and the inadequacy of all ordinary explanations, by taking Forrestier's account of the causes of it, drawn up in the year of its first occurrence.

Although this earliest writer on the sweat recognized its distinctive type quite clearly, making no confusion between it and the plague, yet he referred both diseases to the same set of causes ; and in his section on the causes of the sweat he merely reproduces the conventional list of nuisances which occurs in nearly all treatises on the plague before and after his time. There was little variation from that list, as it is given in the last chapter from a plague-book of the 14th century, down even to the reign of Elizabeth ; thus it is reproduced almost word for word in Bullein's *Dialogue on the Fever Pestilence* written in 1564 (the year after a great plague), and it is so uniform in Elyot's *Castle of Health*, in Phaer's, and in all the other hygienic manuals of the time, that it might almost have been stereotyped. This was the causation which Forrestier transferred bodily to the sweat in his manuscript of 1485 ; almost the same causation had been given in the old essay of the bishop of Aarhus on the plague, actually printed in London in 1480.

"The causes of this sickness," he says, " be far and nigh. The far causes —they be the signs or the planets, whose operation is not known of leeches and of phisitions ; but of astronomers they be known...The nigh causes be the stynkynge of the erthe as it is in many places...For these be great causes of putrefaction : and this corrupteth the air, and so our bodies are infect of that corrupt air....And it happeneth also, that specially where the air is changed into great heat and moistness, they induceth putrefaction of humours, and namely in the humours of the heart ; and so cometh this pestilence, whose coming is unknown, as to them that die sodenley, &c."

Among the causes of the corruption he specially mentions the following, which probably had a real existence in the London of that time, although he is merely reproducing a stock paragraph of foreign origin :

"And of stinking carrion cast into the water nigh to cities or towns,—as the bellies of beasts and of fishes, and the corruption of privies—of this the water is corrupt. And when as meat is boiled, and drink made of the water, many sickness is gendered in man's body ; and [so] also of the casting of stinking waters and many other foul things in the streets, the air is corrupt ; and of keeping of stinking matters in houses or in latrines long time ; and then, in the night, of those things vapour is lift up into the air, the which doth infect the substance of the air, by the which substance the air corrupts and infects men to die suddenly, going by the streets or by the way. Of the which thing let any man that loveth God and his neighbour amend."

He then mentions a more distant source of corrupt air, apt to be carried on the wind—the corruption of unburied bodies after a battle, which enters into all the plague-writings of the time.

These things were, of course, insufficient to account for the special type of the sweat, or for its sudden outbreak, for the first time in history, in September, 1485. There may have been such favouring conditions in London at the time; something of the kind is indeed implied in Henry VII.'s order against the nuisance of the shambles a few years after; but we require a special factor, without which the unsavoury state of the streets, lanes, yards, and ditches, or the crowded state of the houses, would never have come to an issue in so remarkable an infection as the sweating sickness. Common nuisances were the less relevant to the sweat, for the reason that it touched the well-to-do classes most, the classes who suffered least from the "common infection," or "the poor's plague," and were presumably best housed, or located amidst cleanest surroundings. Even within the narrow limits of Old London there were preferences of locality. If the special incidence of the sweat upon the great households of prelates and nobles, and on the families of wealthy citizens, had rested only on the testimony of Dr Caius, who has a theory and a moral to work out, there might have been some reason for the scepticism of Heberden, who questions whether Caius was not probably in error in saying that the sweat spared the poor and the wretched, because he knows of no parallel instance among infective diseases[1]. But the fact is abundantly illustrated in the details, already given, for each of the five English epidemics; and it is confirmed for the continental invasion of 1529, e.g. by Kock, a parish priest of Lübeck, who says that "the poor people, and those living in cellars or garrets were free from the sickness," and by Renner, of Bremen, who says that it "went most among the rich people[2]." It was, indeed, owing to its being an affliction chiefly of the upper classes that the sweat has been so much heard of. So far as mere numbers went, all the five London epidemics together could not have caused so great a mortality as the plague caused

---

[1] *Increase and Decrease of Diseases.* London, 1801, p. 70.
[2] See the references in Gruner, pp. 444, 448.

in a single year of Henry VII., namely the year 1500, or in a single year of Henry VIII., such as the year 1513. But these great mortalities from plague, amounting to perhaps a fifth part of the whole London population in a single season, fell mainly, although not of course exclusively, upon the poorer class. The bubo-plague, domesticated on English soil from 1348 to 1666, was emphatically the "poor's plague," and, as such, it illustrated the usual law of infective disease, namely that it specially befell those who were the worst housed, the worst fed, the hardest pressed in the struggle, and the least able to find the means of escaping to the country when the infection in the city gave warning of an outbreak on the approach of warm weather.

But *morbus pauperum* is not the only principle of infective disease. There are pestilent infections which do not come readily under the law of poor, uncleanly and negligent living, in any ordinary sense of the words; and there are some communicable diseases which directly contradict the principle that infection falls upon those who engender it by their mode of life. Unwholesome conditions of living may be trusted to engender disease, but it does not follow that the infection so engendered will fall upon those who lead the unwholesome lives; sometimes it falls upon the class who are farthest removed from them in social circumstances or domestic habits, or who are widely separated from them in racial characters. This principle I believe to be not only a necessary complement to the more obvious rule, but to be itself one of wide application. It has been an original theme of my own in former writings, to which I take leave to refer in a note[1]; and, I have now to try here whether it may not suit the rather paradoxical and certainly mysterious circumstances of the sweating sickness on its first outbreak in the autumn of 1485.

If the insanitary state of London were insufficient to explain the engendering of the disease, the next thing is to look for

---

[1] "The Autonomous Life of the Specific Infections," in *Brit. Med. Journ.*, 4 August, 1883; "The Origin of Yellow Fever," in *North American Review*, Sept. 1884; *Illustrations of Unconscious Memory in Disease*, London, 1885, Chapter XIII. "Vicarious Infection."

a foreign source. Suspicion falls at once upon the foreign mercenaries who landed with Henry Tudor at Milford Haven on the 6th of August. Who were these mercenaries? Did they suffer from any contagious disease? Were they likely to have engendered the sweat? Can the infection be traced, in matter of fact, to them? In seeking an answer, it will be necessary to enter somewhat fully into the history of the expedition.

The earl of Richmond's successful expedition in 1485 was his second attempt on the English crown. The first had been made in 1483, when the duke of Gloucester was hardly seated on the throne and the duke of Buckingham was in the field against him. Richmond's army on that occasion had been furnished by the duke of Brittany, and is roughly estimated at 5000 men in 15 ships[1]; the expedition sailed from St Malo in October, encountered a storm in the Channel which scattered the fleet, and drove some of the ships back to the harbours of Brittany and Normandy, so that Richmond, having reached the Dorset coast with only one or two ships, was unable to land in force. He returned to a Norman port, and nothing more is heard of his army of Bretons; during the next two years he appears to have been left with no other following than two or three English nobles, among them the earl of Oxford, who afterwards led a division of his army at Bosworth. After repeated solicitation, he obtained in 1485 a small body-guard (*leve praesidium*) from the regents of Charles VIII. at Paris, a few pieces of artillery, and money to help pay for the transport of 3000 or 4000 men. With these resources he betook himself to Rouen in the summer of 1485 and began to fit out his expedition. It would appear that he found some difficulty in making up his force to the intended full complement, and that he was urged by the impatience of his followers and the chance of a fair wind to leave the Seine with what force he had on the 31st of July. His force of Frenchmen, under his kinsman de Shandé (afterwards earl of Bath), consisted of only 2000 men, crowded on board a few ships. It is a fair inference that the

---

[1] Polydore Virgil, p. 553. Philip de Comines says "three large ships and a considerable body of land forces." (Chroniques du Roy Louis XI. Eng. transl. II. 674.)

men had been recruited in and around Rouen; we are told, indeed, by Mezeray that Normandy was at that time infested by bands of *francs-archers* who had been licensed by Louis XI., and that the ministers of Charles VIII. gave them to Henry Tudor, to the number of 3000, regarding the proposed expedition of the latter as a good opportunity of ridding the province of Normandy of a lawless and disreputable soldiery[1].

These, then, were the mercenaries who landed at Milford Haven on the 6th of August, were at once marched through Wales to Shrewsbury and Lichfield, and took a principal part in the battle of Bosworth on the 22nd of August. They were Normans, who had become so great a pest to their own province that Charles VIII.'s ministers were induced to take up Henry Tudor's cause partly with the intention of ridding French territory of them. Their quality is plainly indicated in the speech just before the battle by Richard III., which had been composed for Hall's chronicle; only they were not Bretons, as the speech makes out; they were Normans, recruited for the expedition in Rouen and the surrounding country.

I have given so much emphasis to the nationality of these mercenaries because the theory of the English sweat turns upon it[2]. More than two centuries after Bosworth Field, about the year 1717, when the English sweat had been long forgotten, an almost identical type of disease began to show itself among the villages and towns of that very region of France, the lower basin of the Seine, where the mercenaries of 1485 had been recruited.

A form of Sweat afterwards endemic in Normandy.

The Picardy sweat, which was first noticed as a disease of the soil about the year 1717, and has continued off and on

---

[1] Mezeray, II. 762. He adds: "the Bretons boast of having also lent aid to this prince." His first expedition was purely with Bretons, but the second was composed mostly if not altogether of Normans.

[2] This point, which is essential to the theory, was originally stated in an article on "Epidemics" in the *Quarterly Review*, Jan. 1887, and there claimed as original. The writer on "Sweating Sickness" in the *Encycl. Brit.* has adopted it as a commonplace; it is obvious enough when pointed out, but Hecker had not done so.

down to recent years, was indigenous to the departments in the basin of the Seine, from the Pas de Calais to Calvados, with Rouen as a centre. Why that strange form of sickness should have sprung up there and continued, now in one town or village now in another, with few blank years for a century and a half, no one can venture to say. It was not the English sweat in all its circumstances; on the contrary it was only rarely epidemic over a large population or a large tract of country at once. It was ordinarily limited to one or two spots at a time, and in the individuals affected it ran a longer course than the English sweat had done. But whenever it did become widely prevalent it also became a short and sharp infection like the English sweat, causing in some years a very considerable number of deaths. Distinctively the Picardy sweat was a somewhat mild sickness of a week or more, seldom fatal, distinctively also of a single town or village, or small group of villages. It was not unknown in some other parts of France, such as the Vosges and Languedoc, in Bavaria and in Northern Italy; but in these other localities it has been much more occasional or even rare. Its distinctive habitat for a century and a half has been the lower basin of the Seine; and there it has been so steady at one point or another from year to year throughout the whole of that period that it may be said to be a disease of the soil, indigenous or domesticated, and depending for its periodic manifestations mostly upon vicissitudes of the seasons, as affecting probably the rise and fall of the ground-water. It has been more a disease of the well-to-do bourgeois class than of the very poor, and it has often shown a preference for the cleaner villages. It has been the subject of a very large number of French writings from the year 1717 down almost to the present date. Strange as this form of disease is, neither its circumstances nor its nosological characters are left in any doubt; it is at once mysterious and perfectly familiar[1].

---

[1] The above account is summarised from the chapter in Hirsch, *Geog. and Histor. Path.* Eng. transl. I. 88.

Theory of the English Sweat.

I have been at some pains to show that Henry Tudor's mercenaries were enlisted in and around Rouen, or, in other words, they came from that very district of France in which the sweat, in a somewhat modified form, began to make its appearance as an endemic malady two hundred and thirty years after. If the sweat had not become an endemic or standing disease there, as if native to the soil, or if it had become equally a disease of all other parts of Europe, as typhoid fever has, the coincidence would have been less striking, and might have been made to appear altogether irrelevant by the long interval of more than two centuries between the one event and the other. If it were a mere coincidence, we should conclude that the same causes which established in Normandy in the 18th century a steady prevalence of a sweating sickness, not unlike the more familiar prevalence of typhoid, had been at work on English soil more than two centuries earlier, not indeed to establish a form of sweating sickness steadily prevalent from year to year in one place or another, like the plague, but to induce five sharp epidemic outbursts, within a period of sixty-six years, four of which outbursts began in London and extended probably over the whole country, while one began in Shrewsbury, travelled by stages to London, and spread all over England. And, as we are ignorant of the things which determine the type of the endemic sweat of Normandy or Picardy down to the present day, we can neither deny nor affirm that there may have been corresponding factors of disease at work in the England of Henry VII. By such a line of reasoning we are brought to a view of the English sweat which precludes all farther inquiry and makes a permanent blank or maze in our knowledge. Let us try, however, whether the facts of the case do not better fall in with the view that the English sweat had a real relation to the seats of the Norman and Picardy sweat, even at a time when that sweat had not come into existence as a definite form of disease, and although the French provinces appear to have been spared the invasion of the epidemic when it overran the rest of Northern Europe in 1529.

C. 18

The means of communication in 1485 was not wanting, namely the Norman soldiery of Henry VII. The tradition of their quality is preserved in the speech composed in Hall's chronicle for Richard III. before the battle of Bosworth, and versified somewhat closely by Shakespeare:

> "A sort of vagabonds, rascals, and run-aways,
> A scum of Bretagnes, and base lackey peasants:
> ...Let's whip these stragglers o'er the seas again;
> Lash hence these over-weening rags of France,
> These famished beggars, weary of their lives."

There is nothing incredible in the supposition that these men had brought a disease into London although they had not themselves presented the symptoms of that disease. Such importations are not unknown; the mystery hanging over them does not make them the less real. A well-known instance is the St Kilda boat-cold, "the wonderful story," as Boswell says, "that upon the approach of a stranger all the inhabitants catch cold," a story which Mr Macaulay, the author of the *History of St Kilda*, had been advised to leave out of his book. " Sir," said Dr Johnson, "to leave things out of a book merely because people tell you they will not be believed, is meanness: Macaulay acted with more magnanimity." The St Kilda influenza has been amply corroborated since then by parallel instances from the more remote islands of the Pacific, and by striking instances in veterinary pathology. Among the latter may be quoted the instance which has been heard of in Shropshire, of "sheep which have been imported from vessels, although themselves in a healthy condition, if placed in the same fold with others, frequently producing sickness in the flock[1]." But there is an instance on a vast scale from the United States, the instance of Texas cattle-fever, which has recurred so often, and has been so closely watched on account of the disastrous loss which it causes, that there is no room left to doubt the reality of that mysterious form of contagion. I shall have to speak very shortly of the malignant fevers of the assizes, which spread from prisoners who were not known to be ill of fever; these incidents

---

[1] Darwin, *Naturalist's Voyage round the World*, pp. 435–6.

are historical from the year 1522, when an epidemic of the kind arose among the court and grand jury at the gaol delivery in the Castle of Cambridge. Lastly the history of yellow fever, as expounded in part in this volume, is an instance of a long-enduring infection arising from the circumstances of the African slave-trade, the negroes themselves having been racially exempt from the fever although they had been the source of the virus.

In all such cases the sickness which ensued among the healthy from contact with strangers had a more or less definite type; and that type in each case must have been determined mainly by the antecedents of the strangers, their racial characters being reckoned among the antecedents as well as their special hardships and their personal habits. In the case of the singular visitation of England in 1485, the strangers were a swarm of disreputable free-booters from Normandy, natives of a soil which developed the sweat as an indigenous malady in the long course of generations. If they themselves had shown the symptoms of the sweat in 1485, one might have said that the circumstances of their passage in crowded ships, of their exhausting march from Wales to Leicestershire, and thence to London, had brought to the definite issue of a specific disease that which was otherwise no more than a habit of body, a constitutional tendency, a disease in the making. But there is no reason to suppose that they themselves incurred the symptoms of the disease at all; it was contact with them in England, particularly in London, that determined the peculiar type of disease in others. Those others were of a different national stock, and for the most part of another manner of life; in their very differences lay their liability, according to well-known analogies. Of course there must have been something material, something more than abstract contact, to cause the sweat in certain Englishmen; and although we cannot image the form of the virulent matter, we are safe to pronounce, in this hypothesis, that it must have come from the persons of the foreign soldiery.

The Habitat of the Virus.

We may go even farther in the way of specific probability, and bring the virus definitely to a habitat in the soil. The English sweat, like the Picardy sweat itself, had certain characters of a soil poison, like the poison of cholera, yellow fever and typhoid fever; only it was not endemic like the two last, but periodic, as well as somewhat volatile in its manner of travelling, like dengue, influenza, and others of the "posting" fevers of former times. This brings us to the singular history of the epidemics of sweat in England,—to the clear intervals of many years and the sudden bursting forth anew. What became of the specific virus from 1485 to 1508, to 1517, to 1528, to 1551, and after?

A fresh importation in each of the epidemic years after 1485 is improbable; certainly the circumstances of Henry VII.'s expedition never occurred again, and the traffic between England and her two French possessions of Calais and Guines had nothing in it at all analogous. Equally improbable is the continuance of the sweat in isolated or sporadic cases from year to year throughout the intervals between the epidemics; the only facts that give any countenance to such a continuous succession are the occasionally mentioned "hot agues," as in 1518, and, on a more extensive scale, in 1539. The seeds or germs of the infection which arose first in London in September, 1485, must have lain dormant in the city until some favouring conditions came round to call them into life. It is impossible to figure such dormancy of the virus except on the hypothesis that it was a soil-poison, having its habitat in the pores of the ground. The periodic activity of all such poisons depends, as we can now say with a good deal of certainty, upon the movements of the ground-water, which in turn depend on the wetness or dryness of seasons. The kind of weather preceding each of the epidemics of the English sweat has been remarked on by writers, but somewhat loosely or erroneously. The peculiarity of the year of the second sweat, 1508, (not 1506 as in Hecker, nor 1507 as in other writers) was a "marvellous" forwardness of vegetation in the month of January, unusual heat from the end of May to the 13th of June, much prized rain on that date, on the 16th, and on the 3rd of July[1], the sweat being heard of first in the Lord Treasurer's household in July. The third year of the sweat, 1517, began with a great frost from the 12th January, so that no boat could go from London to Westminster all the term time[2], while men crossed with horse and cart from Westminster to Lambeth[3]. This great frost would appear to have been without snow, the whole season from September, 1516, to May, 1517, being chronicled as one of unusual drought, "for there fell no rain to be accounted," so that "in some places men were fain to drive their cattle three or four miles to water." The kind of weather following the break-up of the drought is not mentioned, but there is implied of course a certain amount of rain. It was about the end of July or first of August, 1517, that the sweat began in London and the suburbs. The fourth, and perhaps the most severe sweat, that of 1528, followed upon two wet seasons, with one spoiled harvest in 1527 and bad prospects for that of 1528. The winter of 1526–27 had been unusually wet from November until the end of January; then dry weather set in until April; after which the rain began again and continued for eight weeks[4]. The harvest before that seems to have been a partial failure, for early in 1527 corn began to run short in London, and for a week or more there was acute general famine, so that the bread carts coming in from Stratford had to be guarded by the sheriffs and their men all the way from Mile End to their proper market. The high price of corn continued into the summer of 1528. The weather of that summer is not specially recorded for England; but we learn from a diplomatic letter dated, Paris, the 4th of

---

[1] Bernard André's *Annales Henrici VII.* Rolls series, No. 10, p. 120. Under a date in January, 1508, he writes: "Quo quidem die nuncius ab urbe incredibilia dictu, hoc est de primis verni fructibus temporis floridoque frumento visis, referebat." Both Fabyan and the anonymous author of MS. Cotton, Vitellius, A. XVI. (*Chronicle of England from 1 .Hen. III. to 1 Hen. VIII.*) give the winter of 1506–7 as "a wonderful [easy] and soft winter without storms or frost," but fail to remark on the weather of 1507–8.

[2] Wriothesley's Chronicle.   [3] Fabyan, Stow.

[4] Stow's Annals. Hecker, in error, makes out this exceptional season to have been the one immediately preceding the sweat in the summer of 1528.

July, that much rain had fallen and destroyed the corn and vines, so that there were fears of universal decay and dearth through all France[1]. On the 5th July, Henry VIII. requests Wolsey to have general processions made through the realm "for good weather and for the plague," the sweat having already been raging for more than a month. The fifth and last sweat, in 1551, also coincided with an unusually high price of corn, or, in other words, followed one or more bad harvests. In 1550 wheat was at 20 shillings the quarter; at Easter in 1551 the price in London was 26*sh.* 8*d.*; ten or twelve ship loads of rye and wheat from Holland and Brittany were sold under the mayor's direction at a stated but very high price. Meanwhile the sweat was advancing from Shrewsbury to London, where it broke out on the 7th July. The statements of Dr Caius about stinking mists carried from town to town are, like most of his statements, so obviously the product of his uncritical rhetoric that it becomes almost impossible to trust his narrative for matters of fact. But we may go so far as to assume that the first half of 1551 was a season of an unusually moist atmosphere. At all events the fifth season of the sweat, and also the fourth (1528), stand out in the annals as years of scarcity following bad harvests, which had probably failed owing to continuous wet weather.

There is not, on the surface, much uniformity in the weather preceding the epidemics of the sweat in 1508, 1517, 1528 and 1551. In the first of these the winter was mild and the early summer excessively hot and dry; in the second the winter and spring were remarkable for drought, with several weeks of intense black frost in the middle period; in the remaining two the antecedent appears to have been an excessive rainfall. But in all the four we shall find that the law of the sub-soil water, as formulated by the recent Munich school with reference to epidemic outbursts, was exemplified. According to that law, the dangerous products of fermentation arise from the soil when the pores of the ground are either getting filled with water after having been long filled with air, or are getting filled with air after having been long filled with water. It is the range of fluctuation in the ground-water, either downwards or upwards,

[1] *Cal. State Papers*, under the date.

that determines the risk to health; and in two of the years of the sweat, 1508 and 1517, we find that there had been a rise from a very low level of the wells, while in the other two, 1528 and 1551, the wells had begun to fall after standing for a length of time at an unusually high level. If this reading of the somewhat imperfect data can be trusted, it is at one and the same time an explanation of the outbreak of the sweat in the respective seasons, and a confirmation of the hypothesis that the virus of the sweat had its habitat in the ground. That hypothesis is, indeed, supported by so great a convergence of probabilities, both for the English sweat and for the endemic sweat of France[1], that it may be used to explain the seasonal incidence without laying the argument open to the charge of running in a vicious circle.

Whatever had been the kind of weather determining the successive outbreaks of the sweat, it is clear that the favouring circumstances were in general not the same as those of the bubo-plague. The greater outbursts of plague, as we shall see, were in 1500, 1509, 1513, 1531, 1535, 1543, 1547, and other years not sweat-years. It is only in the autumn of 1517 that the plague overlaps somewhat on the sweat, and even then it becomes noticeable mostly in the winter following the decline of the sweat. The two poisons had existed in English soil side by side, but had not come out at the same seasons; also the sweat had been mostly a disease of the greater houses, and the plague mostly of the poorer.

The Extinction of the Sweat in England.

The disappearance of the sweat from England after 1551, or its failure to come out again with the appropriate weather, is one of those phenomena of epidemic disease which might be made to appear less of a mystery by finding several more in the like case. A history of all the extinct types of infective disease would probably bring to light some reason why they had each and all died out. But an epidemic disease leaves no bones behind it in the strata; nor has the astonishing progress of science succeeded as yet in detecting palæozoic bacteria,

[1] Summary in Hirsch, *l.c.*

although that discovery cannot be delayed much longer. Meanwhile we have to make what we can of the ordinary records.
In our own time, so to speak, the sweat became extinct in 1551,
and the plague in 1666; perhaps someone before long may be
able to say that typhus died out (for a time) in Britain in such
and such a year, and smallpox (for good) in such and such
another. The surprising thing is that an infection which came
forth time after time should have one day been missed as if it
were dead. If the sweat had five seasons in England, why not
fifty? Perhaps its career was short because the circumstances of
its origin were transient and, as it were, accidental. But it may
have been also subject to the only law of extinct disease-species
which our scanty knowledge points to—the law of the succession,
or superseding, or supplanting of one epidemic type by another.

Other forms of epidemic fever, in the same pestilential class
as the sweat, were coming to the front in England as well as in
other parts of Europe. Thus, in 1539, a summer of great heat
and drought, "divers and many honest persons died of the hot
agues, and of a great laske through the realm." The hot agues
were febrile influenzas, and the great laske was dysentery.
Again, in the autumn of 1557, there died "many of the wealthiest
men all England through by a strange fever," according to one
writer[1], or, according to another[2], there prevailed "divers strange
and new sicknesses, taking men and women in their heads, as
strange agues and fevers, whereof many died." Jones in his
Dyall of Agues, describes his own attack near Southampton, in
1558, and calls it the sweating sickness.

That epidemic corresponded to a great prevalence of
"influenza" on the continent, which was probably as Protean
or composite as the fevers in England. It would not be correct
to say that these new fevers or influenzas, with more or less of
a sweating type, were the sweat somewhat modified. But they
seem to have come in succession to the sweat, if not to have
taken its place, or supplanted it. The prevalent types of disease
somehow reflect the social condition of the population; they
change with the social state of the country or of a group of
countries; they depend upon a great number of associated

---

[1] Continuator of Fabyan.   [2] Wriothesley, II. 139.

circumstances which it would be hard to enumerate exhaustively. As early as 1522 we have the gaol fever at Cambridge, at a time when Henry VIII.'s attempts to repress crime were come to the strange pass described in More's *Utopia.* These things remain for more systematic handling in another chapter; but in concluding the career of the sweat in England we may pass from it with the remark that it did not cease until other forms of pestilential fever were ready to take its place. The same explanation remains to be given of the total disappearance of plague from England after 1666: it was superseded by pestilential contagious fever, a disease which was its congener, and had been establishing itself more and more steadily from year to year as the conditions of living in the towns were passing more and more from the medieval type to the modern. Meanwhile we have to take up the thread of the plague-history where we left it in the reign of Edward IV.

CHAPTER VI.

PLAGUE IN THE TUDOR PERIOD.

WHEN the town council of York met on the 16th of August, 1485, to take measures on account of Henry Tudor's landing in Wales, their first resolution was to despatch the sergeant to the mace to Richard III. at Nottingham, with an offer of men (they promised 400 for his army at Bosworth), and their second resolution was to send at once for all such aldermen and others of the council as were sojourning without the city on account of "the plague that reigneth[1]." These leading citizens of York had gone into the country to avoid the infectious exhalations within the walls in the summer heats; the plague that reigned in York was the old bubo-plague, which would show itself in a house here or there in any ordinary season, and on special occasions would rise to the height of an epidemic, driving away all who could afford to remove from the pestilent air of the town to the comparatively wholesome country, and taking its victims mostly among the poorer class who could not afford a "change of air." In the three centuries following the Black Death, change of air meant a good deal more than it means now. The infection of the air, or the "intemperies" of the air, at Westminster occasioned (along with other reasons) the prorogation or adjournment to country towns of many parliaments; the infection of the air in and around Fleet Street caused the breaking up of many law terms; and the infection of the air in Oxford colleges was so constant an interruption to the studies of the place in the

[1] Drake's *Eboracum*, (from the town council records).

15th century that Anthony Wood traces to that cause more than to any other the total decline of learning, the rudeness of manners and the prevalence of " several sorts of vice, which in time appeared so notorious that it was consulted by great personages of annulling the University or else translating it to another place[1]." From the old college registers, chiefly that of his own college of Merton, he has counted some thirty pestilences at Oxford, great and small, during the fifteenth century. The reason why the Oxford annals of plague are so complete is that each outbreak, even if only one or two deaths had occurred[2], meant a dispersion of the scholars and tutors of one or more halls and colleges, their removal in a body to some country house, alteration of the dates of terms, and postponement of the public Acts for degrees in the schools. Experience had taught the necessity of such prompt measures. Thus the first sweat, that of 1485, came so suddenly that it killed many of the scholars before they could disperse, " albeit it lasted but a month or six weeks." Hardly had the halls and colleges begun to fill again after the dispersion by the sweat of 1485, when " another pestilential disease," that is to say, the bubo-plague itself, broke forth at the end of August, 1486, in Magdalen parish, and daily increased so much that the scholars were obliged to flee again. In 1491 there was another dispersion ; and in 1493 so severe an outbreak of plague from April to Midsummer that many were swept away, both cleric and laic : Magdalen College removed to Brackley in Northamptonshire, Oriel to St Bartholomew's hospital near Oxford, and Merton to Islip, " instead of Cuxham their usual place of retirement." The disastrous fifteenth century closes with a specially severe plague in 1499–1500, in which perished " divers of this university accounted worthy in these times ;" an accompanying scarcity of grain and consequent failure of scholarships or exhibitions led many students to betake themselves to mechanical occupations. In August, 1503, the plague broke out again in St Alban's Hall ; the principal with all but a few of the students went to Islip, where the

---

[1] *Hist. and Antiq. Univ. Oxford*, I. 651.

[2] At Cambridge, in October, 1578, two deaths from plague in Queens' College "moved many to depart." *Cal. Cecil MSS.* II. under date 13 October.

pestilence overtook them (three weeks having been spent first in mirth and jollity), so that several died and were buried, some at Islip, others at Ellesfield and one at Noke; in October it broke out in Merton College and drove some of the fellows and bachelors to the lodge in Stow Wood, others to Wotton near Cumner, where they remained until the 17th December. These interruptions had been so frequent that of fifty-five halls, only thirty-three were now inhabited, and they "but slenderly, as may be seen in our registers." The town of Oxford shared in the decline; streets and lanes formerly populous were now desolate and forsaken. An epidemic in 1508, which may have been the second sweat, caused another dispersion; then the old bubo-plague again in 1510, 1511, 1512 and 1513, filling up the interval until the summer of 1517, when a "sudor tabificus," the third sweat, "dispersed and swept away most, if not all, of the students." The bubo-plague followed in the winter and spring, especially in St Mary Hall and Canterbury College. Meanwhile cardinal Wolsey had founded Cardinal College (afterwards Christ Church), bringing to it an infusion of new learning from Cambridge and elsewhere; but in 1525, "while this selected society was busy in preaching, reading, disputing and performing their scholastic Acts, a vehement plague brake forth, which dispersed most of them, so that they returned not all the year following or two years after," and Cardinal College "thus settled, was soon after left as 'twere desolate." The same outbreak affected specially the halls or colleges of St Alban, Jesus, St Edmund and Queen's[1].

Oxford was not altogether singular in this experience of plague from year to year or at intervals of three or four years. What Sir Thomas More says of the cities of Utopia was true of the towns of England or of any medieval country in Christendom: "As for their cities, whoso knoweth one of them, knoweth them all; they be all so like one to another, as far forth as the nature of the place permitteth." The limitation as to the nature of the place is not without importance for the frequency and severity of plague; the quantity of standing water around Oxford would certainly appear to have made the epidemics there a more regular

---

[1] Anthony Wood, under the respective years.

product of the soil[1]. But we hear of plague also on the soil of Cambridge, particularly in 1511, when Erasmus was there: on the 28th November he writes from Queens' College to Ammonio in London: " Here is great solitude; most are away for fear of the pestilence," adding rather unkindly, " although there is also solitude when everyone is in residence." It is from such chance references in letters of the time that we can infer the existence of plague throughout England. These references become much more numerous as the sixteenth century runs on, not perhaps because plague was more frequent, but because all kinds of documents are better preserved. The remarkable difference between the reigns of Henry VII. and Henry VIII. in regard to the quantity of extant materials for the construction of history is as keenly felt by the student of epidemics as by the student of high politics. The local records of towns, London included, are still almost valueless for our purpose: even the skilled antiquaries employed by the Historical Manuscripts Commission have hitherto extracted nothing concerning pre-Elizabethan epidemics from the archives of civic council-chambers, and only a little from muniment-rooms such as that of Canterbury Abbey.

The few details that we possess, such as those for the plague at Hull from 1472 to 1478, had been extracted from local records by the authors of town and county histories. Before the end of the sixteenth century the evidence of plague epidemic all over England, as well in provincial towns and in the country as in London, becomes abundant. There may have been really a great increase, but it is much more probable that the increase is for the most part only apparent. It is of some consequence to determine the probability as exactly as possible; and I shall therefore examine with more minuteness than would otherwise have been necessary the evidence as to the existence and amount of plague in London and elsewhere year after year from the accession of the Tudor dynasty in 1485,

---

[1] With reference to a pestilence at Oxford in 1448, Wood says: " occasioned, as 'twas thought, by the overflowing of waters, and the want of a quick passage for them from the ground. Also by the lying of many scholars in one room or dormitory in almost every Hall, which occasioned nasty air and smells, and consequently diseases." *Op. cit.* I. 596.

using chiefly the Calendars of State Papers for my purpose. As in the case of the sweat, we happen to hear of plague in London and elsewhere because the Court was kept away by it; the king's secretaries are informed week after week of the state of health in London, and foreign ambassadors, especially the Venetian envoys, have frequently occasion to mention the hindrance to public business caused by the plague. But for these State papers the historian of epidemics would have little beyond an occasional parish register to build upon. The medical profession in England were not concerned to write or print anything thereon; while there are numerous foreign printed books on the plague (e.g. Forrestier's at Rouen in 1490) there is not one original English treatise until that of Skene of Edinburgh in 1568. That the physicians were well employed by those who could engage their services, and that they did sustain the credit of their profession by the liberal scale of their fees, we have every reason to believe; thus the Venetian envoy writes on 3rd June, 1535, that he had been ill, and that he had expended seven hundred ducats during his illness, "and for so many physicians," so that he had only one ducat remaining. But these thriving practitioners did not write books like their brethren abroad. One of their number, Linacre, who was also a prebendary of Westminster, busied himself with editions of certain writings of Galen. Erasmus mentions him in a letter as one of the Oxford scholars in whose society he found pleasure; but there is in the *Praise of Folly* a reference to a certain grammatical pedant whom Hecker identifies with Linacre. The other physicians and surgeons of the period whose names are known, Butts, Chambre, Borde and the rest of the group in Holbein's picture of Henry VIII. handing the surgeons their charter, have left nothing in print which illustrates the epidemic diseases of the time, and little of any kind of writing except some formulæ of medicines: Borde, who was patronised by Cromwell, is known only as a humorist or satirist. Thus the inquiry must proceed without any of those aids from the faculty which make the history of epidemics on the Continent comparatively easy.

After the disastrous prevalence of plague in England in the reign of Edward IV., culminating in the great epidemic of 1479 in London and elsewhere, we do not hear of the disease again in London until 1487, two years after the first sweat; in that year, on the 14th April, a king's writ from Norwich postponed the business of the Common Pleas and King's Bench until Trinity term, on account of the pestilence in London, Westminster and neighbouring places[1]. The next reference is to the great epidemic of 1499–1500, in London and apparently also in the country. Fabyan, who was then an alderman and likely to know, puts the deaths in London at twenty thousand[2]; Polydore Virgil says thirty thousand[3]; and others say thirty thousand deaths from plague and other diseases together[4]. The smaller total is the more likely to be nearest the mark. There is reason to think that the population of London a generation later was little over 60,000; and it will appear in the sequel that a fourth or a fifth part of the inhabitants was as much as the severest plagues cut off, although it is entirely credible that the Black Death itself had cut off one half.

The enormous mortality in 1499–1500 has left few traces in the records of the City or of the State. Five great prelates died during the plague-year, some of them certainly from it : Morton of Canterbury (a very old man), Langton of Winchester (before he could be transferred to Canterbury), Rotheram of York, Alcock of Ely and Jane of Norwich[5]. Like some of the later plagues in London it lasted through the winter. It was at Oxford in the same years, and casual references in two of the Plumpton letters lead one to infer that it may have been in remote parts of the country also[6].

The infection was still active as late as October, 1501, at Gravesend, and it made some difference to the reception of the

[1] *Materials Illustrative of the Reign of Henry VII.* Rolls ser. 60, II. p. 136.

[2] *Chronicle of England*, sub anno.

[3] *Hist. Angl.*, p. 609 (Basil, 1546). [4] Stow, *Annales.*

[5] In Rymer's *Foedera* all these vacancies of bishoprics are entered under the year 1501, beginning with the see of Canterbury (Morton's) on 9th January, 1501.

[6] *Plumpton Correspondence*, Camden Soc. No. 4, p. 138 : Letter of ? 1499, R. Leventhorpe, of Leventhorpe Hall, Yorkshire, to Sir R. Plumpton : "And sithe I hard say that a servant of yours was decesed of the sicknes, which hath bene to your disease, I am right sorry therefore;" he advises fasting, and trusts "ye sal be no more vexed with that sicknes." In the next letter (cviii) to Sir R. Plumpton from his son :—"Also, sir, I am very sorry that the death seaseth not at Plompton."

young princess Catharine of Arragon, who had come over for
her marriage with Prince Arthur, and became famous in history
as the wife of his brother Henry VIII. The following are
Henry VII.'s instructions, dated October, 1501 :—

> "My lord Steward shall shew or cause to be shewed to the said Princess,
> that the King's Grace, tenderly considering her great and long pain and
> travel upon the sea, would full gladly that she landed and lodged for the
> night at Gravesend ; but forasmuch as the plague was there of late, and that
> is not yet clean purged thereof, the King would not that she should be put
> in any such adventure or danger, and therefore his Grace hath commanded
> the bark to be prepared and arrayed for her lodging[1]."

In 1503 there was plague at Oxford, as we have seen, and at
Exeter, where two mayors died of it in quick succession, and
two bailiffs[2]. The infection was certainly in London in 1504 or
1505 (perhaps in both, and possibly at its low endemic level in
the other years from 1501): for Bernard André mentions casually that he had been absent from the City on account of it[3].

In 1509, the first year of Henry VIII., there was a severe
outbreak of plague in the garrison of Calais, as well as "great
plague" in divers parts of England[4]. In 1511, Erasmus writes
from Cambridge on 17th August, 5th October and 16th October,
making reference to the plague in London; and on the 27th
October, 8th November, and 28th November, Ammonio answers
him that the plague has not entirely disappeared, and again
that it is abated, but a famine is feared, and lastly that the
plague is entirely gone. On the 26th of July the Venetian
ambassador had written that the queen-widow (mother of
Edward V.) had died of plague and that the king, Henry VIII.,
was anxious.

On the 1st November, 1512, Erasmus, on a visit to London,
was so afraid of the plague that he did not enter his own lodging,
and missed a meeting with Colet. The next year, 1513, was a
severe plague-year according to many testimonies. In the
diary of the Venetian envoy from August to 3rd September it is

---

[1] *Hardwicke Papers*, London, 1778, I. 2 (from Harl. MSS.).

[2] Freeman, *Exeter*, in "English Towns" series, p. 99.

[3] *Annales Henrici VII.* Rolls series, p. 88.

[4] The information in the next few pages comes from the *Calendar of State Papers,
Henry VIII., Domestic*, unless otherwise referred to in the notes.

stated that deaths from plague are occurring constantly; two of his servants sickened on the 22nd August, but did not recognize the disease; on the 25th they rose from bed, went to a tavern to drink a certain beverage called "ale," and died the same day: their bed, sheets and other effects were thrown into the sea (? Thames). On the 17th September he writes to Venice that it is perilous to remain in London; the deaths were said to be 200 in a day, there was no business doing, all the Venetian merchants in London had taken houses in the country; the plague is also in the English fleet. In October the deaths are reported by the envoy at 300 to 400 a day; he has gone into the country. On the 6th November and 6th December he writes that plague was still doing much damage. On the 3rd December the rumour of a great prevalence of plague in England had reached Rome. On the 28th November Erasmus writes from Cambridge that he does not intend to come to London before Christmas on account of plague and robbers; and on the 21st December he writes again: "I am shut up in the midst of pestilence and hemmed in with robbers."

One year is very like another, but it will be desirable to continue the narrative a little longer so as to remove any suspicion of constructing history beyond the facts. In February, 1514, Erasmus writes that he had been disgusted with London, deeming it unsafe to stay there owing to plague. In going in procession to St Paul's on the 21st May the king preferred to be on horseback, for one reason "to avoid contact with the crowd by reason of the plague;" he had lately recovered from some vaguely reported "fever" at Richmond. On the 1st July Convocation was adjourned on account of the epidemic and the heat.

Next year, 1515, Erasmus writes from London on the 20th April that he is in much trouble; the plague had broken out and it looked as if it would rage everywhere. On the 23rd April Wolsey sends advice to the earl of Shrewsbury in the country (? Wingfield) to "get him into clean air and divide his household," owing to contagious plague among his servants; on the 28th the earl received from London one pound of manus Christi,—the same remedy that Henry VIII. sent to Wolsey

C. 19

for the sweat—with coral, and half-a-pound of powder preservative.   On the same date "they begin to die in London in divers
places suddenly of fearful sickness."   One of the incidents of
the plague of 1515 which has fixed the attention of chroniclers
was the death of twenty-seven of the nuns in a convent at the
Minories outside Aldgate[1].   Next year, on 14th May (1516), the
sickness was so extreme in Lord Shrewsbury's house at Wingfield
that he has put away all his horse-keepers and turned his horses
out to grass.   In London, on the 21st May, the Venetian
ambassador removed to Putney owing to a case of plague in his
house, and he would not be allowed to see Wolsey until the
30th June, when forty days would have passed since the plague
in his house.

The next summer, 1517, was the season of the third sweat.
It was hardly over when plague began in London in September.
On the 21st the Venetian envoy speaks of having had to avoid
" the plague *and* the sweating sickness;" on the 26th he writes
that the plague is making some progress and he has left London
to avoid it.   On the 15th October the king was at Windsor "in
fear of the great plague."   One writes on 25 Oct., "As far as I can
hear, there is no parish in London free[2]."   On the 16th November
the envoy begs the seignory of Venice to send someone to replace
him as he thinks it high time to escape from "sedition, sweat
and plague."   On the 3rd December the king and the cardinal
were still absent from London on account of the plague; on the
22nd their absence was causing general discontent, the plague
being somewhat abated.   It was not until March, 1518, that the
court approached London; on the 15th the Venetian envoy rode
out to Richmond to see the king, and found him in some trouble,
as three of his pages had died "of the plague."   The court withdrew again to Berkshire, and on the 6th April it was decided by
the king's privy council at Abingdon that London was still
infected and must be avoided, the queen (Catharine of Arragon)
having declared the day before that she had perfect knowledge

[1] *Chronicle of the Grey Friars,* Camden Society, No. liii. 1852, p. 29.   Stow
puts the mortality under the year 1513.

[2] Letter from the Fleet prison, assigned to 1517.   *Hist. MSS. Com.* x. pt. 4.
p. 447.

of the sickness being in London, and that she feared for the king, although she was no prophet. On the 7th April the report of four or five deaths at Nottingham ("as appears by a bill enclosed") was made the ground of postponing a projected visit of the king to the north. The spring was unusually warm, which made the risk of sickness to be judged greater. It is clear that public business was suffering by the prolonged absence of the court from London, and that the existence of infection was being denied. On the 28th April Master More certified from Oxford to the king at Woodstock that three children were dead of the sickness, but none others; he had accordingly charged the mayor and the commissary in the king's name "that the inhabitants of those houses that be and shall be infected, shall keep in, put out wispes and bear white rods, according as your grace devised for Londoners;" this was approved by the king's council, and the question was discussed whether the fair in the Austin Friars of Oxford a fortnight later should not be prohibited, as the resort of people "may make Oxford as dangerous as London, next term" (the law courts sat at Oxford in Trinity term). However, the interests of traders had to be kept in view also. On 28th June, 1518, Pace writes from the court at Woodstock to Wolsey that "all are free from sickness here, but many die of it within four or five miles, as Mr Controller is informed." On the 11th July he writes again from Woodstock that two persons are dead of the sickness, and more infected, one of them a servant to a yeoman of the king's guard; to-morrow the king and queen lodge at Ewelme, and stop not by the way, as the place appointed for their lodging is infected. On the 14th July he writes to Wolsey from Wallingford that the king moves to-morrow to Bisham "as it is time: for they do die in these parts in every place, not only of the small pokkes and mezils, but also of the great sickness." The uncertainty as to what these diseases may have been will appear from the next letter, on the 18th July, from Sir Thomas More: "We have daily advertisements here, other of some sweating or the great sickness from places very near unto us; and as for surfeits and drunkenness we have enough at home." The king had also heard that one of my lady Princess's servants was sick of "a hot ague" at Enfield.

On the 22nd July, the Venetian ambassador writes from Lambeth asking to be recalled: two of his servants had died of the plague, and he himself had the sweating sickness twice in one week. The pope's legate, Campeggio, made a state entry into London about the first of August, but the king and Wolsey were not there to receive him, ostensibly for fear of infection. The king was now at Greenwich, and we hear no more of the fear of infection for a time. In the end of March, 1519, deaths from plague occurred on board one of the Venetian galleys at Southampton. On the 4th August, 1520, the king (at Windsor) has heard that the great sickness is still prevalent at Abingdon and other villages towards Woodstock, and has changed his route ("gystes") accordingly; on 8th August, sickness is reported at Woodstock. The same year some kind of sickness was very disastrous in Ireland.

In the winter of 1521 (2nd November), the sickness continues in London : "it is not much feared, though it is universal in every parish." According to a vague entry in Hall's chronicle the year 1522 was in like manner, "not without pestilence nor death," which may refer to the gaol fever at Cambridge.

Thus from 1511 to 1521 there is not a single year without some reference to the prevalence of plague, the autumn and winter of 1513 having been probably the time of greatest mortality in London. After 1521 or 1522 there comes a break of four or five years in the plague-references, except for a vague mention of plague followed by famine at Shrewsbury in 1525[1]. They begin again in 1526 (from Guildford) and go on until 1532 every year much as in the former period, the year 1528 being mostly occupied with the fourth epidemic of the sweating sickness. On the 4th June, 1529, the legate Campeggio writes from London : "Here we are still wearing our winter clothing, and use fires as if it were January : never did I witness more inconstant weather. The plague begins to rage vigorously, and there is some fear of the sweating sickness." On the 31st August the Venetian ambassador has a person sick of the plague in his house; on the 9th September he has gone to a village near London on account of the plague. On the 18th

[1] Phillips, *History of Shrewsbury*, p. 17.

September the French ambassador in London (Bishop Du Bellay) has plague in his household, and in spite of repeated changes of lodging his principal servants are dead; he has been unable to refuse leave to the others to go home, and is now quite alone, but the danger from the plague is much diminished.

In 1530 the plague is heard of as early as March 23, previous to which date two of the Venetian ambassador's servants had died of it; three more of them died afterwards, and the envoy was forbidden the Court for forty days. Parliament was prorogued on April 26 to June 22, on account of the plague in London and the suburbs, and farther, for the same reason, until October 1. The king was at Greenwich, but even there was not beyond the infection; in the Privy Purse book, there is an entry of £18. 8s. paid "to Rede, the marshall of the king's hall for to dispose of the king's charge to such poor folk as were expelled the town of the Greenwiche in the tyme of the plague." Similar payments are entered on January 13, 1531, April 10, April 26 and November 8[1].

On November 23, 1531, the king was obliged to leave Greenwich on account of the plague, removing to Hampton Court (now a royal palace since Wolsey's fall). In London it had somewhat abated, but, according to a letter of the Venetian ambassador, had been up to 300 or 400 deaths in a week. In mid-winter, the 15th of January, 1532, Parliament was prorogued on account of the insalubrity of the air in London and Westminster. The infection may be assumed to have gone on, according to the analogy of known years, all through the spring and summer, rising to a greater height in the autumn. We next hear of it on the 18th September, 1532, when the Venetian envoy writes from London that the king's journey to Gravesend and Dover would be by water, "as there is much plague in those parts, and there is no lack of it in London. Yesterday at the king's court the master of the kitchen died of it, having waited on his majesty the day before." On the 24th September, "the plague increases daily in London and well nigh throughout the country."

On the 14th October, "the plague increases daily, and

---

[1] *Privy Purse of Henry VIII.,* p. 79.

makes everybody uneasy." On the same date the Privy Council write to the king, who had crossed to Calais accompanied by Mr Secretary Cromwell, for a meeting with the French king, that there is a rumour of the plague increasing, especially at the Inns of Court. On the 18th October Hales, one of the justices, writes to Cromwell that "the plague of sickness is so sore here that I never saw so thin a Michaelmas term." On the 20th, Audeley the Lord Chancellor writes that many die of the plague, the sergeants in Fleet Street have left in consequence, the Inner Temple has broken commons, the lawyers being in great fear. *" The Council have commanded the mayor to certify how many have died of the plague."* That is the first known reference to the London bills of mortality, and was probably the very first occasion of them[1]. By that time the plague had been active in London for more than a month, and had clearly begun to alarm the residents. The result of the Privy Council's order to the mayor of London was a bill on or before the 21st October, showing that 99 persons had died of the plague in the city, and 27 from other causes, the number of deaths from other causes suggesting that this was the bill for a week. On the 23rd the Secretary of State is informed that the sickness is fervent and many die; those who are not citizens are much afeard. On the 25th Sir John Aleyn has assurances for Cromwell (at Calais) from all parts of the country that the whole realm is quiet, but the plague has been more severe than in London. Cromwell's French gardener was alive and well on Saturday afternoon, the 12th, and he was dead of the plague and buried on Monday morning the 14th. On the 27th the death "is quite abated" in London and Westminster, according to one; but according to the Lord Chancellor, on the 28th, the plague increases, especially about Fleet Street. On the 31st October one writes, " I have not seen London so destitute of people as it was when I came there." On 2nd November the death is assuaged and there is good rule kept, for Sir Hugh Vaughan takes pains in his office

---

[1] The reference on p. 290 (note 2) to "no parish in London free," under the date of 25 October, 1517, may imply that bills of mortality had been kept in that epidemic, which was certainly an occasion when Henry VIII. interposed in other ways to check the progress of plague.

like an honest gentleman. On the 9th November the plague is abated. There the correspondence ends, the Court having returned from France. But we may here bring in a certain weekly bill of mortality which has come down among the waifs of paper from that period[1]. It is for the week from the 16th to the 23rd of November, the year not being stated; the experts of the national collection of manuscripts were at one time inclined to assign it to "circa 1512;" but the first that we hear of the mayor being called upon to furnish a bill of plague-deaths is the order by the lords of the Council on or about the 20th October 1532, the first bill having shown 99 deaths in the city from plague and 27 deaths (in the week) from other causes. The extant bill for the week 16th to 23rd November is clearly one of a series; there are no good grounds for assigning it to an earlier date than the year 1532, while there are reasons for not placing it later. There are two other plague-bills extant, for August, 1535, written out in a more clerkly fashion, and bearing the marks of greater experience. The bill for the week in November is more primitive in appearance; and we may fairly take it as one of the series first ordered by the Council in 1532: for that was the most considerable year of the plague immediately preceding the outburst of 1535, to which the more finished bills certainly belong. The week in November, for which it gives the deaths from plague and other causes in the city parishes is later than the dates of the 2nd and 9th, when the plague was "suaged" and "abated;" the bill therefore stands for plague on the decline, or near extinction for the season, its total of plague deaths being 33, and of other deaths 32, as against 99 and 27 respectively in the corresponding week of October. As this, the earliest of a great historical series of London bills of mortality, has a peculiar interest, I transcribe it in full, retaining the original spelling.

Syns the xvith day of November unto the xxiii day of the same moneth ys dead within the cite and freedom yong and old these many folowyng of the plage and other dyseases.

Inprimys benetts gracechurch i of the plage
S Buttolls in front of Bysshops gate i corse
S Nycholas flesshammls i of the plage

---

[1] Lately purchased for the Egerton Collection. No. 2603, fol. 4.

S Peturs in Cornhill i of the plage
Mary Woolnerth i corse
All Halowes Barkyng ii corses
Kateryn Colman i of the plage
Mary Aldermanbury i corse
Michaels in Cornhill iii one of the plage
All halows the Moor ii i of the plage
S Gyliz iiii corses iii of the plage
S Dunstons in the West iiii of the plage
Stevens in Colman Strete i corse
All halowys Lumbert Strete i corse
Martins Owut Whiche i corse
Margett Moyses i of the plage
Kateryn Creechurch ii of the plage
Martyns in the Vintre ii corses
Buttolls in front Algate iiii corses
S Olavs in Hart Strete ii corses
S Andros in Holborn ii of the plage
S Peters at Powls Wharff ii of the plage
S Fayths i corse of the plage
S Alphes i corse of the plage
S Mathows in Fryday Strete i of the plage
Aldermary ii corses
S Pulcres iii corses i of the plage
S Thomas Appostells ii of the plage
S Leonerds Foster Lane i of the plage
Michaels in the Ryall ii corses
S Albornes i corse of the plage
Swytthyns ii corses of the plage
Mary Somersette i corse
S Bryde v corses i of the plage
S Benetts Powls Wharff i of the plage
All halows in the Wall i of the plage
Mary Hyll i corse.

Sum of the plage xxxiiii persons
Sum of other seknes xxxii persons

The holl sum iii^{xx} & vi.

And there is this weke clere iii^{xx} and iii paryshes as by this bille doth appere.

The exec^n of corses buryed of the plage within the cite of London syns &c.

There does not appear to have been any occasion for a continuance of plague-bills beyond the date of the one just given until nearly three years after : we hear, indeed, of a severe epidemic of plague at Oxford in 1533, but nothing of it in London until 1535[1]. It so happens that a pair of London bills of mortality is extant from the month of August in that year. Thus, by a singular coincidence, the only original bills of mortality that have come down (so far as is known) from the sixteenth century, are one from the end of the series in the first year of their execution (1532), and another the very first of the series in the second year of their execution (1535), or in the series ordered on account of the epidemic of plague next following. Of that epidemic also it may be permitted to give somewhat full details, for it is only rarely that we have the chance of realizing the facts in so concrete a way.

In the summer and autumn of 1535 Henry VIII., with the queen (Anne Boleyn), was mostly at his manor of Thornbury in Gloucestershire, Cromwell the principal Secretary of State being either with the king or in his immediate neighbourhood. The absence of the Court occasions numerous letters to be sent from and to London, in which we hear of the plague among other things. Cromwell had four houses in or near London at this time,—at the Rolls in Chancery Lane, at Austin Friars in the City, at the fashionable suburb of Stepney, and at Highbury : besides these he had a fine villa building at Hackney. From his steward or other servants at one or more of these he was in receipt of letters constantly during his absence. A letter from the Rolls on the 30th July informs him that twelve heron-shaws had been sent to him from Kent, and had been received at the Rolls "as the city of London is sorely infected with the plague." Next day another writes that the City is infected but Fleet Street is clean. On the 5th August "the common sickness waxeth very busy in London." On the 7th Lord Chancellor Audeley writes from "my house at Christchurch" (Creechurch, near Aldgate) that he had been expecting Cromwell in London,

---

[1] There was, however, an English translation of a small foreign essay on the plague, of unacknowledged authorship, published at London in 1534 by Thomas Paynel, canon of Merton, a literary hack of the time.

but hears that he will not return for nine or ten days; will therefore go to his house at Colchester meanwhile, as they are dying of the plague in divers parishes in London. Cromwell was naturally desirous to know accurately the state of health in the city, so as to regulate his own movements and perhaps the king's also; he accordingly makes inquiries of his various correspondents. Another letter from London on the 7th August informs him that there is no death at Court, but only in certain places in the city: "I fear these great humidities will engender pestilence at the end of the year, rather after Bartholomew tide than before. If you be near London you must avoid conference of people." On receipt of this Cromwell would appear to have written to the mayor of London, for on the 13th August his clerk at the Rolls replies to him that he had delivered the letter to the lord mayor. On the 16th another of the household at the Rolls writes that the plague rages in every parish in London, but not so bad as in many places abroad: "I will send the number of the dead. The mayor keeps his chamber. Some say he is sick of an ague; others that he was cut about the brows for the megrims, which vexeth him sore. Few men come at him, but women." The bill of mortality which Cromwell had asked for previous to 13th August is extant[1]. It is in two parts: one showing 31 deaths from plague and 31 deaths from other causes in thirty-seven out of one hundred parishes from the 5th to the 12th August, with a list of parishes clear; and the other, headed "14th August" and probably meant to include the former, showing a much heavier mortality and a much shorter list of parishes clear, the whole being endorsed by the mayor, Sir John Champneys, as follows: "So appeareth there be dead within the city of London of the plague and otherwise from the 6th day of this month of August to the 14th day, which be eight days complete, the full number of 152 persons [105 of them from plague]. And this day se'night your mastership [Mr Secretary Cromwell] shall be certified of the number that shall chance to depart in the meantime. Yours as

---

[1] In the Record Office. State Papers, Henry VIII., No. 4633. It has been erroneously calendared by Brewer as a bill of mortality of the sweating sickness in 1528.

I am bound, John Champeneys." This double bill for certain days in August, 1535, is rather more elaborate than, but otherwise not unlike, the above bill, for a week in November, most likely of the year 1532. It will be noticed that the deaths in all the city parishes from other causes than plague are 47 in the bill for eight (or nine) days; 31 in the bill, partly the same, for seven days, and 32 in the earlier bill for seven days, while they are known to have been 27 in another bill of October, 1532, probably also for seven days. These figures, the best to be had, are important for calculating the population of London at the time; they represent quite an ordinary weekly mortality, the deaths from plague being found to be always extra deaths, where we can compare the mortality year after year, as in the London bills of later times.

The weekly bills of mortality called for in the plague of 1535 were sent regularly to the Secretary of State until the end of September—on the 22nd and 30th August, and on the 4th, (and 5th), 11th and 27th September. The one sent on Monday the 30th August showed 157 deaths during the preceding week, of which 140 were put down to plague, leaving only 17 deaths in the week from ordinary causes,—a small number owing perhaps to so many residents having gone to the country. No figures remain from the other bills, but we know from letters that the plague increased considerably in September (e. g. 11th Sept. "By the Lord Mayor's certificate which I send you will see that the plague increases") both in London and in the country, justifying the prediction that it would be worse after Bartholomew-tide; it is not until the 28th October that we hear of the deaths being "well stopped" in London. Some few particulars of this epidemic, and of its revival in 1536, remain to be added before we come to speak of the London bills of mortality in general, of the extent of the City and liberties at this period, of its sanitary condition, and of the public health from year to year.

On the 18th August, 1535, one writes to Cromwell from the Temple that the plague "has visited my house near Stepney where my wife lives." On the 20th August a resident in Lincoln's Inn was seized with plague and conveyed thence by night to a poor man's house right against the chamber of one of Cromwell's household at the Rolls, where he died. " Such as lodge in your gate seldom go out, and will have less occasion if, before great time pass, you will appoint from Endevill, or elsewhere within your rule, some venison for the household, that men may be the better contented with their fare." On the same date Cromwell is informed by his steward at Austin Friars that " the Frenchman next your house that was in St Peter's parish [Cornhill] has buried two, but no more." The plague looked threatening enough to raise the question whether Bartholomew fair should be held at Smithfield this year. Meanwhile the king and court were at Thornbury in Gloucestershire, having arrived there on the 18th August. The town of Bristol was avoided " because the plague of pestilence then reigned within the said town;" but a deputation of three persons was sent to the king to present him with ten fat oxen and forty sheep, and to present the queen, Anne Boleyn, with a gold cup full of gold pieces, an offering known as " queen gold[1]." On the 25th of August the French ambassador proceeded to Gloucestershire to inform Henry VIII. " of the interview of the two queens," but he stopped six miles short of the court, owing to a " French merchant" who followed him having died of plague on the road. On the 4th September the plague in London is aggravated by a scarcity of bread; "what was sold for $\frac{1}{2}d$. when you were here is now $1d$.," and it is so musty that it is rather poisonous than nourishing. On the 6th the season has been unfavourable and there is great probability of famine. On the 13th the Lord Chancellor will stay at his house at Old Ford beside Stratford, on account of the plague in London increasing; he will have to go to Westminster on the 3rd November, with the Speaker and others, to prorogue Parliament, and advises the prorogation to be until the 4th of February, and of the law courts until the eve of All Souls, by which time, by coldness of the weather, the plague should cease. Wheat and rye were at a mark and 16/- the quarter. A letter from Exeter on the 17th September shows the danger of famine to have been great there also[2]. On the 23rd September one of the masons

---

[1] *The Maire of Bristowe, his Kalendar.* Camden Society, 1872, p. 53.

[2] The plague is said to have been in Exeter in 1535 (Freeman, *Exeter*, in English Towns Series).

working at Cromwell's house in Austen Friars is sick of the plague: three corses were buried at Hackney [of men employed at the new house?] last St Matthew's day. In October the king is on his way back from Gloucestershire, but changes his route owing to a death at Shalford and four deaths at Farnham. On the 24th October the bishop of Winchester, on his way to Paris, lost his servant at Calais by the great sickness "wherewith he was infected at his late being in London longer than I would he should:" travelling is cumbrous in the "strange watery weather" in France. In November the pope has heard that England is troubled with famine and pestilence. The curate of Much Malvern writes in November (but perhaps of 1536): "I have buried four persons of pestilence since Saturday, and I have one more to bury to-day. Yesterday I was in a house where the plague is very sore."

The sickness appears to have shown itself again in London as early as April, 1536. On the 2nd of May two gentlemen of the Inner Temple had died of the sickness; on the 15th the abbot of York writes to be excused from attending Parliament "because of the plague which has visited my house near Powles [St Paul's]." In the same summer the election of knights to serve in Parliament for Shropshire could not be held at Shrewsbury because the plague was in the town. In September one of the king's visitors of the abbeys, previous to their suppression, found hardly any place clear of the plague in Somerset, and was much impeded in his work. On the 27th September one of the numerous coronations of new queens in Henry VIII.'s reign (this time Jane Seymour in succession to Anne Boleyn, beheaded in May) was like to be postponed "seeing how the plague reigned in Westminster, even in the Abbey." On the 9th October plague was at Dieppe, thought to have been brought over from Rye. In Yorkshire also, the duke of Norfolk, sent to put down the rebellion in November, 1536, came into close contact with plague; many were dying of it at Doncaster: "Where I and my son lay, at a friar's, ten or twelve houses were infected within a butt's length. On Friday night the mayor's wife and two daughters and a servant all died in one house." Nine soldiers also were dead. At Oxford the plague was active, and the scholars had gone into the country. In London on the 27th November it was dangerous to tarry at Lincoln's Inn "for they die daily in the City." In September, 1536, the small essay on plague by the 14th century bishop of Aarhus, which had circulated in manuscript in the medieval period and was first printed in 1480, was reprinted at London, the regimen, as the title declares, having been "of late practised and proved in mani places within the City of London, and by the same many folke have been recovered and cured[1]." In 1537 there appear to have been a few cases of plague at Shrewsbury, on account of which the town council paid certain moneys[2].

Beyond the year 1538 the domestic records of State are not as yet calendared in such fulness as to bring to light any references to plague in them. It may be, therefore, that the clear interval from 1537 to 1542 is in appearance only. From such sources as are available we can continue the history of plague down to the great London plague of 1563; but it is a history meagre and disappointing after the numerous concrete glimpses and details of the earlier period.

The summer of 1540 was a sickly one throughout England[3]; it introduces us to a different and perhaps new type of disease, "hot agues," with "laskes" or dysenteries, of which a good deal remains to be said in another chapter.

It was in 1539 that Parish Registers of the births, marriages and deaths began to be kept—very irregularly for the most part but in some few parishes continuously from that year. By their means we can henceforth trace the existence of epidemic disease in the country, which might not have been suspected or thought probable. Thus, at Watford from July to September, 1540, there were 47 burials, of which 40 were from "plague." Next year, in the month of October, the burials were 14, a number greatly in excess of the average[4]. In 1543 there was "a great death" in London, which lasted so far into the winter that the

---

[1] There is a copy in the Lambeth Library, No. 432.
[2] Owen and Blakeway, I. 311.
[3] Continuator of Fabyan.
[4] Cussan's *History of Hertfordshire*.

Michaelmas law term had to be kept at St Albans[1]. Another civic chronicle adds that there had been a great death the summer before ; and from an ordinance of the Privy Council it appears that the plague was in London as early as May 21, 1543[2]. The next definite proof of plague in the capital is under 1547 and 1548. On the 15th November in the former year blue crosses were ordered to be affixed to the door-posts of houses visited by the plague. In 1548, says Stow, there was "great pestilence" in London, and a commission was issued to curates that there should be no burials between the hours of six in the evening and six in the morning, and that the bell should be tolled for three-quarters of an hour[3]. A letter of July 19 says that they had been visited by plague in the Temple, and that it still continued[4]. On August 28, the Common Council adjourned for a fortnight by reason of the violence of the plague[5].

These are the London informations for 1547 and 1548, but it would be unsafe to conclude that the other years from 1543 were free from plague. In 1544 it was raging at Newcastle[6], at Canterbury[7] and at Oxford[8], at which last it continued most of the next year, and was considered to be "the dregs of that which happened *anno* 1542." It had been prevalent in Edinburgh previous to June 24, 1545[9]. In April, 1546, there was a severe mortality on board a Venetian ship at Portsmouth, which may have been the plague, as in a similar case at Southampton[10]. In the autumn or early winter of the same year the plague was raging so fervently in Devonshire that the Commissioners for the Musters were obliged to put off their work till it ceased[11]. Within the town of Haddington, which was

---

[1] *A London Chronicle of Hen. VII. and Hen. VIII.* Camden Miscellany, 1859.

[2] *Acts of the Privy Council.* New series, 1542–1547, p. 136.

[3] Stow's *Annales.*   [4] *Cal. Cecil MSS.*, I. 15.

[5] Guildhall Records (Extracts by Furnivall in Appendix to Vicary's *Anatomy.* Early English Text Society).

[6] Brand's *History of Newcastle.*

[7] Hasted's *History of Canterbury*, p. 130 (from parish registers).

[8] Anthony Wood, *op. cit.* II. 74. At Banbury probably about the same year. Beesley's *History of Banbury* (from Brasbridge).

[9] *Register of the Privy Council of Scotland*, I. 5.

[10] *Acts of the Privy Council.* New series, 1542–1547, 28 April, 1546, p. 397.

[11] *Ibid.*, Nov. 13, 1546, p. 552.

held by an English garrison against a large besieging force of French and others, plague broke out in 1547[1]. In 1549 the disease is reported from Lincoln[2]. A letter of November 23, 1550, states that the Princess Mary was driven from Wanstead by one dying of the plague there[3].

The reigns of Edward VI. and Mary, full of trouble as they were in other ways, furnish hardly a single record of plague. The sweating sickness of 1551 we hear of sufficiently; and the pestilent fevers, or influenzas, in 1557–58 are not altogether without record; but of plague down to the 5th year of Elizabeth (1563) there is very little said, and that little not free from ambiguity. Sometime in that interval, or still earlier, must have fallen the pestilence at Northampton, severe enough to require the new cemetery which cardinal Pole, in a deed of March 9, 1557, ordered to be henceforth kept enclosed[4]. Only two of the many centres of sickness in England in 1558 are said to have had the infection of the type, not of fever, but of plague, —Loughborough and Chester. In the Leicestershire town the burials were numerous enough for true plague, and the cause of mortality is so named[5]. In Chester also the sickness is called the plague, and it is added that many fled the town, although the deaths were few[6]. A State paper of February 25, 1559, speaks of the county of Cheshire as "weakened by the prevalence of plague[7]."

The London Plague of 1563.

The activity of the plague in London in 1563 made up for its dormancy in the years preceding. The epidemic of that summer and autumn was one of the most severe in the history of the city, the mortality in proportion to the population having

---

[1] Camden's *Britannia*, ed. Gough, I. 262.   [2] *Ibid.* II. 265.
[3] *Calendar of State Papers.* Domestic series, Vol. x.
[4] *Notes and Queries*, 6th series, III. 477.
[5] Nichols, *Leicestershire*, III. 891 (295 deaths from plague &c. 1555–59.)
[6] Ormerod's *Cheshire*, I. under 1558, with a reference to "Harl. MSS." The Harleian MSS. relating to Chester fill many pages of the catalogue.
[7] *Calendar of State Papers*, Eliz. I. p. 122.

been tremendous. This is the first London plague for which we have the authentic weekly deaths. How they were obtained is not stated, but it was probably by the same means that furnished the plague-bills of 1532 and 1535. John Stow must have had before him a complete set of weekly bills from the beginning of June, 1563, to the 26th of July, 1566, of which series not one is known to be extant; but the totals of the weekly deaths from plague for the whole of that period are among Stow's manuscript memoranda in the Lambeth Library[1]. After the week ending the 31st December, 1563, the weekly deaths are few, many of the weeks of 1564, 1565 and 1566 having only one death from plague, and some of them none. The following are the weekly mortalities during the severe period of the epidemic :

Week ending		Plague-deaths	Week ending		Plague-deaths
1563.	12 June	17	1563.	1 October	1828
	19 ,,	25		8 ,,	1262
	26 ,,	23		15 ,,	829
	3 July	44		22 ,,	1000
	10 ,,	64		29 ,,	905
	17 ,,	131		5 November	380
	23 ,,	174		12 ,,	283
	30 ,,	289		19 ,,	506
	6 August	299		26 ,,	281
	13 ,,	542		3 December	178
	20 ,,	608		10 ,,	249
	27 ,,	976		17 ,,	239
	3 September	963		24 ,,	134
	10 ,,	1454		31 ,,	121
	17 ,,	1626	1564.	7 January	45
	24 ,,	1372		14 ,,	26
				21 ,,	13

Stow's · summary of this epidemic in his *Annales* is as follows: " In the same whole year, i.e. from the 1st January, 1562 [old style] till the last of December, 1563, there died in the city and liberties thereof, containing 108 parishes, of all diseases 20,372, and of the plague, being part of the number aforesaid,

[1] *Three Fifteenth Century Chronicles.* Camden Society, ed. Gairdner, 1880, pp. 123, 144.

C.

17,404; and in out parishes adjoining to the same city, being 11 parishes, died of all diseases in the whole year 3288, and of them of the plague 2732." The weekly totals from June 12 to December 31 which are for the City and liberties, and exclusive of the out parishes, add up to very nearly Stow's total for the whole year, or to 16,802 as against 17,404. Where the discrepancy arises does not appear; it is hardly likely that some 600 plague-deaths would have occurred previous to the second week in June, at which time the weekly mortality had reached only 17. We are able to check one of the weekly totals from an independent source. In an extant letter of the time the following figures for the week from 23rd to 30th July are given, having been taken evidently from the published or posted weekly bill: " Died and were buried in London and suburbs, 399, most young people and youths, of which number of the common plague 320 persons. Number of children born and christened in the same week, 52[1]." "London and suburbs" would mean the 108 parishes of the City and liberties together with the 11 out parishes, so that the difference between Stow's 289 and the above 320 would give the number of plague-deaths in the out parishes for the particular week.

The state of matters in the City is thus referred to in Bullein's *Dialogue* published in 1564:—

Civis.—"Good wife, the daily jangling and ringing of the bells, the coming in of the minister to every house in ministering the communion, the reading of the homily of death, the digging up of graves, the sparring of windows, and the blazing forth of the blue crosses do make my heart tremble and quake." A beggar, in the same *Dialogue*, who had arrived from the country, says:

"I met with wagones, cartes and horses full loden with yong barnes, for fear of the blacke Pestilence, with them boxes of medicens and sweete perfumes. O God! how fast did they run by hundredes, and were afraied of eche other for feare of smityng."

We get one or two glimpses of this great plague from the medical point of view in Dr John Jones's *Dyall of Agues*[2]. The worst locality, he says, was " S. Poulkar's parish [St Sepulchre's]

---

[1] Letter from London to the Earl of Shrewsbury, *Hist. MSS. Com.* VI. 455, a.

[2] Without date, but probably 1564. Watt conjectures 1556, but the book contains references to the fever-epidemic of 1558, and, as above, to the plague of 1563.

by reason of many fruiterers, poor people, and stinking lanes, as Turnagain-lane [so called because it led down the slope to Fleet Ditch and ended there], Seacoal-lane, and such other places, there died most in London, and were soonest infected, and longest continued, as twice since I have known London I have marked to be true." Jones believed in contagion: "I myself was infected by reason that unawares I lodged with one that had it running from him." His other observation is interesting as proving the possibility of repeated attacks of the buboes in the same person, an observation abundantly confirmed, as we shall see, in the London plagues of 1603 and 1665:

"Here now, gentel readers, I think good to admonish all such as have had the plague, that they flie the trust of ignoraunt persons, who use to saye that he who hath once had the plague shal not nede to feare the havinge of it anye more : the whych by this example whyche foloweth (that chaunced to a certayne Bakers wife without Tempel barre in London, Anno Do. 1563) you shall find to be worthelye to be repeated : this sayde wyfe had the plage at Midsommer and at Bartholomewtide, and at Michaelmas, and the first time it brake, the seconde time it brake, but ran littell, the thirde time it appeared and brake not : but she died, notwythstanding she was twyce afore healed."

Two London physicians of some note died of the plague in 1563. One was Dr Geynes, who had brought trouble upon himself by impugning the authority of Galen, perhaps without sufficient reason. Having been cited before the College of Physicians, to whose discipline he was subject, he preferred to recant his heresy rather than undergo imprisonment. He died of plague on 23 July, 1563. Another was Dr John Fryer who had suffered twice for religious heresy, having been imprisoned by queen Mary as a Lutheran, and by queen Elizabeth as a papist. He regained his liberty in August, 1563, but only to die of plague on 21 October, his wife and several of his children having been also victims of the epidemic[1].

Stow ascribes the infection of the city of London by plague in the summer of 1563 to the return of the English troops from Havre, which town queen Elizabeth had boldly attempted to hold, and did actually hold for ten months, from September,

[1] Munk, *Roll of the College of Physicians*, I. pp. 32, 63.

1562, as an English fortress in French territory. Havre was not surrendered until the last days of July, 1563, and no returning troops could have reached London until August, by which time the plague had been raging there for two months. There was no doubt frequent communication between Havre and English ports while the siege lasted; but the sickness in each place can have been no more than coincident. Thus, while there were 17 plague-deaths in London in the week from the 5th to the 12th of June, the 7th of June is the first date on which report was made of sickness in Havre, although there had been cases of illness before. On that date the Earl of Warwick wrote to the Privy Council[1]: "For the want of money the works are hindered and the men discouraged. A strange disease has come amongst them, whereof nine died this morning (and many before) very suddenly." On the same day (7th June, 1563), one writes from Havre to Cecil: "Many of our men have been hurt in these skirmishes, but more by drinking of their wine, which hath cast down a great number, of hot burning diseases and impostumations, not unlike the plague." By the 9th June the deaths were from 20 to 30 a day. On the 12th June, 442 were sick out of a total force (including labourers and seamen) of 7143. On June 16, Warwick points out to the Privy Council that the sickness was aggravated by the want of fresh meat and the soldiers' usual beverages: "therefore their continual drinking of wine, contrary to their custom, has bred these disorders and diseases." On the 28th June the daily mortality was 77; from that date it increased somewhat, and was so serious as to hasten the surrender of the place to the French besieging force in the end of July. On July 27 there was plague in the castle of Jersey, and on August 6 it was very sore in Jersey, especially in the Castle[2].

It would have seemed the more probable to the people of London that the plague of 1563 had been imported across the Channel by reason of the unusually long immunity of the English capital in respect of that infection. A clear interval of

[1] This and other information immediately following are from *Cal. State Papers*. Foreign series.
[2] *Calendar of Cecil MSS.*, under the dates.

a dozen years without an epidemic, or a severe epidemic, was enough to make men forget the long tradition of plague domesticated upon English soil; while there was no scientific doctrine of epidemics then worked out, from which they might have known that the seeds of a disease may lie dormant for years, and that their periodic effectiveness depends upon a concurrence of favouring things, most of all upon extremes of dryness or wetness of the seasons as affecting a soil full of corrupting animal matters.

The plague of 1563 in the capital was accompanied or followed by several provincial outbreaks, of which few details are known. It is mentioned at Derby[1] in 1563, at Leicester[2] in 1563 and 1564 (a shut-up house in 1563, the first plague-burial in St Martin's parish on May 11, 1564), at Stratford-on-Avon, at Lichfield[3] and Canterbury[4] in 1564. But it is little more than mentioned at all those places. In the parish register of Hensley, in the North Riding of Yorkshire, a later incumbent, basing upon "an old writing of 1569," says that the explanation of the year 1563 being a blank in the register was "because in that year the visitation of plague was most hot and fearful, so that many died and fled, and the town of Hensley, by reason of the sickness, was unfrequented for a long season[5]."

Preventive Practice in Plague-time under the Tudors.

Having now traced the history of plague in London and in the provinces down to the beginning of the reign of Elizabeth, and having found it steady from year to year for many years in London, with an occasional terrific outburst, we are naturally led to ask whether the causes of it, or its favouring things, were understood, and whether any steps were taken to deal with it. This will be in effect a review of the earliest preventive practice.

---

[1] Glover's *Hist. of Derbyshire* (21 plague deaths in St Michael's register, May—Aug. 1563).

[2] Nichols; Kelly, in *Trans. Hist. Soc.* VI. 395.

[3] Harwood's *Hist. of Lichfield*, p. 304.

[4] Hasted's *Hist. of Canterbury*, p. 130 (parish registers).

[5] *Notes and Queries*, 2nd series, XI. 69.

That which was most clearly perceived by all was that the plague began to reign in certain years as the summer heats drew on, that the air of London or Westminster became "intemperate," or unwholesome, or infectious, and that it was desirable to get out of such air. Accordingly the one great rule, admitted by all and acted upon by as many as could, was to escape from the tainted locality, or as Wolsey expressed it to the earl of Shrewsbury in 1516, to get them "into clean air." There was no other sovereign prescription but that, and it remained the one great prescription until the last of plague in 1665–6.

Difficult points of casuistry arose out of that steady perception of an indisputable rule. Could flight from a plague-stricken place be reconciled with duty to one's neighbour? How ought a Christian man to demean himself in the plague? The Christian conscience may or may not have been tender on that ground in the medieval period; there is little to show one way or the other, except the occasional hints that we get, as in the Danish bishop's treatise, of an unwillingness to go near the victims of plague. But about the Reformation time those points of casuistry were debated; and one elaborate handling of them, in the form of a sermon by a German ecclesiastic, Osiander, was translated into English in 1537 by Miles Coverdale[1]. It followed, accordingly, that period of plague in London which has occupied the first part of this chapter. The translator remarks that they had been negligent of charity one to another, and he prints this discourse "to the intent that the ignorant may be taught, the weake strengthened, and everyone counselled after his callynge to serve his neighbor."

Osiander's perplexed Christian is in much the same case as Launcelot Gobbo in the play: "'Budge,' says the fiend; 'Budge not,' says my conscience. 'Conscience,' say I, 'you counsel well;' 'Fiend,' say I, 'you counsel well.'" The situation was a naturally complex one, and this is how the good preacher comes out of it:

[1] 'How and whether a Christen man ought to flye the horrible plage of the Pestilence. A sermon out of the Psalme "Qui habitat in adjutorio altissimi," by Andrewe Osiander. Translated out of Hye Almayn into Englishe, 1537.' Copy in the British Museum. The initials M.C. are taken to be those of Miles Coverdale.

"It is not my meaning to forbid or inhibit any man to fly, or to use physick, or to avoid dangerous and sick places in these fearful airs—so far as a man doth not therein against the belief, nor God's commandment, nor against his calling, nor against the love of his neighbour." And yet, shortly after : "Out of such fond childish fear it cometh that not only some sick folk be suffered to die away without all keeping, help, and comfort ; but the women also, great with child, be forsaken in their need, or else cometh there utterly no man unto them. Yet a man may hear also that the children forsake their fathers and mothers, and one household body keepeth himself away from another, and sheweth no love unto him. Which nevertheless he would be glad to see shewed unto himself if he lay in like necessity." He then exhorts the Christian man to remain at the post of duty, by the examples of the clergy and of "the higher powers of the world, who also abide in jeopardy"—certainly not the English experience. "Let him not axe his own reason, how he shall do, but believe, and follow the word of God, which teacheth him not to fly evil air and infect places (which he may well do : nevertheless he remaineth yet uncertain whether it helpeth or no)." The Christian man's perplexities can hardly have been resolved when all was said ; and the following sentence puts the case for quitting the infected place as strongly as it can be put: "For if it were in meat or drink, it might be eschewed ; if it were an evil taste, it might be expelled with a sweet savour ; if it were an evil wind, the chamber might with diligence be made close therefore ; if it were a cloud or mist, it might be seen and avoided ; if it were a rain, a man might cover himself for it. But now it is a secret misfortune that creepeth in privily, so that it can neither be seen nor heard, neither smelled nor tasted, till it have done the harm."

In practice the rule was 'Save who can;' so that whenever the infection promised to become "hot," as the phrase was, there was an adjournment of Parliament and of the Law Courts, a flight of all who could afford it to the country, and an interruption of business, diplomatic and other, which sometimes lasted for months. It was only occasionally, however, that the infection became really hot; in ordinary years a certain risk was run. Thus, in 1426, the plague had been severe enough to cut off the Scots hostages ; but it was not until after their death that the king's council left the city. Again, in 1467, Parliament did not adjourn (on 1st July) until several members of the House of Commons had died of the plague.

Although flight was the sovereign preventive in a great plague-season, it was impracticable in ordinary years when the infection was at its steadier or more endemic level. The endemic level was tolerated up to a certain point. In a long despatch to his government, the Venetian ambassador in London wrote of the plague as follows in 1554[1]:

"They have some little plague in England well nigh every year, for which they are not accustomed to make sanitary provisions, as it does not usually make great progress; the cases for the most part occur amongst the lower classes, as if their dissolute mode of life impaired their constitutions."

Whenever the plague showed signs of overstepping these limits, strenuous efforts were made to keep it in check. It may be questioned whether all that was done in that way made any difference; the great outbursts came at intervals, rose to their height, subsided in a few months, and left the city more or less free of plague until some concurrence of things, or the lapse of time, brought about another epidemic of the first degree. None the less, certain measures were taken to restrain the infection, and these were put in force with mechanical regularity whenever the Privy Council informed the Lord Mayor that the occasion required it. A brief account of them, of their beginnings and their development, will now be given.

The first that we hear of attempts at isolation and notification is in 1518. In April of that year, the Court being in Berkshire or Oxfordshire, Sir Thomas More charged the mayor of Oxford, and the commissary, in the king's name "that the inhabitants of those houses that be, and shall be infected, shall keep in, put out wispes, and bear white rods, as your Grace devised for Londoners[2]." By his Grace is to be understood the king himself; and these measures devised by him—the keeping in, the putting out of wisps on the houses, and the carrying of white rods,—might have been tried as early as the epidemic of 1513, which was a severe one. When two of the Venetian ambassador's servants died of the plague in 1513, their bed, sheets and other effects were thrown into the river. On the 21st of May, 1516, the ambassador removed to Putney owing to a case of plague in his house, and he was not allowed to see cardinal Wolsey until the 30th of June, i.e. until forty days had elapsed. This is perhaps the first mention of the quarantine which the Court rigorously

---

[1] Soranzo to the Senate of Venice. *Calendar of State Papers*, Venetian, v. 541 (18 Aug. 1554).

[2] *Cal. State Papers*, Henry VIII. Domestic.

put in practice against those who had business with it. On the 22nd July, 1518, the same ambassador wrote to Venice from Lambeth that two of his servants had lately died of the plague; and, on the 11th August, again from Lambeth, that the king and Wolsey would not see him because of the plague; "but on the expiration of forty days, which had nearly come to an end, he would not fail to do his duty as heretofore."

On the 25th August, 1535, Chapuys, in a letter to Charles V., gives an amusing account of an attempt made by the French ambassador to see Henry VIII. and Cromwell on diplomatic business. The Court was residing in Gloucestershire owing to plague in and near London (it was at Bristol also), and the ambassador journeyed thither to carry his business through. However he went no nearer than six miles, because a " French merchant" who followed him died upon the road of the plague, as it was feared. The king asked him to put his charge in writing, but the ambassador replied that he had orders to tell it in person, and that he could wait. At length he lay in wait for Secretary Cromwell in the fields where he went to hunt with the dukes of Norfolk and Suffolk, and delivered his charge despite the manifest unwillingness of Cromwell, who came away from the improvised diplomatic interview in no good humour.

The first plague-order of which the full text is extant was issued in the 35th of Henry VIII. (1543). As it contains the germs of all subsequent preventive practice, I transcribe it in full[1].

"35 Hen. VIII. A precept issued to the aldermen:—That they should cause their beadles to set the sign of the cross on every house which should be afflicted with the plague, and there continue for forty days:

"That no person who was able to live by himself, and should be afflicted with the plague, should go abroad or into any company for one month after his sickness, and that all others who could not live without their daily labour should as much as in them lay refrain from going abroad, and should for forty days after [illegible] and continually carry a white rod in their hand, two foot long:

"That every person whose house had been infected should, after a visi-

---

[1] From *Abstract of several orders relating to the Plague.* MS. Addit. (Brit. Museum), No. 4376. Probably the originals of these abstracts are among the Guildhall records. I quote from the most accessible source.

tation, carry all the straw and [illegible] in the night privately into the fields and burn ; they should also carry clothes of the infected in the fields to be cured:

"That no housekeeper should put any person diseased out of his house into the street or other place unless they provided housing for them in some other house :

"That all persons having any dogs in their houses other than hounds, spaniels or mastiffs, necessary for the custody or safe keeping of their houses, should forthwith convey them out of the city, or cause them to be killed and carried out of the city and buried at the common laystall :

"That such as kept hounds, spaniels, or mastiffs should not suffer them to go abroad, but closely confine them :

"That the churchwardens of every parish should employ somebody to keep out all common beggars out of churches on holy days, and to cause them to remain without doors:

"That all the streets, lanes, etc. within the wards should be cleansed :

"That the aldermen should cause this precept to be read in the churches."

Here we see a development of the measures which had been devised for London by Henry VIII. or his minister previous to 1518, and probably in the plague of 1513. The wisps put out on the infected houses are replaced by crosses, which, in the order of 1543, are simply called "the sign of the cross." They are next heard of during the plague of 1547, in a Guildhall record of 15 November[1] :

"Item, for as moche as my Lord Mayer reported that my Lorde Chauncelar declared unto hym that my Lorde Protectour's Grace's pleasure ys, and other of the Lordes of the Counseyll, that certain open tokens and sygnes shulde be made and sett furth in all such places of the Cytie as haue of late been vysyted with the plage "—be it therefore ordained that a certain cross of St Anthony devised for that purpose be affixed to the uttermost post of the street door, there to remain forty days after the setting up thereof.

The cross of St Anthony was a headless cross, and the crutch is supposed to have been painted (in blue) on canvas or board and fixed to the post of the street door. The legend under or over the cross was, "Lord have mercy upon us." Before the plague of 1603, the colour had been changed to red.

The white rods, which had been devised along with the wisps previous to 1518, are mentioned in the order of 1543 as two foot

---

[1] Extracts from the Guildhall Records, by Furnivall, in Appendix to Vicary's *Anatomy of the Body of Man.* Early English Text Society.

long ; they were to be carried for forty days by those who must needs go abroad from plague-stricken houses. We hear of them again, both in France and in England in 1580 and 1581. On the 20th November, 1580, the Venetian ambassador to France writes from the neighbourhood of Paris : "This city, I hear, is in a very fair sanitary condition, notwithstanding that as I entered a city gate, which is close to where I reside, I met a man and a woman bearing the white plague wands in their hands and asking alms ; but some believe that this was merely an artifice on their part to gain money[1]." In the regulations for plague added in 1581 by the mayor of London to the earlier code, the third is : "That no persons dwelling in a house infected be suffered to go abroad unless they carry with them a white wand of a yard long ; any so offending to be committed to the Cage." In the seventeenth-century plagues of London and provincial towns, the white wand was retained as the peculiar badge of the searchers of infected houses and of the bearers of the dead. The white rod or wand carried by inmates of infected houses, had become a red rod in the plague of 1603, just as the blue cross had been changed to red.

The other directions in the order of 1543 are heard of from time to time in the subsequent history of plague—such as the burning of straw, and the cleansing of the streets. The Guildhall record of 15 November, 1547, after directing the blue crosses to be affixed to houses, proceeds :

"And also to cause all the welles and pumpes within their seid wardes to be drawen iii times euerye weke, that is to say, Monday, Wednesday, and Friday. And to cast down into the canelles at euerye such drawyng xii bucketts full of water at the least, to clense the stretes wythall."

Under Elizabeth, the orders as to scavenging become much more stringent, as we shall see. In the plague of 1563, on 29 September, the Common Council appointed "two poor men to burn and bury such straw, clothes, and bedding as they shall find in the fields near the city or within the city, whereon any person in the plague hath lyen or dyed[2]."

[1] *Cal. State Papers*, Venetian, VII. 649.
[2] *Abstract*, &c. in Brit. Mus. MSS., as above.

The curious order as to dogs was based upon the belief that they carried the infection in their hair, just as cats are now believed by some to carry infection in their fur. Brasbridge, in his *Poor Man's Jewel* (1578), gives a case of a glover at Oxford, into whose house a disastrous plague-infection was supposed to have been brought by means of a dog's skin bought in London[1]. The plague-regulations contained the clause against dogs to the last; in the great plagues of 1603, 1625, and 1665, thousands of them were killed, many of them having been doubtless left behind in the exodus of the well-to-do classes. In the corporation records of Winchester[2], there is a minute, undated, but probably belonging to the end of the 16th century, that dogs shall be kept indoors "if any house within the city shall happen to be infected with the plague." A proclamation during the London plague of 1563 is directed against cats as well as dogs, "for the avoidance of the plague:" officers were appointed to kill and bury all such as they found at large[3].

The great London plague of 1563 had revived the old practices and given rise to some new ones. Curates and churchwardens were directed to warn the inmates of houses where plague had occurred not to come to church for a certain space thereafter[4]. The blue crosses were again in great request, being ordered by hundreds at a time in readiness to affix to infected houses[5]. Also it was ordered by the Mayor and Council that the "filthie dunghill lying in the highway near unto Fynnesburye Courte be removed and carried away; and not to suffer any such donge or fylthe from hensforthe there to be leyde[6]." On the 9th of July, 1563, plague having been already at work for several weeks, a commission was issued by the queen in Council, that every

---

[1] The following is the case by which he supports the recommendation to kill dogs in plague-time : "Not many years since, I knew a glover in Oxford who with his family, to the number of ten or eleven persons, died of the plague, which was said to be brought into the house by a dogge skinne that his wife bought when the disease was in the Citie" (*Poor Man's Jewel*, Chapter VIII. London, 1578).

[2] *Transcripts from the MS. Archives*, ed. Bayley, 1856.

[3] News-letter to the Earl of Shrewsbury, *Hist. MSS. Commis.* VI. 455.

[4] *Machyn's Diary*, ed. J. Gough Nichols. Camden Soc., No. 42, p. 310.

[5] *Ibid.* p. 396 (note by Nichols); and Guildhall Records, in Furnivall, *l.c.*

[6] *Abstract*, &c. as above.

householder in London should, at seven in the evening, lay out wood and make bonfires in the streets and lanes, to the intent that they should thereby consume the corrupt airs, the fires to be made on three days of the week[1]. On 30th September, 1563, it was ordered that all such houses as were infected should have their doors and windows shut up, and the inmates not to stir out nor suffer any to come to them for forty days. At the same time, a collection was ordered to be made in the churches for the relief of the poor afflicted with the plague, and thus shut up. Another order was that new mould should be laid on the graves of such as die of the plague. Still another, the first of a long series, was to prohibit all interludes and plays during the infection[2]. On the 2nd December, when the deaths had fallen to 178 in the week, an order was issued by the Common Council that houses in which the plague had been were not to be let. On the 20th January, 1564, there was an order for a general airing and cleansing of houses, bedding and the like. By that time the deaths had fallen to 13 in the week.

The most rigorous measures in this plague were those which queen Elizabeth took for her own safety at Windsor in September. Stow says that "a gallows was set up in the market-place of Windsor to hang all such as should come there from London. No wares to be brought to, or through, or by Windsor; nor any one on the river by Windsor to carry wood or other stuff to or from London, upon pain of hanging without any judgment; and such people as received any wares out of London into Windsor were turned out of their houses, and their houses shut up[3]."

In 1568 a more complete set of instructions to the aldermen of the several wards was drawn up by the Lord Mayor, and a corresponding order for the city of Westminster by Sir William Cecil, Secretary of State, and by the Chancellor of the Duchy. In 1581 some additional orders were issued by the Lord Mayor. The whole of these are here given from a state paper in a later handwriting, probably of the time of James I. or Charles I.[4]

---

[1] Stow's *Memoranda* (Lambeth MS.), Camden Soc., 1880, p. 123.
[2] *Abstract*, &c. as above.   [3] Stow, *ibid*.
[4] Record Office. *State Papers*, Elizabeth, vol. XLVIII., No. 70.

A collection of such papers as are found in the office of his Majesties papers and records for business of state for the preventing and decreasing of the plague in and about London.

A. (City of London, 1568.)

1. First a 'tre from the Mayor of London to every alderman of each warde to charge their Deputys counstables and officers to make search of all houses infected within each parish.

2. To cause all infected houses to bee shutt up and noe person to come forth in twenty dayes after the infection.

3. That some honest discreete person be appoynted to attend each such infected house to provide them of all necessaries at the cost of the M^r of the house if he be able.

4. For the poorer houses infected that the Alderman or his deputy doe cause to make collection for the supply of all necessaries to be charged upon the wealthyer sorte of the same warde or parish.

5. That such as shall refuse to pay what they are assest shall be committed to warde untill they pay it.

6. That all bedding and cloathes and other thinges apt to take infection which were about infected persons bee burnt or such order taken that infection may not be increased by them.

7. Lastly that a bill with 'Lord have mercy upon us' in greate 'tres bee sett over the dore of euery infected house and that the counstables and Beadles have a care to see that the same be not taken downe.

These orders were sett downe by the Mayior of London in the yeere 1568, whereupon queene Elizabeth writeth a letter to Sr William Cycill then secretary and Sr Ambrous Cave, chauncellor of the Duchy to take the like order or any other that they should thinke fitt in the citie of Westminster.

B. (City of Westminster, 1568.)

Orders sett down by Sr William Cycill, Secretary, as High Steward of Westminster and Sr Ambrous Cave, chauncellor of the Dutchy to the Bay-leiffes, Hedburroughs, Counstables and other officers of the sayde Citty.

1. That they should follow the good example of the orders devised and observed by the Mayior and Aldermen of London, and further that all that haue any houses shops or loggings that hath had any infection in them by the space of twenty dayes before the making of these orders shall shutt up all their doares and windoares towards the streetes and common passages for forty dayes next and not suffer after the tyme of the sicknes any person to goe forth nor any uninfected to come in upon payne that euery offender shall sitt seven dayes in the stocks and after that be committed to the common Goale there to remayne forty dayes from the first day of his being in the stocks.

2. That the officers aforesayde with the curate of euery parish and churchwardens doe make such collection of the rest of the parishioners as shall be necessary for the sustenance of such as bee poore infected and shutt up.

3. To discharge all inmates out of all houses that there be noe more persons in one house then be of one family except they be lodgers for a small time.

4. To cause the streetes lanes and passages and all the shewers sinkes (?) and gutters thereof dayly to be made sweete and cleane.

C. (London, 1581.)

There were added by the Mayior of London to the former articles these following in the year 1581.

1. That speciall noatis be taken of such houses infected as sell cloth, silke and other wares and make garments and aparrell for men and women.

2. That euery counstable within his precinct haue at all tymes in readines two honest and discreete women to attend any house infected.

3. That noe person dwelling in a house infected bee suffered to goe abroade unless they carry with them a white wand of a yarde long. Any soe offending to bee committed to the Cage there to remayne untill order shallbe taken by the Mayior or his bretheren.

4. That they suffer not any deade corps dying of the plague to be buryed in tyme of divine service or sermon.

5. To appoynt two honest and discreete matrons within euery parish who shall bee sworne truely to search the body of euery such person as shall happen to dye within the same parish, to the ende that they make true reporte to the clerke of the parish church of all such as shall dye of the plague, that the same clerke may make the like reporte and certificate to the wardens of the parish clerkes thereof according to the order in that behalfe heretofore provided.

If the viewers through favour or corruption shall giue wrong certificate, or shall refuse to serue being thereto appointed, then to punish them by imprisonment in such sorte as may serue for the terror of others.

6. That order be taken for killing of dogs that run from house to house dispersing the plague, and that noe swine be suffered or kept within the citty[1].

Several of these plague-regulations had been in force, as we have seen, from near the beginning of the century. Others, not hitherto mentioned, were also of earlier date. Thus the collec-

---

[1] Endorsed "An abstract of such orders as have been heretofore for the preventing and decreasing of the plague in and about London."

tions for the poor are mentioned in the diary of a London citizen in 1538 and 1539, but not specially in connexion with plague. They are heard of often after the plague of 1563, along with other provisions for the poor which mark the reign of Elizabeth. If we may trust Bullein's *Dialogue* of 1564, a systematic provision became necessary because private charity was no longer to be depended on. In many country towns and parishes, as we shall see, the contributions or compensations to the inmates of shut-up houses in the Elizabethan plagues were paid out of the municipal funds, either those of the affected place or of some "unvisited" neighbouring town. The Act of Parliament which most directly provided for "the charitable relief of persons infected with the plague" was the 1st James I. (1603–4), cap. 31.

A most essential part of the means for controlling plague was the institution of searchers[1]. In the orders of 1543, the aldermen of the wards are directed to send their beadles to affix the sign of the cross to affected houses. But in due course these duties of inspection, notification, isolation and registration passed in London into the hands of the Company of Parish Clerks. The original business of the Parish Clerks was with church music. In the thirteenth century they received a charter of incorporation as the Clerks of St Nicholas, and became associated with that love of choral singing which has always distinguished the English people. Legacies and endowments fell to them for the performance of specific services, or for their encouragement in general. From time to time the Company would appear in a particular parish church to sing a mass. It was the singular history of a Company which gained its greatest name as the Registrars of Births and Deaths in London down to the Registration Act of 1837, to have been not only the first Choral Society but also the first company of stage players. In 1391, says Stow, a play was given by the parish clerks of London at the Skinners' Well beside Smithfield, which continued three days together, the king, queen and nobles of the realm being present. Another play, in the year 1409, lasted eight

---

[1] The searchers are mentioned at Shrewsbury as early as 1539 (Phillips).

days, "and was of matter from the creation of the world, whereat was present most of the nobility and gentry of England[1]."

In the time of Sir Thomas More, a parish clerk meant one who sang in the church choir. When More was lord chancellor, the duke of Norfolk came one day to dine with him at his house at Chelsea, and not finding him at home, went in search of him. He found him, where posterity will long delight to picture him,— in the church "singing in the choir with a surplice on his back." As they walked home arm in arm the duke said to Sir Thomas More: "A parish clerk! a parish clerk! God body, my lord chancellor, you dishonour the king and his office;" whereon the chancellor answered as if he did not take the duke altogether seriously.

The whole strength of the Company of Parish Clerks in those times would attend the funeral of some rich person, as we may read in the sixteenth-century diary of Machyn the undertaker (sometimes the Company chosen to follow the body to the grave was that of the Tallow Chandlers, as in the case of John Stow's mother). It was no great step from their old duties to their new. There were, as we have seen, bills of mortality compiled weekly for all the parishes in the city and liberties as early as 1532 and 1535. It is not said that the Parish Clerks were the collectors of the information, but they were as likely to have been so as any other persons whom the mayor would employ. Bills were also drawn up for a few weeks during the sweating sickness of 1551, and again for an unbroken series of some two hundred weeks from the beginning of the plague of 1563. The figures are preserved from a single weekly bill, 22–28 October, 1574, which must have been one of a series[2]. The next bills known are a series for five years, 1578–83, a plague-period of which more will have to be said in its proper place in the chronology.

The orders of 1581, already given, make mention of the two discreet matrons within every parish who shall be sworn truly to search the body of every such person as shall happen to die within the same parish, of their reporting to the clerk of the

---

[1] *Survey of London, ed. cit.* p. 119.
[2] Holinshed, III. p. 1260.

parish, and of the clerk making report and certificate to the wardens of the Parish Clerks, who would send the weekly certificate for all the parishes to the mayor, and he to the minister of State. That was said to be "according to the order in that behalf heretofore provided." It is probable, therefore, that the searchers became an institution as early as the plague of 1563, or, at all events, at the beginning of the plague-period of 1578–83.

The clerk of the Company in 1665 describes how the discreet matrons were chosen as searchers or viewers of the dead in each parish, and how they were sworn to discharge their duties faithfully[1]. The swearing in took place before the Dean of the Arches, that is to say, in St Mary le Bow church ("St Mary of the Arch") in Cheapside. The motive to bribe them for a wrong report on the cause of death was to avoid the shutting up and all other troubles of a household pronounced infected by the plague. In later times their diagnostic duties became, as we shall see, much more complex ; but down to 1604, when they first brought to the Parish Clerks' Hall "an account of the diseases and casualties" (which classification and nomenclature did not begin to be printed until 1629), they had merely to say whether a death had been from plague or from other cause.

Sanitation in Plantagenet and Tudor times.

Along with all those means, having the object of stopping the spread of infection, the Elizabethan policy did not neglect what we should now consider the more radical means of sanitation. It is usual to bring a sweeping charge of neglect of public hygiene against all old times ; there was so much plague in those times, and so high an average death-rate, that it is commonly assumed that our ancestors must have been wanting in the rudimentary instincts of cleanliness. But, in the first place, one might expect to find that all old periods were not alike ; and more generally it is worth inquiring how far nuisances injurious to the public health were tolerated. This inquiry will

---

[1] John Bell, *London's Remembrancer.* Lond. 1665.

have to be as brief as possible; but it will take us back to the period of plague covered by a former chapter.

Nuisances certainly existed in medieval London, but it is equally certain that they were not tolerated without limit. I have collected in a note the instances reported in a visitation of 17 Edward III. (1343), and in a perambulation of the ground outside the walls in 26 Edward III. (1352). The former related only to the alleys leading down to the river, which were likely enough places for nuisance, then as now[1].

There are several orders of Edward III. relating to the removal of laystalls and to keeping the town ditch clean, which show, of course, that there was neglect, but at the same time the disposition to correct it. It is farther obvious that the connexion between nuisances and the public health was clearly apprehended. The sanitary doctrines of modern times were undreamt of; nor did the circumstances altogether call for them. The sewers of those days were banked-up water courses, or "shores" as the word was pronounced, which ran uncovered down the various declivities of the city, to the town ditch and to the Thames. They would have sufficed to carry off the refuse of a population of some forty or sixty thousand; they were, at all events, freely open to the greatest

---

[1] *Liber Albus Londinensis.* Rolls series, ed. Riley. The following instances occur in the report of the commissioners of 1343: P. 446: A water-gate "obturatur ratione unius gutturi exeuntis de una latrina," etc. P. 449: the Ebbegate obstructed by certain persons named, "qui fecerunt in eadem venella latrinas supra dentes, quarum putredo cadit supra capita hominum transeuntium." Same page: Wendegoslane "obturatur per fimos et garderobas." Same page: Rethersgate obstructed "per fimos et alia hujusmodi foetida." Same page: Dowgate. Two householders named "in eisdem aedificiis diversas latrinas fecerunt, pendentes ultra vicum ejusdem venellae; quarum putredines cadunt supra homines per eandem venellam transeuntes." P. 450: at Queenhithe a "communis latrina." P. 451: at Saltwharf the way to the river obstructed "pulvere et aliis putredinibus in eadem projiciendis." P. 452: Lekynggeslane has two latrinae and is impassable owing to want of paving. Same page: Another venel obstructed by the Earl Marshall; three latrinae in it. In a perambulation of the ground outside the walls, 26 Ed. III. (1552), the following encroachments are noted among others: Outside Ludgate, one has erected a shed (*camera*) 16 ft. × 12¾ ft., and made there "unum profundum puteum et quadratum pro latrina"—a deep well and a latrine-pit together. Also outside Ludgate, William of Wircestre has a house there and two shelters for beasts, and a latrine, and part of the said house is 14 ft. × 7½ ft.

of all purifying agents, the oxygen of the air; and they poisoned neither the water of the town ditch (which abounded in excellent fish within John Stow's memory) nor the waters of Thames. In course of time all the brooks of London were covered in, even the Fleet dyke itself, which used to float barges as far as Holborn bridge; but who shall say that they were more wholesome thereafter, although they were underground? Perhaps the poet of the *Earthly Paradise* has as true an intuition as any when, in reference to the city in Chaucer's time, he bids us

> "Dream of London, small, and white, and clean;
> The clear Thames bordered by its gardens green."

The nuisance that gave most trouble in the medieval and Tudor periods was the blood and offal of the shambles. Several ordinances of Edward III. are directed against it, in one of which (1371) the connexion between putrefying blood soaked into the ground and infectious disease is clearly stated. It is also the principal subject of the first sanitary Act that appears in the Statutes of the Realm, made by the Parliament of Cambridge in the 17th of Richard II. (1388), of which I give the preamble and provisions:

"Item, For that so much Dung and Filth of the Garbage and Intrails as well of Beasts killed as of other Corruptions be cast and put in Ditches, Rivers and other Waters, and also within many other Places within about and nigh unto divers Cities, Boroughs and Towns of the Realm, and the Suburbs of them, that the Air there is greatly corrupt and infect, and many Maladies and other intolerable Diseases do daily happen," both to the residents and to visitors:—therefore proclamation is to be made in the City of London, as in other cities, boroughs and towns "that all they which do cast and lay all such Annoyances, Dung, Garbages, Intrails and other Ordure in Ditches, Rivers, Waters and other places shall cause them to be removed, avoided and carried away betwixt this and the feast of St Michael next following," under a penalty of twenty pounds, mayors and bailiffs to compel obedience. Such offences were not to be repeated, and if any did offend he was liable to be called by writ before the Chancellor "at his suit that will complain[1]."

Despite this statute, the shambles in the parish of St Nicholas within Newgate (adjoining the ground now occupied by Christ's

---

[1] *Statutes of the Realm*, 17 Ric. II.

Hospital, and formerly by the Grey Friars) became an established institution of the city. They were a subject of petition to Parliament in 1488–9, and they were still there to give occasion in 1603 to severe remarks by Thomas Lodge, poet and physician, who practised in Warwick Lane, in their immediate neighbourhood. The Act of 1388, it will be observed, was to be set in motion "at his suit that will complain;" so that there was little more in it than the immemorial remedy from a nuisance at common law.

The reign of Henry V. appears to have been marked by care for the public health, perhaps not greater than in Edward III.'s time, but exceptional, in the records at least, under the later Plantagenets and until the accession of the Tudor dynasty. Among other evidences (some of which may be gathered from Stow's *Survey*) is the ordinance of 1415 (3 Hen. V.) against a nuisance in the Moor, beyond the wall and the ditch on the Finsbury side. The Moor was, in Fitzstephen's words, "a great fen, which watereth the walls on the north side." In 1415 there was a "common latrine" in it, and "sicknesses arose from the horrible, corrupt, and infected atmosphere," issuing therefrom[1]. Its removal was ordered, and in the same year (1415) chaussées were built across the fen, one to Hoxton and another to Islington. The ditch all the way round from the Tower to Blackfriars had been cleansed the year before (1414).

Another statute, 3 Henry VII. (1488–9) cap. 3, may be quoted to show that the slaughter-houses were the chief nuisance, that their effects on health were perceived (as in Edward III.'s time), and that it was necessary to appeal to the king's personal interest in the matter as a motive for redress.

Petition to the King from the parishioners of St Faiths and St Gregories in London, near St Pauls.

"That it was soo that grete concourse of peple, as well of his Roial persone as of other grete Lordes and astates wyth other hys true subgettes often tymes was had unto the said Cathedrall Chirche, and for the moost part through oute the parisshe aforesaide, the whiche often tymes ben gretly

---

[1] Riley, *op. cit.*, p. 614.

ennoyed and invenemed by corrupt eires, engendered in the said parisshes by occasion of bloode and other fowler thynges, by occasion of the slaughter of bestes and scaldyng of swyne had and doon in the bocherie of Seynt Nicholas Flesshamls, whos corrupcion by violence of unclene and putrified waters is borne down thrugh the said parishes and compasseth two partes of the Palays where the Kynges most Roiall persone is wonte to abide when he cometh to the Cathedrall Chirche for ony acte there to be doon, to the Jubardouse [jeopardous] abydyng of his most noble persone and to ouer grete ennoysaunce of the parisshens there, and of other the Kyngis subgettes and straungers that passe by the same ;

Compleynte whereof at dyverse and many seasons almost by the space of xvi yeres contynuelly, as well by the Chanons and petty Chanons of the said Cathedrall Chirche, londlordes there...made to Mayor and aldermen of the city; and noo remedie had ne founden.

...Considering that in few noble cities or towns or none within Christendom, where as travellyng men have labored, that the comen slaughter hous of bestys sholde be kept in ony speciall parte within the walle of the same lest it myght engender Siknesse to the destruccion of the peple."

The King etc. "ordeyned and stablished that no Bocher shall sley within the said house called the Scaldinghouse or within the walls of London."

And the same "in eny citte, Burghe and Towne walled within the Realm of Englonde and in the Towne of Cambridge, the Townes of Berwyk and Carlile only except and forprised."

The popular knowledge of and belief in a high doctrine of contagion are curiously shown by the terms of the Act touching Upholsterers in 1495 (11 Hen. VII. cap. 19).

The Act was intended to prevent beds, feather-beds, bolsters and pillows from being sold in market outside London, "beyond control of the Craft of Upholders." Outside the craft an inferior article was apt to be offered, which was at once a lowering of a good and worthy standard and a danger to health. There were two kinds of corrupt bed-stuffs "contagious for mannys body to lye on," firstly, scalded feathers and dry pulled feathers together ; and secondly, flocks and feathers together. Besides these, quilts, mattresses and cushions stuffed with horse hair, fen down, neat's hair, deer's hair and goat's hair, "which is wrought in lyme fattes," give out by the heat of man's body, a savour and taste so abominable and contagious that many of the King's subjects thereby have been destroyed. These corrupt and unlawful stuffs and wares might indeed be made by any person or persons for their own proper use in their houses, so they be not offered for sale in fairs or markets.

The reign of Henry VIII. is not marked by any ordinances or Acts for the restraint of plague or the like sickness by other than quarantine measures. The common ditch between Aldgate and the postern of the Tower was cleansed in 1519 at the charges of the city; in 1540 the Moor ditch was cleansed: and, not long before, the ditch from the Tower to Aldgate. In 1549 the ditch was again cleansed at the charges of the City Companies[1]. In April, 1552, John Shakespeare, the poet's father, a citizen of Stratford-on-Avon in good circumstances and afterwards mayor of the town, was fined twelve pence (eight to ten shillings present value) for not removing the heap of household dirt and refuse that had accumulated in front of his own door[2]. In the records of the borough of Ipswich[3], scavengers are mentioned in the 32nd of Henry VIII. (1540): they were elected in every parish, and the gatherings of refuse ordered to be carried and laid at four places, namely: Warwick Pitts, College Yard, behind the Ditches next John Herne, and the Dikes in the Marsh. When queen Elizabeth visited Ipswich (in 1561, 1565 and 1577), she rated not only the clergy on the laxity of their behaviour, but also the civic authorities upon the filthy condition of the streets. "A marked improvement," says the borough historian, "certainly took place in Ipswich at this period, as is incontestably shown by the constant exhortations and promulgations of laws for the preservation of cleanliness."

In the *Description and Account of the City of Exeter*, written by John Vowell, or Hoker, chamberlain of the city and member of Parliament for it in the reign of Elizabeth[4], we find the following about the offices and duties of scavengers "as of old."

They are "necessary officers who cannot be wanting in any well-governed city or town, because by them and their service all things noisome to the health of man, and hurtful to the state of the body of the commonwealth, are advertised unto the magistrate, and so they be the means of the redress thereof. And therefore they be called Scavengers, as who saith Shewers or Advertisers, for so the word soundeth." Among other duties they had the oversight of pavements, that they were swept weekly, of slaughter-houses, dunghills and the like, of dangerous buildings and of encroachments upon

---

[1] Stow's *Survey*.   [2] Art. "Shakespeare," *Encycl. Britan.*
[3] Wodderspoon's *Memorials of Ipswich*, p. 285, p. 259.
[4] "Now first printed." Exeter, 1765, p. 181.

the streets, of chimneys, and of precautions against fires (tubs of water to be in readiness at the doors to quench fires and cleanse the streets); and on Sundays they had to attend the mayor of Exeter to the church of St Peter's.

These officers of the municipality discharged their duties, says the Elizabethan writer, "as of old;" from which we may conclude that some such regulation had existed from quite early times. The scavengers are mentioned by Stow at the end of his account of each City ward along with other officers. We have already seen, from the court rolls of the manor of Castle Combe under the year 1427, that villagers were fined or admonished for creating nuisances. A sudden revival of zeal in that way at Castle Combe in the year 1590 may have been due to the vigorous sanitary policy of Elizabeth's government:

"And that the inhabitants of the West Strete doe remove the donge or fylth at John Davis house ende before the feaste of Seynct Andrew th'apostell next, and that they lay no more there within x foote of the wey, sub poena iii s iiii d.

"And that none shall lay any duste or any other fylth in the wey or pitte belowe Cristopher Besas house, sub poena pro quolibet tempore xii d.

"And that none shall soyle in the church yerde nor in any of our stretes, for every defaulte to lose xii d.

"And that the glover shall not washe any skynes, nor cast any other fylth or soyle in the water runnynge by his house, sub poena x s[1]."

There is an interval of a century and a half between the two instances of sanitary vigour adduced from the Castle Combe manor court; but there is no reason to believe that the tradition of common cleanliness ever lapsed altogether, in that or in any other village or town of the country.

Some part of the rather unfair opinion as to the foulness of English life in former times may be traced to a well-known letter by Erasmus to the physician of cardinal Wolsey. There are grounds for believing that Erasmus must have judged from somewhat unfavourable instances.

"We read of a city," says Erasmus, "which was freed from continual pestilence by changes made in its buildings on the advice of a philosopher. Unless I am mistaken, England may be freed in like manner." He then proceeds to go over the

---

[1] Poulett Scrope, *op. cit.* p. 333.

defects of English houses, and to suggest improvements. The houses were built with too little regard to the aspect of their doors and windows towards the sun. Again, they have a great part of their walls filled with panes of glass, admitting light in such wise as to keep out the wind, and yet letting in at chinks of the windows the air as if strained or percolated, and so much the more pestilential by being long stagnant. These defects he would remedy by having two or three sides of a house exposed to the sky, and all glazed windows so made that they should open wholly or shut wholly, and so shut that there might be no access of noxious winds through gaping seams; for if it be sometimes wholesome to admit the air, it is sometimes wholesome to keep it out. Inside the houses Erasmus professes to have seen a shocking state of things—the floors covered with rushes piled, the new upon the old, for twenty years without a clearance, befouled with all manner of filth, with spillings of beer and the remains of fish, with expectoration and vomit, with excrement and urine[1]. Here we have clearly to do with the intelligent foreigner. On the other hand, as far back as the reign of Richard I., Englishmen would appear to have contrasted their own personal habits with those of other nations, much as the summer tourist does now. English youths, it has been said, go through Europe with one phrase on their lips: "Foreigners don't wash." Richard of Devizes implies somewhat the same. A Frankish youth is being advised where to settle in England, Winchester being chosen by excluding the other towns one by one. Bristol, for example, was wholly given over to soap-boilers: everyone in Bristol was either a soap-boiler or a retired soap-boiler; "and the Franks love soap as much as they love scavengers[2]." We may cry quits, then, with Erasmus over the rush-strewn floors. It is clear, also, that the glazed fronts of English houses, which he took exception to, are the very feature of them that Sir Thomas More prided himself upon; in that as in other external things the London of his day seemed

---

[1] *D. Erasmi Epistolar. lib. XXX.* London, 1642, Lib. xxii. Epist. 12 (without date).

[2] Richard of Devizes. Eng. Hist. Soc. p. 60: "Apud Bristolliam nemo est qui non sit vel fuerit saponarius; et omnis Francus saponarios amat ut stercorarios."

to him to leave little to be desired as the capital of Utopia, his chief subjects of remark being the shambles and the want of hospitals for the sick[1].

Thus, when we attempt to clear the sense of our rather mixed notions on the unwholesome life of former times, we must feel constrained to withdraw a great part of the accusation as to nuisances tolerated or scavenging neglected. Most of all was the government of Elizabeth marked by vigour in its attempts to restrain plague, not only by quarantine measures, but also by radical sanitation.

Queen Elizabeth and her Council were baffled by the persistence of plague in London in 1581–82–83; the infection pursued its own course despite all efforts to "stamp it out," so that the letters from the lords of the Council to the mayor begin to assume a somewhat querulous and impatient tone[2]. To a letter of remonstrance, 21st September, 1581, the mayor replied next day that every precaution had been taken. On the 22nd March, 1582, the mayor retorted upon the Court that an artificer in leather, dwelling near Fleet Bridge, had the plague in his house, that his house had been shut up, and he restrained from going out; nevertheless he had access to the Court in the things of his art, both for the queen and her household. On the 1st September, 1582, the plague having greatly increased as appeared by certificate of the number of the dead during the last week, the Privy Council informed the mayor that this was in part "by negligence in not keeping the streets and other places about the city clean, and partly through not shutting up of the houses where the sickness had been found, and setting marks upon the doors; but principally through not observing orders for prevention of the infection heretofore sent to them by the Council." The mayor sent answer the same day that every care had been taken: the streets had been cleansed every other day; the parish clerks had been appointed to see to the shutting up of infected houses, and putting papers

---

[1] William Harrison's *Description of England* (in Holinshed) gives proof enough that the filthy floors described by Erasmus had no existence two generations later, even among the poorer classes.

[2] The correspondence is in *Remembrancia*, under the head of "Plague."

upon the doors; he had also appointed some of his own officers to go up and down the city to view and inform him whether these things had been done.

So much did the Council believe, or affect to believe, that the mayor could control the plague if he carried out their orders, that they used the adjournment of the law courts as a threat to the city. On the 15th October, the Term was announced to be held at Hertford, and all persons from infected London houses were forbidden to repair thither with merchandise, victual, &c.[1]. Then follow in January, 1583, letters touching an impracticable attempt of the Privy Council to have a list printed of all inns and taverns that had been infected within the last two months. The mayor made a catalogue which was pronounced too long. On 21st April, 1583, the infection had much increased, and the lords of the Council again urged upon the mayor to have infected houses shut up, and provision made for feeding and maintaining the inmates thereof. They desired to express her majesty's surprise that no house or hospital had been built without the city, in some remote place, to which the infected people might be removed, although other cities of less antiquity, fame, wealth, and reputation had provided themselves with such places, whereby the lives of the inhabitants had been in all times of infection chiefly preserved. The mayor, on 3rd May, wrote that the Court of Aldermen had published orders for the stay of the plague; but that they were comparatively powerless so long as crowds of the worst sort of people resorted to see plays, bear-baiting, fencers, and profane spectacles at the theatre, and Curtain, and other the like places.

The plague pursued its own course, wholly unaffected, so far as one can see, by everything that was tried. One thing that was not touched by the sanitary policy, was probably more relevant than all else to the continuance of plague—the disposal of the dead. The theoretical importance attached to that as an original cause of plague has been avowed in the chapter on the

[1] From a memorandum of Lord Burghley's, dated Hertford Castle, 21 Nov. 1582, it appears that a survey had shown 577 beds available for strangers in one parish of Hertford, and 451 in another, "so that there are lying two a bed above 2000 people." *Cal. State Papers.* Domestic series, Elizabeth 1581–90, p. 75.

Black Death. We have here to see how the theory of it as a favouring thing for the continuance of the infection squares with the facts in such a city as London under the Plantagenets and Tudors.

The Disposal of the Dead.

Intramural interment was one of the most cherished practices of Christendom so long as the word "intramural" had a literal meaning. Hence the correctness of the imagery used of the Spiritual City:

> "To work and watch, until we lie
> At rest within thy wall."

Probably each of the one hundred and twenty small parish churches of London in the medieval period stood in its small churchyard. In an exceptional time like the Black Death, these proved insufficient for the daily burials: three new cemeteries were enclosed and consecrated outside the walls—two of them in Smithfield and the other at Aldgate. These all soon passed into the hands of friars, and became the grounds of monasteries. The churches or churchyards of monasteries were in great request for burial, but not for common burials, or for burials in a time of epidemic. The 'Vision of Piers the Ploughman' is clear enough that the friars took no large view of their duties; they affected the care of the dead, but only if they were well paid:

"For I said I nold | be buried at their house but at my parish church. | For I heard once how conscience it told | that where a man was christened by kynde [nature] he should be buried, | or where he were parishen, right there he should be graven. | And for I said this to friar, a fool they me held | and loved me the less for my lele speech | ......I have much marveil ot you and so hath many another | why your convent coveteth to confess and to bury | rather than to baptise bairns that ben catechumens."

The reason why the friars paid so much attention to burials was that these rites were the most profitable:

"And how that freris [friars] folowed folke that was riche | and folke that was pore at litel price they sette, | and no corps in their kirk-yerde ne in their kyrke was buried | but quick he bequeath them aught or should help quit their debts."

The friars in the towns would appear, then, to have been as much in request for the disposal of the dead within their precincts as the monks were in the country, both alike taking a certain part of that duty out of the hands of the regular parish clergy. Hence we may assign a good many burials, perhaps mostly of the richer class, as in Stow's long lists of conventual burials, to the various precincts of Whitefriars, Blackfriars, Greyfriars (within Newgate) or Friars Minor (Minories), Carthusians, or other settlements of the religious orders in the city and liberties of London. It is not unlikely that the narrow spaces for burial in and around the old churches in the streets and lanes of the city were already getting crowded, and that the friars naturally acquired a large share of the business of burial because their consecrated houses and enclosed grounds were situated where there was most room, namely in the skirt of the Liberties, or in waste spaces within the walls.

The parish churchyards within the walls became insufficient, not merely because of the generations of the dead, but because they were encroached upon. In 1465 the churchyard of St Mary le Bow in Cheapside was so encroached upon by building of houses that John Rotham or Rodham, citizen and tailor, by his will gave to the parson and churchwardens a certain garden in Hosier-lane to be a churchyard; which, says Stow, so continued near a hundred years, but now is built on and is a private man's house[1]. In like manner there was a colony of Brabant weavers settled in the churchyard of St Mary Somerset, and the great house of the earl of Oxford stood in St Swithin's churchyard, near London Stone. John Stow's grandfather directed that his body should be buried " in the little green churchyard of the parish church of St Michael in Cornhill, between the cross and the church wall, as nigh the wall as may be." For some years previous to 1582, as many as 23 of the city parishes were using St Paul's churchyard for their dead, having parted with their own burial grounds. But in that year (letter of 3 April, 1582[2]) the number of parishes privileged to use St Paul's churchyard was reduced to 13, the ten restrained parishes being provided for in the cemetery gifted to the city in 1569 by Sir

---

[1] Stow's *Survey*.   [2] *Remembrancia*, p. 332.

Thomas Roe, outside Bishopsgate, "for the ease of such parishes in London as wanted ground convenient within the parishes." The state of St Paul's churchyard may be imagined from the words of a remonstrance made two years after, in 1584: "The burials are so many, and by reason of former burials so shallow, that scarcely any grave could be made without corpses being laid open[1]." Twenty years before, in 1564, or the year after the last great plague which we have dealt with, Medicus, one of the speakers in Bullein's *Dialogue of the Fever Pestilence* brings in "the multitude of graves in every churchyard, and great heaps of rotten bones, whom we know not of what degree they were, rich or poor, in their lives."

St Paul's churchyard would appear to have received the dead of various parishes from an early date. There was a large charnel house for the bones of the dead on the north side, with a chapel over it, dedicated to the Virgin and endowed in 1282. Stow says that the chapel was pulled down in 1549, and that "the bones of the dead, couched up in a charnel under the chapel, were conveyed from thence into Finsbury field, by report of him who paid for the carriage, amounting to more than one thousand cart-loads, and there laid on a moorish ground, in short space after raised, by soilage of the city upon them, to bear three windmills. The chapel and charnel were converted into dwelling-houses, warehouses, and sheds before them, for stationers, in place of the tombs." Elsewhere he names Reyne Wolfe, stationer, as the person who paid for the carriage of the bones and "who told me of some thousands of carry-loads, and more to be conveyed." From this we may infer that the graves were systematically emptied as each new corpse came to be buried, according to the principle of a "short tenancy of the soil" which is being re-advocated at the end of the 19th century by the Church of England Burial Reform Association.

The spaces reserved for burial around the newer parish churches in the liberties, such as St Sepulchre's and St Giles's, Cripplegate, were gradually pared down and let out for buildings by the parish. Stow, in his *Survey* of 1598, says that St Sepulchre's church stands "in a fair churchyard, although not so

---

[1] *Remembrancia.*

large as of old time, for the same is letten out for buildings and a garden plot." The records of St Giles's, Cripplegate, show that rents were received by the parish for detached portions of the churchyard in 1648[1].

To take an instance of new city graveyards still re-maining: The old fifteenth-century parishes of St Ewin and St Nicholas in the Flesh Shambles became united in the parish of Christ Church within Newgate, which, under that name, buried many, as we may read in Stow's *Survey.* At length its burial ground was full, and it acquired a not very large plot next to the churchyard of St Botolph's outside Aldersgate. Its neighbour parish within the walls, St Leonard's in Foster Lane, acquired the next conterminous plot for its new burial-ground. All three graveyards are now thrown into one strip of public garden by the removal of the two cross walls which originally kept the ground of each parish separate.

While the graveyards were thus curtailed, and dwelling-houses built close up to them, the mode of burial was none of the safest. To take the instance of the great Cripplegate parish again: some few, like John Milton, would be buried within the church in leaden coffins; others would be laid in the ground of the churchyard in the same way, full burial dues being paid; but many more, for whom the dues were remitted, would be buried in a sheet, with no coffin at all, in the part of the churchyard reserved for the poor[2]. For the parish of St Saviour's, Southwark, the scale of burial dues was as follows: " In any churchyard next the church, with a coffin, 2*s.* 8*d.*; without a coffin, 20*d.*; for a child with a coffin, 8*d.*; without a coffin, 4*d.* The colledge churchyard, with a coffin, 12*d.*; without a coffin, 8*d.*" One of their broadsheets, dated 1580, has a picture of a body ready for burial in a cerecloth, a close fitting covering tied at the head and feet, and neatly finished[3].

[1] Baddeley, *Parish of St Giles, Cripplegate.* Lond. 1888.

[2] *Ibid.*, under date August, 1672, p. 193.

[3] Broadsheets in the collection of the Society of Antiquaries. Cited by W. Rendle, F.R.C.S., *Old Southwark and its People.* London, 1878, p. 198. Mr Rendle, in one place, seems to imply disapproval of this mode of coffinless burial; but in another (p. 225, note) he says it was "a sort of forecast of Mr Seymour Haden's wise proposals." His first thoughts appear to have been the best.

It is not to be supposed that no voices were raised against the overcrowding of the old city churchyards. Intramural burial is one of the many practical topics in Latimer's sermons: in 1552 he denounced the state of St Paul's churchyard as an occasion of "much sickness and disease," appealing to its notorious smells; the citizens of Nain, he said, "had a good and laudable custom to bury their corses without the city, which ensample we may follow[1]." Preaching at Paul's Cross on the 8th of August, 1563, when the plague was already destroying at the rate of five hundred in a week, Turner, commonly called Turner of Boulogne, made two solemn petitions to my lord mayor of London: the one was that the dead of the city should be buried out of the city in the field; the other was that no bell should be tolled for them when they lay at the mercy of God departing out of this present life, "for that the tolling of the bell did the party departing no good, neither afore their death nor after[2]." In the writings on plague, putrefying animal matters, such as carrion or offal, are always mentioned among the causes; but it is only rarely that the ordinary burial of the dead is referred to. In the seventeenth century, the filling of the soil with products of cadaveric decomposition played a greater part in the theory of plague, especially in the writings of Prosper Alpinus, physician to the Venetian consulate at Cairo. Among English books, the treatise on Plague by Dr Gilbert Skene, of Edinburgh (1568), is the only one that is at all clear upon the point. In his fourth chapter, on the places which be most pestilential, he includes the localities "where many dead are buried," the ground there becoming "fat and vaporative;" and in his first chapter, on causes in general, he instances "dead carrions unburied, in special of mankind, which, by similitude of nature, is most nocent to man, as every brutal is most infectant and pestilential to their own kind." But even if these truths had been generally apprehended, religious prescription and usage would have been too strong to allow of radical measures being adopted. The grand provocative of plague was no obvious nuisance above ground, but the loading

---

[1] Sermon on Third Sunday in Advent, 1552.
[2] Stow's *Memoranda.* Camden Society, N. S. XXVIII., 1880, p. 125.

of the soil, generation after generation, with an immense quantity of cadaveric matters, which were diffused in the pores of the ground under the feet of the living, to rise in emanations, more deadly in one season than in another, according as the level of the ground-water and the heat of the earth determined the degree of oxidation, or the formation of the more dangerous half-way products of decomposition.

So little is known of the great plagues of London in 1406–7, 1464, 1479, 1500, and 1513, that we can only conjecture how the dead, to the number perhaps of one hundred in a day at the height of the epidemic, were disposed of—probably in trenches in the fields of Whitechapel, Smithfield and Finsbury, or in such parishes as St Sepulchre's. The skirts of the city were used also to deposit the soil upon. Thus it happened that the ground outside the walls, which came in time to be the densely populated liberties and out-parishes, and the chief seat of all later plagues, had for generations before received the refuse of the city and a large proportion of the bodies of the dead. An instance mentioned by Stow, in 1598, may be taken as standing for many more: "On the right hand, beyond Shoreditch Church toward Hackney, are some late-built houses upon the common soil; for it was a lay-stall."

What remains to be said of localities and circumstances of plague in London will come in with the history of successive epidemics, which we may now resume and carry to the end of the Tudor period.

Chronology of Plague, 1564—1592.

The amount of plague in London for the two or three years next following the great epidemic in the autumn of 1563 is accurately known from Stow's abstracts of the weekly bills of mortality. It was exceedingly little, the deaths being but one or two or three in a week, and often none. The figures come to an end with July, 1566, and it is probable that the bills may not have been made for a time after that. The proposal made by Sir Roger Martyn in a letter of 20th October, 1568, to the earl of Northumberland, that all strangers arriving from over sea should be quarantined at Gravesend, would have been instigated by the known prevalence of plague and other malignant types of sick-

C. 22

ness in Scotland and at various parts of the continent of Europe. It was just in those years, before and after the founding of the Royal Exchange in 1566, that the concourse of merchants to London, especially from the war-troubled Low Countries and France, was greatest.

The revival of plague in London, after the great epidemic of 1563, was probably in 1568. In the city records there are orders relating to searchers, shutting up of houses, and collections for infected households, dated 12 October, 1568 (10 Elizabeth), 27 March and 19 October, 1569. But in 1568 the regulations, like the proposal for quarantine of shipping, may have been made more against the importation of cases from outside than on account of cases actually in London. It is in 1569 that we definitely hear of plague in the capital :—

"The plague of pestilence somewhat raging in the city of London, Michaelmas Term was first adjourned unto the 3rd of November, and after unto Hillary Term next following[1]." This outbreak of the autumn and winter of 1569 must have been considerable : for we find the earl of Essex writing from York on the 30th October to Cecil to say that he would have come to London before " had not the plague stayed him[2]; " and Thomas Bishop, giving account of his movements to the Council, says that he remained in London until the 10th October, " when the plague increasing, I departed[3]."

The year 1570 was one of the more disastrous plague-years on the Continent, that now recur somewhat frequently down to the end of the century. " There was general disease of pestilence," says Stow, " throughout all Europe, in such sort that many died of God's tokens, chiefly amongst the Venetians, of whom there died of that cruel sickness about threescore thousand." In London, on 2nd August, a death in the Tower was put down to plague ; but there is no other evidence of its prevalence in the capital[4]. In the beginning of next winter, 1571, there was plague at Cambridge (letter of 18th November)[5]; and at Oxford in the same year it left such misery, says Anthony Wood, that

[1] Stow, *Annales*, p. 662.   [2] *Cal. State Papers.*   [3] *Cal. Cecil MSS.*

[4] On July 15, 1570, the Duke of Norfolk craved his release from the Tower, on account of the great risk to his bodily health and the infection of the pestilence in that part of the city.   (*Calendar of Cecil MSS.*)

[5] *Report Hist. MSS. Commis.*

divers scholars were forced to beg[1]. In 1573 it reappeared in London, at its usual season, the end of the year: it raged so violently "that the Queen ordered the new Lord Mayor not to keep the usual feast upon his inauguration[2]." The register of St Andrew's parish, at Hertford, bears witness to the flight of Londoners to that favourite refuge; there were numerous burials of the plague in 1573, and in subsequent years, many of them being of London citizens[3]. It was in London again in 1574: a letter of 15 November, to the sheriff and justices of Surrey, orders that they should not allow the people to resort to plays and shows [in Southwark] "at that time of contagion[4]," while the figures from a weekly bill of mortality, which have been preserved, show that the outbreak had been one of the more considerable degree—for the week 22–28 October, in the city and liberties (108 parishes), buried of all diseases, 166, whereof of the plague, 65[5].

The known provincial centres in 1574 were Stamford, Peterborough and Chester. The Stamford visitation was one of a good many that the town suffered from first to last, and must have been a severe one; in one month, from 8 August to 7 September, 40 had been buried of the plague, "and the town is so rudely governed, they have so mixed themselves, that there is none that is in any hope of being clear. It is in seventeen houses, and the town is in great poverty; but that the good people of the country send in victuals, there would many die of famine. St Martin's parish is clear[6]." The corporation records also bear witness to the confusion caused, the new bailiffs having been sworn in before the Recorder in a field outside, instead of in the usual place[7]. Peterborough, which was not far off, is known to have had a visitation, from an entry in the parish register, " 1574, January. Here began the plague[8]." At Chester, "plague began, but was stayed with the death of some few in the crofts[9]."

---

[1] Anthony Wood, *op. cit.*   [2] *Remembrancia,* p. 38.
[3] Turnor's *History of Hertford,* pp. 236, 268.
[4] *The Loseley Manuscripts,* ed. Kempe. London, 1836, p. 280.
[5] Holinshed, III. p. 1240.
[6] Letter to Cecil, *Cal. Cecil MSS.,* II. 106 (under the year 1575).
[7] Corporation records, in *Notes and Queries,* 6th series, II. 524.
[8] *Notes and Queries,* 6th series, II. 390.
[9] Ormerod's *Hist. of Cheshire,* I. Harl. MS. 2177 (a death from plague, 3 Nov. 1574).

The year 1575 is somewhat singular for an epidemic of plague in Westminster, but none in the city of London: the deaths for one week in the former are known[1]; and, as regards the immunity of London, Cecil had removed previous to 16 September, from Westminster to Sir Thomas Gresham's house in the City to avoid the infection[2]. It had been at Cambridge in the winter of 1574–5, and was "sore" in Oxford down to November, 1575.

The same year, 1575, was a season of severe plague in Bristol and other places of the west of England. Some 2000 are said (in the Mayor's Calendar) to have died in Bristol between St James's tide (July 25) when the infection "began to be very hot," and Paul's tide (January 25)[3]. As early as the 11th July, the corporation of Wells had ordered measures against the plague in Bristol; but Wells also appears to have had a visitation, if the 200 persons buried, according to tradition, in the "plague-pit" near the north-eastern end of the Cathedral (besides many more buried in the fields) had been victims of the disease in 1575[4]. At Shrewsbury in that year the fairs were removed on account of plague[5]. From a claim of damages which came before the Court of Requests in 1592, it appears that plague had been in Cheshire in 1576; at Northwich the house of one Phil. Antrobus was infected and most of the family died ; on which some linens in the house, worth not more than 13sh. 4d. were put in the river lest they should be used ; the son, who was a tailor, claimed compensation, through the earl of Derby, sixteen years after[6].

At Hull, in 1576, there was an outbreak, small compared with some other visitations there, in the Blackfriars Gate, the deaths being about one hundred[7]. It is somewhat remarkable to find the borough of Kirkcudbright making regulations in the month of January, 1577, a most unlikely season, to prevent the

---

[1] *Cal. Cecil MSS.*, II. 107:—For the week ending 9 September, 1575, in St Margaret's, 25 deaths (of plague 13), St Martin's 3 of plague, Savoy, none, St Clement's 3 (2 of plague).
[2] Cecil to Earl of Lincoln. *Ibid.* 10 September, 1575.
[3] *The Maire of Bristowe, is Kalendar.* Camden Soc. 1872, p. 59.
[4] Wells corporation MSS., *Hist. MSS. Com.*, I. 107.
[5] Owen and Blakeway.
[6] *Calendar of State Papers*, Domestic, 1591–94, p. 269.
[7] Tickell's *Hist. of Kingston upon Hull*, 1798.

introduction of the plague then raging on the Borders[1]. In September, 1577, there were issued orders to be put in execution throughout the realm in towns and villages infected with the plague. More definitely it is heard of on 21 October at Rye and Dover, and on 3 November, 1577, in London.

We now come to a series of years, 1578 to 1583, for which we have full particulars of the burials in London, from plague and other causes, and of the christenings. These valuable statistics, the earliest known, are preserved among the papers of Lord Burghley, who procured them from the lord mayor of London[2], and are here given in full, having been copied from the MS. in the library of Hatfield House[3].

Abstracts of Burials and Baptisms in London, 1578–1583.

1578

Week ending	Dead	Of plague	Of other diseases	Christened	Week ending	Dead	Of plague	Of other diseases	Christened
Jan. 2	62	7	55	66	July 3	92	34	58	52
9	90	12	78	52	10	99	35	64	48
16	63	14	49	59	17	98	39	59	52
23	95	33	62	59	24	129	63	66	49
30	82	25	57	65	31	100	41	59	59
Feb. 6	88	24	64	51	Aug. 7	132	73	59	76
13	102	25	77	59	14	152	78	74	72
20	100	26	74	77	21	232	134	98	63
27	84	12	72	84	28	205	113	92	58
Mar. 6	79	10	69	58	Sept. 4	257	162	95	84
13	66	9	57	53	11	297	183	114	64
20	75	5	70	57	18	308	189	119	68
27	63	12	51	60	25	330	189	141	72
Apr. 3	96	19	77	64	Oct. 2	370	230	140	76
10	89	25	64	67	9	388	234	154	62
17	102	31	71	66	16	361	234	127	73
24	91	37	54	62	23	281	175	106	58
May 1	109	25	84	44	30	258	130	128	68
8	116	33	83	37	Nov. 6	278	127	151	60
15	141	43	98	48	13	230	116	114	64
22	109	36	73	66	20	172	77	95	66
29	119	34	85	43	27	155	84	71	68
June 5	99	38	61	51	Dec. 4	160	77	83	60
12	91	35	56	41	11	161	65	96	69
19	76	34	42	54	18	129	44	85	62
26	75	18	57	48	25	94	20	74	68
						7830	3568	4262	3150

[1] Records of the Burgh of Kirkcudbright. *Hist. MSS. Commiss.*, IV. 539.

[2] *Remembrancia*, p. 333 (27 Nov. and 6 Dec. 1582).

[3] By permission of the Marquis of Salisbury. The contents of this small volume have not been included in the published Calendar of the Cecil MSS.

1579

Week ending	Dead	Of plague	Of other diseases	Christened	Week ending	Dead	Of plague	Of other diseases	Christened
Jan. 1	100	27	73	54	July 9	62	9	53	66
8	67	13	54	68	16	73	19	54	52
15	75	16	59	74	23	72	12	60	63
22	63	9	54	81	30	72	13	59	67
29	79	19	60	75	Aug. 6	66	12	54	61
Feb. 5	84	23	61	46	13	70	18	52	67
12	81	16	65	63	20	68	12	56	61
19	69	15	54	61	27	63	10	53	58
26	70	10	60	77	Sept. 3	66	14	52	65
Mar. 5	51	6	45	71	10	85	25	60	55
12	61	16	45	72	17	66	11	55	80
19	66	10	56	65	24	44	8	36	63
26	75	13	62	68	Oct. 1	60	9	51	42
Apr. 2	81	19	62	53	8	56	8	48	75
9	82	27	55	79	15	68	14	54	70
16	77	22	55	53	22	49	6	43	71
23	58	10	48	44	29	52	10	42	76
30	71	10	61	57	Nov. 5	47	8	39	66
May 7	64	12	52	51	12	37	2	35	69
14	68	14	54	42	19	60	2	58	84
21	75	12	63	54	26	44	6	38	69
28	78	13	65	47	Dec. 3	43	3	40	78
June 4	66	7	59	56	10	55	4	51	80
11	49	7	42	46	17	49	4	45	70
18	74	14	60	60	24	51	3	48	78
25	65	13	52	45	31	42	3	39	72
July 2	57	11	46	50		3406	629	2777	3370

1580

Week ending	Dead	Of plague	Of other diseases	Baptised	Week ending	Dead	Of plague	Of other diseases	Baptised
Jan. 7	49	1	48	78	Apr. 21	40	1	39	74
14	58	4	54	58	28	43	1	42	75
21	50	5	45	63	May 5	58	1	57	72
28	28	2	26	74	12	54	0	54	69
Feb. 4	54	5	49	81	19	40	2	38	75
11	49	2	47	91	26	44	0	44	72
18	47	3	44	81	June 2	36	1	35	59
25	48	3	45	68	9	41	0	41	54
Mar. 3	52	0	52	77	16	46	2	44	60
10	48	2	46	74	23	55	2	53	59
17	48	1	47	75	30	47	4	43	57
24	52	3	49	68	July 7	77	4	73	65
31	48	2	46	59	14	133	4	129	66
Apr. 7	48	1	47	77	21	146	3	143	61
14	53	1	52	78	28	96	5	91	64

1580 (*Continued*).

Week ending	Dead	Of plague	Of other diseases	Baptised	Week ending	Dead	Of plague	Of other diseases	Baptised
Aug. 4	78	5	73	71	Oct. 20	45	2	43	56
11	51	4	47	53	27	40	3	37	80
18	49	1	48	72	Nov. 3	60	7	53	75
25	63	3	60	62	10	59	5	54	67
Sept. 1	48	0	48	71	17	57	3	54	75
8	35	2	33	69	24	45	2	43	70
13	52	1	51	69	Dec. 1	54	3	51	83
22	52	1	51	95	8	58	1	57	56
29	65	2	63	55	15	53	8	45	59
Oct. 6	35	1	34	63	22	53	4	49	61
13	44	2	42	56	29	89	3	86	66
						2873	128	2745	3568

1581

Week ending	Dead	Of plague	Of other diseases	Baptised	Week ending	Dead	Of plague	Of other diseases	Baptised
Jan. 5	42	5	37	63	July 6	72	9	63	62
12	53	4	49	65	13	69	9	60	64
19	50	1	49	65	20	94	19	75	70
26	46	1	45	59	27	95	24	71	89
Feb. 2	49	2	47	56	Aug. 3	87	23	64	58
9	38	0	38	63	10	130	30	100	75
16	48	0	48	87	17	148	47	101	72
23	56	5	51	52	24	143	43	100	55
Mar. 2	56	0	56	62	31	169	74	95	72
9	60	2	58	74	Sept. 7	186	85	101	54
16	52	2	50	80	14	180	76	114	59
23	41	1	40	89	21	203	86	117	55
30	44	3	41	74	28	218	60	158	88
Apr. 6	42	2	40	39	Oct. 5	205	107	98	74
13	47	1	46	53	12	193	74	119	83
20	37	1	36	41	19	128	42	86	77
27	37	2	35	60	26	125	35	90	88
May 4	47	0	47	52	Nov. 2	115	45	70	85
11	40	1	39	50	9	93	26	67	61
18	46	1	45	59	16				
25	64	13	51	62	23				
June 1	48	4	44	60	30				
8	57	2	55	56	Dec. 7				
15	65	7	58	62	14				
22	57	6	51	73	21				
29	56	7	49	52	28				
						3931	987	2954	2949

[The figures in part wanting, and in part defaced.]

(45 weeks)

1582

(74 Parishes clear, week ending Jan. 4.)

Week ending	Dead	Of plague	Of other diseases	Baptised
Jan. 4	63	11	52	57
11	75	13	62	76
18	79	13	66	73
25	58	13	45	90
Feb. 1	73	5	68	66
8	71	12	59	77
15	76	16	60	88
22	82	10	72	74
Mar. 1	69	11	58	81
8	85	13	72	81
15	77	11	66	71
22	62	11	51	65
29	73	16	57	85
Apr. 5	90	13	77	74
12	78	19	59	63
19	88	22	66	56
26	82	20	62	69
May 3	95	23	72	55
10	68	12	56	62
17	62	11	51	59
24	61	10	51	61
31	57	15	42	65
June 7	67	15	52	49
14	48	11	37	52
21	72	11	61	63
28	57	9	48	62
July 5	60	20	40	54
12	88	25	63	66
19	80	30	50	61
26	99	31	68	65
Aug. 2	101	45	56	68
9	116	42	74	77
16	142	70	72	64
23	148	85	63	67
30	205	111	94	70
Sept. 6	229	139	90	74
13	277	189	88	79
20	246	151	95	76
27	267	145	122	63
Oct. 4	318	213	105	87
11	238	139	99	63
18	289	164	125	74
25	340	216	124	54
Nov. 1	290	131	159	66
8	248	149	99	77
15	202	98	104	70
22	227	119	108	74
29	263	124	139	63
Dec. 6	144	58	86	59
13	155	68	87	—
20	—	—	—	—
27	142	68	74	91
	6762	2976	3786	3433

(51 weeks)

1583

Week ending	Dead	Of plague	Of other diseases	Baptised
Jan. 3	137	50	87	69
10	140	57	83	53
17	160	72	88	67
24	162	59	103	59
31	144	40	104	73

These tables were compiled from weekly bills furnished to the Court, and doubtless drawn up like the bills of 1532 and 1535 to show the deaths from plague and from other causes in each of the several parishes in the City, Liberties and suburbs. It is clear that the results were known from week to week, for a letter of January 29, 1578, says that the plague is increased from 7 to 37 (? 33) deaths in three weeks. But that was not the beginning of the epidemic in London ; it was rather a lull in a plague-mortality which is known to have been severe in the end of 1577, and had led to the prohibition of stage-plays in November[1].

In that series of five plague-years in London, only two, 1578 and 1582, had a large total of plague-deaths. The year 1580 was almost clear (128 deaths from plague), and may be taken as showing the ordinary proportion of deaths to births in London when plague did not arise to disturb it. The baptisms, it will be observed, are considerably in excess of the burials ; and as every child was christened in church under Elizabeth, we may take it that we have the births fully recorded (with the doubtful exception of still-births and "chrisoms "). But while the one favourable year shows an excess of some 24 per cent. of baptisms over burials, the whole period of five years shows a shortcoming in the baptisms of 33 per cent. Thus we may see how seriously a succession of plague-years, at the endemic level of the disease, kept down the population ; and, at the same time, how the numbers in the capital would increase rapidly from within, in the absence of plague. There is reason to think that plague was almost or altogether absent from London for the next nine years (1583 to 1592) ; and it is not surprising to find that the population, as estimated from the births, had increased from some 120,000 to 150,000. The increase of London population under Elizabeth was proceeding so fast, plague or no plague, that measures were taken in 1580 to check it. The increase of London has never depended solely upon its own excess of births over deaths ; indeed, until the present century, there were probably few periods when such excess occurred over a series of years. Influx from the country and from abroad always kept London up to its old level of inhabitants, whatever the death-rate ; and from the early part of the Tudor period caused it to grow rapidly. I shall review briefly in another chapter the stages in the growth of London, as it may be reckoned from bills of mortality and of baptisms. But as the proclamation of 1580, against new buildings, the first

---

[1] 'A sermon preached at Powles Crosse on Sunday, the third of November, 1577, in the time of the Plague' by T. W. London, 1578 (February 20).

of a long series down to the Commonwealth, has special reference
to the plague in the Liberties, and to the unwholesome condition
of those poor skirts of the walled city, this is the proper place
for it:

"The Queen's Majesty perceiving the state of the city of London and
the suburbs and confines thereof to encrease daily by access of people to
inhabit in the same, in such ample sort as thereby many inconveniences are
seen already, but many greater of necessity like to follow...and [having regard]
to the preservation of her people in health, which may seem impossible to
continue, though presently by God's goodness the same is perceived to be in
better estate universally than hath been in man's memory: yet there are
such great multitudes of people brought to inhabit in small rooms, whereof
a great part are seen very poor; yea, such must live of begging, or of worse
means; and they heaped up together, and in a sort smothered with many
families of children and servants in one house or small tenement; it must
needs follow, if any plague or popular sickness should by God's permission
enter among those multitudes, that the same should not only spread itself
and invade the whole city and confines, as great mortality should ensue the
same, where her Majesty's personal presence is many times required;
besides the great confluence of people from all places of the realm by reason
of the ordinary Terms for justice there holden; but would be also dispersed
through all other parts of the realm to the manifest danger of the whole body
thereof, out of which neither her Majesty's own person can be (but by God's
special ordinance) exempted, nor any other, whatsoever they be.

For remedy whereof, as time may now serve until by some further good
order, to be had in Parliament or otherwise, the same may be remedied,
Her Majesty by good and deliberate advice of her Council, and being
thereto much moved by the considerate opinions of the Mayor, Aldermen
and other the grave, wise men in and about the city, doth charge and straitly
command all persons of what quality soever they be to desist and forbear
from any new buildings of any new house or tenement within three miles of
any of the gates of the said city, to serve for habitation or lodging for any
person, where no former house hath been known to have been in memory of
such as are now living. And also to forbear from letting or setting, or
suffering any more families than one only to be placed or to inhabit from
henceforth in any house that heretofore hath been inhabited, etc....Given at
Nonesuch, the 7th of July, 1580[1]."

Among the more special suggestions of the mayor, on the
causes and prevention of plague, previous to this proclamation
were[2]:

---

[1] Strype's ed. of Stow's *Survey*, Bk. IV. p. 34.   Nonsuch was near Epsom.
[2] *Remembrancia of the City of London*, p. 331.

1. The avoiding of inmates in places pretending exemption.
2. The restraining of the building of small tenements and turning great houses into small habitations by foreigners.
3. The increase of buildings in places exempt.
4. The increase of buildings about the Charterhouse, Mile End Fields ; also at St Katherine's along the water side.
5. The pestering of exempt places with strangers and foreign artificers.
6. The number of strangers in and about London of no church.
7. The haunting of plays out of the Liberties.
8. The killing of cattle within or near the city.

The best glimpses that we get of the plague in London in 1578 are in letters to Lord Burghley[1]. On October 22, the Recorder of London, Sir W. Fleetwood, writes to him that he "has been in Bucks since Michaelmas, because he was troubled every day with such as came to him having plague sores about them; and being sent by the Lords to search for lewd persons in sundry places, he found dead corses under the table, which surely did greatly annoy him." It will be seen by the statistics that the deaths from all causes had risen to more than three hundred in a week before Michaelmas—a small mortality compared with that of 1563, or of any other London epidemic of the first degree. From other letters, relating to plague at St Albans, Ware and other places near London, it may be concluded that the citizens had escaped from London to their usual country resorts in plague-time. On August 30 there were said to be sixty cases of plague at St Albans, and on October 13 Ware is said to have been "of late" infected. Plague-deaths are entered also in the Hertford parish registers in 1577 and 1578[2]. On 14 September the infection was in the "Bull" at Hoddesdon (Herts), but the landlord refused to close his house against travellers on their way to the Court. On Oct. 13, 1578, two deaths are reported from Queens' College, Cambridge, "the infection being taken by the company of a Londoner in Stourbridge Fair;" these two deaths had "moved many to depart" from the University[3]. In the same month it was at Bury St Edmunds. Earlier in the year, a letter from Truro (11 April) says that the plague was prevalent in Cornwall.

---

[1] *Calendar of Cecil MSS.*, Part II. under the dates.
[2] Turnor's *Hist. of Hertford*, p. 236.   [3] *Cal. Cecil MSS.*

The epidemic of 1578 at Norwich was relatively a far more serious one than that of the capital, and was traced to the visit of the queen: "the trains of her Majesty's carriage, being many of them infected, left the plague behind, which afterwards increased so and continued as it raged above one and three-quarter years after." From August 20, 1578, to February 19, 1579, the deaths were 4817, of which 2335 were of English and 2482 of "alyan strangers," ten aldermen being among the victims[1]. At Yarmouth, in 1579, two thousand are said to have died of the plague between May-day and Michaelmas[2]. Colchester had plague from December, 1578 to August, 1579[3]. It was at Ipswich and at Plymouth in 1579; the epidemic at the latter must have been severe, if the estimate of 600 deaths, given in the annals of the town, is to be trusted[4]. It was again at Stamford in 1580, as appears from an order of the corporation, September 7, prohibiting people from leaving the town[5]. Other centres of plague in 1580 were at Rye, which was cut off from intercourse with London[6], at Leicester, where an assessment for the visited was appointed by the common hall of the citizens[7], at Gloucester, from Easter to Michaelmas, and at Hereford and Wellington, the musters in October having been hindered by "the great infection of the plague[8]."

On February 4, 1582, six houses were shut up at Dover, and on September 12 there was plague in Windsor and Eton[9]. In the parish register of Cranbrooke (Kent), 18 burials are specially marked (as from plague) in 1581, 41 in 1582, and 22 in 1583[10]. It was much dispersed in the Isle of Sheppey, the year after (1584) from Michaelmas into the winter.

Although the years from the spring of 1583 to the autumn of 1592 appear to have been unmarked by plague in London, they witnessed a good many epidemics along the east coast,

[1] Blomefield, vol. III. ("Norwich," under the date).
[2] *Ibid.* "Yarmouth."   [3] Morant's *Hist. of Essex*, I. 50.
[4] *Hist. MSS. Commission*, IX. 277 b.
[5] *Notes and Queries*, 6th series, II. 524.
[6] *Cal. State Papers.*   [7] Nichols, *Hist. of Leicestershire.*
[8] *Cal. S. P.*
[9] *Cal. State Papers.*   Eliz. 1581–90 (Lemon), pp. 45, 70.
[10] Graunt's *Reflections on Bills of Mortality.*   3rd ed., Lond. 1665, p. 135.

and in a few places elsewhere, of which the particulars are for the most part meagre.

A casual mention is made of plague at Yarmouth in 1584[1]. The town of Boston appears to have had plague continuously for four years from 1585 to 1588. In 1585 houses were shut up[2]; in 1586 a case at Southwell was supposed to have been imported from Boston[3]; in the parish register the burials from plague and other causes in 1587 reach the high figure of 372, and in 1588 they are 200, the average for eight years before being 122, and for twelve years after, only 84. In 1588 one Williams, of Holm, in Huntingdonshire, was sent for to cleanse infected houses in St John's Row, which had been used as pest-houses[4]. Within ten miles round Boston the plague prevailed; at Leake there were 104 burials from November, 1587, to November, 1588, the annual average being 24; at Frampton there were 130 burials in 1586–87, the average being 30; at Kirton there were 57 burials in 1589, and 102 in 1590[5].

Another centre on the east coast was Wisbech. In 1585 it appeared in the hamlet of Guyhirne. In 1586 it entered Wisbech itself, caused the usual shutting up of houses, and so increased in 1587 that there were 42 burials in September and 62 in October[6], being three or four times more than average. It is mentioned also at Ipswich in 1585, and at Norwich in 1588[7]. At Derby, in 1586, there was plague in St Peter's parish[8]. At Chesterfield in November, 1586, there were plague-deaths, and again in May 1587[9]. At Leominster, in 1587, there was an excessive mortality (209 burials)[10].

The other great centre on the east coast in those years was in Durham and Northumberland[11]. In 1587 the infection began to show at Hartlepool, and in the parishes of Stranton and Hart; at the latter village 89 were buried of the plague, one of them an unknown young woman who died in the street.

---

[1] *Hist. MSS. Com.*
[2] Saunders, *Hist. of Boston*, p. 228.
[3] Duke of Rutland's MSS. *Hist. MSS. Com.*, May 24, 1586.
[4] Saunders, *l.c.*
[5] *Notes and Queries*, 2nd series, XI. 497.
[6] Blomefield's *Norfolk*.
[7] *Ibid.* and Gawdy MSS. *Hist. MSS. Com.*
[8] Glover's *Hist. of Derby*, p. 613.
[9] *Archaeologia*, VI. 80.
[10] Townsend's *Hist. of Leominster*, p. 59.
[11] Sykes, *Local Records of Northumberland and Durham*, p. 80.

In 1589 the plague entered Newcastle and raged severely; of 340 deaths in the whole year in St John's parish, 103 occurred in September; the total mortality of the epidemic to the 1st January, 1590, was 1727. Durham also had a visitation in 1589, plague-huts having been erected on Elvet Moor. Those were years of scarcity, the year 1586 having been one of famine-prices.

The great event of the time was the defeat of the Spanish Armada off the French coast from Calais to Gravelines in the last days of July, 1588. A southerly gale sprang up, which drove the magnificent Spanish fleet past the Thames as far as the Orkneys. It was perhaps well for England that the winds parted the two fleets. The English ships, which had come to anchor in Margate Roads to guard the mouth of the Thames, were in two or three weeks utterly crippled by sickness. The disease must have been a very rapid and deadly infection. Lord Admiral Howard writes to the queen: "those that come in fresh are soonest infected; they sicken one day and die the next." In a previous letter to Burghley he writes: "It is a most pitiful sight to see the men die in the streets of Margate. The Elizabeth Jonas has lost half her crew. Of all the men brought out by Sir Richard Townsend, he has but one left alive." The ships were so weak that they could not venture to come through the Downs from Margate to Dover[1]. It is doubtful whether any part of this sickness and mortality was due to plague, which was not active anywhere in the south of England in that year. Want of food and want of clothes, and in the last resort the hardness and parsimony of Elizabeth, appear to have been the causes. Lord Howard begs for £1000 worth of new clothing, as the men were in great want, and Lord H. Seymour writes that "the men fell sick with cold." Dysentery and typhus were doubtless the infections which had been bred, and became communicable to the fresh drafts of men. But in the Spanish ships, beating about on the high seas and unable to land their men or even to help each other, the sickness grew into true plague, so that the broken remnants of the Armada which reached Corunna were like so many floating pest-houses.

In 1590 and 1591, at a clear interval from the Armada year,

[1] *Cal. S. P.*, Domestic, Eliz. ed. Lemon.

there was much plague in Devonshire. The evidence of its having been in Plymouth comes solely from the corporation accounts; at various times in 1590 and 1591 there were paid, "ten shillings to one that all his stuff was burned for avoiding the sickness," a sum of £5. 19s. for houses shut, and a like sum to persons kept in, and sixteen shillings to four men "to watch the townes end for to stay the people of the infected places[1]." The chief epidemics, however, appear to have been at Totness in 1590 and at Tiverton in 1591. The parish register of Totness enters the "first of the plague, Margary, the daughter of Mr Wyche of Dartmouth, June 22, 1590," from which it may be inferred that plague was first at Dartmouth, nine miles down the river, and had ascended to Totness. The following monthly mortalities will show how severe the infection became at Totness in the summer and autumn immediately following[2]:

July 42 (36 of plague, 6 not),
August 81 (80 of plague, 1 not),
September 39 (all of plague),
October 37 (all of plague),
November 25 (24 of plague, 1 not),
December 19 (all of plague),
January, 1591, 10 of plague,
February 1 of plague.

This heavy mortality from plague (246 deaths) was hardly over, when the infection began in March, 1591, at Tiverton. It is said to have been introduced by one William Waulker "a waulking man or traveller." From 1st March, 1591, to 1st March, 1592, the deaths from plague and other causes were 551, or about one in nine of the population[3].

The London Plague of 1592–1593.

The epidemic of plague, which reached its height in the year 1593, began to be felt in London in the autumn of 1592[4], and is

[1] Corporation MSS. of Plymouth. *Hist. MSS. Com.* x. pt. 4, p. 539.
[2] *Notes and Queries*, 6th series, III. 477.
[3] Dunsford's *Historical Memoirs of Tiverton*, p. 38.
[4] *Bill of Mortality for the week ending October* 20, 1603. Broadside in Guildhall Library, with summary, on margin, of the mortalities in 1563 and 1592–93.

said to have caused 2000 deaths before the end of the year. On
the 7th September, soldiers from the north on their way to Southampton to embark for foreign parts had to pass round London
"to avoid the infection which is much spread abroad" in the city.
On the 16th September, the spoil of a great Spanish carrack at
Dartmouth could be brought no farther than Greenwich, on
account of the contagion in London ; no one to go from London
to Dartmouth to buy the goods. It was an ominous sign that
the infection lasted through the winter ; even in mid winter
people were leaving London : " the plague is so sore that none of
worth stay about these places[1]." On the 6th April, 1593, one
William Cecil who had been kept in the Fleet prison by the
queen's command, writes that "the place where he lies is a
congregation of the unwholesome smells of the town, and the
season contagious, so many have died of the plague[2]." From a
memorial of 1595, it appears that the neighbourhood of Fleet
Ditch had been the most infected part of the whole city and
liberties in 1593; "in the last great plague more died about there
than in three parishes besides[3]." The epidemic does not appear
to have reached its height until summer ; on 12th June, a letter
states that " the plague is very hot in London and other places
of the realm, so that a great mortality is expected this summer."
On 3 July the Court " is in out places, and a great part of the
household cut off [? dispensed with]." The infection is mentioned in letters down to November, after which date its public
interest, at least, appears to have ceased.

Of that London epidemic a weekly record was kept by the
Company of Parish Clerks, and published by them, beginning
with the weekly bill of 21st December, 1592. The clerk of the
Company of Parish Clerks, writing in 1665, had the annual bill

---

[1] *Cal. State Papers*, 1591–94, p. 312.   [2] *Ibid.* p. 340.
[3] *Ibid.* 1595–97, p. 45, May 26, 1595:

" Arguments in proof of the advantages to be derived by the City of London
from stopping up the town ditch :—It is the origin of infection, and the only noisome
place in the city. In the last great plague, more died about there than in three
parishes besides ; these fields are the chiefest walks for recreation of the cityzens, and
though the ditch were cast every second year, yet the water coming from the kennel
and slaughter-houses will be very contagious. It is no material defence for the city,
and half the ditch has been stopped these many years."

for 1593 before him, with the plague-deaths and other deaths in
each of 109 parishes in alphabetical order, and the christenings
as well[1]. For the next two years, 1594 and 1595, he appears to
have had before him not only the annual bills but also a complete
set of the weekly bills of burials and christenings according to
parishes. The same documents were used by Graunt in 1662, and
had doubtless been used by John Stow at the time when they
were published. The originals are all lost, and only a few totals
extracted from them remain on record. To begin with Stow's.
The mortality of 17,844 from all causes in 1593 is given as for
the City and Liberties only. But there was already a considerable population in the parishes immediately beyond the
Bars of the Liberties, which were known as the nine out-
parishes, namely those of St Clement Danes, St Giles in the
Fields, St James, Clerkenwell, St Katharine at the Tower, St
Leonard, Shoreditch, St Martin in the Fields, St Mary, Whitechapel, St Magdalen, Bermondsey, and the Savoy. Besides
these there were important parishes still farther out—the Westminster parishes, Lambeth, Newington, Stepney, Hackney and
Islington. Of these, Whitechapel, Stepney, Shoreditch, Clerkenwell and some of the western parishes contributed largely to the
plague-bills of the epidemics next following, in 1603 and 1625,
and it is known from the parish registers of some of them that
they contributed to the mortality of 1593. It is probably to
these parishes that we should ascribe the difference between
the above total of 17,844 (for City and Liberties) and the much
larger total of deaths "in and about London," given on the
margin of a broadside of 1603: "And in the last visitation
from the 20th of December, 1592 to the 23rd of the same month
in the year 1593, died in all 25,886—of the plague in and about
London 15,003." The addition for the parishes beyond the Bars
would thus be 8,042 deaths from all causes, and from plague alone

---

[1] *London's Remembrancer*, by John Bell, Clerk of the Company of Parish Clerks.
London, 1665. He says: "I shall begin with the year 1593, being the first year in
which any account of the christenings and burials was kept. I cannot find any record
of more antiquity than that of this year in the Company of Parish Clerks Hall."
However we can now point to original weekly bills of mortality of 1532 and 1535, to
abstracts of weekly plague-burials in 1563–66, to the figures from one weekly bill of
a series in 1574, and to abstracts of 1578–83.

C. 23

4,541—numbers which will seem not inadmissible if they be compared with the figures for the corresponding parishes ten years after, in 1603, Stepney alone having had 2,257 deaths in that plague-year[1].

For the two years next following 1593, Graunt's book of 1662 has preserved the totals of deaths from all causes and from plague in the 97 old parishes within the walls and in 16 parishes of the Liberties and suburbs; he has omitted the christenings, although he had the figures before him. Taking these along with the figures already given for 1593, we get the following table for three consecutive years :

Year	Plague deaths	Other deaths	Total deaths	Christenings
1593	10,662	7,182	17,844	4,021
1594	421	3,508	3,929	—
1595	29	3,478	3,507	—

The proportion of mortality in 1593 that fell to the old area within the walls is known, from Stow's abstract of the figures, to have been about the same as in the space of the Liberties (8598 in the one, 9295 in the other), the deaths from other causes than plague having been rather more in the latter than within the walls. Probably the population in the Liberties was about equal to that in the City proper, the acreage being rather less in the former, but the crowding, doubtless, greater.

The London plague of 1592–93 called forth two known

---

[1] The total of 25,886 was copied, probably from the broadside of 1603, into an anonymous essay of 1665, called *Reflections on the Bills of Mortality*, the total of plague alone being given as 11,503, evidently by a misprint for 15,003. At the same time a table was given, professing to be of the weekly deaths from all causes, in one column, and from plague in another, from March 13 to December 18, 1593. The column of plague-deaths sums up to 11,110, but the total of 11,503 (which originated in a misprint) is printed at the foot of the column as if that were the summation. The column of deaths from all causes is made to sum up to 25,886, the actual sum being 25,817. But the weekly mortalities in it for those weeks that had little plague are an absurdity for 1593. Whatever the source of this table, it is not genuine for 1593, and was disclaimed by Bell, the clerk of Parish Clerks' Hall, whose essay was written in 1665 to correct that and other errors about former plagues in London.

publications, an anonymous ' Good Councell against the Plague, showing sundry preservatives...to avoyde the infection lately begun in some places of this Cittie' (London, 1592), and the Defensative' of Simon Kellwaye (April, 1593). The dates of these two books show that the alarm had really begun in the end of 1592 and early months of 1593. Kellwaye's book is mostly an echo of foreign writings, the only part of it with direct interest for English practice being the 11th chapter, which "teacheth what orders magistrates and rulers of Citties and townes shoulde cause to be observed." As that chapter sums up the various Elizabethan and other orders, and constitutes a short epitome of sanitary practice, I append it in full :

"Teacheth what orders magistrates and rulers of Citties and townes shoulde cause to be observed.

1. First to command that no stinking doonghills be suffered neere the Cittie.

2. Every evening and morning in the hot weather to cause colde water to be cast in the streetes, especially where the infection is, and every day to cause the streets to be kept cleane and sweete, and clensed from all filthie things which lye in the same.

3. And whereas the infection is entred, there to cause fires to be made in the streetes every morning and evening, and if some frankincense, pitch or some other sweet thing be burnt therein it will be much the better.

4. Suffer not any dogs, cattes, or pigs to run about the streets, for they are very dangerous, and apt to carry the infection from place to place.

5. Command that the excrements and filthy things which are voided from the infected places be not cast into the streets, or rivers which are daily in use to make drink or dress meat.

6. That no Chirurgions, or barbers, which use to let blood, do cast the same into the streets or rivers.

7. That no vautes or previes be then emptied, for it is a most dangerous thing.

8. That all Inholders do every day make clean their stables, and cause the doong and filth therein to be carried away out of the Cittie ; for, by suffering it in their houses, as some do use to do, a whole week or fortnight, it doth so putrifie that when it is removed, there is such a stinking savour and unwholesome smell, as is able to infect the whole street where it is.

9. To command that no hemp or flax be kept in water neere the Cittie or towne, for that will cause a very dangerous and infectious savour.

10. To have a speciall care that good and wholesome victuals and corne be solde in the markets, and so to provide that no want thereof be in the Cittie, and for such as have not wherewithall to buy necessary food, that

there to extend their charitable and goodly devotion ; for there is nothing that will more encrease the plague than want and scarcity of necessary food.

11. To command that all those which do visit and attend the sick, as also all those which have the sickness on them, and do walk abroad : that they do carry something in their hands, thereby to be known from other people.

Lastly, if the infection be in but few places, there to keep all the people in their houses, all necessaries being brought to them. When the plague is staid, then to cause all the clothes, bedding, and other such things as were used about the sick to be burned, although at the charge of the rest of the inhabitants you buy them all new."

The letters of the time give us a glimpse of this plague in London. On November 3, 1593, Richard Stapes writes to Dr Cæsar, judge of the Admiralty Court, residing at St Albans (doubtless to escape the infection): "My next door neighbour and tenant on Sunday last buried his servant of the plague, and since, on the other side of me, my son-in-law has buried his servant; but I cannot say his was the sickness because the visitors reported that the tokens did not appear on him as on the other[1]."

The epidemic of 1592–93 continued in London at a low level into the year 1594, when 421 persons died of the plague in the City and Liberties. Next year the plague-deaths had fallen to 29. Watford and Hertford, two of the most usual resorts of Londoners in a sickly season, were infected by plague from 1592 to 1594, many of the deaths being of refugees from the capital. At Watford there were 124 burials in the first eight months of 1594, a number much above the average, and many of them marked in the register as plague-deaths[2]. At Hertford plague-deaths appear in the registers of All Saints and St Andrew's parishes in 1592 and 1594. But the greatest mortality at Hertford was in 1596; in St Andrew's parish there were 13 burials in March, the average being one or two in the month; the mortality declined until July, in which month there were buried, among others, between the 12th and 26th, five children of one of the chief burgesses (mayor in 1603)[3]. These may or

[1] *Cal. State Papers.* Addenda. Elizabeth.

[2] Cussan's *Hist. of Hertfordshire.*

[3] Turnor's *Hist. of Hertford*, p. 268.

may not have been plague-deaths, the year 1596 having been unhealthy, as we shall see, with other types of sickness.

Meanwhile, in several provincial towns at a greater distance from the capital than the summer resorts in Hertfordshire, there was plague in the end of 1592, at the same time as in London, and in the following years. At Derby, "the great plague and mortality" began in All Saints parish and in St Alkmund's, at Martinmas, 1592, and ended at Martinmas, 1593, stopping suddenly, "past all expectation of man, what time it was dispersed in every corner of this whole parish, not two houses together being free from it[1]." At Lichfield in 1593 and 1594 upwards of 1100 are said to have died of the plague[2]. At Leicester, on the 21st September, 1593, a contribution was levied for the plague-stricken[3]. At Shrewsbury in 1592-3 there was either plague itself or alarms of it[4]; in the parish of Bishop's Castle there was the enormous mortality of 135 in July and August, 1593, and 182 burials for the year, the average being 25[5]. In the same years the infection was in Canterbury, as appears from entries of payments "to Goodman Ledes watchying at Anthony Howes dore...when his house was first infected with the plague," and, the year after, "to those ii pore folkes which were appointed to carry such to burial as died of the plague; and also to the woman that was appointed to sock them[6]." There are also various references to houses visited and to poor persons relieved. Nottingham and Lincoln are also mentioned as having been notoriously afflicted with plague in 1593[7].

A solitary record of plague comes from Cornwall in 1595. On 3rd May a letter from the justices at Tregony to the Privy Council states that the inhabitants, having been charged by the

[1] Glover's *Hist. of Derby*, p. 613.

[2] Harwood's *Hist. of Lichfield*, p. 304.

[3] Nichols, *Leicestershire* (Town records of Leicester); Kelly, in *Trans. Roy. Hist. Soc.* VI. (1877), p. 391 (at least 20 houses shut up).

[4] Owen and Blakeway.

[5] Parish registers in Townsend's *Leominster*, p. 59.

[6] Corporation MSS. Canterbury, in 9th Report of *Hist. MSS. Commission*, pp. 159 a, 160 a, b. "This plague continued from the end of September to the month of January."

[7] Parish Register of Penrith: "A sore plage was in London, Nottinghome, Derbie and Lincolne in the year 1593" (Jefferson's *Cumberland*, I. 19).

justices at the General Sessions to restrain divers infected houses within the borough, were molested in executing these commands, and had made complaint thereof[1].

All that remains to be said of plague in England until the end of the Tudor period (1603) relates exclusively to the provinces; unless the records are defective, London was clear of plague for nine years following 1592–94, just as it was clear for nine years preceding. The year 1597 was one of great scarcity in more than one region of England. At Bristol wheat is quoted at the incredible figure of twenty shillings the bushel; a civic ordinance was made that every person of ability should keep in his house as many poor persons as his income would allow[2]. But it is from the North of England in 1597 that we have more particular accounts of famine and of plague in its train. Writing in January, 1597, the dean of Durham says[3]:

"Want and waste have crept into Northumberland, Westmoreland and Cumberland; many have come 60 miles from Carlisle to Durham to buy bread, and sometimes for 20 miles there will be no inhabitant. In the bishopric of Durham, 500 ploughs have decayed in a few years, and corn has to be fetched from Newcastle, whereby the plague is spread in the northern counties: tenants cannot pay their rents; then whole families are turned out, and poor boroughs are pestered with four or five families under one roof."

On the 16th of January, 1597, he wrote again: "In Northumberland great villages are depeopled, and there is no way to stop the enemy's attempt; the people are driven to the poor port towns." On the 26th of May, the dean again complains that there is great dearth in Durham; some days 500 horses are at Newcastle for foreign corn, although that town and Gateshead are dangerously infected. On the 17th September, Lord Burghley, minister of State, is informed that the plague increases at Newcastle, so that the Commissioners cannot yet come thither (the Assizes were not held at all on account of plague about Newcastle and Durham): foreign traders were

---

[1] *Cal. State Papers.* Addenda. Elizabeth.

[2] Syer's *Memorials of Bristol.* The excessive mortality at Leominster (41 burials in September, 1597) may have been an effect of the famine. (Townsend's *History,* p. 59.)

[3] *Cal. State Papers,* Domestic, 1597, § 10, p. 347.

selling corn at a high price, until some members of the town council produced a stock of corn for sale at a shilling a bushel less[1]. There are no figures extant of the plague-mortality at Newcastle in 1597; but at Darlington the deaths up to October 17 were 340; and in Durham, up to October 27, more than 400 in Elvet, 100 in St Nicholas, 200 in St Margaret's, 60 in St Giles's, 60 in St Mary's, North Bailey, and 24 in the gaol. The whole mortality in St Nicholas parish from July 11 to November 27 was 215. Many of the burials were on the moor. The infection broke out again at Darlington and Durham in September, 1598[2].

Coincident with this severe plague on the eastern side, there was an equally disastrous plague in the North Riding of Yorkshire and in Cumberland and Westmoreland. The plague began at Richmond in the autumn of 1597. In August there were 23 deaths, and in September 42 deaths. The epidemic appears to have reached its height in the summer of 1598, the deaths in May having been 93, in June 99, in July 182 and in August 194. These figures indicate a grievous calamity in so small a place as Richmond. The outbreak which began on the 17th August, 1597, was over in December, 1598. The stress of the epidemic is shown by the fact that the churchyard was insufficient for the burials, many of the dead having been buried in the Castle Yard and in Clarke's Green[3]. Of this severe plague in Cumberland and Westmoreland there are few exact particulars. According to an inscription at Penrith Church, "on the north outside of the vestry, in the wall, in rude characters[4]," the deaths in 1598 were:—

> At Penrith 2260,
> „ Kendal 2500,
> „ Richmond 2200,
> „ Carlisle 1196.

We are able to measure the accuracy of these round totals by the monthly burials for Richmond given above; the months of July and August, 1598, with 182 and 194 deaths respectively, were the most deadly season; and it is hardly conceivable that

---

[1] *Cal. State Papers*, Domestic, 1597, p. 501.   [2] Sykes, *Local Records*, p. 82.
[3] Clarkson's *Hist. of Richmond*.   [4] Camden's *Britannia*, p. 175.

there had been as many as 1800 deaths at Richmond in the months when the epidemic was rising to a height and declining therefrom according to its usual curve of intensity.

Again, the parish register of Penrith gives only 583 deaths from the infection, the inscription on the church wall making them 2260. Perhaps the discrepancy is to be explained by including the mortality in the various parishes of which Richmond, Penrith, Kendal and Carlisle were respectively the centres and market-towns. Thus at Kirkoswald there were buried, according to the parish register, 42 of the pestilence in 1597, and no fewer than 583 in 1598[1],—a number which, if correct, means a death-rate comparable to that of the Black Death itself. Again, in the small parish of Edenhall, 42 were buried of the pestilence in 1598[2]. Appleby, also, is known to have had a severe visitation[3], and so had probably many other parishes.

The Tudor period of plague closes with a severe epidemic at Stamford, which began in the end of 1602. On December 2 the corporation resolved to build a cabin for the plague-stricken, and in January following they levied a fourth part of a fifteenth for the relief and maintenance of people visited with the plague. This epidemic is said to have carried off nearly 600; the parish registers of St George's and St Michael's contain entries of persons "buried at the cabbin of the White Fryers[4]."

Plague in Scotland, 1495–1603.

The history of plague in Scotland subsequent to the medieval period is of interest chiefly as affording early illustrations of the practice of quarantine. We last saw the disease prevailing in or near Edinburgh in 1475, the island of Inchkeith, in the Firth of Forth, being used as a quarantine station. It was doubtless the possession of convenient islands near the capital—Inch Colm and Inch Garvie were both used for the same purpose afterwards—that led the Scots government to follow the example of Venice and other foreign cities at no long interval of time.

---

[1] Jefferson's *Cumberland*, 1. 273. But these are the same figures as for Penrith.
[2] *Ibid.* 1. 391.   [3] Parish register of Penrith, in Jefferson, *l.c.*
[4] *Notes and Queries.* 6th series, 11. 524.

When we next hear of plague in Scotland it is again in connexion with infected persons on the island of Inchkeith and in
the town of Leith, some time between 13th August, 1495, and
4th July, 1496[1].

But these quarantine practices were not confined to the Firth
of Forth. On the 17th May, 1498, the town of Aberdeen was
warned by proclamation of the bell of certain measures to be
taken so as to preserve the town from the pestilence "and
strange sickness abefore," the principal precaution being a
guard of citizens at each of the four gates during the day, and
that the gates be "lockit with lokis and keis" at night. The
"strange sickness abefore" is doubtless the other invasion (of
syphilis) which the aldermen tried to check by an order of
April, 1497; but "the pestilence" in the order of May 1498 must
have been the plague itself[2]. Nothing more is heard of it at
Aberdeen or elsewhere in Scotland in that year. It appears to
have been somewhat general in Scotland in 1499 and 1500.
The audit of burgh accounts, mostly held in June, 1499, was
postponed to January 1500 in some cases, the bailie of North
Berwick explaining that he was prevented by the plague from
coming to the Exchequer[3]. An extra allowance is made to the
comptroller, Sir Patrick Hume, in March 1500, "for his great
labour in collecting fermes in different parts of the kingdom in
time of the infection of the plague." At Peebles, hides and
woolfells were destroyed during the plague of 1499. There was
a renewal of it in 1500, the audit being again delayed until
November. The custumar of Aberdeen brings his account of
the great customs of that burgh down only to the 3rd July, 1500,
"because after that date the accountant, from dread of the
plague, did not enter the burgh of Aberdeen[4]."

It is from the same northern city that our information on
plague in Scotland comes exclusively for the next forty-five
years, not, of course, because its experience was singular, but
because its borough records are known[5].

---

[1] *Exchequer Rolls of Scotland*, X. 594. Edin. 1887.
[2] *Burgh Records of Aberdeen* (Spalding Club), I. 66.
[3] *Exchequer Rolls Scot.*, XI. p. lxviii.
[4] *Ibid.*   [5] *Burgh Records*, pp. 88, 90, 130, 165.

On the 24th April, 1514, various orders were made at Aberdeen against a disease that seems to have been the plague: "for keeping of the town from strange sickness, and specially this contagious pestilence ringand in all parts about this burgh;" and, again, watching the gates (as in 1498) against persons "coming forth of suspect places where this violent and contagious pestilence reigns." Lodges were erected on the Links and Gallow-hill, where the infected or suspected were to remain for forty days. In the following year (1515), sixteen persons were banished from the town for a year and a day for disobeying the orders "anent the plague." On the 27th July, 1530, these orders are renewed "for evading this contagious pestilence reigning in the country." On September 15, 1539 (the year after a plague in the North of England), the plague is called in the municipal orders by a distinctive name: the orders are for avoiding the "contagius infeckand pest callit the boiche, quilk ryngis in diverse partis of the same [realm] now instantly"— the botch being a name given to plague in England also as late as the Elizabethan and Stuart periods.

The years 1545 and 1546 were also plague-years in Scotland. At a council held at Stirling on the 14th June, 1545, the session of the law courts was transferred to Linlithgow "because of the fear of the pest that is lately reigning in the town of Edinburgh[1]." On 10th September, of the same year, the town council of Aberdeen issued orders for evading the pest. On September 18 the plague was in the English army at Warkeshaugh, and it is reported from Newcastle, on 5 October, to be raging on the borders[2]. On March 21, 1546, a house in Aberdeen was shut up for the pest; and there are evidences of its continuance in August, October and December both in that town and "in certain parts of the realm:" on the 11th October the St Nicholas "braid silver" was given for the sustentation of the sick folk of the pest; on the 17th December an Aberdonian named David Spilzelaucht was ordered to be "brint on the left hand with ane het irne" for not showing the bailies "the seiknes of his barne, quilk was seik in the pest[3]." In November, 1548,

---

[1] *Register of the Privy Council, Scotland*, I. 5.
[2] *Cal. S. P.* Scot. (Thorpe).　　　[3] *Burgh Records*, pp. 222, 231, 244, 246.

the plague is at St Johnstone (Perth), and the Rhinegrave, with troops there, sick of it and like to die[1].

In 1564 the Scots Privy Council ordered quarantine for arrivals from Denmark, in the manner that was practised on merchandise for nearly three centuries after. As these early practices in the Forth are curiously like those that used to be practised in the Medway in the eighteenth century, I shall quote a part of the order of the Scots Privy Council, dated, Edinburgh, September 23, 1564[2]:

" That is to say, becaus maist danger apperis to be amangis the lynt, that the samyn be loissit, and houssit in Sanct Colm's Inche, oppynout, handillet and castin forth to the wynd every uther fair day, quhill the feist of Martimes nixt to cum, be sic visitouris and clengearis as sal be appointit and deput thairto be the Provest, Baillies and Counsall of the burgh of Edinburgh upoun the expensis of the marchantis, ownaris of the saidis gudis. And as concerning the uther gudis, pik, tar, irine, tymmer, that the samyn be clengeit be owir flowing of the sey, at one or twa tydis, the barrellis of asse to be singit with huddir set on fyre, and that the schippis be borit and the sey wattir to haif interes into thame, to the owir loft, and all the partis within to be weschin and clengeit ; and siclike that the marinaris and utheris that sall loase and handill the gudis above written, be clengeit and kepit apart be thameselffis for ane tyme, at the discretioun of the saidis visitouris, and licenses to be requirit had and obtenit of the saidis Provest, Baillies and Counsall before they presume to resort opinlie or quietlie amangis oure Soverane Ladeis fre liegis."

The same autumn another foul ship from the Baltic arrived and entered the port of Leith in evasion of quarantine ; the master and others are to be apprehended and kept in prison until justice be done upon them for the offence[3].

A severe outbreak of plague in Scotland in the year 1568 gave occasion to the first native treatise upon the disease in the English tongue, the essay by Dr Gilbert Skene, at one time lecturer on medicine at King's College, Aberdeen, but probably removed before 1568 to Edinburgh, where he became physician to James VI.[4] The author says that the plague has " lately

---

[1] *Cal. S. P.* Scot. 18 Nov. 1548. The Rhinegrave recovered, and came to Edinburgh on the 26th.

[2] *Reg. P. C. Scot.* 1. 279–81.   [3] *Ibid.* 1. 281–2.

[4] *Ane Breve Description of the Pest*, Edin. 1568. Reprinted, for the Bannatyne Club, by James Skene of Rubislaw. Edin. 1840.

entered" the country, and he is led to write upon it in the vulgar tongue for the benefit of those who could not afford to pay for skilled advice, or could not get it on any terms : " Mede-cineirs are mair studious of their awine helthe nor of the common weilthe." The panic caused by the plague must have been considerable : " Specialie at this time whan ane abhorris ane other in sic maneir as gif nothing of humanitie was restand but all consumit, euery ane abydand diffaent of ane other."

Although Skene's treatise bears numerous traces of the influence of foreign writers on plague, the same being freely acknowledged in the section of prescriptions and regimen, yet the book is much better than a mere compilation. Thus, under the causes of plague, he gives the stock recital of blazing stars, south-winds, corrupt standing waters, and the like ; but in men-tioning, as others do, dead carrion unburied, he adds that the corrupting human body is most dangerous of all " by similitude of nature."

A season favourable to plague is marked by continual wet in the last part of Spring or beginning of Summer, without wind, and with great heat and turbid musty air.

Anticipating a remark by Thomas Lodge in 1603, and a common ex-perience as regards rats in the recent plagues of various parts of India and China, he points out that the mole (moudewart) and serpent leave the earth, being molested by the vapour contained within the bowels of the same. " If the domesticall fowlis become pestilential, it is ane sign of maist dangerous pest to follow." Among the spots that are most pestilential are those near standing water, or where many dead are buried, the ground being fat and vaporative. Of the duration of infection : " na pest continuallie induris mair than three yeris," according to the principle of " rosten ance can not be made raw againe."

The diagnosis, prognosis, and treatment are given fully and in systematic scholarly order. I give the following long extract on the signs and symp-toms of plague, as being the first native account of the disease in this country :

Quhairby corrupt be pest may be knawin.

Thair is mony notis quhilkis schawis ane man infectit be pest. First gif the exteriour partis of the bodie be caulde, and the interiour partis of the bodie vehement hait. As gif the hoill bodie be heavie with oft scharpe punctiounis, stinkand sweiting, tyritnes of bodie, ganting of mowthe, detestable brathe with greit difficultie, at sumtyme vehement fever rather on nycht nor day. Greit doloure of heid with heavynes, solicitude and sadnes of mynd : greit displesour with sowning, quhairefter followis haistelie deth. As greit appetit and propensnes to sleip albeit on day, raving and walking occupeis the last. Cruell inspectioun of the ene, quhilkis apperis of sindre colouris maist variant, dolour of the stomak, inlak of appetite, vehement doloure of heart, with greit attractioun of Air ; intolerable thirst, frequent vomitting of divers colouris or greit appetit by daylie accustum to vomit without effecte : Bitternes of mowth and toung with blaiknit colour thairof and greit drouth : frequent puls small and profund, quhais urine for the maist part is turbide thik and stinkand, or first waterie, colourit thairefter of bilious colour, last confusit and turbide, or at the beginning is zallow inclyning to greine (callit citrine collour) and confusit, thairefter becummis reid without contentis. Albeit sum of thir properteis may be sene in haile mennis water, quhairby mony are deceavit abydand Helth of the patient, quhan sic water is maist manifest sing of deth, because the haill venome and cause conjunit thar with, leavand the naturall partis occupeis the hart and nobillest interioure partis of the body. Last of all and maiste certane, gif with constant fever, by the earis, under the oxstaris, or by the secrete membres maist frequentlie apperis apostumis callit Bubones, without ony other mani- fest cause, or gif the charbunkil apperis hastelie in ony other part, quhilk gif it dois, in the begining, testifies strenthe of nature helth, and the laitter sic thingis appeir, and apperand, it is the mair deidlie. At sumtym in ane criticall day mony accidentis apperis—principalie vomiteing, spitting of blude, with sweit, flux of womb, bylis, scabe, with dyvers others symptomis maist heavie and detestable."

The signs of death in pestilential persons are as follow :

" Sowning, cold sweats, vomiting ; excrements corrupt, teuch ; urine black, or colour of lead. Cramp, convulsion of limbs, imperfection of speech and stinking breath, colic, swelling of the body as in dropsy, visage of divers colours, red spots quickly discovering and covering themselves."

The great plague which was the occasion of Skene's writing, probably the most severe that Edinburgh experienced, entered that city on the 8th September, 1568, having been brought, it was said, by " ane called James Dalgliesh, merchant[1]." A letter of 21st September, from the bishop of Orkney, then in Edin- burgh, to his brother-in-law Sir Archibald Napier of Merchiston, whose house was near the plague-huts erected on the Muir, refers to the infection as then active :

" By the number of sick folk that gaes out of the town, the muir is liable to be overspread ; and it cannot be but, through the nearness of your place and the indigence of them that are put out, they sall continually repair

---

[1] *Diurnall of Occurrences*, in Chambers.

about your room, and through their conversation infect some of your servants." He advises him to withdraw to a house on the north side. "And close up your houses, your granges, your barns and all, and suffer nae man come therein while it please God to put ane stay to this great plague[1]."

The following account of Edinburgh practices in plague-times is given by Chambers[2]:

"According to custom in Edinburgh the families which proved to be infected were compelled to remove, with all their goods and furniture, out to the Burgh-moor, where they lodged in wretched huts hastily erected for their accommodation. They were allowed to be visited by their friends, in company with an officer, after eleven in the forenoon ; anyone going earlier was liable to be punished with death—as were those who concealed the pest in their houses. Their clothes were meanwhile purified by boiling in a large caldron erected in the open air, and their houses were clensed by the proper officers. All these regulations were under the care of two citizens selected for the purpose, and called *Bailies of the Muir;* for each of whom, as for the cleansers and bearers of the dead, a gown of gray was made, with a white St Andrew's Cross before and behind. Another arrangement of the day was 'that there be made twa close biers, with four feet, coloured over with black, and [ane] white cross with ane bell, to be hung upon the side of the said bere, which sall mak warning to the people.'"

The same writer says that the plague lasted in Edinburgh until February, 1569, and that it was reported to have carried off 2500 of the inhabitants. The plague-stricken in the Canongate were sent to huts "on the hill" and money was collected for their support[3].

The plague of 1574 was again chiefly along the shores of the Firth of Forth. It came to Leith on October 14th, it was said by a passenger from England, and several died in that town before its existence was known at large. On October 24th it entered Edinburgh, "brought in by ane dochter of Malvis Curll out of Kirkcaldy[4]." On the 29th October the town council of Glasgow ordered that no one should be allowed to enter from Leith, Kirkcaldy, Dysart, Burntisland and Edinburgh (in respect of Bellis Wynd only), and that no one in Glasgow was to repair

[1] Cited by R. Chambers (*Domestic Annals of Scotland*, I.) from M. Napier's notes to the Spottiswoode Club edition of Spottiswoode's History.

[2] *Op. cit.* I. 53.

[3] *Burgh Records of Canongate.* Maitland Club, Miscellany, II. 313 (in Chambers).

[4] Chambers, I. 94.

to Edinburgh without a pass[1]. Two days after (October 31st) the Scots Privy Council, at Dalkeith, issued an order to check the spreading of the plague landwards "through the departure of sick folk and foul persons:" no one to conceal the existence of plague, and the infected "to cloise thame selffis in[2]." On November 14th the sittings of the Court of Session were suspended owing to pest within some parts of Edinburgh, in Leith, and some towns and parts of the north coast of Fife[3]. In December the Kirk session of Edinburgh appointed an eight days' fast for the plague threatening the whole realm.

In January, 1577, plague is reported to be raging on the English border, causing alarm in Kirkcudbright[4]. On the 19th October, 1579, the king and council are credibly informed that " the infectioun and plague of the pistolence" is not only in divers towns and parts of the coast of England frequented by Scots shipping but also in Berwick and sundry other bounds of the East and Middle Marches of England ; the markets at Duns and Kelso are therefore forbidden, and traders not to repair to infected places or to break bulk of their wares[5]. Next year, 1580, on September 10th, a ship laden with lint and hemp from " Danske," with forty persons on board, including seven Edinburgh merchants, arrived in the Forth, and was quarantined for many weeks at Inchcolm; the master and several others died of plague, and the survivors were transferred in November, some to Inchkeith and some to Inchgarvie, the ship being still at Inchcolm in a leaky state. On November 22 a vessel which had come down the Tay with plague-stricken inhabitants of Perth, some of whom were dead, and with their goods and gear, was ordered to the Isle of May[6].

One of the most serious epidemics of plague in Scotland was from 1584 to 1588. It was said to have been brought to Wester Wemyss, in Fife, by a certain " creare;" but it was in some other places at the same time, and was probably a revival of old seeds of the disease. On July 28th the Privy Council issued orders that beggars and tramps should be kept from wandering about[7].

---

[1] *Burgh Records of Glasgow*, 1573–1581. Maitland Club, p. 27.
[2] *Reg. P. C. Scot.*, II. 415.   [3] *Ibid.* p. 419.   [4] *Hist. MSS. Com.*, IV. 539.
[5] *Reg. Scots P. C.*, III. 229.   [6] *Ibid.*   [7] *Ibid.* III. 679.

On the 24th September, 27th October, 4th November, and the 11th December, the Privy Council issued order after order to stop all traffic, unless by licence, from Fife, Perth, and other places north of the Forth; sails were to be taken out of the ferry-boats at all ferries except Burntisland and Aberdour, and eventually at these also, Leith and Pettycur being left free[1]. For Perth we have some particulars of this great outbreak. From the 24th September, 1584, to August, 1585, there died 1437 persons, young and old[2]. It was also in Dysart and other parts of Fife through the winter of 1584–85[3].

The infection appeared at Edinburgh about the 1st of May, 1585, in the Flesh Mercat Close by the infection of a woman who had been in St Johnstone (Perth) where the plague was[4]. On the 18th May orders were issued to Edinburgh to remove all filth, filthy beasts and carrion forth of the highways, and the same to be cleansed and kept clean. On the 23rd June the coining-house was removed to Dundee, and the Court of Session transferred to Stirling[5]. The plague next broke out in Dundee, whence the mint was removed to Perth. At St Andrews it appeared in August, 1585, and became a severe epidemic, causing the dispersion of the students, and continuing so long that the miserable state and poverty of the town are in part ascribed, in a petition of March 24, 1593, to the plague[6]. Upwards of four hundred are said to have died of it there[7]. The state of sickness was much aggravated by wet harvest weather. In Edinburgh it continued through the winter until January, 1586, sometimes carrying off twenty-four in a single night: "the haill people, whilk was able to flee, fled out of the town; nevertheless there died of people which were not able to flee, fourteen hundred and some odd" (Birell). James Melville, riding in November from Berwick to Linlithgow, entered Edinburgh by the Water-Gate of the Abbey at eleven o'clock in the forenoon and rode up

[1] *Reg. Scots P. C.* s. d.
[2] *Chronicle of Perth*, Bannatyne Club, p. 4, and Chambers, I. 154.
[3] *Reg. Scots P. C.*, III. 727.
[4] Calderwood's *Hist. of Kirk of Scotland*, IV. 366: "It was first known to be in Simon Mercerbank's house." Birell's *Diary* (1532–1605) in Chambers, I. 157.
[5] *Scots P. C.*, III. 746.   [6] *Ibid.* V. 56.
[7] Moysie, in Chambers, I. 157.

"through the Canongate, and in at the Nether Bow through the great street of Edinburgh to the West Port, in all whilk way we saw not three persons, sae that I miskenned Edinburgh, and almost forgot that I had ever seen sic a town[1]." The same year it was unusually severe at Duns[2]. In the winter of 1586-7, "the pest abated and began to be strangely and remarkably withdrawn by the merciful hand of God, so that Edinburgh was frequented again that winter, and at the entry of the spring all the towns, almost desolate before, repeopled, and St Andrews among the rest[3]."

In the harvest of 1587 "the pest brake up in Leith, by opening up of some old kists," and in Edinburgh about the 4th November. It continued in those two towns till Candlemas, 1588[4]. On April 26, 1588, the infection is reported anew from Edinburgh, threatening the law session[5]. In October, 1588, it was at Paisley, causing alarm in Glasgow[6].

On the 8th August, 1593, a ship from an English port, with persons and goods suspected of the plague, was quarantined at Inchcolm[7]. Four years after, on the 6th August, 1597, "the pest began in Leith[8]." Twelve days after, August 18, the Privy Council declared that divers inhabitants of sundry towns near Edinburgh were infected, and that the disease was suspected to be in the capital itself[9]. Many fled from Edinburgh, but the epidemic was over by the end of harvest[10].

In the winter of 1598, the plague which was in Cumberland extended to Dumfries, and caused great decay of trade, and even scarcity of food[11]. On the 12th October, 1600, a petition

---

[1] *The Diary of Mr James Melville*, 1556-1601. Bannatyne Club. Edin. 1829, p. 153.

[2] Marioreybank's *Annals*, in Chambers.

[3] Melville's *Diary*, p. 162.

[4] Melville, p. 173; Calderwood, cited by Chambers; *Cal. Cecil Papers*, III. 298, 310.

[5] *Cal. Cecil Papers*, III. 321.   [6] *Memorabilia of Glasgow*, in Chambers.

[7] *Scots Privy Council.*   [8] Birell, in Chambers.

[9] *Scots P. C.*   [10] Calderwood, v. 655.

[11] Two men sent to buy nolt in Galloway for the needs of the borough of Dumfries were stopped, with 38 head of cattle, by the provost and others of Wigton, at the Water of Crie, the cattle being impounded at Wigton for eight days so that they became lean. A hundred merks compensation was demanded. *Scots Privy Council*, v.

from Dundee declares that the plague of the pest had " entered and broken up within the town of Findorne[1]." Findhorn had been only one of several places infected in that locality ; for in December, the Kirk session of Aberdeen ordered a fast " in respect of the fearful infection of the plague spread abroad in divers parts of Moray[2]."

On the 24th November, 1601, the parishes of Eglishawe, Eastwood, and Pollok, in Renfrewshire, and the town of Crail in Fife are declared infected, and ordered to be shut up. On the 28th of the same month it was in the barony of Calderwood, and on the 21st December, in Glasgow. It increased daily in Crail in January, 1602, and suspects were put out on the muir, so that they wandered to sundry parts of Fife. It still continued in Glasgow, and had appeared at Edinburgh before the 4th of February : the town council built shielings and lodgings for the sick of the plague in the lands of Schenis (Sciennes) belonging to Napier, of Merchiston, without his leave, having ploughed up the old plague-muir, and let it for their profit: against the plague-shelters Napier protested on the 11th March. By the 1st of May it had ceased in Edinburgh, and a solemn thanksgiving was held on the 20th (Birell). A ship owned in Crail arrived in the Forth on 30th July, 1602, from " Danske," with three or four dead of the plague, and was quarantined at Inchkeith. In April, 1603, James VI. left for England, to assume the English[3] crown, with which event we resume in another chapter the eventful history of Plague under the Stuarts.

Meanwhile, in the foregoing records of plague in Scotland, the absolute immunity of Aberdeen in the latter half of the sixteenth century is remarkable. It does not depend on any imperfection of the records; for, under the year 1603, the borough register contains this entry[4]: " It has pleasit the guidness of God of his infinite mercy to withhauld the said plague frae this burgh this fifty-five years bygane "—that is to say, since the

---

Scots P. C., VI. 164.

[2] *Aberdeen Kirk Session Records*, Spalding Club, 1846, Calderwood (cited by Chambers, I. 319) says that the year 1600 was one of famine, and that there was also a great death of young children, six or seven being buried in Edinburgh in a day.

[3] *Scots Privy Council*, VI. under the respective dates.   [4] *Burgh Records*.

winter of 1546–47, when David Spilzelaucht was burned on the left hand with a hot iron for concealing a case of plague in one of his children. The northern city may have owed its immunity to various causes ; but there can be no question of the Draconian rigour of its decrees against the plague. Following the example of queen Elizabeth at Windsor in 1563, the magistrates in May, 1585, when Perth, Edinburgh and many other places in Scotland were suffering severely from plague, erected three gibbets, "ane at the mercat cross, ane other at the brig of Dee, and the third at the haven mouth, that in case ony infectit person arrive or repair by sea or land to this burgh, or in case ony indweller of this burgh receive, house, or harbour, or give meat or drink to the infectit person or persons, the man be hangit and the woman drownit."

Plague in Ireland in the Tudor period.

The accounts of plague in Ireland in the Tudor period are not many, but some of them are of interest. The province of Munster is said to have had a pestilence raging in it in 1504, evidently not a famine-fever, for the dearth, and mortality therefrom, came in 1505[1]. There is no doubt as to the reality of the next plague in Ireland, in 1520.

The earl of Surrey writes from Dublin to Wolsey, on the 3rd August, 1520: "There is a marvellous death in all this country, which is so sore that all the people be fled out of their houses into the fields and woods, where they in likewise die wonderfully ; so that their bodies be dead like swine unburied." On the 23rd July he had already written that there was sickness in the English pale ; and on the 6th September he wrote again that the death continued in the English pale[2]. It is perhaps the same epidemic, or an extension of it, that is referred to as the plague raging in Munster in 1522[3]. On the same authority, "a most violent plague" is said to have been in the city of Cork in 1535, and "a great plague" in the same in 1547. The earlier of those dates corresponds probably to a season of ill-health in

---

[1] Smith's *Cork*, II. 34.   [2] *Cal. State Papers.* Domestic.
[3] Smith's *Cork*, on the authority of MS. annals.

Ireland generally: "1536. This year was a sickly, unhealthy year, in which numerous diseases, viz. a general plague, and smallpox [i.e. a disease with an Irish name supposed to be smallpox], and a flux plague, and the bed-distemper prevailed exceedingly[1]." In a State letter from Ireland September 10, 1535, the prevalence of "plague" is mentioned[2].

In the winter of 1566-7, a remarkable outbreak of plague occurred among the English troops quartered around the old monastery of the Derry, at the head of Loch Foyle, where Londonderry was afterwards built. The men were landed there in October, and by November "the flux was reigning among them wonderfully." On December 18 and January 13, many of the soldiers are dead, the rest are discontented, and provisions are short. On February 16, the sickness continues, "in this miserable place," and on March 26, the death at the Derry is said to be by cold and infection: the survivors to be removed to Strangford Haven[3]. Only 300 men were fit for service out of 1100, and several officers of rank were dead. The men's quarters had been built over the graveyard of the ancient abbey, and the infection of plague was ascribed at the time to the emanations from the soil[4]. The scarcity was general in Ireland that winter, and was attended by great mortality. Sir Philip Sydney, the lord deputy, writes to the queen on April 20, 1567: "Yea the view of the bones and skulls of your dead subjects who, partly by murder, partly by famine, have died in the fields is such that hardly any Christian with dry eye could behold[5]."

In 1575 there was a severe and wide-spread outbreak of plague, the localities specially named being Wexford, Dublin, Naas, Athy, Carlow, and Leighlin. The city of Dublin was as if deserted of people, so that grass grew in the streets and at the

---

[1] *Annals of Loch Cé.* Rolls ed., II. 289.

[2] Brabazon to T. Cromwell. *Cal. State Papers.* Irish.

[3] *Cal. State Papers.* Irish, 1566-7.

[4] *State Papers* (Record Office), Irish, 1567, No. 54. Letter from Lord Treasurer Winchester and Ed. Baeshe, to the Lord Deputy. Mr Froude's summary of it is that "the clammy vapour had stolen into their lungs and poisoned them," and again, "the reeking vapour of the charnel house." I have had difficulty in deciphering the letter, but I can make out "being a graveyard where all their buriall," etc.

[5] *Cal. State Papers.* Irish.

doors of churches; no term was held after Trinity, and prayers
were appointed by the archbishop throughout the whole province[1]. The extremity of the plague in Ireland was such that
the English troops sent by way of Chester and Holyhead had
difficulty in finding a safe place to land[2]. Whether that outbreak
had been connected with the military operations (as afterwards
in Cromwell's time), the information does not enable us to judge;
but Chester and other places near, in direct communication with
Ireland, had been visited with plague the year before (1574).

[1] Thady Dowling, p. 41.
[2] *Cal. State Papers.* Domestic. Sept. 1, 1575.

CHAPTER VII.

GAOL FEVERS, INFLUENZAS, AND OTHER FEVERS IN THE TUDOR PERIOD.

THE Common Gaols of England date from the Council of Clarendon, in 1164, by the articles of which the limits of civil and ecclesiastical jurisdiction were fixed, and the quarrel between archbishop Becket and Henry II. reduced to terms. In obedience to Article VII. of the Council, gaols were built, the chief among them having been at Canterbury, Rochester, Huntingdon, Cambridge, Malmesbury, Sarum, Aylesbury, and Bedford[1]. Little is heard of the unwholesomeness of prison life until the medieval period is nearly over—not indeed because the prisons were better managed than they were later. "In the year 1385," says Stow, "William Walworth gave somewhat to relieve the prisoners in Newgate; so have many others since." One benefactor brought a supply of water into Newgate; another, the famous Whittington, left money actually to rebuild the gaol, which was done in 1422. For several years before that, Newgate had been notorious. An ordinance of 7 Henry V. (1419) for the re-establishment of the debtor's prison at Ludgate, so that debtors need not have to go to Newgate gaol, was made in compliance with a petition which said that, in " the hateful gaol of Newgate, by reason of the fetid and corrupt atmosphere, many persons committed to the said gaol are now dead[2]." The greatest mortality must

---

[1] Stubbs, in his edition of Roger of Howden (Rolls series, No. 51, II. 249), on the evidence of the Pipe Roll of 1166.

[2] *Memorials of London in the 13th, 14th and 15th centuries*, ed. Riley.

have been, according to Stow, in 1414, when the gaolers of Newgate and Ludgate died, and sixty-four prisoners in Newgate[1].

More than a century after, in 1522, there occurred the first of a series of gaol-fever tragedies, which were well calculated to produce the effect ascribed by Aristotle to scenic tragedy, provided only the workings of cause and effect had been more apparent. The first of these historical Black Assizes occurred on the occasion of the gaol delivery at the Castle of Cambridge in Lent, 1522. The facts, which appear to be given nowhere but in Hall's *Chronicle* (of almost contemporary authority), are less fully related than for some of the later instances of the same strange visitation; but there is no mistaking the air of reality and the generic likeness.

Cambridge Black Assizes.

In the 13th year of Henry VIII. at the Assize held in the Castle of Cambridge in Lent, "the justices and all the gentlemen, bailiffs and other, resorting thither, took such an infection, whether it were of the savour of the prisoners, or of the filth of the house, that many gentlemen, as Sir John Cut, Sir Giles Arlington, Knights, and many other honest yeomen, thereof died, and almost all which were present were sore sick, and narrowly escaped with their lives[2]."

It is to be observed that nothing is said of the prisoners being infected: they were brought from the dungeons to stand their trial in due course, and the gentlemen and yeomen attending the court officially or as jurors, or otherwise, were poisoned by their presence. This early chronicle indicates as the cause, "the savour of the prisoners, or the filth of the house;" and Bacon, in touching upon that class of incidents nearly a century later, indicates "the smell of the gaol," but says nothing of cases of fever among the prisoners, having no warrant in the evidence for doing so.

Before we come to consider the condition of England in the

---

[1] Stow's *Survey of London*, pop. ed. (1890), p. 66.
[2] Hall's *Chronicle*, ed. of 1809, p. 632.

Tudor period, with the policy of Henry VIII. for the repression of beggary and crime, and the appearance of "new fevers" or "strange fevers" and "laskes" in the chronicles and other records of the time, it will be desirable to make out as accurately as possible the clinical type of the Assizes fever, and its circumstances. For that purpose we must turn to the next recorded outbreak on the occasion of the Assizes at Oxford in 1577, which happens to have been somewhat fully described as a memorable event in the register of Merton College. The entry in the Merton register appears to have been made within a few weeks of the event[1].

Oxford Black Assizes.

The Assizes met on the 5th and 6th July, 1577, in the Castle and Guild Hall. Those only fell ill, whether in Oxford itself or after leaving, who had been present at the Assizes. The two judges (Robert Bell, Chief Baron of the Exchequer and John Barrham, sergeant-at-law), the sheriff of the county, two knights, eight squires and justices of the peace, several gentlemen and not a few of their servants, the whole of the grand jury with one or two exceptions—these all had not long left Oxford when they were seized with illness and died (*statim post fere relictam Oxoniam mortui sunt*). In Oxford itself, on the 15th, 16th and 17th July, some ten or twelve days after the Assizes, about three hundred fell ill; and in the next twelve days there died ("*ne quid errem*") one hundred scholars, besides townsmen not a few. Five died in Merton College, including one fellow, the names of four being given who died on the 24th, 27th, 28th and 29th July. Every college, hall, or house had its dead. Women were not attacked, nor indeed the poor; nor did the infection spread to those who waited on the sick or came to prescribe for them.

---

[1] This account of the Black Assizes at Oxford in 1577 was brought to light, like so many other things from the register of Merton, first by Anthony Wood in his *Hist. and Antiq. of the Univ. of Oxford* (ed. Gutch, II. 189). It was copied in full, from the original Latin text, in 1758, by John Ward, LL.D., and sent to the Royal Society, in whose *Phil. Trans.* (vol. L. p. 699) it is printed, with remarks, by Tho. Birch, D.D., Sec. R. S.

Only those who had been present at the Assizes caught the fever. The symptoms are described as follows :

The patients laboured under pain both of the head and of the stomach ; they were troubled with phrensy, deprived of understanding, memory, sight, hearing and their other senses. As their malady increased, they took no food, could not sleep, and would not suffer attendants or watchers to be near them ; their strength was remarkable, even in the approach of death ; but if they recovered they fell into the extreme of weakness. No complexion or constitution was spared ; but those of a choleric habit were most obnoxious to the disease. The affected persons suddenly became delirious and furious, overcoming those who tried to hold them ; some ran about in courts and in the streets after the manner of insane persons ; others leapt headlong into the water. The spirits of all the people were crushed ; the physicians fled, and the wretched sufferers were deserted. Masters, doctors, and heads of houses left almost to a man. The Master of Merton remained, *longe omnium vigilantissimus,* ministering sedulously to the sick. The pharmacies were soon emptied of their conserves, oils, sweet waters, pixides and every kind of confection.

This sudden epidemic, which began on the 15th—17th July, did not last long ; within the space of one month the city was restored to its former health, so that one wonders, says the registrary of Merton, to see already so many scholars and so many townsmen abroad in the streets and walks.

The infection was suspected by many, says the same eye-witness, to have arisen either from the fetid and pestilent air of thieves brought forth from prison, of whom two or three died in chains a few days before (*quorum duo vel tres sunt ante paucos dies in vinculis mortui*), or from the devilishly contrived and obviously papistical spirits called forth " e Lovaniensi barathro," and let loose upon the court secretly and most wickedly.

The latter explanation arose out of the heated feelings of the time against papist plotters, and has no farther interest. But the statement that two or three of the prisoners had died in chains a few days before has a great interest, as showing the kind of treatment to which they had been subjected while await-ing the gaol delivery. A strange confirmation of the truth of the statement came to light many years after. When John Howard visited the Oxford gaol in 1779, in the course of his humane labours on behalf of the prisoners, he was told by the gaoler that, some years before, wanting to build a little hovel and digging up stones for the purpose from the ruins of the court, which was formerly in the Castle, he found under them a complete skeleton with light chains on the legs, the links very small. "These," says Howard, "were probably the bones of a malefactor who died in court of the distemper at the Black Assize[1]."

Next to the Merton register's account, we may take that of Thomas Cogan, a graduate in medicine of Oxford, sometime fellow of Oriel, but probably removed to Manchester previous to 1577. Wherever Cogan got his information, he acknowledges no source of the following in his *Haven of Health*, 1589 :

"What kind of disease this should be which was first at Cambridge [in 1522] and after at Oxford, it is very hard to define, neither hath any man (that I know) written of that matter. Yet my judgment is, be it spoken without offence of the learned physicians, that the disease was *Febris ardens*, a burning fever. For as much as the signes of a burning ague did manifestly appear in this disease, which after Hollerius be these : Extreame heate of the body, vehement thirst, loathing of meate, tossing to and fro, and un-quietnesse, dryness of the tongue rough and blacke, griping of the belly, cholerick laske, cruell ake of the head, no sound sleepe, or no sleepe at all, raving and phrensie, the end whereof, to life or death, is bleeding at the nose, great vomitting, sweate or laske. And this kind of sicknesse is one of those rods, and the most common rod, wherewith it pleaseth God to brake his people for sin...And this disease indeed, as it is God's messenger, and sometimes God's poaste, because it commeth poaste haste, and calleth us quickly away, so it is commonly the Pursuivant of the pestilence and goeth before it....And certainly after that sodaine bane at Oxford, the same yeare, and a yeare or two following, the same kind of ague raged in a manner over all England, and tooke away very many of the strongest sort, and in their lustiest age, and for the most part, men and not women nor children, culling them out here and there, even as you should chuse the best sheepe out of a flocke. And certaine remedy was none to be found....And they that took a moderate sweate at the beginning of their sickness and did rid their stomachs well by vomit sped much better. Yet thanks be to God hitherto no great plague hath ensued upon it."

Besides these medical particulars, he gives certain dates and numbers. It began, he says, on the 6th of July, from which date to the 12th of August next ensuing there died of the same

---

[1] Howard, *The State of the Prisons in England and Wales.* 3rd ed., Warrington, 1784, p. 342.

sickness five hundred and ten persons, all men and no women :
the chiefest of which were the two judges, Sir Robert Ball, lord
chief baron, and maister Sergeant Baram, maister Doile the
high sheriff, five of the justices, four councillors at law and an
attorney.   The rest were jurors and such as repaired thither.

An account not unlike Cogan's is given by Stow in his
Annales (p. 681);

"The 4, 5 and 6 dayes of July were the assizes holden at Oxford, where
was arraigned and condemned one Rowland Jenkes for his seditious toung,
at which time there arose amidst the people such a dampe, that almost all
were smothered, very few escaped that were not taken at that instant : the
Jurors died presently.   Shortly after died Sir Robert Bell, lord chief
baron, Sir Robert de Olie, Sir William Babington, maister Weneman,
maister de Olie, high sheriff, maister Davers, maister Harcurt, maister
Kirle, maister Phereplace, maister Greenwood, maister Foster, maister Nash,
sergeaunt Baram, maister Stevens, and there died in Oxford 300 persons,
and sickned there but died in other places 200 and odde, from the 6th of
July to the 12th of August, after which died not one of that sicknesse, for
one of them infected not another, nor any one woman or child died thereof."

Stow's account differs from that of the Merton College register
in several important particulars.   The latter is explicit that the
sickness appeared among the scholars and townsmen of Oxford
on the 15th, 16th and 17th of July, or after an interval of ten days
or more, and that the deaths amongst those who had come to
Oxford on Assize business did not occur in Oxford but on their
return home.   On the other hand, Stow makes out the Oxford
people to have been smothered by the damp which arose in the
court itself: "very few escaped that were not taken ill at that
instant ;" next come the deaths of the jurors, and "shortly after"
those of the judges and other high officials, whose names are
given by Stow more fully than by anyone.   His total of deaths,
the same as Cogan's, is 300 in Oxford and 200 and odd of
persons who had left Oxford, and his dates, "from the 6th of
July to the 12th of August," are also the same as Cogan's.

Wood's account is for the most part taken from the Merton
register and in part from the very different version in Stow's
Annals ; but he has the following new matter: "Above 600
sickened in one night, as a physician that now lived in Oxford
attesteth, and the day after, the infectious air being carried into

the next villages, sickened there an hundred more[1]." That, of course, is very unlike the Merton College account, which is explicit that no one caught the fever who had not been in the court. The Oxford physician whose authority is given for the six hundred cases in Oxford in one night, and the extension next day to villages around, is Dr George Ethredge, or Ethryg, a physician and learned Greek scholar living in Oxford at the time and keeping a boarding-house, called George Hall, for the sons of Catholic gentlemen. In 1588 he published a small volume of comments upon some books of Paulus Aegineta, which is the authority given by Wood[2]. On discovering the passage, one finds that it was not 600 in one night, but "sexaginta" or 60, and that the occasion on which more than sixty were taken ill at once in a single night at Oxford, and nearly a hundred next day in the adjacent villages, "whither the infected air had by chance been borne," was not that of the gaol-fever in 1577 but of the sweating sickness in 1551. An extension in the atmosphere to the villages around is just what would have happened in the sweating sickness, a disease in that as in other respects closely analogous to influenza. Ethredge says that, on the particular occasion, "hardly any of the Oxford people died"—a statement which should of itself have prevented Wood's mistake, even if the reference to the same disease having "at the same time" cut off the two sons of the duke of Suffolk "at Cambridge" (therefore a less healthy place than Oxford where hardly any died) had not quite clearly pointed to the sudor Britannicus, which is actually named in the context ("sic enim vocant")[3].

Although, in the passage quoted, it is the sweating sickness

[1] *Hist. and Antiq. Univ. Oxford*, ed. Gutch, II. 188–192.

[2] Georgius Edrichus, 'In Libros aliquot pauli Aeginetae Hypomnemata quaedam.' Londini apud Tomam East 1588 (without pagination).

[3] The passage which Anthony Wood thought to relate to the gaol fever at Oxford in 1577 is the following, under the heading "De morbis publicé grassantibus :" "Publice grassari morbos vidimus Oxonii, et una nocte simul plus sexaginta agrotasse (*sic*) novimus, et in vicinis postridie pagis, eo forte aëre delato, fere centum. Quod etiam eodem tempore, regnante tum Edwardo sexto, Cantabrigiae evenit, cum duo simul liberi ducis inclyti Suffolchiae ibi morerentur. Nec tamen Oxonienses ulli fere interierunt, quod coeli constitutio apud nos quam ibi salubrior sit. Sed iis ita succurrendum morbis putamus, ut Brittanico sudore (sic enim vocant) opitulari solemus."

at Oxford in 1551 that Ethredge refers to, he does also refer to the gaol fever of 1577 in another passage which has hitherto escaped notice.

In the section of his book next following, entitled "De Curatione morborum populariter grassantium, et de Peste," he says that he had used a certain prescription of aloes, ammoniacum and myrrh rubbed together in wine, for himself as well as for others in a serious contagion, "quae fuit in martiali sede cum ibi essem," and also, with happy effect, upon many "in the most cruel pest at Oxford which carried off Judge Bell and ever so many more ; one gentleman, I could not persuade to try this medicine, whom therefore I commended to God, and four days after he was dead. Concerning that pestilential fever, many colloquies took place between me and two most learned physicians ; and, as to the kind of this contagion, we all agreed (*manibus et pedibus in hanc sententiam itum est*) in a sentence which I quoted from Valescus, who sayeth thus : Those sicknesses are dangerous in such wise that the physicians may be for the most part deceived ; for we see a good hypostasis in the urine, and some other good signs, yet the sick person dies "—a remark which often recurs in the early writings on plague.

It has taken longer than usual to determine the matter of fact as to the fever of the Oxford Black Assizes, because an erroneous version passes current on respectable authority ; but enough has perhaps been said to enable us to pass from the matter of fact to the matter of theory[1].

The theory of the gaol fever at Oxford, in 1577, was not attempted by any writer at the time, nor indeed has it been so

[1] Anthony Wood, as we have seen in the text, put together his version of the fever of 1577 from the Merton College register, from Stow's *Annals*, and from Ethredge's reference to the sweat of 1551. In 1758, John Ward, LL.D., copied the passage in the Merton register and sent it to the Royal Society ; whose secretary, the Rev. Dr Thomas Birch, appended to it in the *Philosophical Transactions* some annotations—"copying," as Carlyle said of him with reference to some Cromwell matter, " from Wood's *Athenae* ; and has committed—as who does not ?—several errors," his annotations being " sedulous but ineffectual "—to the extent of fixing on the original correct narrative an accretion of mistakes (600 for 60, sweating sickness for gaol fever, &c.). Trusting to the respectable Birch, Bancroft in his *Essay on the Yellow Fever, with observations concerning febrile contagion &c.* (Lond., 1811) has based a theory that the Oxford epidemic was not typhus at all. Murchison (*Continued Fevers of Great Britain*, 2nd ed. 1873, p. 103) has also been misled, and has found himself therefore at a disadvantage in answering Bancroft's empty verbalisms about the invariable reproduction of typhus from some previous case. F. C. Webb, in a paper "An Historical Account of the Gaol Fever," *Trans. Epidem. Soc.* for 1857, p. 63, has not used the Oxford case for any argumentative purpose, but he has, like the others, given the facts erroneously. He gives no particulars of the Exeter Black Assize.

in later times; but the significance of the outbreak has been recognized and admitted.   An Oxford scholar, Dr Plot, writing just a century after (1677) mentions the statement that a "poisonous steam" broke forth from the earth, having probably in his mind Stow's imaginative explanation, that a damp arose amongst the people and smothered them, very few escaping that were not taken at that instant.   Plot then proceeds :—

"But let it not be ascribed to ill fumes and exhalations ascending from the earth and poysoning the Air, for such would have equally affected the prisoners as judges, but we find not that they dyed otherwise than by the halter, which easily perswades me to be of the mind of my lord Verulam (*Nat. Hist.* cent. x. num. 914) who attributes it wholly to the smell of the Gaol where the prisoners had been long, close, and nastily kept."

We know, indeed, from the register of Merton that "two or three of the prisoners died in chains a few days before," which is a sufficient indication of the state they were kept in, but is no warrant for Anthony Wood's free rendering of the words : "of whom two or three, *being overcome with it* [i.e. with the "nasty and pestilential smell of the prisoners"] died a few days before the Assizes began."   Two or three prisoners died in their chains with symptoms undescribed ; and although typhus among the inmates of gaols has often occurred, it has also been wanting in many cases where the filth and misery might have bred it in the prisoners themselves[1].

Bacon's judgment on the case, referred to above, was based upon a strict scrutiny of the evidence, and does not transcend the evidence.   He attributes the infection that arose in the court to "the smell of the gaol;" and so as not to assume a smell which does not appear to have attracted any particular notice at the time, he is careful to explain in what sense he means the smell of the gaol:

[1] Howard, *On Lazarettos in Europe*, &c. Warrington, 1789, p. 231 : "But as I have found, in some prisons abroad, cells and dungeons as offensive and dirty as any I have observed in this country, where however the distemper was unknown, I am obliged to look out for some additional cause of its production.   I am of opinion that the sudden change of *diet* and lodging so affects the *spirits* of *new* convicts that the general causes of putrid fever exert an immediate effect upon them.   Hence it is common to see them sicken and die in a short time with very little apparent illness." The last words are important.

" The most pernicious infection," he says, " next the plague, is the smell of the jail, when prisoners have been long and close and nastily kept ; whereof we have had in our time experience twice or thrice ; when both the judges that sat upon the jail, and numbers of those that attended the business or were present, sickened upon it and died. Therefore it were good wisdom, that in such cases the jail were aired before they be brought forth.......

" Leaving out of question such foul smells as be made by art and by the hand, they consist chiefly of man's flesh or sweat putrefied; for they are not those stinks which the nostrils straight abhor and expel, that are most pernicious ; but such airs as have some similitude with man's body, and so insinuate themselves and betray the spirits[1]."

Exeter Black Assizes.

The next Black Assizes occurred at Exeter in 1586, nine years after the Oxford tragedy. The Exeter incident has had the fortune to be chronicled by a person as competent as was the writer in the Merton College register in the former case, namely by John Hoker *alias* Vowell, chamberlain of the city, and its representative in Parliament, a lawyer of good education, who must have been conversant with all the circumstances, and wrote his account within six months. He is known as the chief contributor to the second edition of Holinshed's *Chronicle,* in which the history is brought down to 1586, his name appearing on the title-page. It is in that work that he inserted his account of the Exeter Black Assizes, written in October, 1586. The margin bears the words:

" The note of John Hooker *alias* Vowell ;" and the text of the note is as follows[2] (III. pp. 1547-8) :—" At the assizes kept at the citie of Excester, the fourteenth daie of March, in the eight and twentieth yeare of hir majesties reigne, before Sir Edmund Anderson, Knight, lord chief justice of the common pleas, and sargeant Floredaie, one of the barons of the excheker, justices of the assises in the Countie of Devon and Exon, there happened a verie sudden and a strange sickenesse, first amongst the prisoners of the Gaole and Castell of Exon, and then dispersed (upon their triall) amongst sundrie other persons ; which was not much unlike to the sickenesse that of

---

[1] *Sylva Sylvarum, or A Natural History.* In ten centuries. Cent. 10, §§ 914-15. Spedding's ed. II. 646.

[2] Holinshed's *Chronicle.* New edition by Hoker, London, 1587, pp. 1547-8.

late yeares happened at an assise holden at Oxford, before Sir Robert Bell, Knight, lord chiefe baron of the excheker, and justice then of that assise...

The origin and cause thereof diverse men are of diverse judgment. Some did impute it, and were of the mind that it proceeded from the contagion of the gaole, which by reason of the close aire and filthie stinke, the prisoners newlie come out of a fresh aire into the same are in short time for the most part infected therewith ; and this is commonlie called the gaole sickenesse, and manie die thereof. Some did impute it to certain Portingals, then prisoners in the said gaole. For not long before, one Barnard Drake, esquire (afterwards dubbed Knight) had beene at the seas, and meeting with certeine Portingals, come from New-found-land and laden with fish, he tooke them as a good prize, and brought them into Dartmouth haven in England, and from thense they were sent, being in number about eight and thirtie persons, unto the gaole of the castell of Exon, and there were cast into the deepe pit and stinking dungeon[1].

These men had beene before a long time at the seas, and had no change of apparell, nor laine in bed, and now lieing upon the ground without succor or reliefe, were soone infected ; and all for the most part were sicke, and some of them died, and some one of them was distracted ; and this sicke-nesse verie soone after dispersed itselfe among all the residue of the prisoners in the gaole ; of which disease manie of them died, but all brought into great extremities and were hardly escaped. These men, when they were to be brought before the foresaid justices for their triall, manie of them were so weak and sicke that they were not able to goe nor stand ; but were caried from the gaole to the place of judgement, some upon handbarrowes, and some betweene men leading them, and so brought to the place of justice.

The sight of these men's miserable and pitifull cases, being thought (and more like) to be hunger-starved than with sickenesse diseased, moved manie a man's heart to behold and look upon them ; but none pitied them more than the lords justices themselves, and especially the lord chief justice himselfe ; who upon this occasion tooke a better order for keeping all prisoners thenseforth in the gaole, and for the more often trials ; which was now appointed to be quarterlie kept at every quarter sessions and not to be posted anie more over, as in times past, untill the assises.

These prisoners thus brought from out of the gaole to the judgment

---

[1] These statements by Hoker, chamberlain of Exeter, are sufficiently circumstantial ; but they do not quite suit the theory of a writer in the *Dict. Nat. Biog.*, under "Drake, Sir Bernard" that the ship was "a great Portugal ship," called the Lion of Viana, with an English master, taken by Bernard Drake in Brittany. No doubt such a capture is stated in the *Cal. State Papers*, 1585, p. 295 (the reference given), Sir W. Raleigh's ship the "Jobe" being included in the same petition ; but nothing is said of Dartmouth as the port to which the two vessels were brought, or of Exeter as the place where their captains were imprisoned. It is of importance for the theory of the Exeter gaol fever to know whether Drake's prisoners were Portuguese fishermen or not, and Hoker may be supposed to have known.

place, after that they had been staied, and paused awhile in the open aire, and somewhat refreshed therewith, they were brought into the house, in the one end of the hall near to the judges seat, and which is the ordinarie and accountable place where they do stand to their triales and arraignments. And howsoever the matter fell out, and by what occasion it happened, an infection followed upon manie and a great number of such as were there in the court, and especially upon such as were nearest to them were soonest infected. And albeit the infection was not then perceived, because every man departed, (as he thought), in as good health as he came thither; yet the same by little and little so crept into such as upon whom the infection was seizoned, that after a few daies, and at their home coming to their owne houses, they felt the violence of this pestilent sicknesse ; wherein more died, that were infected, than escaped. And besides the prisoners, manie there were of good account, and of all other degrees, which died thereof ; as by name sargeant Floredaie who then was the judge of those trials upon the prisoners, Sir John Chichester, Sir Arthur Basset, Sir Barnard Drake, Knight[1]; Thomas Carew of Haccombe, Robert Carie of Clovelleigh, John Fortescue of Wood, John Waldron of Bradfeeld and Thomas Risdone, esquires and justices of the peace.

...Of the plebeian and common people died verie manie, and especiallie constables, reeves, and tithing men, and such as were jurors, and namelie one jurie of twelve, of which there died eleven.

This sicknesse was dispersed throughout all the whole shire, and at the writing hereof in the time of October, 1586, it is not altogether extinguished. It resteth for the most part about fourteene daies and upwards by a secret infection, before it breake out into his force and violence."

Here we have the same incubation-period as in the Oxford fever, about fourteen days. But in the Exeter case, we have it clearly stated that an infection arose in the prison from the poor Portuguese sailors or fishermen who had been thrown into " deep pit and stinking dungeon" after their capture on the high seas by Sir Bernard Drake, that the infection attacked the other prisoners, that many of the prisoners died and all were brought to extremities, and that those who stood their trial were then in a most feeble state, although they seemed to the pitying spectators to be more starved than diseased.

So far as concerned the infection in the Assize Court, among the lawyers, county gentry, and officials, jurors and others, it was of the same tragic kind as at Oxford in 1577 and at Cambridge

---

[1] The author of the misadventure. He succeeded in getting home to Crediton, where he died on the 12th April, four weeks after the Assizes began.

in 1522, and, as we shall see, on several occasions in the eighteenth century. But the Exeter case has some features special to itself. Within the gaol were both English felons and thirty-eight Portugals, who had become subject to capture on their way home from the banks of Newfoundland with boat-loads of stock-fish, and to treatment as felons, because Spain and England were at war. Within the gaol there seems to have been also a gradation of misery, a deep pit and stinking dungeon, "in the lowest deep a lower deep," to which were consigned the men of foreign breed, the Portugals. It was among them that deaths first occurred, in what special form we know not. From them an infection is clearly stated by Hoker to have spread through the gaol at large, and to have made many of the prisoners so weak that they had to be carried into court. This is quite unlike what we read of in the Cambridge and Oxford cases, in neither of which was illness noted in the prisoners or asserted of them, although at Oxford two or three had died in chains a few days before. In the Exeter case there were three circles of the damned instead of two only: nay there were four. Farthest in were the Portugals, next to them were the native English felons, then came those present on business or pleasure at the Assizes, and lastly there were the country people all over Devonshire for many months after. We must take all those peculiarities of the Exeter gaol-fever together, and explain them one by another. It was a somewhat elaborated poison. It had passed from the foreign prisoners to the English, and in the transmission had, as it were, consolidated its power; hence, when the prisoners did give it to those who breathed their atmosphere in court, the infection did not limit itself to them, as it certainly did at Oxford and, so far as anything is said, at Cambridge also, and as it usually does in typhus-fever; but it became a volatile poison, it developed wings and acquired staying power, so that its effects were felt over the county of Devon for at least six months longer.

Poverty and Vagrancy in Tudor England.

The Black Assizes of Cambridge (1522), of Oxford (1577), and of Exeter (1586) cast, in each case, a momentary and vivid light upon the state of England in the Tudor period as late as the middle of the reign of Elizabeth. It has been pointed out in a former chapter that prices and wages were favourable to the cultivators of the soil in the fifteenth century, that the English yeomanry sprang up in that period, that village communities and trading towns prospered although their morals were none of the best, and that the civil wars of York and Lancaster were so far from injuring the domestic peace of England that they even secured it. It was the observation of Philip de Comines, more than once quoted before, that England had the "peculiar grace" of being untroubled at large by the calamities of her civil wars, because kings and nobles were left to settle their quarrels among themselves. "Nothing is perfect in this world," says the French statesman, who did not like independence of spirit among the lower orders. But he recognizes the fact as peculiar to England in the fifteenth century; and there can be little doubt about it.

The civil wars were hardly over when the troubles of the common people began. Here, if anywhere, is the turning-point brought into Goldsmith's poem of "The Deserted Village:"

> A time there was, ere England's griefs began,
> When every rood of ground maintained its man.

Deserted villages became a reality in the last quarter of the fifteenth century, and throughout the century following. We hear of this depopulation first in the Isle of Wight, where it affected the national defence and therefore engaged the attention of the State. Two Acts were passed in 1488—9, cap. 16 and cap. 19 of 4 Henry VII. The first declares that "it is for the security of the king and realm that the Isle of Wight should be well inhabited, for defence against our ancient enemies of France; the which isle is late decayed of people, by reason that many towns and villages have been let down, and the fields

25—2

dyked and made pastures for beasts and cattle." The second relates that

> "Great inconveniences daily doth increase by desolation and pulling down and wilful waste of houses and towns, and laying to pasture lands which customably have been used in tilth, whereby idleness, ground and beginning of all mischiefs, daily do increase ; for where in some towns two hundred persons were occupied and lived by their lawful labours, now be there occupied two or three herdsmen, and the residue fall into idleness." The remedy enacted is that no one shall take a farm in the Isle of Wight which shall exceed ten marks, and that owners shall maintain, upon their estates, houses and buildings necessary for tillage.

An instance of the same depopulation is given by Dugdale in Warwickshire : seven hundred acres of arable land turned to pasture, and eighty persons thrown out of employment causing the destruction of sixteen messuages and seven cottages. An instance of the same kind has already been quoted from the neighbourhood of Cambridge as early as 1414 ; but it is not until the settlement of the dynastic quarrels and jealousies, partly on the victories of Edward IV. at Barnet and Tewkesbury in 1471, and completely after the victory of Henry Tudor at Bosworth in 1485, that agrarian troubles became general. Then began the famous *enclosures*—enclosures both of the "wastes" of the manors, and of the open cultivated fields of the manors in which all the orders of villagers had their share of tenancy.

A few years after, in 1495, the number of vagabonds and beggars had so increased, of course in consequence of the enclosures, that a new Act was required, cap. 2 of the 11th of Henry VII. "Considering the great charges that should grow for bringing vagabonds to the gaols according to the statute of 7 Richard II., cap. 5, and the long abiding of them therein, whereby it is likely many of them would lose their lives:" therefore to put them in the stocks for three days and three nights upon bread and water, and after that to set them at large and command them to avoid the town, and if a vagabond be taken again in the same town or township, then the stocks for *four* days, with like diet. The deserving poor, however, were to be dealt with otherwise, but in an equally futile manner. In 1503–4, by the 19th of Henry VII. cap. 12, the period in the stocks was reduced to one day and one night (bread and water as before), probably in order that all vagabonds might have their turn.

The most correct picture of the state of England under Henry VII. and Henry VIII. is given by Sir Thomas More. The passages in his *Utopia*, relating to the state of England may be taken as veracious history. A discussion is supposed to arise at the table of Morton, archbishop of Canterbury, who was More's early patron, and who died in 1500. "I durst boldly speak my mind before the Cardinal," says the foreign observer of our manners and custom, Raphael Hythloday; and then follows an account of the state of England which lacks nothing in plainness of speech.

"But let us consider those things that chance daily before our eyes. First there is a great number of gentlemen, which cannot be content to live idle themselves, like drones, of that which other have laboured for : their tenants I mean, whom they poll and shave to the quick by raising their rents (for this only point of frugality do they use, men else through their lavish and prodigal spending able to bring themselves to very beggary)— these gentlemen, I say, do not only live in idleness themselves, but also carry about with them at their tails a great flock or train of idle and loitering serving-men, which never learned any craft whereby to get their living. These men, as soon as their master is dead, or be sick themselves, be incontinent thrust out of doors....And husbandmen dare not set them a work, knowing well enough that he is nothing meet to do true and faithful service to a poor man with a spade and a mattock for small wages and hard fare, which being daintily and tenderly pampered up in idleness and pleasure, was wont with a sword and a buckler by his side to strut through the street with a bragging look, and to think himself too good to be any man's mate.

Nay, by Saint Mary, Sir, (quoth the lawyer), not so. For this kind of men must we make most of. For in them, as men of stouter stomachs, bolder spirits, and manlier courages than handicraftsmen and ploughmen be, doth consist the whole power, strength and puissance of our army, when we must fight in battle."

So much for the serving-men of the rich, apt to be discarded to swell the ranks of poverty and crime. But further :—

"There is another cause, which, as I suppose, is proper and peculiar to you Englishmen alone.—What is that? quoth the Cardinal.—Forsooth, my lord, quoth I, your sheep that were wont to be so meek and tame, and so small eaters, now, as I hear say, be become so great devourers and so wild that they eat up and swallow down the very men themselves. They consume, destroy and devour whole fields, houses and cities. For look in what parts of the realm doth grow the finest and therefore dearest wool, these noblemen and gentlemen, yea and certain abbots, (holy men, no doubt), not contenting themselves with the yearly revenues and profits that were wont to grow to their forefathers and predecessors of their lands, nor being content that they live in rest and pleasure, nothing profiting yea much annoying the weal public leave no ground for tillage; they inclose all into pastures; they throw down houses; they pluck down towns and leave nothing standing, but only the church to be made a sheep-house. And as though you lost no small quantity of ground by forests, chases, lawns, and parks, these holy men turn all dwelling-places and all glebe-land into desolation and wilderness. Therefore the one covetous and insatiable cormorant and very plague of his native country may compass about and inclose many thousand acres of ground together within one pale or hedge; the husbandmen be thrust out of their own, or else either by cunning and fraud, or by violent oppression they be put besides it, or by wrongs and injuries they be so wearied that they be compelled to sell all. By one means, therefore, or by other, either by hook or crook, they must needs depart away, poor silly wretched souls, men, women, husbands, wives, fatherless children, widows, woeful mothers with their young babes, and their whole household small in substance and much in number as husbandry requireth many hands. Away they trudge, I say, out of their known and accustomed houses, finding no place to rest in. All their household stuff, which is very little worth, though it might well abide the sale, yet being suddenly thrust out, they be constrained to sell it for a thing of nought. And when they have wandered abroad till that be spent, what can they then else do but steal, and then justly, pardy! be hanged, or else go about a begging. And yet, then also they be cast in prison as vagabonds, because they go about and work not; whom no man will set a work, though they never so willingly profer themselves thereto."

Thus were the gaols filled. The policy of Henry VIII. was to hang for petty theft—"twenty together upon one gallows." And yet the lawyer, the defender of the king's firm rule, "could not choose but greatly wonder and marvel, how and by what evil luck it should come to pass that thieves nevertheless were in every place so rife and rank."

These descriptions of the state of England were written about 1517, and the recitals in various Acts of Henry VIII. bear them out. Thus, in 1514 and 1515 (6 Hen. VIII. cap. 5, and 7 Hen. VIII. cap. 1), the towns, villages and hamlets, and other habitations decayed in the Isle of Wight are to be re-edified and re-peopled. In 1533-4 (25 Hen. VIII. cap. 13), there is a more comprehensive Act against the aggrandisements of pasture-farmers, "by reason whereof a marvellous multitude of the people of this realm be not able to provide meat, drink and clothes necessary for themselves, their wives, and children, but be so discouraged with misery and poverty that they fall daily to theft, robbery, and other inconvenience, or pitifully die for hunger and cold." Some greedy and covetous persons have as many as 24,000 sheep: no one to keep above 2,000 sheep under the penalty of 3*s*. 4*d*. for every sheep kept by him above that number. Ten years after comes the well-known Act relating to the decay of towns[1] (35 Hen. VIII. cap. 4).

Besides these recitals in Acts of Parliament, we have other glimpses of the causes of agrarian distress. Thus, in a letter of June 24, 1528, from Sir Edward Guildford to Wolsey: Romney Marsh is fallen into decay; there are many great farms and holdings in the hands of persons who neither reside on them, nor till, nor breed cattle, but use them for grazing, trusting to the Welsh store cattle[2].

In Becon's *Jewel of Joy*, written in the reign of Edward VI. the same condition of things is described:

" How do the rich men, and specially such as be sheepmongers, oppress the king's liege-people by devouring their common pastures with their sheep, so that the poor people are not able to keep a cow for the comfort of them and of their poor family, and are like to starve and perish for hunger, if there be not provision made shortly...Rich men were never so much estranged from all pity and compassion toward the poor people as they be at this present time...They not only link house to house, but when they have gotten many houses and tenements into their hands, yea whole townships, they suffer the houses to fall into utter ruin and decay, so that by this means whole towns are become desolate and like unto a wilderness, no man dwelling there except it be the shepherd and his dog." The interlocutor in the dialogue answers: "Truth it is. For I myself know many towns and villages sore decayed; for whereas in times past there were in some town an hundred households, there remain not now thirty; in some fifty, there are not now ten; yea (which is more to be lamented) I know towns so wholly decayed that there is neither stick nor stone, as they say....And the cause of all this wretchedness and beggary in the common weal is the greed of gentlemen which are sheepmongers and graziers[3]."

---

[1] Sir George Nicholls, in his *History of the English Poor Law*, 1854, I. 113, threw out the suggestion that the decay was in the old walled towns, and that it was compensated by the rise of populations on less hampered sites. This theory has been adopted by some later writers.

[2] *Calendar of State Papers*. Domestic, Hen. VIII.

[3] Becon's *Works*, 3 vols. II. fol. 15–16.

Again, in Bullein's *Dialogue of the Fever Pestilence* (1664), the groom Roger who accompanies the citizen and his wife to the country, in the direction of Barnet, points out an estate on which the rents had been raised; the fields had been turned into large pastures, and all the houses pulled down save the manor house: "for the carles have forfeited their leases and are gone a-begging like villaines, and many of them are dead for hunger."

Vagabonds, beggars, valiant beggars, sturdy beggars, and ruffelers continue to occupy the pages of the Statute Book for many years. In 1530–31 (a long and elaborate Act), and in 1535–6, they are to be repressed by the stocks, by whipping, and ear-cropping; "and if any ruffeler, sturdy vagabond, or valiant beggar, having the upper part of the right ear cut off as aforesaid, be apprehended wandering in idleness, and it be duly proved that he hath not applied to such labours as have been assigned to him, or be not in service with any master, that then he be committed to gaol until the next quarter sessions, and be there indicted and tried, and, if found guilty, he shall be adjudged to suffer death as a felon." A still more distracted Act was made by the Lord Protector in 1547 (1 Ed. VI. cap. 3): if the vagabond continue idle and refuse to labour, or run away from work set him to perform, he is to be branded with the letter V, and be adjudged a slave for two years to any person who shall demand him, to be fed on bread and water and refuse-meat, and caused to work in such labour, "how vile soever it be, as he shall be put unto, by beating, chaining, or otherwise." If he run away within the two years, he is to be branded in the cheek with the letter S, and adjudged a slave for life; and if he run away again he is to suffer death as a felon. Similar provisions are made for "slave-children;" while the usual exceptions are brought in for the impotent poor. The above statute remained in force for only two years, having been from the first a monstrous insult to the intelligence of the nation, and never applied. It was succeeded by two meek-spirited Acts, 3 and 4 Ed. VI. cap. 16, and 5 and 6 Ed. VI. cap. 2, in which the impotent poor are provided for:—collectors in church to "gently ask and demand alms for the poor." By the 1st of Mary, cap. 13, the collections for the poor were made weekly. When Elizabeth came to the throne, greater pressure was put upon the well-to-do to support the poor: by the Act of 5 Eliz. cap. 3 (1562–3) those who obstinately refused voluntary alms might be assessed. A more important Act of Elizabeth was that of her 14th year (1572–3) cap. 5, "For the Punishment of Vagabonds and for Relief of the Poor and Impotent." A vagabond, as before, is to be whipped, and burnt on the ear; for a second offence to suffer death as a felon "unless some honest person will take him into his service for two whole years;" and for a third offence to suffer death and loss of lands and goods, as a felon, without allowance of benefit of clergy or sanctuary. Aged and infirm poor, by the same Act, are to be cared for by "overseers of the poor" in every parish, and to have abiding places fixed for them. In 1575–6 (18th Eliz. cap. 3), the Act of 1572–3 was amended and explained: "collectors and governors of the poor" are to provide a stock of wool, hemp, iron etc. for the poor to work upon, and "houses of correction," or Bridewells, are to be built—one, two or more in every county for valiant beggars or such other poor persons as refuse to work under the overseers or embezzle their work. The last and greatest poor-laws of Elizabeth's reign were those of her 39th year (1597–8) caps. 3 and 4 and her 43rd year (1601) cap. 2. These remained the basis of the English poor-law down to a recent period. Overseers of the poor are appointed in every parish—the churchwardens *ex officio* and four others appointed by the justices in Easter week: the overseers to meet once a month in the parish church after divine service on the Sunday: contributions to be levied by the inhabitants of any parish among themselves, or the parish or hundred to be taxed by the justices, failing the contributions, or, if the hundred be unable, then the county to be rated "in aid of" the parishes.

These being the developments of the poor-law and the law against vagabonds to the end of the Tudor period, we may now return to our particular illustrations, and more especially to the illustrations from popular sickness.

Under the year 1537, one of the citizen chroniclers of London has an entry, "Began a collection for the poor, and a great number cured of many grievous diseases through the charity thereof." Under 1540, he records that "the collection for the poor people ceased[1]." Preaching before Edward VI. on the fourth Sunday in Lent, 1550, Thomas Lever, Master of St John's College, Cambridge, said: "O merciful Lord! what a number of poor, feeble, halt, blind, lame, sickly—yea with idle vagabonds and dissembling caitiffs mixed among them, lie and creep, begging in the miry streets of London and Westminster[2]." In May, 1552, Ridley wrote to Cecil that the citizens were willing to provide for the poor "both meat, drink, clothing and firing;" but they lacked lodging, and he wanted the king to give up Bridewell "to lodge Christ in," or in other words, the poor "then lying abroad in the streets of London."

Coming to the middle of Elizabeth's reign, in the year 1579 we find, in an essay dedicated to the queen by Dr John Jones upon general topics of health and morals, an account of poverty and crime which reads little better than Sir Thomas More's for 1517. In his 31st chapter on "The great cost that the commonwealth is at daily in relieving the poore: Of the number of them that are yeerly executed," he speaks of the new poor-rate as "a greater tax than some subsidies," and as a "larger collection than would maintain yeerly a good army;" and, of the felons as "a mightier company of miserable captives than would defend a large country, as in the records of the Clerks of the Peace and of the Assize may easily be seen."

Even from the outset, the poor-rate does not appear to have met the difficulty:

"And yet housekeepers be but little less discharged, if ye note the continual resort of the needy, especially in the country and towns that be incorporate, the poor (as they say) not much the more aided, as by the moan they make to travellers may be easily gathered, nor theft and wickedness the less practised. For what misery it is to see condemned at one assize in a little shire thirty-nine, notwithstanding the clemency of the Judges, and three hundred and odd in one Diocese to do penance or fine for their loose living in a year. But these be the meanest sort only, for the others scape as though it were in them no offence. And in one gaol of prisoners three hundred and upwards at one time, whereof a great part perhaps may be through negligence of justice or cruelty, that otherwise might be punished answerably to the offences lawfully."

[1] Continuation of Fabyan's *Chronicle.*
[2] Greyfriars *Chronicle*, Camden Soc. LIII., 1852. Preface by J. G. Nichols, xxiv.

He then refers to the Bridewells "so charitably and politicly appointed by the late Act of Parliament, although not yet in every shire erected." The Act of Parliament was that of 1572 and the Bridewells were the houses of correction for vagrants, the first type of workhouses, and so named after the Bridewell in Fleet Street, which was given by Edward VI. from being a royal residence to be a refuge of the poor. So far as fever was concerned, it mattered little whether the Bridewell were a poorshouse or a prison, for in later times gaol fever and workhouse fever were both synonyms for typhus.

It would not have been surprising to find this enormous extent of pauperism, vagrancy and crime attended by the distinctive *morbus pauperum*, typhus-fever. But we are here concerned only with the evidence, and not with antecedent probabilities. The records are, of course, very imperfect. The gaol-fevers of Cambridge, Oxford and Exeter attracted much notice because they touched the governing class. There may have been much more gaol-fever unrecorded. Hoker, in his account of the Exeter fever, does indeed say: "and this is commonly called the gaol sickness, and many die thereof;" and, in a petition to the Crown, March, 1579, the Queen's Bench prison in Southwark is said to contain twice its complement, there is in it a disease called "sickness of the house," and near a hundred had died of that sickness in the prison during the previous six years[1]. We shall not be able to give colour to our epidemiological history by other such instances from the Tudor period[2]; even for plague itself, the records of particular out-

---

[1] Strype's ed. of Stow's *Survey of London.*

[2] In the Rolls of the Middlesex Sessions (Middlesex Record Society), there occur numerous entries of inquests on deaths in the gaol of Newgate from the 25th year of Elizabeth: a few of these are from plague; but by far the larger number are from "the pining sickness," a malady which sometimes cut off several prisoners in the same few days and after a brief illness. In one of these epidemics (Dec. 1586—Feb. 1587), a single case is called "pestilent fever," the other seven being "pining sickness." Next year, June 19, there is a case of bloody flux, and, on June 24, a case of "pining sickness." The other periods when the disease so named was epidemic in Newgate were Feb.—May, 1595, June and July, 1597, March, 1598, and March—April, 1602. The pining sickness was probably a generic term, and may have included chronic disease; there is a solitary case entered as ailing for as long a period as eight months,

breaks are meagre and almost certainly only a part of the whole. The epidemics which shall occupy us for the rest of this chapter are those that had a general prevalence over the country on two or three occasions, the same general prevalence of fever that recurs at shorter intervals in the Stuart period and in the eighteenth century.

Hitherto we have attempted to work out the history of epidemics in Britain without reference to the epidemics in other countries, except in the case of the Black Death, which had remarkable antecedents in the remote East, and in the case of the English Sweat of 1528, which overran a great part of the Continent in 1529 and 1530. To have attempted a parallel record of epidemics abroad would have served inevitably to confuse the vision; for the annals of pestilence in all Europe would have been from year to year an unrelieved record of sickness and death, an unnatural continuance or sequence, from which the mind turns away. The several countries of Europe, and the several cities, had each their turn of plague; but they had each, also, their free intervals, sometimes very long intervals, as we have seen in the case of Aberdeen with no plague for nearly two generations in the sixteenth century. The epidemiography of each country should therefore be kept apart; and

the usual duration of the sickness being one, two, or three days up to three or four weeks.

This place will serve to notice the strange teaching about "parish infection" which has received currency among the writers of good repute as authorities. Guy (*Public Health*, Lectures, 1870, I. 23) says the gaol distemper was an old offender known as the *sickness of the house*: "I think I recognize it in the London Bills from 1606 to 1665 as the *Parish Infection*." The column of figures in the London Bills which has been taken to show the weekly prevalence of a disease, otherwise unheard of, "parish infection," really shows the number of "parishes infected." The earlier bills showed, in the corresponding column, the number of parishes clear ("parish. clere" or "paroch.clere"). By adding up the number of parishes infected in each of the 52 weeks of a bad plague-year, a total of some thousands is got, and that total has been taken to be the annual mortality from "parish infection"—a pure myth. The original author of this singular mistake appears to have been Marshall, in his *Mortality of the Metropolis*, London, 1832, p. 67. Of the "parish infection," he says: "The disease below is specified by Mr Bell in his *Remembrancer* [1665]; it is probably the same as exhibited under the name of spotted fever." What Bell "specifies" is not another disease, but the number of parishes in the City and suburbs infected with the plague in each week of the year.

within a given country care should be taken to prevent the illusion of universal sickness, which is apt to be created in the bringing of scattered centres of disease (such as plague) together in the same page.

But there are instances of what are called pandemics, or universal epidemics, of sickness. The Black Death was one such, covering a period of perhaps four years in Europe, from 1347 to 1350, the curve of the disease in each locality lasting about six months. With the beginning of the modern period we come to more frequent pandemics, not of plague, but of minor or milder forms of pestilential infection. On the continent of Europe these were in part related to the state of war, which may be taken as beginning with the invasion of Italy by Charles VIII. of France in 1494. Typhus-fever, or war-fever with famine-fever, now begins to be a familiar form of sickness —in 1498, 1505, 1510, 1528, and so on. Other forms are putrid sore throat, dysentery, and varieties of fever included under influenza. The various forms were apt to occur together or in succession, so that epidemiography has a "Protean" character. This epidemic Proteus is at once a great difficulty and a most instructive fact. It opens up the very old doctrine of "epidemic constitutions" of the air, which to many moderns savours of unscientific vagueness; and it brings us face to face with degrees or kinds of infectiveness which are, in matter of fact, more wonderful or more incomprehensible than the deadlier infections, such as the plague or Asiatic cholera. The most familiar instance of the kind is influenza.

Influenza.

Influenza enters undoubtedly into the Protean infections of the sixteenth century, and is itself no small part of the Proteus. But what is influenza? The name is comparatively modern— Italian of the 18th century—and appears to mean defluxion or catarrh, not in the familiar sense only, but as derived from the comprehensive pathological doctrine of humours: thus the Venetian envoy in London called the sweat of 1551 an "influsso." It is open to us to include much or little under influenza; but the name itself, having its root in an obsolete doctrine of humours, can never be made exact or scientific. Usage has applied it to all universal colds and coughs; and it has been applied capriciously to some universal fevers, but not to others. There are two tolerably clear references to its prevalence in England before the peculiarly unwholesome state of Europe began with the modern age. Under the year 1173, the chronicle of Melrose enters "a certain evil and unheard-of cough" (*tussis quaedam mala et inaudita*), which affected everyone far and near, and cut off many.

One of the St Albans chroniclers, an unknown writer who kept a record from 1423 to 1431 (reign of Henry VI.), has the following entry under the year 1427: "In the beginning of October, a certain rheumy infirmity (*quaedam infirmitas reumigata*) which is called '*mure*' invaded the whole people, and so infected the aged along with the younger that it conducted a great number to the grave[1]." A good deal is said in this brief passage, and all that is said points to influenza—the rheumy nature of the malady, the universality of incidence, presumably the suddenness and brief duration, the deaths among the aged and the more juvenile. It is known also that a similarly general malady was prevalent the same year in Paris, where it bore the name of *ladendo*; the particulars given in the French record of it leave no doubt that it was influenza.

The singular name of *pestilentia volatilis* given by Fordoun to two epidemics in Scotland in his own lifetime, one which began at Edinburgh in February, 1430 (1431 new style), and the other at Haddington in 1432, suggests that they may have been influenzas, but there is nothing more than the name to indicate their nature. Those years are not known to have been years of

[1] *Annales Monastici*, Rolls series, No. 19. Chronicle by an unknown author (St Albans) temp. Hen. VI., 1422–31 :—"Quaedam infirmitas reumigata invasit totum populum, quae *mure* dicitur : et sic senes cum junioribus inficiebat quod magnum numerum ad funus letale deducebat."

In the Report of the Irish Local Government Board, Medical Department, 1890, influenza is identified under the name "slaedan," or prostration, which was epidemic in Ireland in 1326 or 1328, the same epidemic being called "murre" in the *Annals of Clonmacnoise*. The use of the word "mure" in the St Albans Chronicle is just a century later. Murrain (or *morena* in Latin chronicles) is probably the modern survival of "mure" or "murre."

influenza in any other country of Europe: the record of the malady passes direct from 1427 to 1510. There was certainly a great wave of influenza over Europe in 1510, under the names of *cocqueluche* and *coccolucio*. It is said to have come up from the Mediterranean coasts and to have extended to the shores of the Baltic and North Seas; its prevalence in Britain is likely enough, and is indeed asserted in one foreign account, but there is no known native notice of it. Abroad, it had the usual character of suddenness, simultaneity and universality, and the symptoms of heaviness, prostration, headache, restlessness, sleeplessness, and for some time after a violent paroxysmal cough, like whooping-cough. None died except some children; in some it went off with a looseness, in others by sweating[1]. The mention of sweating in the influenza epidemic of 1510 is not without importance. It may serve to explain a remark by Erasmus, in a letter of 25th August, 1511, from Queens' College, Cambridge, that his health was still rather doubtful "from that sweat" (*a sudore illo*[2]); the sweat can hardly have been the sweating sickness of 1508, three years before, but the still unsettled health of Erasmus in 1511 may perhaps have been the dregs of the influenza of 1510.

The next great European epidemic of influenza was in 1557, for which I shall produce medical evidence of England sharing in it, probably during that year and certainly in the one following. But the intervening years afford some notices of sickness in England, which was neither so severe as plague at one end of the pestilential scale nor altogether mild at the other, being forms of illness which contemporaries pronounced to be "new" and "strange," and appear to have been of the nature of pestilent fever and dysentery.

Neither typhus nor dysentery was really new to England in the sixteenth century; on the contrary, they were (with putrid sore throat and lientery) the common types of disease in the

---

[1] I take this summary from Short (*Chronology*, etc. I. 204), who omits his authority, probably the foreign writers to whom he is usually indebted in the earlier period. The first part of Theophilus Thompson's *Annals of Influenza* (Sydenham Society) is little else than extracts from Short, and therefore of foreign origin.

[2] *Cal. State Papers.* Domestic, *sub dato.*

great English famines which came at long intervals, as described in the first chapter. But on the continent of Europe typhus and dysentery and putrid sore throat (*angina maligna*) began with the modern age to appear as if capriciously, and independently of such obvious antecedents as want, although some of the epidemics of typhus and dysentery were clearly related to the hardships of warfare[1]. Typhus, indeed, was a disastrous malady on the Continent in those years, notably in 1528 in Spain, where it was known as " las bubas," and in France, where it was called " les poches "—both names relating to the spots on the skin, and both more strictly applicable to the eruptions of the lues venerea, which was then also rampant.

Apart from the gaol fever at Cambridge in 1522, the first mention of those new epidemics in England since the end of the medieval period is under the year 1540 : " This said xxx and two year [of Henry VIII.] divers and many honest persons died of the hot agues and of a great lask throughout the realm[2]." The " lask " was dysentery, (Stow, in chronicling the epidemic in his much later *Annales* calls it " the bloody flux"), and the " hot agues," according to later references under that name, appear to have been influenza in the sense of a highly volatile typhus[3]. All that we know of the circumstances of this epidemic is that the summer was one of excessive drought, that wells and brooks were dried up, and that the Thames ran so low as to make the tide at London Bridge not merely brackish but salt.

[1] Thus in the continuation of Fabyan's Chronicle under the year 1512, the Marquis of Dorset, sent into Spain with 10,000 men, is said to have "returned in winter by reason of the flix (dysentery)." And in Hall's *Chronicle* (ed. of 1807, p. 523), we have particulars of the very serious sickness in his army in Biscay; owing to their diet being largely of garlic and fruits, and their drink being hot wines in hot weather, "there fell sick 3000 of the flix, and thereof died 1800 men."

[2] Continuator of Fabyan's *Chronicle*, sub anno. There is an almost identical entry in *A London Chronicle of Henry VII. and Henry VIII.* (Camden Miscellany, vol. v. 1859), but under the year 1539, in a hot and dry summer. The most discrepant date and designation of the epidemic of those years are those given in Hardiman's *History of Galway* (p. 40): "This charitable institution [St Bridget's Hospital] was fortunately completed in the year 1543, when the sweating sickness broke out, and raged with great violence, destroying multitudes of the natives, and particularly the tradesmen of the town."

[3] The term "hot ague" occurs as early as 1518, in a letter of 18 July (*Cal. State Papers*).

The spring and summer of 1551 were the seasons of the last outbreak of the sweat in England, which curiously coincided with another epidemic of influenza (*cocqueluche*) in France. The years from 1555 to 1558 were a sickly period for all Europe, the diseases being of the types of dysentery, typhus, and influenza. The most authentic particulars are given under the years 1557 and 1558; and those for England, which specially concern us, are now to be given. Wriothesley, a contemporary, enters under the year 1557: "This summer reigned in England divers strange and new sicknesses, taking men and women in their heads; as strange agues and fevers, whereof many died[1]." Under the year 1558, the continuator of Fabyan's chronicle says: "In the beginning of this mayor's year died many of the wealthiest men all England through, of a strange fever[2]."

Some light is thrown upon the sickness, general throughout England in 1557–8, also by Stow in his *Annales*. Before the harvest of 1557 corn was at famine prices, but after the harvest wheat fell to an eighth part of the price (5*s*. the quarter), the penny wheaten loaf being increased from 11 oz. to 56 oz.! In the harvest of 1558, he goes on, the "quartan agues continued in like manner, or more vehemently than they had done the last year passed, where-through died many old people and specially priests, so that a great number of parishes were unserved and no curates to be gotten, and much corn was lost in the fields for lack of workmen and labourers[3]." Harrison, canon of Windsor, says that a third part of the people of the land did taste the general sickness, which points to influenza[4].

---

[1] Wriothesley, *A Chronicle of England during the reigns of the Tudors* (1457–1559). Camden Society, II. 139.

Anthony Wood also enters for Oxford, under 1557, "A pestilential disease to the settling of some and the driving away of many; the causes of which proceeding from the eating of green fruit, the Commissary commanded that none should be sold in the market or elsewhere in Oxford."

[2] Fabyan's *Chronicle*, p. 711.

[3] Stow's *Annales*, ed. Howse, p. 631. Speed also has a paragraph, unusual with him, on the state of health in the year of Queen Mary's death (1658), in which the mortality among the clergy is specially mentioned.

[4] Extracts from Harrison's MS. *Chronologie* by Furnivall, in Appendix to *Elizabethan England*. Camelot series, 1890, p. 267. His famine prices, and the enormous fall of them after harvest, are the same as given by Stow.

C.   26

The year 1557 was certainly remarkable on the continent of Europe as a year of widely prevalent "pestiferous and contagious sickness," which was described by numerous medical writers. That universal epidemic, or pandemic, is usually counted as one of the great historical waves of influenza; and in the annals of that wonderful disease it stands the first which was well recorded by competent foreign observers, including Ingrassias, Gesner, Rondelet, Riverius, Dodonaeus, and Foreest. The corresponding sickness in England in 1557 (still more severe in 1558), which carried off many of the wealthiest men, and made so great an impression that it is noticed by Stow and Speed, has missed being noticed by English physicians, with a single exception, and that a casual one. If the continental physicians had not been copious in writing on several occasions when our English physicians were silent, such as the epidemic of syphilis in 1494-6, the English sweat of 1529, and the influenza of 1557-8, it might appear ungracious to remark upon the scanty literary productiveness of the profession in the Tudor period. Whoever attempts medical history for England will soon feel our deficiency in materials, and become disposed to envy the easier task of the foreign historian. The academical physicians of the time hardly ever wrote. The men who wrote on medicine were laymen like Sir Thomas Elyot, who justified his interest therein by the example of men of his own rank like Juba, king of Mauritania, and Mithridates, king of Pontus; or they were irregular practitioners desirous to advertise themselves; or book-sellers' hacks like Paynel; or such as Cogan, a schoolmaster and a physician in one. The modern reader will be surprised at the common burden of the prefaces of medical (and perhaps other) books in the Tudor period,—the intolerable nuisance of "pick-faults," "depravers," and cavillers, who sat in their chairs and criticised; and if the modern reader happen to be in quest of authentic facts, he can hardly fail to sympathise with Phaer, when he addresses the academical dog-in-the-manger with the Horatian challenge: "Si quid novisti rectius istis, candidus imperti; si non, his utere mecum."

It is possible, however, to collect a few particulars of the prevalent sickness of 1558 in England from casual notices of it.

Thus, it comes into a letter to the queen, of September 6, by Lord St John, governor of the Isle of Wight, from his house at Letley, near Southampton: sickness affected more than half the people in Southampton, the Isle of Wight and Portsmouth (those places being filled with troops under St John's command), and the captain of the fort at Sandown was dead[1]. Curiously enough we get an intimate glimpse of this epidemic from a book published some years after, the *Dyall of Agues* by Dr John Jones. In his chapter "Of the Sweating Fevers" (chapter xiv), after illustrating from Galen the proposition that a sweat may not be critical and wholesome, but τυφώδης or typhus-like, attending the seizure from its outset and "the same said sweat little or nothing profiting," he proceeds to point his remarks by his own experience:

"I had too good experience of myself in Queen Mary's reign, living at Lettlé in my good lord's house, the right honourable Lord St John, beside Southampton, the which, notwithstanding the great sweat, it was long after before I recovered of my health, so that the said sweat did nothing profit."

He then proceeds to compare the sweat, almost certainly the epidemic mentioned in St John's despatch of 6th September, 1558, with the sweating sickness of 1551:

"So in our days, even in King Edward VI.'s reign, it brought many to their long home, as some of the most worthy, the two noble princes of Suffolk, imps of honour most towardly, with others of all degrees infinite many; and the more perished no doubt for lack of physical counsel speedily[2]."

The next that we hear of this epidemic of the autumn of 1558, is in a despatch from Dover, 11 p.m. 6th October: the writer has "learnt from the mayor of Dover that there is no plague there, but the people that daily die are those that come out of the ships, and such poor people as come out of Calais, of the new sickness[3]." A despatch of 17th October, 1558, from one of the commissioners for the surrender of Calais, Sir Thomas Gresham, at Dunkirk, to the Privy Council, says that he "returned hither to write his letter to the queen, and found

---

[1] *State Papers*, Record Office.
[2] John Jones, M.D. *The Dyall of Ague*, London, 1564?
[3] *Calendar of State Papers.* Foreign, II. 1558, p. 398.

Sir William Pickering very sore sick of this new burning ague.
He has had four sore fits, and is brought very low, and in danger
of his life if they continue as they have done[1]."

Here we have the same term "new sickness" and "new
burning ague" as in the two English chronicles under the year
before—the "strange and new sicknesses" which "took men
and women in their heads," and the "strange agues and fevers."
The very general prevalence in Southampton, Portsmouth and
the Isle of Wight suggests influenza; the symptom of sweating
described by Jones for his own case during that prevalence is in
keeping with what we hear of the influenzas of the time from
foreign writers, and so is the long and slow convalescence; the
fact of one person having had four sore fits of "this new
burning ague" is more like influenza than typhus.

The severe mortalities in the autumn of 1558 at Loughborough and Chester are put down to "plague," and they may,
of course, have been circumscribed outbursts of the old bubo-
plague. If, however, they were part of the general prevalence
of hot or burning agues, which we may take to have been
influenza or a very volatile kind of typhus, they would indicate
a degree of fatality in the latter somewhat greater than more
recent influenzas have had. A high death-rate is, indeed,
demonstrable for the year 1558, from parish registers, by comparing the deaths in that year with the deaths in years near it,
and by comparing the deaths with the births in 1558 itself.

The registers of christenings and burials, which had been
ordered first in 1538, were kept in a number of parishes from
that date; and from 1558, when the order for keeping them was
renewed by queen Elizabeth, they were generally kept. Dr
Thomas Short, a man of great industry, about the middle of last
century obtained access to a large number of parish registers,
and worked an infinite number of arithmetical exercises upon
their figures[2]. His abstract results or conclusions are colourless
and unimpressive, as statistical results are apt to be for the
average concrete mind; nor can they be made to illustrate the

---

[1] *Calendar of State Papers.* Foreign, II. 1558, p. 400.
[2] *New Observations, Natural, Moral, Civil, Political and Medical, on City, Town
and Country Bills of Mortality.* By Thomas Short, M.D., London, 1750.

epidemic history of Britain with the help of his companion volumes, 'A General Chronological History of the Air, Weather, Seasons, Meteors etc[1].', for these extraordinary annals are for the most part loosely compiled from foreign sources, bringing into one focus the most scattered references to disease in any part of Europe, and that too without criticism of authorities but often with surprising credulity and inaccuracy. That so much statistical or arithmetical zeal and exhaustiveness (in the work of 1750) should go with so total a deficiency of the critical and historical sense, (in the work of 1749) is noteworthy, and perhaps not unparalleled in modern times. Short's history is mostly foreign, but his statistics, which are English, may be used to illustrate and confirm what can be learned of sicknesses in England in the ordinary way of historical research.

Thus, the period from 1557 to 1560 stands out in Short's table as one of exceptional unhealthiness both in country parishes and in market towns, the unhealthiness being estimated by the excess of burials over christenings.

Country Parishes.

Year	Registers examined	Unhealthy Parishes	Baptised in same	Buried in same
1557	16	7	62	181
1558	26	11	171	340
1559	34	12	145	252
1560	38	6	100	162
1561	41	1	19	32

Market Towns.

Year	Registers examined	Unhealthy Towns	Baptised in same	Buried in same
1557	4	2	262	381
1558	4	2	104	159
1559	5	3	102	149
1560	8	3	134	201
1561	8	3	276	399
1562	8	1	58	71

Short's collection of parish registers appears to have represented many English counties, although there is no clue to their identity in the tables from which these figures are taken. The

---

[1] 2 vols. London, 1749.

heavy mortalities in the registers correspond exactly to the epidemic years as otherwise known, and may be said to bear witness to the extent or generality of the epidemic infection.

The next that we hear of malignant fevers in England is the outbreak at Oxford in 1577, following the Assizes. Anthony Wood says of it: "Some thought that this Oxford mortality was the same that Leonard Fuchsius styles sudor Anglicus." Cogan, a contemporary, says :

"And certainly after that sudden bane at Oxford, the same year and a year or two following, the same kind of agues raged in a manner all over England, and took away very many of the strongest sort in their lustiest age, and for the most part men and not women nor children, culling them out here and there, even as you should choose the best sheep out of a flock. And certain remedy was none to be found....And they that took a moderate sweat at the beginning of their sickness, and did rid their stomachs well by vomit, sped much better."

This is partly confirmed by Short's abstracts of the parish registers. Thus in 1580, of sixty registers examined, ten showed unhealthiness, the births being to the deaths as 248 to 284. In 1582, seven country parishes were markedly unhealthy, the births being to the deaths as 140 to 244. In market towns the incidence is not so striking : in 1580, four towns out of sixteen examined showed an unhealthy birth-rate, 237 births to 276 deaths. It is in 1583 that the disparity becomes greatest in these towns : three out of the sixteen in the list were notably unhealthy, the deaths being 1062 and the births 467. But it is the obvious defect of Short's method that we have no means of knowing whether that mortality may not have been largely from plague, and not from fever or other form of epidemic sickness.

The only year between 1558 and 1580 in Short's tables, which stands out as decidedly unhealthy both in country parishes and market towns is 1570, while the years from 1573 to 1575 are less healthy than the average. Those were years of war, and of war-typhus, on the Continent, as the foreign writings show, but there are no records of the kind of sickness in England.

One glimpse of the prevalence of those fevers of 1580–82 is

got from a letter of the earl of Arundell to Lord Burghley, October 19, 1582. The earl had left his house in London because it was so "beset and encompassed" by plague; while, as to his country house: "The air of my house in Sussex is so corrupt even at this time of the year as, when I came away, I left xxiv sick of hot agues." He therefore begs the loan of the bishop of Chichester's house till such time as the vacancy in the see should be filled up[1].

The widespread volatile sicknesses of 1557–8 and 1580–2, which are grouped under the generic name of influenza, were related in time to great epidemics of the far more deadly bubo-plague. These plague outbursts were less noticeable in England than abroad. Thus in 1557 there were most disastrous epidemics of true bubo-plague in several towns of the Low Countries, and in 1580 there was at Cairo one of the worst epidemics in the whole history of plague from its beginning. The years preceding 1580 were also plague-years in many parts of Europe (Padua, Mantua, Venice, Messina, Palermo, Lisbon, Brussels). Those years were also the occasion of the first great and disastrous epidemics of diphtheria (*garottillo*) in Spain. Then come the epidemics of typhus; and at the far end of the pestilential scale the flying waves of influenza. A relation of influenza to other prevalent infections has been one of the theories of its nature, especially the relation to epidemics of Asiatic cholera.

In that view influenza looks as if it were a volatile product, a swifter and more superficial wave on the top of some slower and more deadly earth-borne virus. As the old writers said, it was a *levis corruptio aeris*, a diluted virus as it were, mild in proportion to its volatility and swiftness, but in universality equalling in its own milder way the universality of the plague of Justinian's reign or of the Black Death.

Now, the same century and the same state of society which witnessed the most remarkable of those flying ripples of infection over the whole surface of Europe witnessed also some waves of infection which did not travel so far, nor were mere influenzas. The English sweat travelled over England in that

---

[1] *Calendar of Cecil MSS.*, II. 525.

way; it was called the posting sweat, because it posted from town to town: thus in 1551 it suddenly appeared one day in Oxford, and next day it was in the villages around, as if carried in the air; in like manner it posted to Devonshire, to Leicestershire, to Cheshire, and doubtless all over England, like the influenzas of recent memory. And while the English sweat was thus flying about in England, influenza was flying about the same year (1551) in France, a country which never suffered from any of the five sweating sicknesses of 1485–1551. Again, the influenza in England in 1558 had the symptom of sweating so marked that it was compared to the true sweat of 1551 by Dr Jones, who himself suffered from it. Also the influenza of 1580 all over Europe had so much of a sweating character that in some places they said the English sweat had come back. Lastly, the gaol-fever of Oxford in 1577 was thought by some to present the symptoms described by Leonard Fuchs for *sudor Anglicus;* and Cogan, an English medical writer then living, specially mentions the phenomenon of sweating (as well as the intestinal profluvium called a "lask)," both at Oxford and in the more widely prevalent diseases of that year and the years following. The gaol-fever of Exeter in 1586 illustrates still another side of the question; it diffused itself—probably by other means than contact with the sick—all over the county of Devon, and had not ceased six months after it began in the month of March at Exeter. The Devonshire diffusion was like the spreading circles in a still pool. The spread of influenza was like the flying ripples on a broad surface of water. The spread of plague, on the occasions when it was universal, was like the massive rollers of the depths, the onward march of cholera from the East having, in our own times, illustrated afresh the same momentum.

In using hitherto the name of influenza for the universal fevers in England in 1557–58 and in 1580–82, I have done so because those years are usually reckoned in the annals of influenza. But the name is at best a generic one, and need not commit us to any nosological definition. I shall have to deal at more length with this question in the tenth chapter, when speaking of the fevers of 1657–59 described by Willis and

Whitmore, two competent medical observers ; in those years the vernal fever was a catarrhal fever, or influenza proper, while the fever of the hot and dry season, autumnal or harvest-fever, was a pestilential fever, a spotted fever, a burning ague, a contagious malignant fever.   There were also differences in their epidemological as well as in their clinical characters, the influenza wave being soonest past.   But so far as regarded universality of diffusion and generality of incidence, both types were much alike.

Molineux, writing in 1694, a generation after Willis, "On the late general coughs and colds," brought into comparison with them another epidemic which he had observed in Dublin in the month of July, 1688: "The transient fever of 1688...I look upon to have been the most universal fever, as this [1693] the most universal cold, that has ever appeared[1]."

When we come to the 18th century, to great epidemics not only in connexion with famine in Ireland, but also in England, we shall find the same diffusiveness associated with the clear type of disease which we now call typhus.   Influenza is the only sickness familiar to ourselves which shows the volatile character, and we are apt to conclude that no other type of fever ever had that character.   But, without going farther back than the 18th century we shall find epidemics of spotted typhus resting like an atmosphere of infection over whole tracts of Britain and Ireland, town and country alike ; and even if we give the name of influenza to the epidemical "hot agues" with which we are here immediately concerned, in the years 1540, 1557–8, and 1580–82, we may also regard them as in a manner corresponding to, if not as embracing, the types of fever that prevailed from time to time over wide districts of country in the centuries following.

The term "ague," often used at the time, is no more decisive for the nosological character than the term "influenza." Ague originally meant a sharp fever (*febris acuta*, ὀξύς), and in Ireland, from the time of Giraldus Cambrensis down to the 18th century, it meant the acute fever of the country, which

---

[1] *Phil. Trans.* XVIII. 103.

has not been malarial ague, in historical times at least, but
typhus. "Irish ague" was in later times a well-understood
term for contagious pestilential fever or typhus. In the *Dyall
of Agues* by Dr John Jones (1564?), just as in the writings of
Sydenham a century later, intermittents were mixed up with
continued fevers which had nothing malarial in their cause or
circumstances. Thus, Jones has a chapter on "Hot Rotten
Agues," which he identifies with the synochus or continued fever
of the Greeks; in another chapter on "The Continual Rotten
Ague," he locates the continued fevers within the vessels and the
"interpolate" without their walls, and proceeds:

> "It happeneth where all the vessels, but most chiefly in the greatest
> which are annexed about the flaps of the lungs and spiritual members, all
> equally putrefying, which often happeneth, as Fuchsius witnesseth, of
> vehement binding and retaining the filth in the cavity or hollowness of the
> vessels, inducing a burning heat. Wherefore, this kind of fever chanceth
> not to lean persons, nor to such as be of a thin constitution and cold tem-
> perament, nor an old age (that ever I saw), but often in them which abound
> with blood and of sanguine complexion, replenished with humour, fat and
> corpulent, solemners of Bacchus' feasts,—gorge upon gorge, quaff upon
> quaff—not altogether with meat or drink of good nourishment but of omnium
> gatherum, as well to the destruction of themselves as uncurable to the
> physician, as by my prediction came to pass (besides others) upon a gentle-
> man of Suffolk, a little from Ipswich, who by the causes aforesaid got his
> sickness, and thereof died the ninth day, according to my prediction, as his
> wife and friend knoweth."

Again, in his eighth chapter, ' Of the Pestilential Fever, or
Plague, or Boche [Botch]," he remarks upon the varying types
of pestilential diseases, mentioning among other national types
the English sweat :

> "As we, not out of mind past, with a sweat called stoupe galante, as that
> worthy Doctor Caius hath written at large in his book *De Ephemera
> Britannica*," adding the remark that here concerns us :—"and sethence
> [since then], with many pestilential agues, and, lastly of all, with the pesti-
> lential boche [botch or plague rightly termed]." These continued fevers,
> pestilential agues, or hot rotten agues, Jones distinguishes from quotidians,
> tertians and quartans. Of the last he says: "and when quartans reign
> everywhere, as they did of no long years past; of the which then I tasted
> part, besides my experience had of others,"—probably the fevers of 1558,
> elsewhere called by him the sweating sickness, and by Stow called "quartan
> agues." He mentions also quintans, which he had never seen in England,

"but yet in Ireland, at a place called Carlow, I was informed by Mr Brian Jones, then there captain, of a kerne or gentleman there that had the quintain long."

Not only the term "ague," but also the terms "intermittent," "tertian," and more especially "quartan," can hardly be taken in their modern sense as restricted to malarial or climatic fevers. An intermittent or paroxysmal character of fevers was made out on various grounds, to suit the traditional Galenic or Greek teaching; but the paroxysms and intermissions were not associated specially with rise and fall of the body-temperature. The curious history of agues, and of the specialist ague-curers, properly belongs to the time of the Restoration, when Peruvian bark came into vogue, and will be fully dealt with in the first chapter of another volume.

The last years in the Tudor period that stand out conspicuously in the parish registers for a high mortality, not due to plague, are 1597-8. The year 1597 was a season of influenza in Italy, and perhaps elsewhere in Europe; so that the epidemic in England that year may have been the same, but more probably was famine-fever. In the parish register of Cranbrooke the deaths for the year are 222, against 56 births; and 181 of the deaths are marked with the mark which is supposed to mean plague proper. The register of Tiverton has 277 deaths, against 66 births, but it is almost certain that the cause of the excess was not plague, of which the nearest epidemic in that town was in 1591. In a country parish of Hampshire, with a population of some 2700, the deaths in 1597 were 117, against 48 births, the mortality being about twice as great as in any year from the commencement of the register in 1569, and after until 1612[1]. In the north of England the type of disease in 1597-8 was plague proper.

The parish register of Finchley has a remarkable entry under the year 1596 which introduces us to other considerations: "Hoc anno moriebantur de dysenteria xix," the whole number of burials for the year having been 28. Next year, 1597, there are 23 deaths from dysentery, the burials in all having been 48—an enormous mortality compared with the average of the parish.

[1] Graunt, *Reflections on the Bills of Mortality*, 3rd ed. 1665.

The year 1597, if not also 1596, was a year of great scarcity, apparently all over England ; in Northumberland, Durham, and Cumberland, the scarcity was attended by plague proper ; but in other parts of England, it would seem, by other types of sickness, of which dysentery was one.

One of the 16th century English names used for flux was the obsolete word lask, which occurs often enough in writings of the period to suggest that the malady was common ; it is some-times called a choleric lask (cholera morbus), or a vehement lask, as in Elyot's *Castel of Health* and in Cogan's *Haven of Health*. Lasks, or lienteries, or dysenteries have not been dealt with in a chapter by themselves because the records of them are too few and meagre, so far as we have gone in the history ; but it may be convenient to bring together here the better known instances. In the period of famine-sicknesses, dysentery and lientery must have been common types, the latter being specially mentioned by Rishanger of St Albans for the year 1294. Trokelowe, another St Albans chronicler, writing of the famine-sickness of 1315–16, uses the singular phrase "morbus enim dysentericus ex corruptis cibis fere omnes maculavit" and says it was followed by "acuta febris vel pestis gutturuosa." Dysentery from corrupt food is again specially named for the year 1391. The "wame-ill" was the prevalent type of sickness in the great Scots famine of 1439, a year of famine in England and France. When we next hear of it in English history it is among the troops of the marquis of Dorset in Gascony and Biscay in 1512, some 1800 of them having died of "the flix." Then comes the "great lask throughout the realm" in 1540, associated with "strange fevers." The sickly years 1557–58 and 1580–82 had probably some dysentery, or lientery, either as primary maladies or as complications of the fevers : Cogan's generalities imply as much for 1580–82, and we know that the corresponding sickly period a century after (1657–59) was so characterised in the description by Willis. The fatal infection in the fleet after the defeat of the Spanish Armada, in August, 1588, was probably dysentery and ship-fever. Many other instances of the kind remain to be given in the chapter on the sicknesses of voyages and colonial settlements.

Dysentery begins to be heard of more frequently in the Stuart period, as a malady of London. It is a prominent item, along with summer diarrhoea, in the London bills of mortality from the year 1658, under the name "griping of the guts," and is occasionally mentioned in letters from London about the same years. The dysentery of London in 1669 was the subject of Sydenham's observations, who says that it had been rarely seen in the preceding ten years[1]. On the other hand he speaks of "the endemic dysentery of Ireland," although he is not sure as to its type or species[2]. Statements as to the Irish "country disease," are as old as Giraldus Cambrensis[3]; but as the whole question of dysentery is intimately bound up with that of typhus-fever, I shall reserve consideration of its prevalence in Ireland on the great scale, as well as of the annual mortality from it in the London bills of the 17th century, until that section of the work in which fevers and the maladies akin to them come into the first rank as if in lieu of the plague.

---

[1] *Opera*, ed. Greenhill, p. 160.   [2] *Ibid.* p. 169.

[3] Giraldus Cambrensis, Rolls series, No. 21, vol. v. *Topogr. Hiberniae*, p. 67 :—
"Advenarum, tamen, una hic fere est passio et unica vexatio. Ob humida namque nutrimenta, immoderatum ventris fluxum vix in primis ullus evadit." Flux among the English troops in Ireland in 1172 is mentioned by Radulphus de Diceto, *Imag. Histor.* I. 348.

NOTE. A sweating character in the "hot agues" or fevers of the Elizabethan period, in those of 1580–82 as well as in those of 1557–58, is asserted in several passages in the text. It is noteworthy that in *Measure for Measure*, one of Shakespeare's early comedies, the bawd says : "Thus, what with the war, what with the sweat, what with the gallows, and what with poverty, I am custom-shrunk" (Act I. Scene 2).

CHAPTER VIII.

THE FRENCH POX.

ONE great epidemic disease of the first Tudor reigns, which brought consternation and distress to multitudes, makes hardly any appearance in the English records of the time, and no appearance at all in the writings of the English profession. Long after, in 1576, William Clowes, surgeon to St Bartholomew's Hospital, first broke the professional silence about *lues venerea* in England, and in his larger work of 1579 he gave a number of startling facts and figures of its then prevalence in London. But the great epidemic outburst of that disease in Europe began in the last years of the 15th century; its ravages on the epidemic scale are supposed to have lasted for twenty or thirty years from 1494; and its subsequent prevalence is assumed, not without reason, to have been of a milder type and within narrower limits. We hear of it, in England, from the political side, at the time when popular arguments were wanted against the Romish mass-priests and against the monasteries and the orders of friars. In the practical reasoning of Englishmen the scandalous lives of priests, monks and friars made the strongest argument for the policy which the king had adopted towards Rome; and it so happened in those very years that a scandalous life was betrayed, and made odious in more than sentiment, by bearing an outward and visible sign. The epidemic of *morbus Gallicus* arose at an unfortunate time for the pretensions of Rome, or, perhaps, it was itself part of the march of events. In Simon Fish's *Supplication of Beggars,*

which was compiled in 1524 and was read to Henry VIII. shortly
after, the weightiest plea is the charge of scandalous conduct
resting upon the priests. In the inquisitions which preceded
the suppression of the monasteries, the same plea is, justly or
unjustly, brought to the front in the case of one abbey after
another. So close did the association of a scandalous vice
and its attendant disease become with the priesthood that
James I., writing long after concerning the sentiments of his
mother, Mary the queen of Scots, represents her as forbidding
the archbishop "to use the spittle" in his own baptism, for the
reason that she would not have "a pokie priest to spet in her
child's mouth[1]." These, says king James, were "her owne very
words ;" at all events, "a pocky priest" may be accepted as a
phrase of the time. The fact that the epidemic of syphilis in
England was used to discredit Romish priests is one of the few
indications that we have of its existence in this country. Wide
and deep as the commotion must have been which it caused, it
found hardly any more permanent expression than the private
talk of the men of those days. It was otherwise on the Continent. There, indeed, a copious literature sprang up, of which
some thirty works remain, from the essay of Conrad Schellig of
Heidelberg, printed without date or place, but ascribed to the
year 1494 or 1495, down to the elaborate survey of the disease
by Nicolas Massa of Venice in 1532. The single work extant
in England from that, the earliest and greatest, period of the
disease, is a poor piece of manuscript in the Sloane collection,
translated from some foreign author, and entitled, "The tretese
of the pokkis: and the cure by the nobull counsell of parris[2]."
One of its cases is that of a man, aged forty, with two broad
and deep, corroding and painful sores on his leg ; another is of
a bishop of Toledo, who had "pustules" and nocturnal pains
"as if the bones would part from the flesh." The vague
meaning of the term pox is shown in one phrase, "paynes, viz.
aches and pokkis."

[1] *Works of James I.*, p. 301.
[2] *Sloane MS.* (Brit. Mus.) No. 389, folios 147–153. It bears no date, but is
marked in the catalogue "xv and xvi cent.," as if belonging either to the end of the
fifteenth century or the beginning of the sixteenth.

It was nothing unusual abroad to give cases, and to authenticate them with the names of the sufferers.   Thus Peter Pinctor, physician to the pope Alexander Borgia, in a notorious but exceedingly scarce work published in 1500, enters fully into the truly piteous case of the cardinal bishop of Segovia, major-domo of the Vatican, "qui hunc morbum patiebatur cum terribilibus et fortissimis doloribus, qui die ac nocte, praecipue in lecto, quiescere nec dormire poterat," as well as into the case of Peter Borgia, the pope's nephew, "in quo virulentia materiae pustularum capitis corrosionem in pellicaneo [pericranio] et in craneo capitis sui manifeste fecit[1]."

Contrasted with the copious writing and recording of cases abroad, the English silence is remarkable.   The origin of our first printed book on the subject is characteristic.   A literary hack of the time, one Paynel, a canon of Merton Abbey, had translated, among other things, the *Regimen Salernitanum*, a popular guide to health several hundred years old.   Going one day into the city to see the printer about a new edition, he was asked by the latter to translate the essay on the cure of the French pox by means of guaiacum (or the West-Indian wood) "written by that great clerke of Almayne, Ulrich Hütten, knyght."   For, said the printer, "almost into every part of this realme this most foul and peynfull disease is crept, and many soore infected therewith."   Ulrich von Hütten's personal experience of the guaiacum cure was accordingly translated from the Latin, in 1533, and proved a good venture for the printer, several editions having been called for[2].   The translation has no notes, and throws no light on English experience.   It is not until 1579, when Clowes published his essay on the morbus

---

[1] Hensler, who reproduced in 1783 (*Geschichte der Lustseuche*, App. p. 53) these and other particulars from one of the two remaining copies of Pinctor's work (in the possession of Professor Cotunni of Naples), collated with the other copy in the Garelli library at Vienna, finds in the concluding dedication of the book to Alexander Borgia a sinister meaning, as if the supreme pontiff had been himself a victim of the *grande maladie à la mode;* it is easier, he says, to extricate the sense than the syntax of the passage.

[2] There was another edition in 1539, and several more following.   Paynel also added a short section, "A Remedy for the Frenche pockes," to his book entitled, *A Moche Profitable Treatise against the Pestilence.*   Translated into English by Thomas Paynel, chanon of Martin [Merton] Abbey, London, 1534.

Gallicus, that we obtain any light from the faculty upon the prevalence of the malady in England. Meanwhile it remains for us to collect what scraps of evidence may exist, in one place or another, of this country's share in the original epidemic invasion during the last years of the 15th century.

Earliest Notices of the French Pox in Scotland and England.

The first authentic news of it comes from the Council Register of the borough of Aberdeen under the date 21st April, 1497[1] :—

"The said day, it was statut and ordanit be the alderman and consale for the eschevin of the infirmitey cumm out of Franche and strang partis, that all licht weman be chargit and ordaint to decist fra thar vicis and syne of venerie, and all thair buthis and houssis skalit, and thai to pas and wirk for thar sustentacioun, under the payne of ane key of het yrne one thar chekis, and banysene of the towne."

The next news of it is also from Scotland, from the minutes of the town council of Edinburgh, wherein is entered a proclamation of James IV., dated 22 September, 1497[2] :—

"It is our Soverane Lords Will and the Command of the Lordis of his Counsale send to the Provest and Baillies within this bur[t] that this Proclamation followand be put till execution for the eschewing of the greit appearand danger of the Infection of his Leiges fra this contagious sickness callit the *Grandgor* and the greit uther Skayth that may occur to his Leiges and Inhabitans within this bur[t]; that is to say, we charge straitly and commands be the Authority above writtin, that all manner of personis being within the freedom of this bur[t] quilks are infectit, or hes been infectit, uncurit, with this said contagious plage callit the *Grandgor*, devoyd, red and pass fur[t] of this Town, and compeir upon the sandis of Leith at ten hours before none, and their sall thai have and fynd Botis reddie in the havin ordanit to them be the Officeris of this bur[t], reddely furneist with victuals, to

---

[1] *Extracts from the Council Register of the Burgh of Aberdeen*, 1398–1570. Edited for the Spalding Club [by Dr John Stuart], vol. I. 1844, p. 425.

[2] *Phil. Trans.*, vol. 42 (1743), p. 420: "Part of a Letter from Mr Macky, professor of History, to Mr Mac Laurin, professor of Mathematics in the University of Edinburgh, and by him communicated to the President of the Royal Society; being an Extract from the Books of the Town Council of Edinburgh, relating to a Disease there, supposed to be Venereal, in the year 1497."

C. 27

have thame to the *Inche* [the island of Inch Keith in the Firth of Forth], and thair to remane quhill God proviyd for thair Health : And that all uther personis the quilks taks upon thame to hale the said contagious infirmitie and taks the cure thairof, that they devoyd and pass with thame, sua that nane of thair personis quhilks taks sic cure upon thame use the samyn cure within this bur' in pns nor peirt any manner of way. And wha sa be is foundin infectit and not passand to the *Inche*, as said is, be *Mononday* at the Sone ganging to, and in lykways the said personis that takis the sd Cure of sanitie upon thame gif they will use the samyn, thai and ilk ane of thame salle be brynt on the cheik with the marking Irne that thai may be kennit in tym to cum, and thairafter gif any of tham remains, that thai sall be banist but favors[1]."

Sir James Simpson, with his indefatigable research over antiquarian points[2], has brought together evidence of payments from the king's purse to persons infected with the " Grantgore" at Dalry, Ayrshire, in September, 1497, at Linlithgow on 2nd October, 1497, at Stirling on the 21st February, 1498 ("at the tounne end of Strivelin to the seke folk in the grantgore"), at Glasgow (also "at the tounn end") on 22nd February, 1498, and again at Linlithgow, 11th April, 1498. He quotes also from a poem of William Dunbar, written soon after 1500, on the conduct of the Queen's men on Fastern's e'en, the terms "pockis" and "Spanyie pockis." From Sir David Lyndsay's poems, of much later date, and from other references, he makes out that "grandgore" or "glengore" was the usual name in Scotland down to the 17th century. Grandgore means *à la grande gorre,* which is the same as *à la grande mode.* This name was given for a time in France to the great disease of the day, but it was soon superseded by *vérole.* Scotland is the only country where "grandgore" became established as the common name of the pox.

Before leaving the Scots evidence, two other ordinances may

---

[1] Simpson (*l. c.*) quotes the Proclamation from the original minute-book, almost in the above spelling; it is in Vol. I. of the *Town Council Records,* fol. 33–34, and is entitled in the rubric " Ane Grangore Act."

[2] "On Syphilis in Scotland in the Fifteenth Century," *Trans. Epidem. Soc.* N. S. I. (1862), p. 149. Two of the entries are published in the *Criminal Trials of Scotland,* I. 117 ; the others were collected for Simpson by Mr Joseph Robertson from the High-Treasurer's Accounts in the Register House, Edinburgh. These accounts have since been published in the Rolls series (vol. I. 356, 361, 378 (*his*), 386).

be quoted from the town council records of Aberdeen. In a long list of regulations under date the 8th October, 1507, there occur these two[1] :—

> " Item, that diligent inquisitioun be takin of all infect personis with this strange seiknes of Nappillis, for the sauetie of the town ; and the personis beand infectit therwith be chargit to keip thame in ther howssis and uther places, fra the haile folkis."
>
> " Item, that nayne infectit folkis with the seiknes of Napillis be haldin at the common fleschouss, or with the fleschouris, baxteris, brousteris, ladinaris, for sauete of the toun, and the personis infectit sall keip thame quyat in thar housis, zhardis, or uther comat placis, quhill thai be haill for the infectioun of the nichtbouris."

" Sickness of Naples" is a reference to the well-known diffusion of the disease all over Europe by the mercenaries of Charles VIII. of France, dispersing after the Italian war and the occupation of Naples.

For England the first known mention of the pox is several years later than the Scots references, although that proves nothing as to its actual beginning in epidemic form. In the book of the Privy Purse Expenses of Elizabeth of York, queen of Henry VII., there is an entry under the date of March 15, 1503, of a sum of forty shillings paid on behalf of John Pertriche " oon of the sonnes of mad Beale ;" which sum appears to have been what the youth cost her majesty for board, clothes, education, and incidental expenses, during the year past. The various items making up the sum of forty shillings are: his diets " for a year ending Christmas last past," a cloth gown, a fustian coat, shirts, shoes and hose, " item, for his learning, 20*d.* item for a prymer and saulter 20*d.* And payed to a surgeon which heled him of the Frenche pox 20*s.* S$\overline{m}^{a}$ 40*s.*" It will be observed that the surgeon's bill was as much as all his other expenses for the year together[2].

The London chronicler of the time is alderman Robert Fabyan ; but although Fabyan, writing in the first years of the 16th century, uses the word " pockys " to designate an illness of

---

[1] *Op. cit.* I. 437.

[2] *Privy Purse Expenses of Elizabeth of York.* Edited by Nicolas, London, 1830, p. 104.

Edward IV. during a military excursion to the Scots Marches in
1463, or long before the epidemic invasion from the south of
Europe, he says nothing of that great event itself.   There is a
record, however, of one significant measure taken in the year
1506, the suppression of the stews on the Bankside in Southwark.   These resorts were of ancient date, and for long paid
toll to the bishop of Winchester.   In 1506 there were eighteen
of them in a row along the Surrey side of the river, a little above
London Bridge ; they were wooden erections, each with a stair
down to the water, and each with its river front painted with a
sign like a tavern, such as the Boar's Head, the Cross Keys, the
Gun, the Castle, the Crane, the Cardinal's Hat, the Bell, the
Swan, etc.   These houses, says Stow, were inhibited in the year
1506, and the doors closed up ; but it was not long ere they were
set open again, the number being at the same time restricted to
twelve[1].   They had been suppressed once before, at the earnest
demand of the citizens, in the reign of Henry IV., and it appears
from a sermon of Latimer's that they were again suppressed
about the year 1546.   Thus Shakespeare had several pre-
cedents in London for the situation which he creates in a foreign
city, in *Measure for Measure*.

   The next reference that I find to it is an oblique one, by
Bernard André in his *Annals of Henry VII*.   On the occasion
of mentioning the sweating sickness of 1508, he says the latter
disease occurred first in England about four-and-twenty years
before, and that it was "followed by a far more detestable
malady, to be abhorred as much as leprosy, a wasting pox which
still vexes many eminent men" (multos adhuc vexat egregios
alioquin viros tabifica lues[2]").   Bernard André's association of
the pox with the sweating sickness, as of one new disease following another, is in the same manner as the reference to it by
Erasmus.   In a letter from Basle, in August, 1525, to Schiedlowitz,
chancellor of Poland, he discourses upon the sickliness of seasons

---

   [1] Stow's *Survey of London*, "Bridge Ward Without." He ascribes these informations to "Robert Fabian," both in the text and in the margin.   The statement is
certainly not made in Fabyan's *Chronicle of England* under the year 1506, or other
year of the decade, nor is it indexed as occurring in some earlier connexion.
   [2] Bernard André's Works.   Rolls series, No. 10.

and the mutations of diseases[1] : Until thirty years ago England was unacquainted with the sweat, nor did that malady go beyond the bounds of the island. In their own experience they had seen mutations :—"nunc pestilentiae, nunc anginae, nunc tusses; sed morbum morbus, velut ansam ansa trahit; nec facilé cedunt ubi semel incubuere." He then proceeds :

"But if one were to seek among the diseases of the body for that which ought to be awarded the first place, it seems to my judgment that it is due to that evil, of uncertain origin, which has now been for so many years raging with impunity in all countries of the world, but has not yet found a definite name. Most persons call it the French pox (*Poscas Galleas*), some the Spanish. What sickness has ever traversed every part of Europe, Africa and Asia with equal speed? What clings more tenaciously, what repels more vigorously the art and care of physicians? What passes more easily by contagion to another? What brings more cruel tortures? Vitiligo and lichens are deformities of the skin, but they are curable. This lues, however, is a foul, cruel, contagious disease, dangerous to life, apt to remain in the system and to break out anew not otherwise than the gout."

Whether it was from some mistaken theory of contagiousness or for other reasons, a fellow of Merton was ordered to leave in 1511 because he had the French pox[2]. In the English history nothing appears above the surface until the beginning of the movement against the papal supremacy and in favour of Reformation. That was a time of public accusations of all kinds, and among the rest of opprobrious references to the pox. In Simon Fish's *Supplication of Beggars*[3], which was written in 1524, certain priests are thus hyperbolically spoken of:

"These be they that have made an hundred thousande ydel hores in your realme, which wold have gotten theyr lyvinge honestly in the swete of their faces had not there superfluous riches illected them to uncleane lust and ydelnesse. These be they that corrupte the hole generation of mankynd in your realme, that catch the pockes of one woman and beare it to another, ye some one of them will boste amonge his felowes that he hath medled with an hundreth wymen."

---

[1] *Erasmi Epistolae,* folio. London, 1642, p. 1789 e.

[2] Anthony Wood, *Hist. Univ. Oxford,* ed. Gutch, I. 514. Freind (*Hist. of Physic,* Pt. II. p. 345) says that the French pox is mentioned in the will of Colet, dean of St Paul's, 1518.

[3] *The Supplication of Beggers* compyled by Symon Fyshe. Anno MCCCCCXXIIII. Lond. 1546.

In the year 1529, there is a more painful and most undignified charge. In the Articles of Arraignment of Wolsey in the House of Peers, the sixth charge is :

"The same Lord Cardinall, knowing himself to have the foul and contagious disease of the great pox, broken out upon him in divers places of his body, came daily to your Grace [the King], rowning in your ear, and blowing upon your most noble Grace with his perilous and infective breath, to the marvellous danger of your Highness, if God of his infinite goodness had not better provided for your Highness. And when he was once healed of them, he made your Grace believe that his disease was an impostume in his head, and of none other thing[1]."

Among the glimpses of contemporary manners in Bullein's *Dialogue of the Fever Pestilence* (1564), there is one referring to the pox; Roger, the groom, soliloquizes thus: "her first husband was prentice with James Elles, and of him learned to play at the short-knife and the horn thimble. But these dog-tricks will bring one to the poxe, the gallows, or to the devil[2]." Bullein, in his more systematic handbook to health, promises to treat of the pox fully, but omits to do so. In one place he refers to the wounds of a young man who fell into a deep coal-pit at Newcastle as having been healed "by an auncient practisour called Mighel, a Frencheman, whiche also is cunnynge to helpe his owne countrey disease that now is to commonly knowen here in England, the more to be lamented : But yet dayly increased, whereof I entinde to speake in the place of the Poxe." But the only other reference is (in the section on the "Use of Sicke Men and Medicine,") to certain drugs "which have vertue to cleanse scabbes, iche, pox. I saie the pox, as by experience we se there is no better remedy than sweatyng and the drinkyng of guaiacum," etc[3].

A good instance of the oblique mode of reference to the malady occurs in another dialogue by a surgeon, Thomas Gale[4].

---

[1] *Parliamentary History*, I. 494.

[2] Bullein's *Dialogue of the Fever Pestilence*, 1564. Early English Text Society, Extra series, 1888, p. 122.

[3] Bullein's *Bulwarke of Defence against all Sicknes, Sornes, and Woundes*, etc., 1562, foll. 2, 68.

[4] *Certain Works of Chirurgerie newly compiled and published by T. Gale.* London, 1563.

The pupil who is being instructed tables the subject of "the morbus," which he farther speaks of as "a great scabbe;" whereupon Gale pointedly takes him to task for the affectation of "the morbus;" any disease, he says, is the morbus; what you mean is the morbus Gallicus.

About the same date, 1563, a casual reference is made to the wide prevalence of the pox by John Jones in his *Dyall of Agues*. In illustration of the fact that various countries originate different forms of pestilence, as the Egyptians the leprosy, the Attics the joint-ache, the Arabians swellings of the throat and flanks, and the English the sweating sickness, he instances farther, "the Neapolitans, or rather the besiegers of Naples, with the pockes, spread hence to far abroad through all the parts of Europe, no kingdom that I have been in free—the more pity[1]."

English Writings on the Pox in the 16th Century.

The first original English writer on the pox was William Clowes. In his treatise[2] of 1579, dedicated to the Society of the Barbers and Chirurgions, he says that he had been bold "three years since to offer unto you a very small and imperfect treatise of mine touching the cure of the disease called in Latine *Morbus Gallicus,* the which, forasmuch as it was at that time rather wrested from me by the importunitye of some of my frendes, upon certain occasions then moving, than willingly of my selfe published, it passed out of my handes so sodeinly and with so small overlooking or correction," that he now in 1579 reissues it in a revised and corrected form.

"The Morbus Gallicus or Morbus Neapolitanus, but more properly Lues Venera, that is the pestilent infection of filthy lust, and termed for the most part in English the French Pocks, a sicknes very lothsome, odious, trouble-some and daungerous, which spreadeth itself throughout all England and overfloweth as I thinke the whole world." He then characterises the vice "that is the original cause of this infection, that breedeth it, that nurseth it,

---

[1] *Dyall of Agues*, cap. VIII. "Of the Pestilential fever, or plage, or boche."

[2] William Clowes, *A short and profitable Treatise touching the cure of the disease called (Morbus Gallicus) by unctions*, London, 1579.

that disperseth it." In the cure of the malady he has had some reasonable experience, and no small practice for many years. According to the following passage, St Bartholomew's Hospital, to which Clowes was surgeon, was three parts occupied by patients suffering from this malady:—

"It is wonderfull to consider how huge multitudes there be of such as be infected with it, and that dayly increase, to the great daunger of the common wealth, and the stayne of the whole nation: the cause whereof I see none so great as the licentious and beastly disorder of a great number of rogues and vagabondes: The filthye lyfe of many lewd and idell persons, both men and women, about the citye of London, and the great number of lewd alehouses, which are the very nests and harbourers of such filthy creatures; By meanes of which disordered persons some other of better disposition are many tymes infected, and many more lyke to be, except there be some speedy remedy provided for the same. I may speake boldely, because I speake truely: and yet I speake it with very griefe of hart. In the Hospitall of Saint Bartholomew in London, there hath bene cured of this disease by me, and three (3) others, within this fyve yeares, to the number of one thousand and more. I speake nothing of Saint Thomas Hospital and other howses about this Citye, wherein an infinite multitude are dayly in cure....For it hapneth in the house of Saint Bartholomew very seldome but that among every twentye diseased persons that are taken in, fiftene of them have the pocks." Like the earlier writers on the Continent he recognizes that the disease is communicated in more ways than one; he speaks of "good poor people that be infected by unwary eating or drinking or keeping company with those lewd beasts, and which either for shame will not bewray it, or for lack of good chirurgions know not how to remedy it, or for lack of ability are not able otherwise to provide for the cure of it."

In so far as Clowes follows his own experience, he is under no illusion as to the nature and circumstances of the French pox. But he goes on to append a pathology of the disease, which is taken from foreign writers and reflects the bewilderment of the faculty over the constitutional effects of the malady. As Erasmus said, in the letter quoted, it went all through the body, "not otherwise than the gout." When it was first observed, it appeared to be constitutional from the outset. More particularly it covered the skin with "pustules" or "whelks" as if it had been a primary eruption like variola, to which it was compared; hence the names "great pox" and "small pox." It was not until long after that our present pathology of primary, secondary and tertiary effects was worked out; in the earliest writings the constitutional effects were referred to an "inward cause," as Clowes says, to some idiopathic corruption of the humours having the liver for their place of elaboration, or *minera morbi.* Thus the learned explanation of the malady, which Clowes adopts from foreign writers more skilled than himself in such disquisitions, has no organic unity with his own common-sense observations. In his *Proved Practice* he defers still farther to the academical view, as given in the treatise of John Almenar, a Spanish physician[1].

Although Clowes, in 1579, testifies to the very wide prevalence of the disease, to so great an extent, indeed, that it occupied the hospitals more than all other diseases put together, yet there is reason to think that it had by that time lost the terrible severity of its original epidemic type. The usual statement is that the disease abated both in extent and in intensity within twenty or thirty years of the Italian outbreak among the soldiery in 1494–96. A contemporary and ally of Clowes, John Read, of Gloucester, published in 1588 a volume of translations, from the Latin manuscript of the English surgeon of the 14th century, John Ardern, on the cure of fistulas, and from the treatise on wounds, etc. by the Spanish surgeon Arcaeus (Antwerp, 1574)[2]. In the latter he finds the following passage, which seems to describe the *morbus Gallicus* on its first appearance :—

"The French disease did bring with it a kind of universal skabbe, oftentimes with ring wormes, with the foulness of all the body called vitiligo and alopecia, running sores in the head called acores, and werts of both sortes, and many times with flegmatic or melancholic swellings or ulcers corrosive, filthie and cancrouse, and also running over the body, together with putrifying of the bone, and many times also accompanied with all kind of grief, with fevers, consumptions, and with many other differences of diseases."

Read's own remarks draw an explicit contrast between the disease on its first appearance and in his own later experience. Everyone knows now, he says, how to treat the French pox,

---

[1] 'A Prooved Practice for all young Chirurgeons, concerning burning with gunpowder, and woundes made with Gunshot, Sword, Halbard, Pike, Launce or such other. Hereto is adjoyned a Treatise of the French or Spanish Pocks, written by John Almenar, a Spanish Phisician. Also a commodious collection of Aphorismes, both English and Latine, taken out of an old written coppy. Published for the benefit of his country by William Clowes, Maister in Chirurgery.' New ed., 1591.

[2] *A most excellent and compendious Method,* etc. London, 1588.

" the disease daylie dying and wearing away by the exquisite cure thereof"—which may be taken to mean, at least, a notable mitigation of the constitutional effects[1]. The treatment, however, must have been much less effective then than now. Clowes speaks of a class who " either for shame will not bewray it, or for lack of good chirurgions know not how to remedy it, or for lack of ability are not able otherwise to provide for the cure of it." The expense of a cure would have been considerable, to judge by the case given above from an account-book of the year 1503. Unable to employ "good chirurgions," the poorer class would resort to quacks, of whose practice, in that and other diseases, we have some glimpses both from Clowes in London and from Read in Gloucester and Bristol. Of one irregular practitioner Clowes says, " He did compound for fifteen pound to rid him within three fits of his ague, and to make him as whole as a fish of all diseases." There was still a lower order of empirics, whom Clowes disdained to contend with :

"Yet I do not mean to speak of the old woman at Newington, beyond St George's Fields, unto whom the people do resort as unto an oracle; neither will I speak of the woman on the Bankside, who is as cunning as the horse at the Cross Keys; nor yet of the cunning woman in Seacole Lane, who hath more skill in her cole-basket than judgment in urine, or knowledge in physic or surgery"—nor of many others who are compared to "moths in clothes," to "canker," and to "rust in iron."

Read gives an account of a travelling mountebank, which is too graphic to be omitted :

"In this year, 1587, there came a Fleming into the city of Glocester named Woolfgange Frolicke, and there hanging forth his pictures, his flags, his instruments, and his letters of mart with long lybells, great tossells, broad scales closed in boxes, with such counterfeit shows and knacks of knavery, cozening the people of their money, without either learning or knowledge. And yet for money got him a licence to practise at Bristow. But when he came to Gloceter, and being called before some being in authority by myself and others, he was not able to answer to any one point

---

[1] Read uses, among other terms, one that has played a great part in the modern pathology of syphilis. Among the points to be noticed are,—"if recent or old, if the ulcers or whelks be many, whether pustulous matter or *gummie* substance appear."

in chirurgerie; which being perceived, and the man known, the matter was excused by way of charity, to be good to straungers."

One of the most systematic and detailed surgical treatises of the time, John Banister's book on the "general and particular curation of ulcers" (1575), is significant for the indirect way in which it refers to the lues venerea.

Thus at folio 25, "the malignant ulcer called cacoethes" is described without anything said of a venereal origin, but the specific guaiacum is given among the remedies. The same is the case on the 31st and 32nd leaves, which treat of "filthie and putrefied ulcers," guaiacum being again prescribed. At folio 51, on ulcers of the mouth, it is said, "If it proceed a morbo venereo, then first begin with due purgation, and prescribe the party a thin diet with the decoction of guaiacum, and use ointments requisite for that disease, strengthening the inner parts. Use twice a day a sublimated water, as is afore written, to touch the ulcer with lint rolled therein :

> Rec. Aqua Rosar.⎱ an. two
>   & Plantag.⎰ ounces,
>   Sublimati i dragme.

Boil them in a glass bottel till the sublimate be dissolved."

On fol. 57, he describes "ulcers of the privie parts," among which are corroding ulcers, but without reference to the lues. It is in the section headed, "To prepare the humours" (fol. 61) that the most explicit reference occurs: "When the ulcers proceed through the French pockes, a thinne diet must be used, with the decoction of guaiacum or use universall unctions ex Hydrargyro[1]."

In 1596 there appeared Peter Lowe's essay on *The Spanish Sickness*[2], which is purely a product of experience abroad, his own or of others, and is mainly doctrinal or theoretical. The other properly English works on the subject are all subsequent to the Restoration, and do not come into the period of this volume, nor, from an epidemiological point of view, into this work at all.

The evidence as to the wide prevalence of the pox in high

---

[1] John Banister, 'A needefull new and necessarie treatise of Chyrurgerie, briefly comprehending the generall and particular curation of ulcers...drawn forth of sundrie worthy writers...Hereunto is annexed certaine experimentes of mine owne invention.' London, 1575.

[2] Peter Lowe, *An easie, certaine and perfect method to cure and prevent the Spanish sicknes*, Lond. 1596. For an account of the book see *The Life and Works of Maister Peter Lowe*. By James Finlayson, M.D. Glasgow, 1889.

and low becomes abundant in the writings and memorials of the reign of James I. The effects of the disease, as they would have been commonly remarked at this period, are summed up in a well-known passage in *Timon of Athens*. It would serve no purpose to collect the numerous references from Puritan sermons, moral and descriptive essays, plays, and letters of the time. An anonymous work of the year 1652 actually couples "the plague and the pox," and shows "how to cure those which are infected with either of them[1]." One more piece of evidence may be given for London in the year 1662, or the beginning of the Restoration period,—a date which brings us down a century and a half from the epidemic invasion with which we are more immediately concerned; but the information for 1662 will serve to show how the existence of the disease was still viewed *sub rosa*, and it may help one to realize what its prevalence and its serious effects on the public health must have been continuously in the generations before, and most of all in the generation which experienced the full force of it as an epidemic[2].

The London bills of mortality, setting forth the several causes of death, were first printed in 1629. The entry of the French pox is in them from the beginning, and the annual total of deaths set down to it is considerable, approaching a hundred in the year. But according to Graunt, who made the bills of mortality the subject of a critical study in 1662[3], they were defective or incorrect in their returns of deaths due to the pox :—

"By the ordinary discourse of the world, it seems a great part of men have, at one time or other, had some species of this disease...whereof many complained so fiercely, etc." He then explains, with reference to the deaths entered as due to it in the bills of mortality: "All mentioned to die of the French pox were returned by the clerks of St Giles' and St Martin's in the

---

[1] *A Treatise concerning the plague and the pox, discovering as well the means how to preserve from the danger of these infectious contagions, or how to cure those which are infected with either of them.* London, 1652.

[2] Burnet (*History of his own Time*, 1. 395–6, Oxford, 1823) retails a good deal of unsavoury gossip concerning the disease in noble and princely personages after the Restoration.

[3] *Natural and Political Observations upon the Bills of Mortality.* By Captain John Graunt, F.R.S. Preface dated from Birchin Lane, January, 1662.

Fields only, in which place I understand that most of the vilest and most miserable houses of uncleanness were; from whence I concluded that only *hated* persons, and such whose very noses were eaten off were reported by the searchers to have died of this too frequent malady"—the rest having been included under the head of consumption.

Origin of the Epidemic of 1494.

The French pox, as it was called in England (also the great pox and simply the pox), or the Spanish pox, as it was called in France, or the sickness of Naples, or the grandgore, is one of the epidemic diseases concerning which it seems fitting to say something of the antecedents, in addition to what has been said of its arrival as an epidemic in this country, and of its prevalence therein. But this will have to be said very briefly, and without entering upon the pathology or ultimate nature of the disease.

The numerous foreign writings upon it during the first years of its spread over Europe are all singularly at a loss to account for its origin. One of the earlier guesses was that it arose out of leprosy, as if a graft or modification of that medieval disease, replacing it among the maladies of the people. The occasion of that hypothesis seems to have been the lax diagnosis of leprosy itself, a laxity which goes as far back as Bernard Gordonio and Gilbert, if not farther back. Many things were called *lepra* which were not elephantiasis Graecorum, and among those things the lues venerea in the Middle Ages was undoubtedly included. At a time when true leprosy was disappearing or had already disappeared from Europe, a new form of disease, which came suddenly into universal notice although by no means then first into existence, seemed to be the successor of leprosy, evoked out of it, and even caught from the leprous by contagion. That is the view of Manardus, in a passage quoted in the sequel,—that syphilis began in certain most particular circumstances at Valencia, in Spain, the source of all the subsequent contamination of Europe having been a certain soldier of fortune who was *elephantiosus* or leprous. In the infancy of a science it is natural to assign to some such single and definite source a new phenomenon which was really called forth by a concurrence of causes[1].

Another guess of the same kind was the famous theory, which found a truly learned defender in Astruc last century and has had supporters more recently, that the lues venerea came from the New World with the returning ships of Columbus. There never was any considerable body of facts, consistent as regards times and places, in support of that theory; and, on antecedent grounds, the objection to it was that it is as difficult, to say the least, to conceive of the origin of such a disease among the savages of Hispaniola as among the natives of Europe. "Here or nowhere is America" is the proper retort to all such visionary theories put upon the distant and the unknown. The American theory is now hopelessly dead; the more that the New World became known, the less did syphilis appear to be indigenous to it: indeed the disease followed the track of Europeans, and those parts of the American continent, north and south of the Isthmus, which were longest in being reached by the civilisation of the Old World, were also longest in being reached by the lues venerea[2].

The name "sickness of Naples," which occurs in the Aberdeen records as early as 1507, indicates the common opinion of the laity as to the origin and means of diffusion of the strange malady. In the passage above quoted from Jones's *Dyall of Agues*, it will be seen that he refers it to "the besiegers of Naples." The besiegers of Naples were the mercenaries of Charles VIII. occupying it in the beginning of the year 1495, although there was no real siege. The new disease was at the time, rightly or wrongly, traced to them while they occupied Italy, and its diffusion over Europe was justly traced to their dispersion to their several countries at the end of the campaign. There is medical testimony that the malady appeared in 1495 among the Venetian and Milanese troops which were banded against Charles VIII. at the siege of Novara. Marcellus

---

[1] The origin of syphilis from leprosy has been maintained in a modern work by Friedr. Alex. Simon, *Kritische Geschichte des Ursprungs, der Pathologie und Behandlung der Syphilis, Tochter und widerüm Mutter des Aussatzes.* Hamburg, 1857-8.

[2] Hirsch, *Geographical and Historical Pathology* (Translated), ii. 67, 68, 81.

Cumanus, of Venice, who was surgeon to the forces, thus speaks of the event, in certain *Observationes de Lue Venerea* which he wrote on the margin of Argelata's work on Surgery[1]:

"In Italy, in the year 1495, owing to celestial influences, I have myself seen, and do testify that, while I was in the camp at Novara with the troops of the Lords of Venice and of the Lords of Milan, many knights and foot-soldiers suffered from an ebullition of the humours, producing many pustules in the face and through the whole body; which pustules commonly began under the prepuce or without the prepuce, like a grain of millet-seed, or upon the glans, attended by considerable itching. Sometimes a single pustule began like a small vesicle without pain, but with itching. Being broken by rubbing, they ulcerated like a corrosive *formica*, and a few days after, troubles began from pains in the arms, legs and feet, with great pustules. All the skilled physicians had difficulty in curing them....Without medicines, the pustules upon the body lasted a year or more, like a leprous variola." He then gives many other details of symptoms and treatment.

For the year after, 1496, two German writers, who were not surgeons but occupied with affairs of state, Sebastian Brant (author of the *Ship of Fools*) and Joseph Grünbeck, have described the disease, apparently in connexion with the troops serving in Italy under Maximilian I. against the invading army of Charles VIII. Thus, there is sufficient evidence that the malady in its first two or three years of epidemic prevalence, was associated with a state of war on Italian soil, in the persons of French troops (and mercenaries of all nations), of Venetian and Milanese troops, and of the German troops of the Emperor.

But the German writers are clear that the disease did not originate on Italian soil, at the siege of Naples or elsewhere. Thus Brant in his poem of 1496 assigns to it an origin in France, and a dispersion within a year or two over all Europe[2]:

"Pestiferum in Lygures transvexit Francia morbum,
Quem *mala de Franzos* Romula lingua vocat.
Hic Latium atque Italos invasit, ab Alpibus extra
Serpens, Germanos Istricolasque premit;
Grassatur mediis jam Thracibus atque Bohemis
Et morbi genus id Sarmata quisque timet.
Nec satis extremo tutantur in orbe Britanni
Quos refluum cingit succiduumque fretum.
Quin etiam fama est, Aphros penetrasse Getasque
Vigue sua utrumque depopulare polum."

[1] In Hensler, p. 14, and Appendix, p. 11.   [2] *Ibid.*, App. p. 15.

Grünbeck, who wrote briefly on the disease in 1496, returned
to the subject at much greater length in 1503, when he was
secretary to the Emperor Maximilian, his later treatise, *De
Mentulagra, alias Morbo Gallico*, being, indeed, among the best
that the epidemic called forth.   Hensler doubts whether Grünbeck was himself in Italy, so as to observe the ravages of the
disease among the troops of the Emperor (including Venetians
and Milanese) at the sieges of Pisa and Leghorn in the summer
of 1496, and among the opposing troops of Charles VIII.   Be
that as it may, the following is from Grünbeck's description[1]:

"O! quid unquam terribilius et abominabilius humanis sensibus occurrit!
Difficile est dictu, creditu fere impossibile, quanta foeditatis, putredinis et
sordium colluvione, quantisque dolorum anxietatibus nonnullorum militum
corpora involuerit.   Aliqui etiam a vertice ad usque genua quodam horrido,
squalido, continuo, foedo et nigro *scabiei* genere, nulla parte faciei, (solis
oculis exemtis), nec colli, cervicis, pectoris vel pubis immuni relicta, percussi, ita sordidi abominabilesque effecti sunt, qui ab omnibus commilitonibus
derelicti, ac etiam in plano et nudo campo sub dio emarescentes, nihil
magis quam *mortem* expetiverunt...At his omnibus nihil vel parum profici-
entibus, et morbo ipso non contento hoc hominum numero, ut eos solos
tantis passionum cruciatibus afficeret, venenum contagiosum in multos
spectantes Italos, Teutones, Helveticos, Vindelicos, Rhaetos, Noricos,
Batavos, Morinos, Anglicos, Hispanos, et alios quos belli occasio in copias
conscripserat, transfudit....Interea temporis, per clandestinam Gallorum
abitionem, exercitus fuerunt dissoluti,"—Grünbeck himself proceeding with
some merchants to Hungary and thence to Poland[2].

[1] In Hensler, Appendix, p. 66.
[2] The rise of the pox in the Italian wars, with its dispersion over all Europe,
comes into "The Smallpox, a Poem" by "Andrew Tripe, M.D.," London, 1748:

"Whip! thro' both camps, halloo! it ran,
Nor uninfected left a man...
Hence soon thro' Italy it flew
Veiled for a while from mortal view,
When suddenly in various modes,
It shone display'd in shankers, nodes,
Swell'd groins, and pricking shins, and headaches
And a long long long string of dread aches...
From thence with every sail unfurl'd
It traversed almost all the world...
Until at length this Stygian fury
Worked its foul way to our blest Drury,
Where still Lord Paramount it reigns,
Pregnant with sharp nocturnal pains," etc.

How came this terrible infection to be among the troops of all nations on Italian soil in the years 1494, 1495 and 1496? Sebastian Brant clearly states that the French brought it with them, and that it spread first over Liguria. Grünbeck says that it was seen *primo super Insubriam,* or the Milanese, on which it rested like a dense cloud, until it was scattered by the winds over the whole of Liguria, and so found its way into the armies in Italy. Beniveni, of Florence, who wrote in 1498, says that it came to Italy from Spain, and from Italy was carried to France. Thus we have a theory of a Spanish origin, of a French origin, and perhaps also of a native Italian origin—all agreeing that Italy during the state of war from 1494 to 1496 was the theatre of its first ravages on the great scale, and the source from which the disease was brought to all the countries of Europe by the returning soldiery.

The solution of the difficulty is to be looked for in the inquiries after still earlier notices of the *lues venerea.* It is beyond the purpose of this book to enter upon that large subject, farther than has already been done with the object of proving the generic use of the medieval term *lepra.* It is now accepted by competent students of medical history that the same disease, with all varieties or modes of primary, secondary or tertiary, existed in antiquity and in the Middle Ages, although secondaries and tertiaries may not have been ascribed to their primary source. But what specially concerns us here is the question whether the malady was anywhere beginning to be more noticeable in the years immediately preceding the great military explosion on Italian soil. On that point there is some evidence from more than one source, that the malady was sufficiently prevalent in the south of France to be a subject of remark previous to the French expedition to Italy, that it had found its way to the ports of Spain (Barcelona and Valencia), and that the troops of Charles VIII., if not also that youthful monarch himself, carried it across the Alps into Liguria, and so gave it that start on Italian soil which the state of war for the next two years raised to the power of a virulent and diffusive epidemic[1].

[1] I do not include among the good evidence the often quoted letter of Peter

C. 28

The best piece of evidence of its prevalence in Languedoc and its spreading thence to the adjoining coast of Spain is found in a letter of the 18th April, 1494 (four months before Charles VIII. entered Italy), written by Nicolas Scyllatius just after arriving at Barcelona[1]. The province of Narbonne, he says, a part of France adjoining Spain, now sent forth another vice. Women felt it most; it infected neighbours by contact; it has lately invaded Spain, hitherto untouched by it. "I was horrified," he continues, "on first landing at Barcelona; for I met with many of the inhabitants who were seized by that contagion. On my inquiring of the physicians (for with these I held converse during nearly all that journey), they assured me that the new *lues* had been derived from truculent France." In keeping with this entirely credible testimony is the statement of Torella, a native of Valencia, who wrote one of the earlier essays on the new disease ("De Pudendagra") in November, 1497. The disease first broke out, he says, in Auvergne in 1493 (incepit, ut aiunt, haec maligna aegritudo anno 1493 in Alervnia), and so came in the way of contagion to Spain and the Islands [to Sardinia, where he was bishop, and to Corsica], and to Italy, creeping in the end over all Europe, and, if one may so speak, over the whole globe[2].

Torella thus confirms the Barcelona traveller so far as regards importations from the south of France to the neighbouring ports, the former writer naming Auvergne as the endemic seat of the malady, whereas the latter gives Narbonne. Another piece of evidence, that the pox was in Valencia, as well as in Barcelona, before the expedition of Charles VIII., is found in a story told by Manardus of Ferrara (1500), a story which is wholly improbable so far as concerns the origin of syphilis, at a stated time and place, out of a case of leprosy,

Martyr to a professor of Greek at Salamanca, under the date of "nonis Aprilis, 1488," in which "morbus Gallicus" is used as well as the Spanish name "las bubas." It seems to me certain that the date should be 1498, or something else than 1488, the correspondence having gone on until 1525. The same kind of misdating occurs among the printed letters of Erasmus.

[1] This letter is printed in his *Opuscula*, Papiae, 1496. Attention was first called to it by Thiene, in his essay confuting the doctrine of the West-Indian origin of syphilis.

[2] In Hensler, App. p. 108.

but is entirely credible so far as regards the grossness of its
circumstances :

"Coepisse hunc morbum per id tempus, dicunt, quo Carolus, Francorum
rex, expeditionem Italicam parabat: coepisse, autem, in Valentia, Hispaniae
Taraconensis insigni civitate, a nobili quodam scorto, cujus noctem elephantiosus quidam, ex equestri ordine miles, quinquaginta aureis emit ; et cum
ad mulieris concubitum frequens juventus accurreret, intra paucos dies supra
quadringentos infectos ; e quorum numero nonnulli, Carolum Italiam pe-
tentem sequuti, praeter alia quae adhuc vigent importata mala et hoc
addiderunt[1]."

The evidence that follows is not so explicit, but it has
strong probability. The progress of Charles VIII. from France
to Italy in the autumn of 1494 has been told by Philip de
Comines in his *Cronique du Roy Charles VIII.*, first printed at
Paris in 1528, nineteen years after the author's death. De
Comines accompanied his master, the French king, as far as
Asti; he was then sent on a mission to Venice, and rejoined the
king at Florence. But De Comines, who was no gossip, omits
one interesting fact near the beginning of the journey to Italy,
which has been preserved for us in a contemporary work (1503)
called *La Cronique Martiniane*, or chronicle of all the popes
down to Alexander Borgia lately deceased[2]. This chronicle
relates as follows concerning Charles VIII.'s journey:—"Il se
arresta premierement aucuns jours a Lyon, doubteux s'il passe-
roit les mons, car il y estoit detenu pour les delices et plaisances
de la cité et pour les folles amours de aucunes gorrieres lyon-
noises. Mais quant l'air devint pestilent, il s'en tyra à Vienne,
cité de Daulphinè." His great army had already passed the
Alps and arrived in the country of Asti: it is said to have
consisted, in round numbers, of 3600 men-at-arms, 6000 bowmen, 8000 pikemen, and 8000 with arquebuses, halberds, two-
handed swords, or other arms, together with a heavy artillery
train of 8000 horses. A large part of this force were Swiss ;
another part were Gascons[3].

[1] Manardus, *Epist. Med.* lib. VII. epist. 2. Basil, 1549, p. 137 (as cited by
Hirsch). The first letter of Manardus "de erroribus Sym. Pistoris de Lypczk circa
morbum Gallicum," was printed in 1500 (Hensler, p. 47).

[2] I quote it from Hensler, *Geschichte der Lustseuche die zu ende des xv Jahr
hunderts in Europa ausbrach.* Altona, 1783, Appendix, p. 109.

[3] Mezeray, *Histoire de France*, II. 777.

Charles VIII. left Vienne on the 23rd of August, and crossed Mont Genèvre on the 2nd September, whence he proceeded direct by Susa and Turin, joining his army at Asti on September 9. At Asti, says De Comines, he had an illness, which caused that minister to delay setting out on his mission to Venice for a few days. The original printed text of De Comines' *Chronique* (Paris, 1528), says that the author remained at Asti a few days longer " because the king was ill of the smallpox (*de la petite verolle*) and in peril of death, for that the fever was mixed therewith ; but it lasted only six or seven days, and I set out upon my way." The next edition has no change but " in great peril of death" (*en grant peril de mort*), instead of merely " in peril." Now, where did this diagnosis of *petite verolle* come from ? Nothing is said of smallpox being prevalent at the time among the troops or along their route. The name *petite verolle* itself did not exist in 1494; it came into existence with *grosse verolle*, having being made necessary by the latter ; and the first that we hear of *grosse verolle* is when the Italian campaign was over and the pox was raging in Paris, the Parlement of Paris, on the 6th of March, 1497, having made an ordinance against a certain contagious malady " nommée *la grosse verole*," which had been in the kingdom and in the city of Paris since two years. Probably Comines deliberately wrote "*petite verolle*" in his manuscript, having composed the latter subsequent to 1498, or at a time when the terms *verolle*, or *grosse verolle*, and *petite verolle*, were passing current and were known in their respective senses. The causes or circumstances of the king's malady at Asti are not enlarged upon by De Comines, farther than that he makes a somewhat disjointed remark, that all the Italian wines of that year were sour and that the season was hot, which would have had as little to do with the one kind of pox as with the other. Nor is anything said of smallpox spreading among those near the king[1].

The whole sequence of events, from the " folles amours " of

[1] The diagnosis in De Comines' text appears to have struck the editors of the chief edition of his work, that of 1747; for they have appended a footnote to the passage, which is a superfluity unless it be meant to express surprise: "Charles VIII. malade de la petite vérole à l'age de vingt-deux ans."

Lyons to the sharp sickness at Asti, has suggested to historians, who have no medical theory to advocate, that it was not really *petite vérole* that the king suffered from, but *grosse vérole.* Martin says that Charles VIII. recommenced at Asti his Lyons follies and that he became violently sick, " of the smallpox, says one, or, perhaps, of a new malady which began to show itself in Europe," meaning syphilis. To show that such infection was already possible, he quotes an ordinance of the provost of Paris April 15, 1488, enjoining "the leprous" to leave the capital. This is very like Edward III.'s order to the London "lepers" a century and a half earlier, in which the reasons given (the frequenting of stews, the pollution of their breath, &c.) point somewhat clearly to the nature of their "leprosy." An order for the banishment of "lepers" from Paris in 1488 must have been occasioned by some unusual risk of contamination, just as the London order of 1346 would have been. It is in that sense that the French historian regards it; the ordinance, he says, "concernait probablement déjà les syphilitiques confondus avec les lépreux[1]."

De Comines, who is the authority for the diagnosis of smallpox, had inserted the word *petite* before *verolle* for reasons best known to himself. I shall show in the next chapter, upon smallpox and measles in England, that the ambiguous teaching of the faculty as to the nature and affinities of the pox proper within the first years of its epidemic appearance gave a ready opportunity of calling the *grosse vérole* by the name of *petite vérole* in circumstances where it was polite, or prudent, or convenient so to do. The only importance of a correct diagnosis of the king's malady is that the case of one would have been the case of many.

The indications all point to a somewhat unusual prevalence of *lues venerea* previous to the autumn of 1494, in the luxurious provinces of southern France as well as in the capital. Beyond doubt, the malady had already spread by contagion to the great Spanish ports nearest the Gulf of Lyons. The expedition of Charles VIII. passed through that region on its route over the Alps. According to Sebastian Brant, it was the French who

---

[1] Martin, *Histoire de France*, VII. 257, 283.

brought the disease into Liguria, and, according to Grünbeck, it issued, *Gallico tractu, ab occidentali sinu*, gathered like a dense cloud *super Insubriam* (the Milanese), and was thence dispersed, as if by the winds, over the whole province of Liguria.

But for the circumstances of the military expedition of 1494, and the state of war in Italy for two years after, it is conceivable that the unusual prevalence in France of a very ancient malady would have had little interest for Europe at large, although the cities on the nearest coast of Spain appear to have already shared the infection. That unusual prevalence in the south of France has in it nothing of mystery; the period was the end of the Middle Ages, distinguished by a revival of learning, of trade and commerce,—a revival of most things except morals. But, assuming that there was such unusual prevalence above the ancient and medieval level, it may still seem unaccountable that a great European epidemic, of a most disastrous and fatal type, should have been engendered therefrom.

There are, however, many parallel cases, on a minor scale from modern times, of a peculiar severity of type, of inveteracy, and of communicability by unusual ways, having been cultivated from commonplace beginnings, among unsophisticated communities about the Baltic and Adriatic, the people being without resident doctors and unfamiliar with such a disease and its risks. These have been collected and analyzed by Hirsch, whose conclusion is that "the mode of origin, and the character of these endemics of syphilis, appear to me to furnish the key to an understanding of the remarkable episode of the disease in the 15th century,—an episode which entirely resembles them as regards its type, and differs from them only as regards extent[1]."

Referring the reader for farther particulars to the work quoted, I shall leave the antecedents of the epidemic of pox in the end of the 15th century to be judged of according to the probabilities thus far stated.

---

[1] *Handbook of Geographical and Historical Pathology.* Translated by C. Creighton, 3 vols. London, 1883-86, II. 92-98.

CHAPTER IX.

SMALLPOX AND MEASLES.

WITH our modern habit of seeking out the matter of fact, of going back to the reality and of reconstructing the theory, it is not easy for us to understand how completely the medieval world of medicine was enslaved to authority and tradition even in matters that were directly under their eyes. It was thought a great thing that Linacre, of Oxford, in the first years of the 16th century, and Caius, of Cambridge, some fifty years later, should have gone back to Galen for their authority, passing over the Arabians who had been the interpreters of classical medicine all through the Middle Ages. Their editions of forgotten medical works of the Graeco-Roman school were a step forward in scholarship, and they opened the way to the first-hand observations of disease which really began some hundred years after with the writings of Willis, Sydenham and Morton. But smallpox and measles were not Galenist themes, they were peculiarly Arabian; and the very moderate share that England took in the medical Revival of Learning made no difference to the paragraphs or chapters on those diseases that were circulating in the medieval compends. While the Arabian or Arabistic writers of Spain, of Salerno, and of Montpellier were the depositaries and interpreters of the Galenic teaching, they were also the first-hand authorities upon some matters of specially Arabian experience, of which smallpox and measles were the chief. Whatever was said of those two epidemic maladies abroad, in the systematic works of Gordonio and Gilbert, and in the later compilation of Gaddesden in England, was not only of Arabian origin, but it was all that was known of them. Rhazes, the original Arabic writer on smallpox and measles about the beginning of the 11th century, supplied both the doctrine and the experience. His observations and reasonings, altered or added to by his later countrymen, passed bodily into the medical text-books of all Europe. The interest in the treatise of Rhazes was so great that it was printed in 1766 by Channing, of Oxford, in Arabic with a Latin translation, and in an English translation from the original by Greenhill, of Oxford, in 1847.

In the literature we took over smallpox from the Arabians; but had we no native experiences of the disease itself, and, if so, when did it first appear in this country? One can hardly attempt an answer to these questions even now without stirring up prejudice and embittered memories. It has been the fate of smallpox, as an epidemological subject, to be invested with bigotry and intolerance. Whoever has maintained that it is not as old as creation has been suspected in his motives; anyone who shows himself inclined to put limits to its historical duration and its former extent in Britain is clearly seeking to belittle the advantages that have been derived during the present century from vaccination.

The wish to establish the antiquity of the smallpox in Europe has been as strong as the wish to overthrow the antiquity of the great pox. While undoubted traces of the latter in early times have been covered over with the generic name of leprosy, the vaguest reference to "pustules" or spots on the skin have been turned by verbalist ingenuity to mean devastating epidemics of smallpox. I am here concerned only with Britain, and must pass over the much-debated reference by Gregory of Tours to epidemics in the 6th century, the period of the Justinian plague. But in England the epidemic which stands nearest in our annals to the great plague of the 6th century, the widespread infection described by Beda as having begun in 664 and as having continued in monasteries and elsewhere for years after, has been claimed by Willan as an epidemic of smallpox[1]. Willan,

---

[1] *Miscellaneous Works of the late Robert Willan, M.D., F.R.S., containing an Inquiry into the Antiquity of the Smallpox, Measles, and Scarlet Fever, etc.* Edited by Ashby Smith, M.D., London, 1821.

with all his erudition, was a dermatologist, and acted on the maxim that there is nothing like leather. His contention in favour of smallpox has been referred to in the first chapter, dealing with the plague described by Beda, and need not farther concern us. It is not in England that we find evidence of smallpox in those remote times but in Arabia.

Smallpox in the Arabic Annals.

For our purpose the evidence on the antiquity of smallpox in China and India may be accepted, and for the rest left out of account. The Arabian influence is nearer to us, and is the only one that practically concerns us. Coming, then, to the history of smallpox in its prevalence nearest to Europe, we find a definite statement of the disease appearing first among the Abyssinian army of Abraha at the siege of Mecca in what was known as the Elephant War of A.D. 569 or 571. The best of the Arabic historians, Tabari[1], writes : "It has been told to us by Ibn Humaid, after Salima, after Ibn Ischâg, to whom Ja'gûb b. Otha b. Mughira b. Achnas related that one had said to him, that in that year the smallpox appeared for the first time in Arabia, and also the bitter herbs,—rue, colocynth [and another]." The tradition is by word of mouth through several, after the Semitic manner, but it need not on that account be set aside as worthless. So far as concerns the bitter herbs, it is said to be against probability ; but as regards the new form of epidemic sickness, there is no such objection to it.

The Arabic legend, as given by Tabari is as follows: "Thereupon came the birds from the sea in flocks, every one with three stones, in the claws two and in the beak one, and threw the stones upon them. Wherever one of these stones struck, there arose an evil wound, and pustules all over. At that time the smallpox first appeared, and the bitter trees. The stones undid them wholly. Thereafter God sent a torrent which carried them away and swept them into the sea. But Abraha and the remnant of his men fled : he himself lost one member after

[1] Th. Nöldeke, *Geschichte der Araber und Perser, nach Tabari.* Leyden, 1879, pp. 218, 219.

another." In a former passage, the calamity of Abraha is thus given : " But Abraha was smitten with a heavy stroke ; as they brought him along in the retreat, his limbs fell off piece by piece, and as often as a piece fell off, matter and blood came forth." To illustrate this account by Tabari, his recent editor, Nöldeke, cites the following from an anti-Mohammedan poem: " Sixty thousand returned not to their homes, nor did their sick continue in life after their return." One of the elephants which dared to enter the sacred region is said to have been also wounded and afflicted by the smallpox.

In this narrative of Abraha's disaster, says Nöldeke, there is a mixture of natural causation and of purely fabulous miracle ; a real and sufficient account of the cause of the Abyssinian leader's discomfiture, namely, an outbreak of smallpox, had been blended with legendary tales. That the disease was smallpox is made probable by the continuity of the Arabic name; under the same name Rhazes, the earliest systematic writer, describes the symptoms, pathology and treatment of what was unquestionably the smallpox afterwards familiar in Western Europe. Why it should have originated on Arabian soil in an invading army from Africa, is a question that would require much knowledge, now beyond our reach, to answer conclusively.

Theory of the nature of Smallpox.

The nature of the disease should, however, be borne in mind always in the front of every speculation as to the origin of its contagious and epidemic properties. It involves no speculative considerations to pronounce smallpox a skin-disease, of the nature of lichen turned pustular. It is a skin-disease first, and a contagious or epidemic malady afterwards; its place among diseases of the skin is indeed fully acknowledged by derma- tologists. Apart from its contagiousness it conforms to the cha- racters of other cutaneous eruptions : its outbreak is preceded by disturbed health, including fever ; when the eruption comes out the fever is so far relieved ; and as in some other eruptions which are not contagious the constitutional disturbance is in proportion to the area of the skin involved. Even the peculiar scars or pits which it leaves behind in skins of a certain texture or in the more vascular regions, such as the face, are not unknown in non-contagious skin-diseases; nor does its other peculiarity, the offensive odour of many pustules, seem unaccountable in a skin-disease native to tropical countries.

Eruptions on the skin are in many cases the outcome of constitutional ill-health; for example, the eczema of gout. Also where the whole body is infected, as in syphilis, there are skin-eruptions, which may be pimples (lichenous) or scales, or rashes, or, as in the first great outburst of syphilis, " pustules" so general over the body that those who were casting about for the nosological affinities of the new malady, saw no better place for it than Avicenna's group of *alhumata*, which included smallpox and measles. That a skin-eruption of the nature of smallpox should have come out as a constitutional manifestation, and that a number of persons should have exhibited it together for the same internal reason, are both credible suppositions, although necessarily unsupported by historic evidence. Let us suppose that the Abyssinian army before Mecca endured some ordinary discomfort of campaigning, that, in the uniformity of their life, numbers together had fallen into the same constitutional ill-health just as numbers together have often fallen into scurvy, and that an eruption of the skin, proper to the tropics, was part of it. What we have farther to suppose is that the constitutional eruption became catching from the skin outwards, so to speak,—that it could be detached from its antecedents in the body, and could exist as an autonomous thing, so that it would break out upon those who had none of its underlying constitutional conditions, but had been merely in contact with such as had developed it constitutionally or from within. Such detachment of a constitutional eruption from its primary conditions is little more than constantly happens when a skin-disease like eczema, or acne, persists long after its provocation, or the disordered health which called it forth, is removed. The inveteracy or chronicity of some skin-diseases is itself a form of autonomy, but a form of it which does not transcend the individual, just as, among infections themselves, cancer does not transcend the individual or propagate itself by contagion[1]. But there exists a closer probable analogy for a secondary eruption becoming a self-existent or independent infective disease. The instance in view is no more than probable, and may easily be disputed by those who have sufficient prepossessions the other way; but there is no theory that suits so well the negro disease of yaws as that it is a somewhat peculiar secondary of syphilis, which is now able to be communicated as an exanthem detached from the primary lesions on which it had depended originally for its existence.

All the evidence, historical and geographical, points to the several varieties of the black skin (or yellow skin) as the native tissues of smallpox. It is not without significance that a disease of the negroes which was observed by English doctors not long ago in the mining districts of South Africa led to a sharp controversy whether it was smallpox or not: according to some, it was a constitutional eruption; according to others it was a contagious infection. Such phenomena are not likely to be seen in our latitudes; but the original smallpox itself was not a disease of the temperate zone[2].

I shall not carry farther this line of remark as to the probable circumstances in which a pustular eruption, among the Abyssinians before Mecca, or among other Africans or other dark-skinned races in other places and at other times, had

---

[1] The term "autonomy" in the foregoing is used according to the exposition which I originally gave of it in an address to the British Medical Association (1883) on "The Autonomous Life of the Specific Infections" (*Brit. Med. Journ.*, Aug. 4, 1883). The semi-independence of constitutional states has been dealt with in my book, *Illustrations of Unconscious Memory in Disease.* London, 1885.

[2] The South-African controversy, which became acute, was carried on in journals of the colony (the *South African Medical Journal* about 1883 and 1884 is a likely source of information), but some echoes of it were heard in letters to the *British Medical Journal*, 1884. A few years ago a similar diagnostic difficulty arose, not in an African race, but among the inmates of a Paris hospital. In the smallpox wards of the Hôpital St Antoine, a number of cases occurred, one of them in a nurse, another in an assistant physician, of a particular skin-disease, which was either discrete or confluent, lasted about ten days, and was attended by fever up to 40° C. or 41° C. Yet these cases were discriminated from smallpox; they were diagnosed, and have been recorded, as an epidemic of ecthyma. (Du Castel, *Gazette des Hôpitaux*, 1881, No. 122, quoted in the *Jahresbericht.*)

become epidemically contagious in the familiar way of small-pox. One has to learn by experience that there is at present no hearing for such inquiries, because a certain dominant fashion in medicine prefers to relegate all those origins to the remotest parts of the earth and to the earliest ages (practically *ab aeterno*), and there to leave them with a complacent sense that they have been so disposed of. That is not the way in which the study of origins is carried out for all other matters of human interest. Yet diseases are recent as compared with the species of living things; some of them are recent even as compared with civilized societies. Epidemical and constitutional maladies touch at many points, and depend upon, the circumstances of time and locality, and upon racial or national characters. Perhaps their origins will one day be made a branch of historical or archaeological research.

European Smallpox in the Middle Ages.

The present extensive prevalence of smallpox among the Arabs may or may not date from the Elephant War of A.D. 569. Its prevalence also in Abyssinia, so widely in modern times that almost everyone bears the marks of it, may have no con-tinuous history from the return of Abraha's expedition. But the history of smallpox in the West comes to us through the Saracens, and there can be no question that the disease is at the present day peculiarly at home in all African countries, and most of all in the upper basin of the Nile, where, as Pruner says, "it appears as the one great sickness[1]." It is a remark of Freind, whose erudition and judgment should carry weight, that "the Saracens first brought in this distemper, and wherever their arms prevailed, this spread itself with the same fury in Africa, in Europe, and through the greatest part of Asia, the eastern part especially[2]." Our inquiry here does not extend beyond England, so that the extremely disputable question of the amount and frequency of smallpox in the European

[1] *Krankheiten des Orients.* Erlangen, 1847, p. 127.
[2] *History of Physic*, II. 190.

countries conquered or invaded by the Saracens in the Middle Ages need not be raised[1].

So far as concerns England, smallpox was first brought to it, not by the Saracen arms, but by Saracen pens. The earliest English treatise on medicine, the *Rosa Anglica* of Gaddesden, has the same chapter "De Variolis [et Morbillis]" as all the other medieval compends—in substance the same as in the earlier work of Gilbert, and in all the other Arabistic writings earlier or later. The *Rosa Anglica* was a success in its day, partly, no doubt, by reason of its style being more boisterous than that of Gilbert's or Gordonio's treatises, partly, also, on account of its blunt indecency in certain passages. Guy de Chauliac, of Avignon, one of the few original observers of the time, had heard of the *Rosa Anglica*, and was curious to see it ; but he found in it "only the fables of Hispanus, of Gilbert, and of Theodoric," and he rather unkindly fixed upon it the epithet of "fatuous." What de Chauliac had probably heard of was Gaddesden's occasional claims to originality ; and these we shall now examine so far as they concern smallpox.

One of Gaddesden's variations from the stock remarks on smallpox is his explanation of why the disease was called variola : it is called variola, says he, because it occurs *in diverse*

---

[1] Gruner, a learned professor of Jena, who made collections of works or passages relating to syphilis and to the English sweat, published also in 1790 a collection of medieval chapters or sentences on smallpox, "De Variolis et Morbillis fragmenta medicorum Arabistarum," including the whole of Gaddesden's chapter but omitting the earlier and more important chapter from Gilbert. Gruner correctly says at the end of his extracts : "while the Arabists write thus, they seem to have followed their Arabic guides, and to have repeated what they received from the latter." This is obvious from the text of the chapters themselves : some quote more often than others from Avicenna, Rhazes and Isaac; but it is clear that they all base upon the Arabians. The substance is the same in them all; it is a merely verbal handling of Arabic observation and theory. There are no concrete experiences or original additions, from which one might infer that they were familiar at first hand with smallpox and measles. Häser, however, seems to take these chapters in the medieval compends as evidence of the general prevalence of smallpox in Europe in the Middle Ages. As he finds little writing about smallpox when modern medical literature began, he is driven into the paradox that epidemics of smallpox had actually become rarer again in the sixteenth century (III. p. 69). But the sixteenth-century references to smallpox, although they are indeed scanty, are at the same time the earliest authentic accounts of it in Western Europe.

parts of the skin (quia in cute diversas partes occupant). This is an ingenious improvement upon Gilbert, who says that it is called variola from the variety of colours (*et dicitur variola a varietate coloris*)—sometimes red, sometimes white, or yellow, or green, or violet, or black. Another remark attributed (by Häser at least) to Gaddesden as original, is that a person may have smallpox twice; but Gaddesden, in a later paragraph, shows where he got that from: "And thus says Avicenna (*quarto* Canonis), that sometimes a man has smallpox twice— once properly, and a second time improperly." The most famous of Gaddesden's originalities is his treatment by wrapping the patient in red cloth; for that also Häser ascribes to him. But Peter the Spaniard, the Hispanus of de Chauliac's reference given above, is before him with the red-cloth treatment also, while he is candid enough to quote Gilbert: "Any cloth dyed in purple," says Hispanus, "has the property of attracting the matter to the outside."

Gilbert's reference is as follows: "Old women in the country give burnt purple in the drink, for it has an occult property of curing smallpox. Let a cloth be taken, dyed *de grano.*" Bernard Gordonio, also, says: "Thereafter let the whole body be wrapped in red cloth." There was probably Arabic authority for that widely diffused prescription, as for all the rest of the teaching about smallpox. But Gaddesden does improve upon his predecessors in boldly appealing to his own favourable experience of red cloth:—"Then let a red cloth be taken, and the variolous patient be wrapped in it completely, as I did with the son of the most noble king of England when he suffered those diseases (*istos morbos*); I made everything about his bed red, and it is a good cure, and I cured him in the end without marks of smallpox."

With reference to this cure, it has to be said, in the first place, that the object of the red cloth was to draw the matter to the surface[1], and that it had nothing to do with the pre-

---

[1] This intention is most clearly expressed by Valescus de Tharanta: "Then let him be wrapped in a woollen cloth of Persian, or at least of red, so that by the sight of the red cloth the blood may be led to the exterior and so be kept at no excessive heat, according to the tenour of the sixth canon [of Avicenna]." *Apud* Gruner, p. 46.

vention of pitting. The means to prevent pitting was usually to open the pustules with a golden needle; that is the Arabian advice, and all the Arabists copy it. Gaddesden among the rest copies it, but he does not say that he practised it on the king's son. If he had said so, we might have believed that the disease was actually one bearing pustules which could be opened by a needle. What he says, in the earliest printed text (Pavia, 1492) is that, while the king's son was "suffering from those diseases," he caused him to be wrapped in red cloth, and the bed to be hung with the same, and that he cured him without the marks of smallpox. Gaddesden was not altogether an honest practitioner; on the contrary he was an early specimen of the quack *in excelsis*. According to the learned and judicious Dr Freind, "his practice, I doubt, was not formed upon any extraordinary knowledge of his faculty;" and again, "He was, as it appears from his own writings, sagacious enough to see through the foibles of human nature; he could form a good judgment how far mankind could be imposed upon; and never failed to make his advantage of their credulity[1]." The opportunity of diagnosing variola in the king's son, and of curing it by red cloth, so as to leave no pits, was one that such a person was not likely to let slip. "It is a good cure," he says; and we may go so far with him as to admit that it must have been impressive to the royal household to have heard some sharp sickness of the nursery called by the formidable name of variola, and to have seen it cured "*sine vestigiis.*"

Measles in Medieval Writings.

In the writings of the Arabians and of their imitators, the so-called Arabists, measles and smallpox are always taken together. The usual distinction made between them is that *morbilli*, or measles, come from the bile, whereas *variolae*, or smallpox, come from the blood, that the former are small, and that they are less apt to attack the eyes. The reference in Gaddesden is of the usual kind, but it is complicated by the

---

[1] *History of Physic*, Pt. II. p. 280.

introduction of a third term, *punctilli*, which Gruner, however, takes to be merely a synonym for *morbilli*. As Gaddesden's passage is of some importance for the history of the familiar name of the disease in England, I shall translate it at length, so far as it can be made into sense :—

"Variolae are so called, as if variously choosing the skin itself, because in the skin they occupy divers parts, by apostematising and infecting ; they are caused by corruption of blood, and therein they differ from morbilli and punctilli.

Morbilli are small apostemata in the skin generated of bile ; and they are a diminutive of apostematous diseases because they occupy less space by reason of the sharpness of choleric matter. They are in fact variolae of choleric matter, and the smallest of pustules. But punctilli are infections commonly sanguineous, as if they had arisen from a fleabite, only they remain continually. And punctilli are of two kinds, large and small. Of the small I have already spoken [under the name of morbilli ?]. But the large are broad, red and opaque infections in the legs of poor and wasting persons, (*pauperum et consumptuorum*), who sit as if continually at the fire without boots ; and they are called in English *mesles*[1]."

The rest of Gaddesden's chapter on smallpox and measles contains nothing that is not to be found in Avicenna or in any medieval compend on medicine. But the passage quoted is of interest as using the old word "mesles" to mean one of the two forms of *morbilli* or *punctilli*. We are here enabled to see a little way into the confusion of mind which attended the medievalists in their verbalist dealing with disease. The syntax of Gaddesden's sentence implies that the broad, red and opaque infections on the legs of poor and wasted persons were called in English *mesles*. In other writers, both before and after his date, the name of mesles or mesels or meseals was given, not to a form of disease, but to a class of sufferers from disease. It is the name applied to the inmates of leper-houses by Matthew Paris (circa 1250)—*miselli* and *misellae*, being diminutives of *miser*[2]. It is the word used for the same class in the Norman-French entries in the Rolls of Parliament in the reign of Edward I. fixing the taxation of leper-houses : if the head of the house was himself a *meseal*, the hospital was to

---

[1] *Rosa Anglica.* Papiae, 1492.
[2] *Chronica Majora.* Rolls ed. V. 452.

pay nothing, but if the head were a whole man, the hospital
had to pay[1].   The same use of mesles, as meaning the leprous,
in the generic sense, occurs several times in the 14th century
poem, 'The Vision of Piers the Ploughman[2].'   Thus, Christ in
His ministrations,

> "Sought out the sick and sinful both,
> And salved sick and sinful, both blind and crooked ;
> And comune women converted, and to good turned.
> Both meseles and mute, and in the menysoun bloody,
> Oft he heled such.   He ne held it for no mystery,
> Save tho he leched Lazar that had ylain into grave."

Or again :

> "Ac old men and hore that helpless ben of strength,
> And women with child that worche ne mowe,
> Blind and bedred and broken their members,
> That taketh their mischief mekely, as meseles and other."

It is this old English word "mesles," meaning the leprous
in the generic sense, that Gaddesden brings into his Latin text
in connexion with *morbilli* (or *punctilli*).   It is useless to look
for precision in such a writer; but if his introduction of "mesles"
in the particular context mean anything at all, it means that the
English word represented a variety of *morbilli*,—the large, broad
and opaque variety.   That it should have occurred to him to
bring these blotches or spots on the legs of poor people even
remotely into relation with the *morbilli* of the Arabians,
probably means that Gaddesden had a merely verbal acquaintance with the latter, or that he knew them only in
books.   It is certainly improbable that anyone, even in the
Middle Ages, who had ever seen a case of measles should
bracket that transitory and insubstantial mottling of the skin,
with the large, broad and "obscure" spots (or nodules, or
what else) on the legs of poor and wasted persons, which
were called, in the vernacular, mesles.   But Gaddesden, though
a verbalist and a plagiary, was a great name in medicine, a
name usually joined (as in Chaucer) with more solid reputations
than his own.   If he identified "mesles" with a variety of

---

[1] *Rolls of Parliament.*
[2] Early English Text Society's edition by Skeat.   Passus xvi. (108), and Passus vii.

morbilli (which variety no one but himself seems to have heard of), it was an easy transition for the name in English usage to become what it now is, measles meaning *morbilli,* in the correct and only real sense of the latter[1].

History of the name "Pocks" in English.

Gaddesden's case of *variola* which he cured without pitting by means of red cloth stands alone in English records until the 16th century; probably he was as little able to diagnose variola as *morbilli,* and it is more than probable that he would not have scrupled to call some infantile malady by the book-name *variola,* on the principle of "omne ignotum pro terribili," when there was

[1] Trench, in his *Select Glossary,* has adopted the derivation of measles from *misellus,* without apparently knowing that John of Gaddesden had actually used "mesles" for a form of *morbilli.* The derivation of measles from *misellus* has been summarily rejected by Skeat, who thinks that "the spelling with the simple vowel *e,* instead of *ae* or *ea,* makes all the difference. The confusion between the words is probably quite modern." Perhaps I ought not to contradict a philologist on his own ground; but there is no help for it. I know of four instances in which the simple vowel *e* is used in spelling the name of the disease that is associated with smallpox, the English equivalent of *morbilli.* In a letter of July 14, 1518, from Pace, dean of St Paul's to Wolsey (*Cal. State Papers,* Henry VIII. II. pt. 1), it is said, "They do die in these parts [Wallingford] in every place, not only of the small pokkes and mezils, but also of the great sickness." In the *Description of the Pest* by Dr Gilbert Skene, of Edinburgh (Edin. 1568, reprinted for the Bannatyne Club, 1840, p. 9), he mentions certain states of weather "quhilkis also signifeis the Pokis, Mesillis and siclik diseisis of bodie to follow." And if a Scotsman's usage be not admitted, an Oxonian, Cogan, says, "when the small pockes and mesels are rife," and another Oxonian, Thomas Lodge, in his *Treatise of the Plague* (London, 1603, Cap. iii.) says: "When as Fevers are accompanied with Small Poxe, Mesels, with spots," etc. On the other hand, Elyot, in the *Castel of Health* (1541), Phaer in the *Book of Children,* (1553), Clowes in his *Proved Practice,* and Kellwaye (1593) write the word with *ea.* There is, indeed, no uniformity, just as one might have expected in the sixteenth century. Again, Shakespeare (*Coriolanus,* Act III., scene 1) spells the word with *ea* where it is clearly the same word that is used in *The Vision of Piers the Ploughman* in a generic sense and in the spelling of "meseles:"—"Those meazels which we disdain should tetter us." Lastly, there are not two words in the Elizabethan dictionaries, one with *e* signifying lepers, and another with *ea* signifying the disease of *morbilli.* In Levins' *Manipulus Vocabulorum,* we find "ye Maysilles"=*variolae,* but there is no word "mesles"=*leprosi.* There was only one word, with the usual varieties of spelling; and in course of time it came to be restricted in meaning to *morbilli,* Gaddesden's early use of "mesles" in that sense having doubtless helped to determine the usage.

29—2

anything to be gained by so doing. There is no independent evidence that smallpox or measles existed in England in the 14th and 15th centuries. There are extant various medieval prescription-books, in which remedies are given for all the usual diseases. If the name of *variola*, or any English form of it, occur therein, we should draw the same inference as from the prescriptions for maladies of children such as "the kernels," and "the kink" (or whooping-cough)[1]. In the Anglo-Saxon "leechdoms," which have been collected in three volumes, the word *poc* occurs once in the singular in the phrase "a poc of the eye" (probably a hordeum or sty of the eyelid), and once in the plural (*poccan*) without reference to any part of the body and with no indication that a general eruption was meant. Willan, indeed, has found in a manuscript of uncertain date a Latin incantation against disease, in which the words *lues, pestis, pestilentia*, and *variola* occur; at the end of it is written in Anglo-Saxon an invocation of certain saints to "shield me from the *lathan poccas* and from all evil[2]." This looks as if *poccas* had been the Anglo-Saxon translation of *variola*. But it remains to be seen in what sense the word "pokkes" was used in the earliest English writings.

In the 'Vision of Piers the Ploughman' (passus XX) the retribution of Nature or "Kynde" upon the wickedness of the times is thus mentioned:

"Kynde came after with many keen sores,
As pokkes and pestilences, and much people shent ;
So kynde through corruptions killed full many."

In the lines immediately preceding there occur some other names, equally generic:

"Byles and boches and brennyng agues
Frensyes and foul evils, foragers of kynde."

[1] *Harl. MS.*, No. 2378. So far as I have observed, there is no prescription for "mesles," or for smallpox under its Latin name or under any English name that might correspond thereto. Moulton's *This is the Myrror or Glasse of Helth* (? 1540), which reproduces these medieval prescriptions with their headings, is equally silent about smallpox and measles.
[2] Willan's *Miscellaneous Works*. "An Inquiry into the Antiquity of the Smallpox, Measles, and Scarlet Fever." London, 1821, p. 98. The MS. is Harleian, No. 585.

" Boche" is botch,—the name given to the plague as late as the Stuart period, from its chief external sign, the bubo; and "byles" is merely the Latin *bilis = ulcus*. "Pokkes" may be the Anglo-Saxon word; but it is known that many of Langland's colloquialisms are of Norman or French origin, and in that language there is a term *poche*, which is not far from the English "boche." Whether "poche" be the same as "boche" or not, "pokkes and pestilences" may be taken to be synonyms for "byles and boches." The generic or elastic use of such terms received a striking illustration in 1528, when spotted fever (typhus), perhaps mixed with plague, became exceedingly common among French and Spanish troops. Among the French the disease was called *les poches* and among the Spaniards *las bubas*[1], although both names had been assigned to syphilis at the time of its epidemic outburst in the end of the 15th century. In those times diseases were called by their external marks; so that diseases essentially most unlike, but having certain spots, or blemishes, or botches, or pustules of the skin in common, were called by a common name. The plague itself was known by certain spots on the breast or back called tokens: hence the figure of John Stow and others that "many died of God's tokens."

There was certainly laxity of naming to that extent in the case of modern languages. As to Willan's inference from the medieval incantation, it is by no means clear that *variola* in medieval Latin may not have been used generically also; although, in the school of Salerno it appears to have had its meaning fixed, in the Arabic sense of smallpox, from the time of Constantinus Africanus, who introduced the teaching of Bagdad into that school about the year 1060.

The next use of "pokkes" that I have found is in a manuscript chronicle of England down to the year 1419[2], one of the series known as the chronicle of the Brute (from its commencing with the mythical landing of Brutus in England after the siege of Troy); this manuscript, known as the "Fruit of Times," was

---

[1] Sandoval, cited by Hecker, *Der Englische Schweiss.* Berlin, 1834, p. 80.
[2] MS. Harl., 1568.

afterwards printed at the St Albans press about 1484[1], the history being carried down to Edward IV., and the passage in question reproduced exactly as it stands in the handwriting. Under the 40th year of Edward III. (1366) there is the following entry:

"Ther fell also such a pestalence that never none such was seen in no man's tyme or lyf, for many men as they were gone to bede hole and in gude poynte sodanly thei diede.   Also that tyme fell a sekness that men call ye pokkes, slogh both men and women thorgh ther enfectyne."

It is clearly the same passage that occurs condensed in the chronicle of William Gregory, mayor of London, which was written probably in 1451–52[2].   Under the 40th of Edward III., after referring to a " grete batille of sparows " just as the earlier chronicle does, he proceeds: "Also the same yere men and bestys were grettely infectyd with pockys, wherfore they dyde, bothe men and bestys."   The variation of "men and beasts," instead of men and women, is curious, and suggests that there may have been a common source for the story.   The chronicle contemporary with 1366, which is of best authority, was that kept at St Albans Abbey; but it gives nothing under that year. Shortly after 1361, however, and probably about 1362 or 1363 it has a singular entry, which may have been the source of these references to "pockys."   The Latin may be translated thus: "Numbers died of the disease of lethargy prophesying troubles to many; many women also died of the flux; and there was a general murrain of cattle[3]."   Here we have men, women, and cattle; also lethargy, flux, and murrain; and it is conceivable that later compilers of English chronicles may each have used this contemporary Latin entry of composite events to put their own gloss upon it, or to amplify the history into what each conceived to be the probable meaning.   But the most singular enlargement was that made by Holinshed in his chronicle of

---

[1] There is a fine copy of the earliest printed version in the British Museum, with "Sanctus Albanus" for colophon.   The same text was reprinted often in the years following by London printers—in 1498, 1502, 1510, 1515 (twice), and 1528.

[2] Camden Society, ed. Gairdner, 1876, p. 87.

[3] Walsingham, *Hist. Angliae,* I. 299.   Also *Chronicon Angliae a quodam Mo-nacho, sub anno* 1362.

1577. Having copied word for word, sparrows and all, the entry under the year 1366 in the "Fruit of Times" (as printed at St Albans about 1484), he takes leave to amend the sense in the part that chiefly concerns us—he changes "pockys" into "smallpocks," and "men and women" into "men, women, and children[1]." Holinshed was dealing with an event two hundred years before his own time, and had no more first-hand knowledge of it than we have; but his authority has been accepted for the fatal prevalence of smallpox in 1366 by modern writers on the history of that disease, such as James Moore[2], who have not sought for the contemporary authority nor exercised a critical judgment upon the lax ways of verbalist compilers. Thus is history made—but not so easily unmade.

One other reference to "pockys" has to be noticed before we leave the philological part of the subject and come to the unambiguous history of the realities. Fabyan, in his *Chronicle* written not long before his death in 1512, says that Edward IV. during an expedition to the Scots Marches "was then vysyted with the syknesse of pockys[3]." It is futile to conjecture what the king's illness may really have been. The word in Fabyan's time had already acquired a technical sense, which it has ever since retained; but that well-understood meaning was some twenty years later than the year 1474 (although the disease itself doubtless existed all through the Middle Ages); while, in its earlier generic sense, as in the 'Vision of Piers the Ploughman,' it seems to have meant botches or other tokens of pestilential disease. In a Latin glossary of English words, published a hundred years after[4], "a pocke" is still defined as *phagedaena*, and "the French pocke" as *morbus Gallicus*, while "smallpox" is not given at all.

---

[1] "Also manie died of the smallpocks, both men, women and children."

[2] *History of the Smallpox*, 1817. Blomefield, also, in his *History of Norfolk*, quotes the passage about "pockys" correctly from the "Fruit of Times," applies it to Norwich, to which city it had no special relation, and then says that this is the first mention of "small pocks."

[3] Fabyan's *Chronicle*. Ed. Ellis, p. 653.

[4] Levins, *Manipulus Vocabulorum*, 1570. Camden Society's edition, column 158.

Smallpox in England in the 16th Century.

The earliest references to smallpox in England, apart from the probably incorrect one by Gaddesden early in the 14th century, occur in letters of the years 1514 and 1518. Another letter of 1514 will serve to bring out the ambiguity of the names given to diseases at the time. On June 30, 1514, Gerard de Pleine writes from London to Margaret of Savoy that he had been asked by the bishop of Lincoln why the marriage between the princess Mary and Louis XII. had been broken off (it took place shortly after), and by another great peer whether Louis XII. "avoit eu les pocques," which last sentence has a marginal note in the printed collection of letters: "c'est la petite verole[1]." But *les pocques* in a letter written from London in 1514 did not mean the smallpox. In a letter of March 3, 1514, Peter Martyr writing in Latin from Valladolid to Ludovico Mendoza, says that the King of England has had a fever, and that the physicians were afraid it would turn to the pustules called *variolae*, but he is now well again and rises from his bed[2]. This illness of Henry VIII. happened at Richmond previous to 7th February. Although in the letter quoted there was only a fear that the illness might have turned to the pustules called smallpox, yet in the instructions of Henry VIII. to Spinelly, English ambassador in the Low Countries, sent in February, the twelfth item instructs him to say that the English king has lately been visited by a malady "nommée la petitte verolle[3]."

Four years after, on July 14, 1518, Pace writes to Wolsey from Wallingford, where the court then was, that the king was to leave next day for Bisham "as it is time; for they do die in these parts in every place, not only of the small pokkes and mezils, but also of the great sickness[4]."

---

[1] *Lettres du Roy Louis XII.* Brusselle, 1712, IV. 335.

[2] *Cal. State Papers.*

[3] " Item, que à son grand desplaisir il ait esté naguaires mal disposé d'une maladie nommée la petitte verolle, dont à present, graces à Dieu, il est recouvert et passé tout dangier." *Lettres du Roy Louis XII.*, IV. 260. Brusselle, 1712.

[4] *Cal. State Papers.*

These are the earliest known instances of the use of the words *pocques, variola, petite verolle*, "small pokkes and mezils," as applied to particular cases of sickness, in correspondence from or relating to England. The remarks to be made upon the early usage are: first, that the word *pocques*, as used by one writing in French from London in 1514, did not mean smallpox, but pox; second, that the first authentic mention of smallpox happens to have been in the French form—"une maladie nommée la petitte verolle;" third, that, in the political gossip of the time the opinion of the physicians regarding the illness of the young king is given as of a fever which they feared might have turned to the pustules called "*variolae*;" and fourthly, that in the very first mention of the disease *variola* by an English name "small pokkes," the name is modelled on the French, being coupled with the old English name "mezils." It is impossible to infer from these references anything as to the amount of smallpox in England at the time, or even to be sure of the correctness of the diagnosis. The lax usage as between "pox" and "smallpox" is shown in a book of the year 1530 called 'Prognosticacions out of Ipocras and Avicen,' in which a brief reference to *variola* in the Latin original is translated "to prognosticate of the pockes."

In Sir Thomas Elyot's *Castel of Health*, published in 1541, children after their first infancy are said to suffer from a number of maladies, and in "England commonly purpyls, meazels and smallpockes." That is perhaps the first use of the terms in a systematic work on medicine, not indeed by one of the faculty, but by a layman. About the same time we hear of smallpocks in an infant of noble family: a letter of May 26, 1537, from Charles duke of Suffolk to Cromwell, written from Hoxun in Suffolk, excuses his not repairing to Lincolnshire, as the king had ordered, on the ground that "his son fell sick of the smallpox and his wife of the ague[1]." "His son" was Henry Brandon, born September 18, 1535, so that he was then an infant of some twenty months; he is the same that died, with his younger brother, of the sweating sickness in July 1551.

The reference to smallpocks and meazels by Elyot in his

[1] *Cal. State Papers.*

Castel of Health is repeated in the almost contemporary *Book of Children* by Thomas Phaer. Whether Phaer translated that also " out of the French tongue" as he did the *Regiment of Life*, with which it is bound up in the edition of 1553, we have nowhere any information. In a list of forty infirmities of children, the 32nd in order is " small pockes and measels." A later passage in the *Book of Children* shows how much, or how little, intelligent meaning Phaer attached to these terms : " Of smallpockes and measels. This disease is common and familiar, called of the Greeks by the general name of exanthemata, and of Plinie papulae et pituitae eruptiones. It is of two kinds :—varioli, ye measils ; morbilli, called of us ye smal pocks. They be but of one nature and proceed of one cause. The signs of both are so manifest to sight that they need no farther declaration ;"—but he does add some signs, such as " itch and fretting of the skin as if it had been rubbed with nettles, pain in the head and back etc. : sometimes as it were a dry scab or lepry spreading over all the members, other whiles in pushes, pimples and whayls running with much corruption and matter, and with great pains of the face and throat, dryness of the tongue, hoarseness of voice, and, in some, quiverings of the heart with sownings." He then gives the four causes, three of them being intrinsic states of the humours, and the fourth " when the disease commenceth by the way of contagion, when a sick person infecteth another, and in that case it hath great affinity with the pestilence." The treatment is directed towards bringing out the eruption ; all occasions of chill are to be carefully avoided. More special directions are given for cases in which " the wheales be outrageous and great ; " also, " to take away the spots and scarres of the small pockes and measils," a prescription of some authors is given, to use the blood of a bull or of a hare.

The whole of Phaer's section on smallpox and measles bears evidence of a foreign source, namely the same stock chapter from which Kellwaye drew most of his section upon the same two diseases appended to his book on the plague in 1593. Not only does Phaer speak of smallpox and measles conjointly as leaving spots and scars, but he actually renders *variolae* by measles, and *morbilli* by smallpox. Phaer was more of a literary compiler than a physician with original knowlege of diseases and their pathology. But he is not singular among the Tudor writers in taking measles to be the equivalent of *variolae*. William Clowes, of St Bartholomew's Hospital, one of the most experienced practitioners of his time, does the same. His *Proved Practice for all Young Chirurgeons* has an appendix of Latin aphorisms "taken out of an old written coppy," to each of which aphorisms Clowes has added an English translation: in the aphorism on *variolae*, that term is translated "measles," the name of "smallpox" nowhere occurring in the book. Clowes's translation is exactly in accordance with the English-Latin glossary of the time by Levins (1570). Levins was an Oxford fellow who had graduated in medicine and afterwards become a schoolmaster, just as Cogan, of *The Haven of Health*, had done. He wrote the *Pathway of Health*, and also compiled the *Manipulus Vocabulorum*. His definitions in the latter may be taken, therefore, to stand for the medical usage of the time. In this glossary, "ye maysilles" is rendered by *variole*, while the name of "smallpox" is omitted altogether, "a pocke" having its Latin equivalent in *phagedaena*, and "ye French pocke" in *morbus Gallicus*. In the Elizabethan dictionary by Baret, "the maisils" is defined as "a disease with many reddish spottes or speckles in the face and bodie, much like freckles in colour;" and that was the disease which the English profession then understood to be the same as the *variolae* of medieval writers.

I leave readers to draw their own conclusions, whether there was much or little smallpox or measles in England in the Tudor period. They may be reminded that Pace, dean of St Paul's, in a letter from Berkshire in 1518, asserts the fatal prevalence of "smallpox and mezils," and that the duke of Suffolk called the illness of his infant son by the name of smallpox in 1538. They may be farther helped to a conclusion by the following curious instance which has been recorded by John Stow.

Among the miscellaneous collections of that antiquary preserved in the Lambeth Library[1], there is a narrative of the troubled conscience of Master Richard Allington, esquire, a

---

[1] Edited by Gairdner for the Camden Society, 1880.

gentleman who appears to have lent money at high interest. Believing himself to be dying on November 22, 1561, he summoned to his bedside at eight in the evening the Master of the Rolls ("Sir John of the Rolls"), two doctors of the law and two other lawyers.

> He began : "Maisters, seinge that I muste nedes die, which I assure you I nevar thought wolde have cum to passe by this desseease, consyderinge it is but the small pockes, I woulde therefore moste hertely desyre you in the reuerence of God and for Christes passions sake to suffer me to speake untyll I be dede, that I may dyscharge my conscens" etc. He then explains that "no man had so especial tokens of God's singular grace, and so litele regarded them as I have done," and goes on to mention particular acts of usury and to offer restitution to the amount of some hundred pounds or more. It had occurred to him to do so the second night after he fell sick, being in perfect memory lying in his bed broad awake, but with puppets dancing around him. After entrusting the lawyers at his bed side with these restitutions, he asked the Master of the Rolls to read to him certain of the penitential Psalms which the sick man had selected as appropriate. "And then he thought he should have died, but then broth being given unto him, he revived again and fell to prayer and gave himself wholly to quietness;" and there the narrative ends.

It appears from a reference in Stow's *Survey of London* that he did die in 1561, and that his widow was left well off: for she afterwards built one of the finest of the new houses that were now beginning to line the highway of Holborn almost as far out as St Giles's in the Fields.

This is the first recorded case of smallpox in English. According to the patient's own view, smallpox was not usually a formidable disease, nor does it appear that the Master of the Rolls and four other eminent lawyers (Dr Caldwell, Dr Good, Mr Garth, and Mr Jones) had been apprehensive of catching it. One finds no other evidence of the existence of smallpox in London or elsewhere in England until it is mentioned in a letter of 1591 and in the essay of Kellwaye, 1593, which asserts the occurrence of "smallpox and measles" in almost the same language as Phaer's earlier *Book of Children* and for the most part under the same foreign inspiration. From Scotland we have a single reference in Dr Gilbert Skene's essay on the plague, published in 1568, from the terms of which one may suppose that he is giving his own experience. The season, he says, will sometimes foretell the plague, as well as other diseases:

> " Siclyk quhen pokis or sic pustulis are frequent, not onlie amangis barnis, but also amangis those quha be of constant or declynand aige—greit frequent south and south-vest vyndis." In a similar passage on the previous page he couples "pokis, mesillis and siclike diseisis of bodie[1]."

In a letter of August 26, 1591, written to a member of queen Elizabeth's court, it is said: "Hir Higness wold you should remove from that place where the smalle pocks were, to take the fresh and clere ayre, the better to purge ye from the infection[2]."

In 1593 we come to the first systematic English essay on the disease, appended to the treatise on the plague by Simon Kellwaye[3]. The author is otherwise unknown as a medical writer, but he is commended in a preface by George Baker, a court surgeon, for his "good and zealous intent and sufficiencie in his profession." In appending an essay on smallpox to a treatise on the plague he follows the example of the Salernian treatise of Alphanus, which also affords him most of his systematic materials in both diseases, filtered through Ambroise Paré and other writers. Kellwaye claims, however, to have incorporated native experience: "which work I have collected and drawn from sundry both auncient and later writers, the which being shadowed under the calm shroud of auncient consent and strengthened with the abundant sap of late experience (as well mine own as others) I here present the same." In the treatise on the plague (fol. 2) he mentions smallpox as among the forerunners or prognostics of that disease:

> " When the smalle poxe doth generally abound both in young and old people." In the separate essay on the smallpox (fol. 38), its interest is again that of a forerunner or sequel of the plague, according to the foreign teaching of the time:

> " For that oftentimes those that are infected with the plague are in the end of the disease sometimes troubled with the smallpockes or measels, as also by good observation it hath been seen that they are forerunners or

---

[1] Bannatyne Club's reprint, 1840, pp. 9–10.

[2] *The Loseley Manuscripts.* Edited by Kempe. London, 1836, p. 315.

[3] *A Defensative against the Plague......whereunto is annexed a short treatise of the small Poxe, how to govern and help those that are infected therewith.* London, 1593.

warnings of the plague to come, as Salius and divers other writers do testify, I have thought good and as a matter pertinent to my former treatise" etc.

He proceeds : " I need not greatly to stand upon the description of this disease because it is a thing well known unto most people." It begins with a fever ; then shortly after there arise small red pustules upon the skin throughout all the body, which come forth more or less intermittently ; " In some there arise many little pustules with elevation of the skin, which in one day do increase and grow bigger, and after have a thick matter growing in them, which the Greeks call exanthemata or ecthymata ; and after the Latins variola, in our English tongue the smallpockes; and here some writers do make a difference betwixt variola and exanthemata : for, say they, that is called variola when many of those pustules do suddenly run into a clear bladder, as if it had been scalled, but the other doth not so ; yet are they both one in the cure." He recognizes the contagious property of the disease, calling it "hereditable :" " For we see when one is infected therewith, that so many as come near him (especially those which are allied in the same blood) do assuredly for the most part receive the infection also." His *Practica* are taken almost entirely from the Arabian writers, as filtered through Gaddesden, one of them being the prevention of pitting by opening the pocks with a gold pin or needle. He had heard, however, " of some which, having not used anything at all, but suffering them to dry up and fall of themselves without picking or scratching, have done very well, and not any pits remained after it." He then refers to complications, such as ulcerations of the skin, soreness and ulcerations of the mouth (*aphthae*), soreness of the tonsils, and glueing together of the eyelids, all of which are stock paragraphs in the foreign writers of the time and are probably transferred from the latter. Also he goes a considerable way towards the separation of measles from smallpox, which was not fully effected in England until the century following : " What the measels or males are :—many little pimples which are not to be seen but only by feeling with the hand are to be perceived ; they do not maturate as the pocks doth do, nor assault the eyes" etc.

About ten years after Kellwaye's essay, there began, in 1604, the classification of the deaths in London by the Company of Parish Clerks : but it was not until 1629 that their weekly and annual bills were regularly printed. In the first printed bills, " Flox, smallpox and measles" appear as one entry. The meaning of "flox" seems to be explained by Kellwaye's remark : " And here some writers do make a difference betwixt variola and exanthemata ; for, say they, that is called variola when many of those pustules do suddenly run into a clear bladder as if it had been scalled, but the other doth not so." That is the distinction between confluent smallpox and discrete ;

and the most probable explanation of "flox" is that it stands for the confluent kind, or for the pustules that run together into a clear bladder.

Smallpox in the 17th Century.

The gradual rise of smallpox to prominence in England about the end of the Elizabethan period and in the first years of the Stuarts cannot fail to strike anyone who is occupied with the English records of disease as a whole. Smallpox and measles may have been, and almost certainly were, observed in England in the earlier part of the 16th century; but they make no such figure in the records, domestic and other, as they do from the beginning of the 17th century onwards. Perhaps the first mention of smallpox, in English literature proper, occurs in a collection of lyrical poems published in 1602[1]. In some verses "Upon his Ladies sicknesse of the Small Pocks," the poet, Th. Spilman, apostrophises the "cruel and impartial sickness" and asks,—

> Are not these thy steps I trace
> In the pure snow of her face?

> Th' heavenly honey thou dost suck
> From her rose cheeks, might suffice;
> Why then didst thou mar and pluck
> Those dear flowers of rarest price?

In two letters of Dr Donne, dean of St Paul's, written probably a few years before his death in 1631, reference is made to the smallpox in London. In the one he says:

"At my return from Kent to my gate, I found Peg had the pox: so I withdrew to Prickham and spent a fortnight there. And without coming home, when I could with some justice hope that it would spread no farther amongst them (as I humbly thank God it hath not, nor much disfigured her that had it), I went into Bedfordshire" etc.

[1] Francis Davison's *Poetical Rapsodie*. The poem of Spilman occurs at p. 189 of the edition of 1611. In the piratical edition of 1621, after Davison's death, "small" is left out before "Pocks," and Spilman's name omitted at the foot of the verses. The printer's error has had the singular effect of leading Dr Farmer, the writer on Shakespeare, to conclude that the word "pox" in the Elizabethan period meant smallpox even in imprecations such as "a pox on it."

This dread of smallpox infection is quite unlike anything that we meet with in the earlier 16th-century domestic memorials; in them it is only the infection of the plague that comes in. Donne's other reference is to the sickness of my lord Harrington: "a few days since they were doubtful of him; but he is so well recovered that now they know all his disease to be the pox and measles mingled[1]."

Cases of smallpox among the upper classes are occasionally mentioned in the letters written by Chamberlain to Carleton in the reigns of James I. and Charles I.[2]. On December 17, 1612, "The Lord Lisle hath lost his eldest son, Sir William Sidney, by the smallpox, which were well come out." On December 31, the same year, Carleton, writing from abroad, mentions that the duke of Mantua had died of the smallpox about three weeks since, of which he buried his only son not three weeks before. Also on December 31, Chamberlain writes to him, that the Lady Webbe was sick of the smallpox, of which, he says in another letter, she died: "She was grown a very proper woman, but loved the town too well, which in a short time would have drawn her and her husband dry as well in purse as in reputation." It is the year 1614 that is given (by Horst) as the worst season of smallpox all over Europe and the East; England is mentioned by the foreign writer as among the countries affected, but there is no trace of an epidemic in our own records. On April 20, 1616, Chamberlain mentions the case of the duke of Buckingham, the favourite; "he hath been crazy of late, not without suspicion of the smallpox, which, if it had fallen out, *actum est de amicitia.* But it proves otherwise." Buckingham's illness, for which he took much physic, produced an imposthume on his head (an effect which followed in the more notorious illness of Wolsey), and he is elsewhere said to be suffering from the *morbus comitialis.* The suggestion of smallpox appears to be the same euphemism which was resorted to in the cases of other exalted personages.

On August 21, 1624, having written of the great mortality

[1] Sir Tobie Matthews' *Letters* (1577–1655), London, 1660. (1) Donne to Mrs Cockaine, p. 342; (2) Donne to Sir R. D——, both without date.
[2] *Court and Times of James I.*

from fevers, Chamberlain adds: "Lady Winwood, hearing that her only daughter was fallen sick of the smallpox at Ditton and that they came not out currently," had gone to her. On December 18, 1624, "the Lady Purbeck is sick of the smallpox, and her husband is so kind that he stirs not from her bed's feet." In the first week of June, 1625, the famous composer Orlando Gibbons died at Canterbury, not without suspicion of the plague[1], but according to another opinion of the smallpox[2].

With the year 1629, the causes of death in London began to be published by Parish Clerks' Hall in a rough classification, smallpox being a regular item from year to year. For the first eight years the deaths from "flox, smallpox, and measles" were as follows:

1629	72	1631	58	1633	72	1635	293
1630	40	1632	531	1634	1354	1636	127

The greatest epidemic, it will be seen, was in 1634[3]. For the years 1637–1646, the figures are lost (owing to Graunt's omitting them in his Table of 1662, for want of room). But it is known from letters that the autumn of 1641 was a season of severe smallpox as well as plague. Thus on August 26, "both Houses grow very thin by reason of the smallpox and plague that is in the town, 133 dying here this week of the plague, and 118 of the smallpox, 610 in the whole of all diseases." On September 9, a letter from Charing Cross says: "Died this week of the plague 185, and of the smallpox 101." The plague mortality continues to be mentioned in subsequent letters, but the references to smallpox cease[4]. On July 16, 1642, one excuses his attendance on some State business because he is sick of the smallpox[5].

About the Restoration the references to smallpox become more numerous[6]. A letter of January 4, 1658 (1659), speaks of

[1] *Court and Times of Charles I.* (Chamberlain to Carleton), I. 28.

[2] Anthony Wood.

[3] For Chester also, in the parish register of Trinity Church (Harl. MS. 2177) there is a note opposite 1636: "for this two or three years divers children died of smallpox in Chester."

[4] *Cal. State Papers.*   [5] *Ibid.*

[6] *Hist. MSS. Commission*, V. 146, 151, 156, 168, 174, 201. See also the Diaries of Pepys and Evelyn.

C.   30

"much sickness in the town [London], especially fevers, agues and smallpox." On February 7, 1660, the earl of Anglesey is dead of the smallpox. In September, 1660, Lord Oxford had a severe attack and recovered; at the same time the duke of Gloucester, on the 8th September, was diagnosed by the doctors to have "a disease between the smallpox and the measles; he is now past danger of death for this bout, as the doctors say." However he died on 14th September, in the tenth day of the disease, with remarkable evidences (post mortem) of internal haemorrhage, having bled freely at the nose a few hours before his death. The eruption had "come out full and kindly" at the beginning, so that it was not the ordinary haemorrhagic type. On the 20th December, 1660, the princess Henrietta goes to St James's for fear of the smallpox. On the 16th January, 1660 (? 1661), "the princess is recovered of the measles." Letters from a lady at Hambleton to her husband in London, May 26, 1661, speaks of smallpox raging in the place, and in the house of her nearest neighbour, her own children having the whooping-cough. In the bills of mortality of those years the deaths in London from smallpox and measles were as follows:

1647	139	1652	1279	1657	835	1662	768
1648	401	1653	139	1658	409	1663	411
1649	1190	1654	832	1659	1523	1664	1233
1650	184	1655	1294	1660	354	1665	655
1651	525	1656	823	1661	1246	1666	38

These figures bring us down to the period of Sydenham, who was the first accurate observer of smallpox in London. With his writings, and with those of Willis and Morton, we begin a new era in the history of epidemics in England. We find, for the first time in the history, an adequate discussion of the epidemiological and clinical facts by the ablest men in the profession. But, as the new era is at one and the same time marked by the cessation of plague and by the enormous increase of various fevers, as well as of smallpox, it falls without the limits of this volume, making, indeed, the appropriate beginning of the new kind of epidemic history which is characteristic of England from the Restoration and the Revolution down to the end of the 18th century. It is clear, from the instances above given, that smallpox was already at the beginning of the 17th century becoming a pest among the upper classes. But to anyone who studies the history over continuous periods it is equally clear that its prominence was then something new and that the horror and alarm which it caused became greater as the 17th century approached its close. And so as not to leave the history of smallpox at this point with a wrong impression of its general virulence, it may be added that Dr Plot, writing of Oxfordshire in 1677, says: "Generally here they are so favorable and kind, that be the nurse but tolerably good, the patient seldom miscarries[1]."

Smallpox in Continental Writings of the 16th century.

It would be beside the purpose of this work to follow the history of smallpox and measles on the continent of Europe. But it will be necessary to say a few words on the contemporary foreign writings upon these diseases, as it is chiefly teaching from a foreign source that we detect in the English authors of the 16th century.

It might be inferred from the classical work of Fracastori[2], published in 1546, that smallpox and measles were frequent and familiar diseases in the author's experience at Verona. At the same time it is clear that even he, original observer as he was, is in places merely repeating the old statements of the Arabian writers. Thus his statement that everyone has smallpox or measles sooner or later, is the old Arabian tradition or experience, usually joined to the explanation that the cause of that universality was the nourishment of the foetus by the retained and impure menstrual blood, so that all children had to free their constitutions of a congenital impurity sooner or later. So far as Fracastori's originality comes in, it is clear that he does not regard smallpox and measles as serious troubles. In his second chapter he says:

"First we must treat of those contagious maladies which, although contagious, are not called pestilential, because, for the most part, they are

---

[1] *Natural History of Oxfordshire.* Oxford, 1677, p. 23.
[2] *De contagione et contagiosis morbis*, etc. Venet. 1546.

salubrious. Of such are variolae and morbilli. By variolae are understood those which are called also varollae by the common people, from their likeness, I suppose, to the pustules called vari. By morbilli are understood those which the common people style fersae, so-called perhaps from *fervor*. But of these the Greeks do not appear to have treated under any other name than exanthemata. They happen principally in children, rarely in men, most rarely in old people. But they seem to befall all men once in life, or to be apt to befall them unless a premature death removes the individual. In boys the malady is more benign than in adults. For the more part, as already said, they are salubrious, since this ebullition of the blood is something of a purification of the same. It afflicts more or less according to the density of the blood and as the vice is apt or not to be separated from it. If the blood be more pituitous, the pustules are variform, white, round and full of a kind of mucus ; but if it be more bilious the pustules break forth more of a dry sort. Where the disease has happened once it is not apt to recur ; but there are cases where it has happened more than once."

In the brief account by Fracastori, all the points are stated for measles and smallpox together ; and the opinion is twice put forward that an attack was salubrious as purifying the blood or as freeing it from some vice—an opinion which is still popularly held.

It is not until the latter half of the 16th century that we come to real epidemiological records of smallpox on the Continent,—the works by Donatus on smallpox and measles at Mantua in 1567, and by Betera upon epidemics at Brescia in 1570, 1577 and 1588, in which the more malignant types of smallpox were seen[1]. The treatise most used was that of Alphanus, published at Naples in 1577[2]; it was on plague and pestilential fever, with an appendix on smallpox. Either it or Ambroise Paré's chapters seem to have furnished the greater part of the English essay by Kellwaye on the plague and smallpox.

In Ambroise Paré's references to smallpox there occurs one singular line of remark which will serve to bring us back to etymology and to the great pox[3]. The *petite vérole*, he says,

[1] Titles in Häser, III. 383.

[2] *Opus de peste......necnon de variolis*, Neap. 1577.

[3] *Les œuvres de M. Ambroise Paré.* 5th ed., Paris, 1598, Books XIX. and XX. The chapters on Plague, Smallpox, etc., were originally published, according to Häser, in 1568.

has a resemblance to the *grosse vérole* as sometimes attacking the bones. He had seen that in smallpox cases not only in 1568 but on other occasions : and he gives the details of two cases of smallpox, apparently with periostitis and necrosis, which he compares to cases of the great pox. To express in one word the meaning of such cases, he says, the smallpox and *rougeolle*, not having been well purged, give rise to various troublesome accidents, as the great pox does. One cannot read Paré's chapters on the *grosse vérole* and the *petite vérole* without detecting an inclination to compare them or class them together in nosological characters. The comparison or classification is by no means explicit ; but it seems to be in his thoughts, and he would seem, accordingly, to have held until a late period of the 16th century a view of the two diseases which was not unusual at the beginning of that century (as in the treatise of Pinctor and in the accounts of the dreadful mortality of Indians in Hispaniola and Mexico[1]), and was expressed in the popular names given to each disease in France and in England.

[1] See Purchas, *Pilgrimes*, III. 996, where syphilis and smallpox are included together as "infectious or pestilentiall pocks," Ramusio being given as the authority for the smallpox and Oviedo for the great pox.

CHAPTER X.

PLAGUE, FEVER AND INFLUENZA FROM THE ACCESSION OF THE STUART DYNASTY TO THE RESTORATION.

THE last period of plague in England, from 1603 to its extinction in 1666, was as fatal as any that the capital, and the provincial towns, had known since the 14th century. The mortalities in London in 1603, 1625, and 1665 are the greatest in the whole history of the City's epidemics, not, perhaps, relatively to the population, but in absolute numbers. The capital was growing rapidly, having now become the greatest trading community in Europe. The dangers which were foreseen in the proclamation of 1580, of an extension of the City's borders beyond civic control, had been realized. The old walled city, like Vienna down to a quite recent date, remained both the residential quarter and the centre of trade and commerce: the original suburbs, which were in the Liberties or Freedom of the City, were the slums—the fringe of poverty covered by the poorest class of tenements, unpaved and without regular streets, but penetrated by alleys twisting and turning in an endless maze. The City was not, indeed, without a good deal of building of the same class, especially in the parish of St Stephen, Coleman Street, the most populous parish within the walls. But what was an occasional thing in the City where gardens and other open spaces had been built upon, was the rule in the parishes beyond the walls. It was in the Liberties and outparishes that the plague of 1603 began: its origin in 1625 is less certain; but there can be no question as to the gradual progress of the Great Plague of 1665 from the west end of the town down Holborn and the Strand to the City, to the great parishes on the north-east and east, and across the water to Southwark. From one point of view we may represent the later plagues as incidents in the transition from the medieval to the modern state of the capital—a transition which proceeded slowly and is still unfinished so far as concerns the forms of municipal government. The history of the public health of London is, for nearly two centuries, the history of irregular and uncontrolled expansion, of the failure of old municipal institutions to overtake new duties. Perhaps if Wren's grand conception of a New London after the fire of 1666 had been taken up and given effect to by Charles II., the Liberties and suburbs might have been joined more organically to the centre and have benefited by the municipal traditions of the latter. The history of the public health in London during the latter part of the 17th century and the whole of the 18th might in that case have been a less melancholy record. That history falls within our next volume; but as it began with the expansion of London under Elizabeth and the Stuarts, this is the place to review the growth of the City from the time when it broke through its medieval limits.

The Growth of London in the Tudor and Stuart Periods[1].

The accession of James I. to the English crown in 1603 corresponds in time with the pretensions of London to be the first city in Europe. "London," says Dekker, in *The Wonderfull Yeare*, "was never in the highway to preferment till now. For she saw herself in better state than Jerusalem, she went more gallant than ever did Antwerp, was more courted by amorous and lustie suitors than Venice (the minion of Italy); more lofty towers stood about her temples than ever did about the beautiful forehead of Rome; Tyre and Sydon to her were like two thatcht

---

[1] For details of the increase of London population, with the sources of evidence, I beg to refer to my essay, " The Population of Old London," *Blackwood's Magazine*, April, 1891.

houses to Theobals, the grand Cairo but a hogsty." That is, of course, in Dekker's manner; but it can be shown by figures that London took a great start in the end of Elizabeth's reign and grew still faster under James.

From Richard I. to Henry VII., London was the medieval walled city, as Drayton says, "built on a rising bank within a vale to stand," with a population between 40,000 and 50,000. Without the walls lay a few city parishes or parts of parishes, including the three dedicated to St Botolph outside Aldgate, Bishopsgate and Aldersgate, respectively, and St Giles's without Cripplegate, all of these being at the gates or close to the walls. On the western side, however, lay an extensive but sparsely populated suburb, which was erected in 1393 into the Ward of Farringdon Without; it extended westward from the city wall as far as Temple Bar, Holborn Bars and West Smithfield, and was divided into the four great parishes of St Sepulchre's without Newgate, St Andrew's, on the other side of Holborn valley, St Dunstan's in the West (about Chancery Lane and Fetter Lane), and St Bride's, Fleet Street.

The earliest known bills of mortality, in 1532 and 1535, from which a population of some 62,400 might be deduced, show that the St Botolph parishes, St Giles's without Cripplegate and the four great parishes in the western Liberties (or, more correctly, in the ward of Farringdon Without) had one-third of the whole deaths, and presumably about one-third of the whole population. In the few memoranda left of the plague-bills of 1563, we find evidence that the population had increased to some 93,276, of which about a sixth or seventh part, or some 12,000 to 15,000 was in the "out-parishes," or in the parishes not only beyond the walls, but beyond the Bars of the Freedom. The most valuable series of statistics for Elizabethan London are those which give the christenings and burials for five years from 1578 to 1582; from those of the year 1580, which was almost free from the disturbing element of plague, a population of some 123,034 may be deduced by taking the birth-rate at 29 per 1000 living and the death-rate at 23 per 1000, or in each case at a favourable rate corresponding to the large excess of births over deaths.

There is not enough left of the introduction to these old manuscript abstracts of weekly births and deaths to show how many parishes they relate to, or what is the proportion for each division of the capital. But, as the earlier series of bills of mortality from 1563 to 1566 included the City, the Liberties and the out-parishes, it is probable that the series from 1578 to 1582 had done the same. The crowding of the Liberties with a poor class of tenements, and the extension of the out-parishes, are otherwise known from the preamble to the proclamation of 1580, which prohibited all building on new sites within three miles of the City wall. The next figures are for the years 1593, 1594, and 1595, which show a population increased to about 152,000.

From the figures of the plague-year, 1593, it appears that the mortality within the walls, both from plague and from ordinary causes, had now become the smaller half, or somewhat less than that "without the walls and in the Liberties,"—a phrase which is used loosely, even in some official bills, for both Liberties and suburbs. In 1604 we have the exact proportions of deaths in the City, in the Liberties and in the out-parishes respectively :

	96 parishes within walls	16 parishes in Liberties	8 parishes out of the Freedom	Total
All deaths	1798	2465	956	5219
Plague deaths	280	368	248	896
Christenings	—	—	—	5458

The sixteen parishes of the Liberties are now decidedly ahead of the ninety-six old City parishes, while the eight out-parishes have some 18 per cent of the whole mortality. The population is best reckoned from the 6504 baptisms of the year after, 1605, by which time the disturbance of the enormous mortality in 1603 had ceased to be felt; at a birth-rate of 29 per 1000, the population would be some 224,275. The proportions in 1605, from the bills of mortality for the year, are 33·8 per cent. in the City, 50 per cent. in the Liberties, and 16·2 per cent. in the out-parishes ; so that the City would have contained in that year about 76,000, the Liberties about 114,000, and the out-parishes about 37,000. To those numbers we should have to add some 20,000 or 30,000 for Westminster, Stepney, Lambeth, Newington, etc.

According to Graunt's contemporary estimate for 1662, the population had grown to 460,000, or to rather more than double that of 1605; and whereas the proportion in 1605 was two-sixths in the City, three-sixths in the Liberties and one-sixth in the out-parishes, he makes it in 1662 to have been one-fifth in the City, three-fifths in the Liberties (including Southwark) and the out-parishes nearest to the Bars, and one-fifth in the out-parishes of Stepney, Redriff, Newington, Lambeth, Islington and Hackney, with the city of Westminster. Thus, whereas in 1535 the City had two-thirds of the whole estimated population, in 1662 it had one-fifth; but with its one-fifth in 1662 it was twice as crowded as with its two-thirds in 1535, the comparatively open appearance given to it by gardens in various localities, as on Tower Hill, having entirely gone.

As early as the plague of 1563, the Liberties were observed to be first infected, and to retain the infection longest; that is alleged of St Sepulchre's parish by Dr John Jones, from personal knowledge. The history of the plague of 1593 is imperfectly known; but it is clear from Stow's summation of the deaths during the year, that more died of plague in the Liberties and suburbs than in the City. Of the next plague, that of 1603, we know that it did begin in the Liberties and was prevalent in those skirts of the City for some time before it entered the gates. "Death," says *The Wonderfull Yeare*, "had pitcht his tents in the sinfully polluted suburbs...the skirts of London were pitifully pared off by little and little; which they within the gates perceiving," etc. Then the plague, represented as an invading force, "entered within the walls and marched through Cheapside," the wealthier inhabitants having escaped meanwhile.

The London Plague of 1603.

The most useful document for the London plague of 1603 is a printed Bill of Mortality which is in the Guildhall Library. The bill, which is in the form of a broadside, is for the week

13–20 October, and purports to be a true copy, according to the report made to the king by the Company of Parish Clerks, and printed by John Winder, printer to the honourable City of London[1]. It is necessary to be thus particular, because the clerk of the Company of Parish Clerks in the end of 1665 (between the Plague and the Fire) published an account of all the statistics of former plagues preserved in his office, and emphatically denied that the Parish Clerks gave in an accompt for the year 1603 ; they did not resume their series after 1595, he says, until 29th December, 1603. But the clerk was mistaken, as even the most prim of officials will sometimes be. The printed bill which has come down to us gives the usual weekly return of deaths from all causes in one column and those from plague in another, for each of the 96 parishes within their walls, each of the 16 parishes in the Liberties and each of 8 out-parishes. On the right hand margin it gives also a summary statement of the deaths in " the first great plague in our memory " that of 1563, which is the same as in Stow's *Annales*, and of the deaths in the next great plague, that of 1593, which differs considerably from Stow's. It then goes on to give the sum of the figures of the year 1603 from 17th December, 1602, and carries the deaths per week from 21st July down to date, the 20th of October, adding some information for the parishes which kept separate bills, namely, Westminster, the Savoy, Stepney, Newington Butts, Islington, Lambeth and Hackney. This extant weekly bill was probably one of a series ; for Graunt, in his book of 1662, cites various figures of weekly baptisms throughout the year 1603 which would appear to have been taken from the bills for the respective weeks. But the returns had not been made regularly from all the parishes within the Bills from the beginning of the year 1603. The reason why the weekly figures are not recapitulated farther back than the week ending July 21, is that the outparishes had not sent in their returns until that week. From another source, we know the figures for the City and Liberties from March 10 to July 14, and from the same source we obtain the totals for all parishes within the Bills from

---

[1] Broadside in the Guildhall Library, bound up in a volume labelled *Political Tracts*, 1680.

October 19 to the end of the year. By putting these figures into one table, we may represent the mortality of 1603, not indeed completely, as follows:

Weekly Mortalities in London during the plague of 1603.

Week ending	City and Liberties.		Out parishes.		Totals.	
	All causes.	Plague.	All causes.	Plague.	All causes.	Plague.
March 17	108	3				
24	60	2				
31	78	6				
April 7	66	4				
14	79	4				
21	98	8				
28	109	10				
May 5	90	11				
12	112	18				
19	122	22				
26	112	30				
June 2	114	30				
9	134	43				
15	144	59				
23	182	72				
30	267	158				
July 7	445	263				
14	612	424				
21	867	646	319	271	1186	917
28	1312	1025	398	354	1710	1379
Aug. 4	1700	1439	537	464	2237	1901
11	1655	1372	410	361	2065	1733
18	2486	2199	568	514	3054	2713
25	2343	2091	510	448	2853	2539
Sept. 1	2798	2495	587	542	3385	3037
8	2583	2283	495	441	3078	2724
15	2676	2411	433	407	3109	2818
22	2080	1851	376	344	2456	2195
29	1666	1478	295	254	1961	1732
Oct. 6	1528	1367	306	274	1834	1641
13	1109	962	203	184	1312	1146
20	647	546	119	96	766	642
27					625	508
Nov. 3					737	594
10					545	442
17					384	257
24					198	105
Dec. 1					223	102
8					163	55
15					200	96
22					168	74

These figures may be accepted as real, so far as they go; and they give a total (37,192 from all causes, whereof of the plague, 30,519) which is nearly the same as that usually taken, *e.g.* by Graunt, for the mortality of the whole year in all London (37,294 from all causes, whereof of the plague, 30,561). But it is clear that important additions have to be made. In the first place, no deaths are included for the weeks previous to March 10. In the second place, no deaths are included from the out-parishes (within the Bills), previous to July 14. In the third place, no deaths at all are included from Westminster, Stepney, Newington, Lambeth, etc. These omissions have to be kept in mind when the plague of 1603 is compared with those of 1625 and 1665, for which the figures are fully ascertained; and we possess various data from which to supply them approximately. One great addition, with nothing conjectural in it, is for the seven parishes outside the general bill of mortality, Stepney being the largest : they kept their own bills, and the figures from them, for the principal part of the year, are given on the margin of the broadside, as quoted below[1]. Another unconjectural addition is the mortality from all causes in the City and Liberties from December 17, 1602, to March 10, 1603, which was 1375, having been mostly non-plague deaths. All these deaths, actually known, bring the total for the year up to 42,945 whereof of the plague about 33,347. The farther

[1] "The time when it began in the City of Westminster and these places following :
"Buried in Westminster from 14 July to 20 October, in the whole number 832, whereof of the plague 723. Buried in the Savoy from the 1st of June to the 20th of October, in the whole number 182, whereof of the plague, 171. Buried in the parish of Stepney from the 25th of March to the 20th of October, in all 1978, whereof of the plague, 1871. Buried at Newington-buts from the 14th of June to the 20th of October, in all 626, whereof of the plague, 562. Buried at Islington 201 in all, 170 of plague; at Lambeth 373 in all, 362 of plague; at Hackney 192 in all, 169 of plague. Buried in all within the 7 several places last aforenamed 4378, whereof of the plague, 3997. The whole number that hath been buried in all [to 20th October], both within London and the Liberties, and the 7 other severall places last before mentioned is 39,380, whereof of the number of the plague, 32,609."

From the parish registers the burials for the whole year are known : Stepney, 2257; Lambeth, 566; Islington, 322; Hackney, 321 (of plague 269).

In Stow's *Annales*, the mortality of 1603 is given as follows :—"There died in London and the liberties thereof from the xxiii day of December 1602 unto the xxii day of December 1603, of all diseases 38,244, whereof of the plague 30,578."

additions, which can only be guessed, are the mortality from all causes in the eight out-parishes (within the Bills) previous to July 14, and the mortality in the seven other suburban localities (Westminster, Stepney, etc.) before and after the dates stated in the note for each.   Only the former of these additions would have been a considerable figure, the plague being already at 271 deaths a week when the reckoning begins.   Thus the totals, 42,945 burials from all causes, and from plague alone, 33,347, are well within the reality.

Some details are extant of the incidence of the disease in particular parishes at certain dates.   Thus, in the great parish of Stepney, which extended from Shoreditch to Blackwall, 650 plague-deaths, and 24 from other causes, took place in the single month of September; so that, if the plague began in Stepney about the 25th of March, it had not come to a head until autumn.   In St Giles's Cripplegate, the burials entered in the parish register for the whole year are 2879, the highest mortality having been in the beginning of September, when the burials on three successive days were 36, 26 and 26[1].   In the week 13 to 20 October, for which the printed bill is extant, the proportions of the City, Liberties and 8 out-parishes respectively were, for the week, 351, 296, and 119.   Of the parishes without the walls, the most infected were, in their order at that date, St Sepulchre's, St Saviour's, Southwark, St Andrew's, Holborn, St Giles's, Cripplegate, St Clement's Danes, St Giles's in the Fields, St Olave's, Southwark, St Martin's in the Fields, St Mary's, Whitechapel and St Leonard's, Shoreditch.   For St Olave's, Southwark, we have some particulars of the plague from the minister of the parish.

In a dialogue conveying various instructions on the plague[2], to his parishioners of St Olave's, James Bamford states that 2640 had died in that parish from May 7 to the date of writing (October 13), and that the burials had fallen from 305 in a week to 51, and from 57 in a day to 4.   St Olave's was a typical parish of the new London.   It extended eastwards along the

---

[1] Baddeley, *l. c.*

[2] *A short Dialogue concerning the Plague Infection.*   Published to preserue Bloud through the blessing of God.   London, 1603.

Surrey bank of the river from London Bridge, and had been almost all built within the half-century since the purchase of the Borough of Southwark by the City from the Crown in 1550. In Stow's *Survey* of 1598 the parish is thus described: "Then from the bridge along by the Thames eastward is St Olave's Street, having continual building on both the sides, with lanes and alleys, up to Battle Bridge, to Horsedown and towards Rotherhithe some good half mile in length from London Bridge"—the Bermondsey High Street running south from the Horsleydown end of it. St Olave's Church, he continues, stood on the bank of the river, "a fair and meet large church, but a far larger parish, especially of aliens or strangers, and poor people." A mansion of former times, St Leger House, was now "divided into sundry tenements." Over against the church, the great house that was once the residence of the prior of Lewes, was now the Walnut Tree inn, a common hostelry.

London was now so extensive in area that it becomes of interest to know in what part of it the plague broke out, and in what course the infection proceeded. These things are known for the plague of 1665; but for that of 1603 they cannot be ascertained precisely. Dekker is emphatic that it began in the suburbs. The earliest reference to it in the State papers is under the date of April 18, when the Lord Mayor wrote to the Lord Treasurer to inform him of the steps taken to prevent the spread of the plague in the counties of Middlesex and Surrey. "The parishes in Middlesex and Surrey" was an expression which afterwards came to mean a group of twelve out-parishes beyond the Bars of the Freedom, including St Giles's in the Fields, Lambeth, Newington and Bermondsey, Stepney, White-chapel, Shoreditch and Clerkenwell, Islington, Hackney and two others. The phrase used by the mayor may not have had so definite a meaning in 1603, but he can hardly have intended it to apply to the City and Liberties of London, although those were the only divisions of the capital directly under his own jurisdiction. The parish which is associated with the earliest date, in the summary of the epidemic in the broadside of 1603, is Stepney, where the record of deaths from plague and other causes begins from 25th March. It would perhaps be safe to conclude that the plague of 1603 began at the extreme east in Stepney, as that of 1665 certainly did at the extreme west in St Giles's in the Fields.

An examination of the Table shows that the eight out-parishes had reached a higher plague mortality relative to their population on July 21, than the parishes within the bars of the Freedom : but the maximum of deaths falls in both divisions about the same week. We may take it that the plague broke out in one of the suburbs ; and as Dekker speaks of the flight having been westwards, the evidence points on the whole to an eastern suburb, perhaps Whitechapel or Stepney. March is clearly indicated by various things as a time when plague-deaths began to attract notice ; and that date of commencement is corroborated by the following passage from the essay of Graunt, based, it would seem, upon a series of weekly bills :—

"We observe as followeth, viz. First, that (when from December 1602 to March following there was little or no plague) then the christenings at a medium were between 110 and 130 per week, few weeks being above the one or below the other ; but when the plague increased from thence to July, that then the christenings decreased to under 90.... (3) Moreover we observe that from the 21st July to the 12th October, the plague increasing reduced the christenings to 70 at a medium. Now the cause of this must be flying, and death of teeming women" &c.—the total christenings of the year 1603 having been only 4789, as against some 6000 in the year before the plague, and 5458 in the year after it.

This prevalence of plague in the suburbs and liberties of the City in the spring of 1603 coincides with great political events. Queen Elizabeth died at Richmond on the 24th of March, and was buried at Westminster on the 28th of April ; according to Dekker, "never did the English nation behold so much black worn as there was at her funeral." The approach of king James from Scotland appears to have caused an outburst of gaiety, his accession to the crown, according to the same writer, having led to a marked revival of trade : "Trades that lay dead and rotten started out of their trance.... There was mirth in everyone's face, the streets were filled with gallants, tabacconists filled up whole taverns, vintners hung out spick and span new ivy-bushes (because they wanted good wine), and their old rain-beaten lattices marched under other colours, having lost both company and colour before." James made a slow progress from Scotland, paying visits on the way. He arrived at Theobalds, near Cheshunt, on the 3rd of May, and was at Greenwich before the end of the month. On May 29, a proclamation was issued commanding gentlemen to depart the court and city on account of the plague. On June 23, the remainder of Trinity law term was adjourned. On July 10, a letter (one of the series between J. Chamberlain and Dudley Carleton) says: " Paul's grows very thin [the church aisles where people were wont to meet to exchange news], for every man shrinks away. Our pageants are pretty forward, but most of them are such small-timbered gentlemen that they cannot last long, and I doubt, if the plague cease not sooner, they will riot and sink where they stand." The Coronation was shorn of its full splendour. On July 18, it was announced that, as the king could not pass through the City—the traditional route being from the Tower to Westminster—all the customary services by the way are to be performed between Westminster Bridge and the Abbey. The ceremony, thus shortened, took place on July 25. On August 8, it was ordered that all fairs within fifty miles of London should be suspended, the more important being Bartholomew fair at Smithfield, and Stourbridge fair near Cambridge. The new Spanish ambassador was unable to approach the king, who moved from place to place,—Hampton Court, Woodstock and Southampton.

These are the traces left by this great epidemic in the state papers of the time. As in the case of the sweating sickness of 1485, which was in London while the preparations were going on for Henry VII.'s coronation, we should hardly have known from public documents that the City was in a state of panic. But in 1603 we are come to a period when other sources of information are available. It remains to put together what descriptions have come down to us of the City of the Plague.

The most graphic touches are those left by Thomas Dekker, the dramatist, of whom it has been said that " he knew London

as well as Dickens[1]." To describe first the condition of the
" sinfully polluted suburbs," he takes a walk through the still and
melancholy streets in the dead hours of the night.   He hears
from every house the loud groans of raving sick men, the
struggling pangs of souls departing, grief striking an alarum,
servants crying out for masters, wives for husbands, parents for
children, children for their mothers.   Here, he meets some
frantically running to knock up sextons; there, others fearfully
sweating with coffins, to steal forth dead bodies lest the fatal
handwriting of death should seal up their houses.   This would
have been an evasion of the order, dating from 1547, that no
bodies were to be buried between six in the evening and six
in the morning—an order which was exactly reversed in the
plague of 1665.

When morning comes, a hundred hungry graves stand
gaping, and everyone of them, as at a breakfast, hath swallowed
down ten or eleven lifeless carcases ; before dinner, in the same
gulf are twice so many more devoured, and before the sun takes
his rest these numbers are doubled,—threescore bodies lying
slovenly tumbled together in a muck-pit[2] ! One gruesome story
he tells of a poor wretch in the Southwark parish of St Mary
Overy, who was thrown for dead upon a heap of bodies in the
morning, and in the afternoon was found gasping and gaping
for life.   Others were thrust out of doors by cruel masters, to
die in the fields and ditches, or in the common cages or under
stalls.   A boy sick of the plague was put on the water in a
wherry to come ashore wherever he could, but landing was
denied him by an army of brown-bill men that kept the shore,
so that he had to be taken whence he came to die in a cellar.
The sextons made their fortunes, especially those of St Giles's,
Cripplegate, of St Sepulchre's, outside Newgate, of St Olave's

---

[1] *The Wonderfull Yeare* 1603, *wherein is shewed the picture of London lying sicke of
the Plague.* London, 1603.

[2] In his *Seven Deadly Sins of London* (1606) he returns to the mode of burial in
the plague : "All ceremonial due to them was taken away, they were launched ten
in one heap, twenty in another, the gallant and the beggar together, the husband saw
his wife and his deadly enemy whom he hated within a pair of sheets." As an after
effect of this mode of interment, "What rotten stenches and contagious damps would
strike up into thy nostrils !"

in Southwark, of St Clement's at Temple Bar, and of Stepney. Herb-wives and gardeners also prospered; the price of flowers, herbs, and garlands rose wonderfully, insomuch that rosemary, which had wont to be sold for twelve pence an armful, went now for six shillings a handful.

While plague was thus raging in the poor skirts of the City, "paring them off by little and little," the well-to-do within the walls took alarm and fled, "some riding, some on foot, some without boots, some in slippers, by water, by land, swarm they westwards. Hackneys, watermen and waggons were not so terribly employed many a year; so that within a short time there was not a good horse in Smithfield, nor a coach to be set eyes on." But they might just as well have remained as trust themselves to the "unmerciful hands of the country hard-hearted hobbinolls." The sight of a Londoner's flat-cap was dreadful to a lob: a treble ruff threw a whole village into a sweat. A crow that had been seen on a sunshiny day standing on the top of Powles would have been better than a beacon on fire, to have raised all the towns within ten miles of London for the keeping her out. One Londoner set out for Bristol, thinking not to see his home again this side Christmas. But forty miles from town the plague came upon him, and he sought entrance to an inn. When his case was known, the doors of the inn "had their wooden ribs crushed to pieces by being beaten together; the casements were shut more close than an usurer's greasy velvet pouch; the drawing windows were hanged, drawn, and quartered; not a crevice but was stopt, not a mouse-hole left open." The host and hostess tumbled over each other in their flight, the maids ran out into the orchard, the tapster into the cellar. The unhappy Londoner was helped by a fellow-citizen who appeared on the scene, and was carried to die on a truss of straw in the corner of a field; but the parson and the clerk refused him burial, and he was laid in a hole where he had died. According to Stow, Bamford, and Davies of Hereford, such experiences of fugitive Londoners were repeated every-where in the country, and Dekker gives several other tales of the same sort "to shorten long winter nights."

Meanwhile, Dekker goes on, the plague had entered the gates

of the City and marched through Cheapside; men, women, and children dropped down before him, houses were rifled, streets ransacked, rich men's coffers broken open and shared amongst prodigal heirs and unworthy servants. Every house looked like St Bartholomew's Hospital and every street like Bucklersbury: ("the whole street called Bucklersbury," says Stow, "on both sides throughout is possessed of grocers, and apothecaries towards the west end thereof"), for poor Mithridaticum and Dragon-water were bought in every corner, and yet were both drunk every hour at other men's cost. "I could make your cheeks look pale and your hearts shake with telling how some have had eighteen sores at one time running upon them, others ten or twelve, many four and five ; and how those that have been four times wounded by this year's infection have died of the last wound, while others, hurt as often, are now going about whole." Funerals followed so close that three thousand mourners went as if trooping together, with rue and wormwood stuffed into their ears and nostrils, looking like so many boars' heads stuck with branches of rosemary. A dying man was visited by a friendly neighbour, who promised to order the coffin ; but he died himself an hour before his infected friend. A churchwarden in Thames Street, on being asked for space in the churchyard, answered mockingly that he wanted it for himself, and he did occupy it in three days.

One more extract from Dekker will bring us back to the strictly medical history :

"Never let any man ask me what became of our Phisitions in this massacre. They hid their synodical heads as well as the proudest, and I cannot blame them, for their phlebotomies, losinges and electuaries, with their diacatholicons, diacodions, amulets and antidotes, had not so much strength to hold life and soul together as a pot of Pinder's ale and a nutmeg. Their drugs turned to durt, their simples were simple things. Galen could do no more good than Sir Giles Goosecap. Hippocrate, Avicen, Paracelsus, Rasis, Fernelius, with all their succeeding rabble of doctors and water-casters, were at their wits' end ; for not one of them durst peep abroad."

Only a band of desperadoes, he goes on, some few empirical madcaps—for they could never be worth velvet caps—clapped their bills upon every door. But besides the empirical desperadoes, who dared the infection for the sake of the golden harvest, some few physicians and surgeons remained at their post, or at least put out essays with prescriptions and rules of regimen. Three such books on the plague were published in London in 1603, of which the most notable was one by Dr Thomas Lodge[1], a poet like Dekker himself, but of the academical school to which Dekker did not belong. The passage quoted about the impotence of the faculty is perhaps aimed at these books, which all abound with the sayings and maxims of Hippocrates, Galen, Avicenna, and the like, Lodge also quoting the more obscure name of Fernelius, which Dekker has not failed to seize upon.

Lodge confirms the statement about the empirical desperadoes clapping their bills upon every post. One of them, "who underwrit not his bills," posted them close to Lodge's house in Warwick Lane, so that the physician was taken by the populace to be himself the advertiser. He was besieged with applicants for his cordial waters, and wrote his book to make his own position clear, being "aggrieved because of that loathsome imposition which was laid upon me to make myself vendible (which is unworthy a liberal and gentle mind, much more ill-beseeming a physician and philosopher), who ought not to prostitute so sacred a profession so abjectly." Farther confirming Dekker about the greed of the quacks as well as about the strictly business-like attitude of the regular profession, he speaks of "my poor countrymen left without guide or counsel how to succour themselves in extremity ; for where the infection most rageth, there poverty reigneth among the commons, which, having no supplies to satisfy the greedy desires of those that should attend them, are for the most part left desolate to die without relief." The reader must wonder, he says, "why, amongst so many excellent and learned physicians of this city, I alone have undertaken to answer the expectation of the multitude, and to bear the heavy burthen of contentious critiques and depravers." The explanation was that the regular faculty had for the most part gone out of town, along with

---

[1] *A Treatise of the Plague.* By Thomas Lodge, Doctor in Phisicke. London, 1603. It has been reprinted, among Lodge's other works, by the Hunterian Club of Glasgow, 1880.

magistrates, ministers and rich men. Bamford, the minister of St Olave's, Southwark, who remained at his post, has no excuse to offer for magistrates or for his clerical brethren, but he is extremely fair to the doctors: "As for physicians, I only propound this question: Whether they be bound in conscience to be resident, in regard of their profession and ability to do good, or they may use their liberty for themselves and (as they think) for their lives, in regard they are no public persons and live (not by a common stipend but) by what they can get."

Dr Lodge, who dated his book from Warwick Lane on August 19, or when the epidemic would have been at its height, had already won laurels in the field of poetry and romance. He was an Oxonian (Trinity College, 1573) and one of a set with Marlowe and Greene. "At length his mind growing serious," says Anthony Wood, "he studied physic," travelling abroad for the purpose and graduating M.D. at Avignon. He had great success in practice, especially among Catholics, to whom he was suspected of belonging. He died of the plague, during the next great epidemic of 1625, at Low Leyton in Essex. His book on the plague would be entitled to a place in medical literature if only that its style is above the average of medical compositions. I cannot forbear quoting the following collect for its structure and euphony:

" But before I prosecute this my intended purpose, let us invocate and call upon that divine bounty, from whose fountain head of mercy every good and gracious benefit is derived, that it will please him to assist this my labor and charitable intent, and so to order the scope of my indevour, that it may redound to his eternal glory, our neighbours' comfort, and the special benefit of our whole country ; which, being now under the fatherly correction of Almighty God, and punished for our misdeeds by his heavy hand, may through the admirable effects and fruits of the sacred art of physic, receive prevention of their danger, and comfort in this desperate time of visitation. To him therefore, King of kings, invisible and only wise, be all honor, majesty and dominion, now and for ever. Amen."

It is only in dealing with the more public aspects of the plague that Lodge shows any individuality. So far as concerns causes, prognostications, symptoms, remedies, preventives, and precautions, there is little in his essay which is not to be found in the older plague-books, such as the 14th century one of the bishop of Aarhus, his anatomical directions for blood-letting being word for word the same as the bishop's. Some of his points are the same as in Skene's Edinburgh essay of 1568, such as the indication of plague about to begin which is got from rats, moles and other underground creatures forsaking their holes. To keep off the infection he advises the wearing of small cakes of arsenic in the armpits, where the buboes usually came. That Paracelsist practice is known to have been tried at Zurich in 1564; it was one of the matters of dispute between the Galenists and the chemical physicians. During the plague of 1603, Dr Peter Turner published a curious tract in defence of it [1].

From a Venetian gentleman Lodge obtained also the formula of a preservative from infection, which contained, among other things, tormentilla root, white dittany, bole Armeniac and oriental pearl: "The gentleman that gave me this assured me that he had given it to many in the time of the great plague in Venice, who, though continually conversant in the houses of those that were infected, received no infection or prejudice by them."

In his chapter on "The Order and Police that ought to be held in a City during the Plague-time," he advises the removal of the shambles from within the walls to some remote and convenient place near the river of Thames, to the end that the blood and garbage of beasts that are killed may be washed away with the tide. Lodge lived just on the other side of Newgate Street from the shambles, and could speak feelingly about them, as many more had done since Edward III.'s time. The nobles of Arles, he says, had acted so on the advice of

---

[1] *The opinion of Peter Turner, Doctor in Physicke, concerning Amulets or Plague-Cakes, whereof perhaps some hold too much and some too little.* London, 1603, p. 10. Turner held high offices at the College of Physicians, and died in 1614. There was another physician of the name, also a dignitary of the College, Dr George Turner, whose widow was the notorious Mrs Anne Turner, executed for having been an instrument in the poisoning of Sir T. Overbury. Scott has drawn from her the character of Mrs Suddlechop, in *The Fortunes of Nigel*, a work invaluable for realizing the London of King James. The reference in the Earl of Northumberland's accounts, under date Feb. 6, 1607, to a Dr Turner, who was paid ten shillings for a "pomander" against the plague, would suit either Dr Peter or Dr George (*Hist. MSS. Commis.* VI. 2, 29).

Valenolaes, having built their slaughter-houses to the westward of the city upon the river of Rhone. The chief interest of the book is in the sections on preventing the spread of infection. He quotes an instance from Alexander Benedetti of Venice, of a feather-bed, slept on by one in the plague, having been laid aside for seven years, "and the first that slept upon the same at the end of the same term was suddenly surprised with the plague." His directions for the cleansing of houses, bedding, clothes, &c. are minute and thorough (Chapter XVII.) [1]. Modern readers will find his views on isolation and compulsory removal to hospital worth noting. The Pest House, which had been lately built in the fields towards Finsbury, was then the only special hospital to which patients in the plague could be removed, and its accommodation was not great; the burials at it in the nine weeks from July 21 to September 22, 1603, were respectively 18, 18, 12, 21, 12, 6, 5, 10 and 10. The Bridewell near Fleet Street appears also to have admitted a small number of plague-cases, the burials from it in the five weeks from August 18 to September 22, having been respectively 8, 5, 17, 7 and 19. There was also a pest-house in Tothill fields, for the Westminster end of the town. Servants appear to have been mostly sent to these refuges. Lodge saw that the principle of compulsory removal of the sick had no chance without more hospital accommodation (as Defoe also insisted in reviewing the plague of 1665), and he proposes a plan for a pest-house with "twenty-eight to thirty separate chambers on the upper floor, and as many beneath." He is humanely alive to the hardships of compulsory isolation:

"For in truth it is a great amazement, and no less horror, to separate the child from the father and mother, the husband from his wife, the wife from her husband, and the confederate and friend from his adherent and friend; and to speak my conscience in this matter, this course ought not to be kept before that, by the judgment of a learned physician, the sickness be resolved on. And when it shall be found it is infectious, yet it is very needful to use humanity towards such as are seized. And if their parents or friends have the means to succour them, and that freely, and with a good heart they are willing to do the same, those that have the charge to carry them to the

---

[1] A letter from Hampstead, August 27, 1603, speaks of "the imprudent exposure of infected beds in the streets." (*Cal. State Papers.*)

pest-house ought to suffer them to use that office of charity towards their sick, yet with this condition that they keep them apart and suffer them not to frequent and converse with such as are in health. For, to speak the truth, one of the chiefest occasions of the death of such sick folks (besides the danger of their disease) is the fright and fear they conceive when they see themselves devoid of all succour, and, as it were, ravished out of the hands of their parents and friends, and committed to the trust of strangers....And therefore in this cause men ought to proceed very discreetly and modestly."

Another London essay of the same year, by " S. H. Studious in Phisicke " is a much slighter production. The author writes in a superior strain and offers advice " unto such Chirurgeons as shall be called or shall adventure themselves to the care of this so dangerous sickness," one piece of advice being not to let blood except at the beginning of the seizure, and to take then five ounces of blood in the morning, and three ounces more at three in the afternoon, repeating the depletion next day at discretion. He states also the theory of the plague-bubo : it was a way made by nature to expel the venomous and corrupt matter which is noisome unto it. He advises the practice of incising the bubo and of helping it to suppurate, which was the treatment in the Black Death of 1348–49: if nature be "weak and not able to expel the venom fast enough, by insensible transpiration the venom returneth back to the heart and so presently destroyeth nature [1]."

It is significant of the state of medical practice and literature in England at the end of the Elizabethan period that the only other treatise which the plague of 1603 is known to have called forth was a mystification [2] under the name of one Thomas Thayre, chirurgian, " for the benefite of his countrie, but chiefly for the honorable city of London," elaborately dedicated to the Lord Mayor of the year (by name), the Sheriffs and the Aldermen, to whom " Thomas Thayre wisheth all spirituall and temporal blessings." It proves on examination to be a very close reproduction, with some omissions at the end and a

[1] *A New Treatise of the Pestilence, etc. the like not before this time published, and therefore necessarie for all manner of persons in this time of contagion.* By S. H. Studious in Phisicke. London, 1603.

[2] This mystification was pointed out in a note to " Thayre" (the 1625 edition) in the printed Catalogue of the Library of the Royal Medical and Chirurgical Society.

few additions, of the old Treatise of the Pestilence by Thomas Phayre or Phaer, first published in 1547, and was probably the venture of some bookseller or literary hack. The original treatise of Phayre had been reprinted last in 1596, "latelye corrected and enlarged by Thomas Phayre," although that writer must have been dead many years. A reprint of some of "Dr Phaer's" remedies and preservatives, without date, is conjecturally assigned to the year 1601. The original work of Henry VIII.'s time was also a literary compilation, in some parts copied verbatim from the 14th century book by the Danish bishop of Arusia, and bears not a trace of first-hand observation. Yet it had the fortune to be reprinted once more, in 1722, by a physician W. T., who remarked that, as the writers on plague in his own time "usually transcribe from others," he wished to set before them a specimen "of such as have written on a disease of which they were eye-witnesses."

Two printed addresses on the plague by London ministers are extant: one by Henoch Clapham, "to his ordinary hearers," which is merely a sermon, in the form of an epistle, to improve the occasion[1]; and the other by James Bamford, rector of St Olave's, Southwark, in the form of a dialogue, and full of practical and sensible advice[2]. Bamford's tract is especially directed against "that bloody error which denieth the pestilence to be contagious; maintained not only by the rude multitude but by too many of the better sort;" and its chief medical interest lies in the reasons with which he confutes that deadly heresy :—

"Do not the botches, blains and spots (called God's tokens) accompanied with raving and death, argue a stranger [*sic*] infection than that of the leprosy, to be judged by botches and spots? [the infectiousness of leprosy being proved by revelation, Lev. xiii.]. Doth not the ordinary experience of laying live pigeons to plague-sores and taking them presently dead away, and that one after another, demonstrate mortal infection? In that the plague rageth and reigneth especially amongst the younger sort, and such as do not greatly regard clean and sweet keeping, and where many are

---

[1] *An Epistle discoursing upon the present Pestilence, teaching what it is and how the people of God should carrie themselves towards God and their neighbours therein.* Reprinted, with some Additions, by Henoch Clapham. London, 1603.

[2] *A Short Dialogue, etc., ut supra.*

pestered together in alleys and houses—is not this an argument of infection? Thousands can directly tell where, when, and of whom they took the infection....Persons of a tender constitution or corrupt humours sooner take the plague than ·those of a strong constitution and sound bodies. The infirmities of many women in travail, and other diseases, turn into the plague. We see few auncient people die in comparison of children and the younger sort.

"Lastly, of those that keep a good diet, have clean and sweet keeping, live in a good air, use reasonable and seasonable preservatives, and be not pestered many in one house, or have convenient house-room for their household—we see few infected in comparison of those that fail in all these means of preservation and yet will thrust themselves into danger."

The plague of London in 1603 called forth also a poem by John Davies, a schoolmaster of Hereford. It is called "The Triumph of Death; or the Picture of the Plague, according to the Life, as it was in A.D. 1603 [1]." The description is by no means so concrete as the title would have us believe, and might, indeed, have been taken, most of it, at second-hand from Dekker:—

> "Cast out your dead, the carcass-carrier cries,
> Which he by heaps in groundless graves inters....
> The London lanes, themselves thereby to save,
> Did vomit out their undigested dead,
> Who by cart-loads are carried to the grave,
> For all those lanes with folk were overfed."

He mentions that the prisoners in the gaols were comparatively exempt from plague [2]. One line suggests the great size that the plague-buboes sometimes reached:

> "Here swells a botch as high as hide can hold."

Perhaps his particulars of the plague in the provinces, in 1603 and following years, are from his own knowledge. Both the Universities, he says, were forsaken.

> "Each village free now stands upon her guard....
> The haycocks in the meads were oft opprest
> With plaguy bodies, both alive and dead,
> Which being used confounded man and beast."

One incident he vouches for (in a marginal note) as having

---

[1] In a volume with other pieces. London, 1605.
[2] But several warders in the Tower died of it. (*Cal. State Papers*, Sept. 16, 1603.)

occurred at Leominster : A person with the plague was drowned
to prevent infection, by the order of Sir Herbert Croft, one of
the Council of the Marches of Wales.

The Plague of 1603 in the country near London.

Most of the country parishes nearest to London had plague-
burials in 1603, doubtless from the escape of infected Londoners
to them and from the spreading of the infection.   In several of
these parish registers[1] the plague-deaths in 1603 are more than
in the time of the Great Plague of 1665 : there is a note in the
Croydon register that " many died in the highways near the
city."   The following table shows the mortalities, great and
small.

	Burials from all causes.	Burials from plague.		Burials from all causes.	Burials from plague.
Barking	381	—	Hackney	321	269
Battersea	23	—	Hampstead	7	—
Beckenham	24	—	Isleworth	75	—
Bromley	26	—	Islington	322	—
Cheam	13	9	Kensington	32	—
Chigwell	28	—	Lambeth	566	—
Chiselhurst	62	—	Lewisham	117	—
Clapham	20	mostly plague	Romford	122	—
Croydon	—	158	Stratford	130	89
Deptford	235	—	Streatham	36	—
Ealing	136	—	Tottenham	79	44
Edmonton	145	85	Twickenham	—	67
Eltham	52	17	Wandsworth	—	100
Enfield	253	129	Wimbledon	21	—
Finchley	51	38			

A comparison of these figures with those of 1665 will show
that the northern parishes, Islington and Hackney, as well
as parishes farther out in the country, such as Enfield,
had more plague-deaths in 1603 than in the time of the
Great Plague.   Also Barking, Stratford and Romford on the
one side, and Lewisham, Eltham and Croydon on the other, had

---

[1] In Lysons, *Environs of London.*

heavier mortalities in the earlier year. It would appear, indeed, that the infection in the country near London had been attracting notice before the plague in the capital caused any alarm. On April 18, 1603, the lord mayor wrote to the Privy Council concerning the steps that had been taken " to prevent the spread of the plague in the counties of Middlesex and Surrey." On July 20, 1603, the king issued a warrant to the constables and others of the hundred of Twyford in Kent, to levy a special rate on certain parishes to relieve the sufferers by a grievous plague in the villages of West Malling, East Malling, Offham, and seven others[1]. Such rates were usually levied when an epidemic was nearly over; so that the outbreak in Kent must have been at least as early as that in London.

The towns and villages of Hertfordshire, which were favourite resorts of Londoners in plague-time, had their share of the visitation in 1603. At Great Amwell, there were 41 burials in the year, of which 19 were of the plague between August 19 and November 28, 6 of them in one day. Doubtless the registers of other parishes in the home counties would show a similar history if they were searched[2].

Annual Plague in London after 1603.

Before following the plague of 1603 into the provinces, it will be convenient to give the history of the infection in London for the next few years. There was little plague in 1604 and not much in 1605; but in 1606 the infection again became active, and continued at its endemic level for some five or six years. The following table, from the weekly bills of mortality, shows how regularly the infection came to a height in the autumn year after year, as if it had been a product of the soil[3] :

---

[1] *Hist. MSS. Com.* x. pt. 4, p. 5.

[2] E.g. plague at Datchet (*Notes and Queries*, 3rd ser. VI. 217).

[3] John Bell, *London's Remembrancer.* London, 1665 [1666].

Table, from the Weekly Bills of Mortality (London), showing the increase of Plague in Autumn, for five successive years.

	1606	1607	1608	1609	1610
Total deaths from plague in the year	2124	2352	2262	4240	1803
Weekly deaths in					
July	25	27	16	60	38
	33	33	26	57	45
	50	37	24	58	45
	46	51	50	91	40
	66	43			
August	67	77	45	100	47
	75	69	70	126	50
	85	76	79	101	73
	85	71	73	150	60
				177	99
Sept.	116	105	123	141	96
	105	121	136	158	89
	92	114	107	210	86
	87	177	143	144	72
			147		
Oct.	141	150	103	154	63
	106	113	131	177	79
	117	110	124	131	59
	109	82	102	55	49
	101	68			
Nov.	68	66	109	84	58
	41	55	72	69	40
	78	46	69	67	22
	72	21	70	59	42
				51	39

In Dekker's *Seven Deadly Sins of London,* published in 1606, he returns to the subject of the plague. He says that it still slays hundreds in a week, a statement which will be seen to be an exaggeration by reference to the Table. But, on another point, Dekker would have been correctly informed. The play-houses, he says, stand empty, with the doors locked and the flag taken down. The policy of forbidding plays during plague-time, or when the infection threatened to be active, was advocated by the Puritan clergy as early as 1577, and had been in force in the plague of 1563. "Plaies are banished for a time out of London," says Harrison in 1572, "lest the resort unto them should ingender a plague, or rather disperse it being already begonne¹." In a sermon preached at Paul's Cross on Sunday, November 3, 1577, in the time of the plague, by T. W., on the text "Woe to that abominable, filthy and cruel city," the preacher exclaims, " Behold the sumptuous theatre-houses, a continual monument of London's prodigal folly! But I understand they are now forbidden because of the plague²." By the year 1581 the lord mayor had become a zealous supporter of the Puritan demands for the stopping of plays in the City and in the Liberties³. In July(?), 1603, James I. granted a licence to players for performances in the Curtain and Boar's Head theatres, "as soon as the plague decreases to 30 deaths per week in London⁴." In the beginning of winter, 1607, on the subsidence of plague, the theatres were permitted to be opened, so that the "poor players," might make a living; but as the plague revived in 1608, and became still more serious in 1609, it is tolerably certain that the theatres were shut during the whole summer and autumn of those years.

Those years, from 1606 to 1610, when the actor's and dramatist's profession was seriously hindered by the fear of plague, correspond to a blank period in the personal history of Shakespeare. It has been conjectured that he retired from London for a time, before his final retirement to Stratford-on-Avon. At all events his occupation, if not gone, was greatly interfered with in every one of the years from 1603 to 1610, excepting perhaps the years 1604 and 1605, which would hardly have come within the limit of 30 plague-deaths in a week. In 1604 his name is joined in a patent with that of Laurence Fletcher for the Globe theatre. Plays continued to be acted in the plague-years, before the court or in the houses of the nobility; but the applause of the pit and gallery would have been wanting. *Macbeth,* which is supposed, from its subject, to have been written to celebrate the accession of the king of Scots to the English crown was not put on the stage until 1610 or 1611.

---

¹ Extracts from *Harrison's MS. Chronologie* by Furnivall in Appendix (p. 268) to *Elizabethan England.* Camelot Series, 1890.

² *A Sermon preached at Powles Crosse,* etc. London, 1578.

³ *Remembrancia* (numerous extracts from the City records, under "Plays").

⁴ *Cal. State Papers,* Addenda, James I. p. 534.

King Lear was given before the court at Christmas 1606. One of the quartos of *Troilus and Cressida*, published in 1609, with the author's name, has a note to say that "this new piece had never been staled with the stage, never clapper-clawed by the palms of the vulgar;" but another edition of the same year (1609) omitting the preface, bears on the title that the piece had been played at the Globe theatre by the king's servants, from which it is inferred that it had been acted in the interval between the two editions of 1609. After 1610, and continuously so until 1625, there was no plague in London to interfere with the business of actors and play-writers, just as the period from 1594 to 1603 was a clear interval. The earlier time of freedom was the great period of the drama in London. The disastrous plague of 1603 and the successive unhealthy summers and autumns until 1610 seriously interfered with it, and seriously interfered, also, with Shakespeare's active share in the production of plays on the stage. Whatever writing he did after that would have been with a less certain prospect of representation, or, one may say, was not done under the same direct influence of playhouse atmosphere which inspired his earlier comedies and historical plays.

Plague in the Provinces in 1603 and following years.

Returning now to 1603, to follow the infection into towns and villages in the provinces, we find first that the plague had been active in some provincial parts of England for several months before it broke out severely in London in 1603. At Chester the great epidemic, referred to in the sequel, began in September, 1602. At Stamford, an epidemic which eventually carried off nearly 600 is heard of first on December 2, 1602, when the corporation resolved to build a "cabbin" for the plague-stricken, and again in January, 1603, when a fourth part of a fifteenth was levied for their relief and maintenance[1].

At Oxford, which was one of the towns earliest and most

---

[1] *Notes and Queries*, 6th series, II. 524. The mortality is stated on the authority of the parish registers of St George's and St Michael's, the dead having been "buried at the cabbin of Whitefryers."

severely smitten, after London, the disease was first seen in July, 1603, and was supposed to have been spread abroad by the "lewd and dissolute behaviour of some base and unruly inhabitants." In September the colleges broke up, having made a collection for the relief of the plague-stricken town's people before leaving. The Michaelmas term was prorogued until December 5, but very few came to the congregation, the plague not ceasing until February. Anthony Wood says:

"The truth is, the times were very sad, and nothing but lamentation and bemoanings heard in the streets. Those that had wealth retired into the country, but those that were needy were, if not taken away by death, almost starved, and so consequently ready to mutiny against their superiors for relief." All the gates of colleges and halls were constantly kept shut day and night, a few persons being left in them to keep possession. The shops of the town were closed, none but the attendants on the sick or the collectors for them were to be seen stirring abroad, the churches were seldom or never open for divine service.

The plague having ceased in February most of the scholars came back, and in April the infection broke out again, but was prevented from spreading. The court was at Oxford in 1604, and plague broke out after it left, the infected being sent, as before, to the house in Portmead and to the cabins. Among the deaths was that of the Principal of Hart Hall, apparently in August. It broke out once more in March, 1605, but did not spread, whether owing to the measures that were taken or to natural causes may remain doubtful[1]. From that date Oxford had a twenty years' immunity, until 1625. The Cambridge annals are less full, partly, perhaps, because none of the colleges kept a register on the plan of that of Merton College; but it appears from a letter assigned to 1608 that the Visitor of King's College had been unable to come to the college to exercise his much-needed authority, "in regard of the infection[2]."

The severity of plague in 1603 among the provincial towns and country parishes is known accurately for only a few of them. From a considerable number more there is evidence of

[1] There is *An Account of the Plague at Oxford,* 1603, in the Sloane MS. No. 4376 (14), extracted from the register of Merton College, which had also been the source of Anthony Wood's account, as summarised in the text.
[2] *Cal. State Papers.* Addenda, 1580–1625.

outbreaks of one degree or another. Thus at Canterbury, the
accounts of the corporation contain entries of sums paid for
watching shut-up houses, for carrying out the dead, and the
like, during twenty-four weeks in 1603-4[1]. At Exeter, a pest-
house had to be provided, and the fairs were not kept[2]. Similar indications of plague come from Winchester[3], Colchester[4],
Ipswich[5], Norwich[6], Boston[7], and Newcastle[8]. The register of a
parish in Derbyshire (Brimington) contains plague-deaths in the
end of 1602[9].

For Chester there are full particulars of a great plague. It
began in September, 1602, in a glover's house in St John's Lane,
where 7 died, and kept increasing until the weekly deaths
reached 60. In 1603 there died of the plague 650, and of other
diseases 61. In 1604 the plague-deaths were 986, of which 55
were in one week. From October 14, 1604, to March 20, 1605,
812 died, and about 100 more until the 9th January, 1606, when
the infection ceased for a time. Cabins outside the city were
erected for the plague-stricken. In some houses, especially of
sailors, five or six of the same family died in the course of two or
three weeks[10].

It appears to have been in Nantwich and Northwych in one
or more of the years 1603-1605, a rate for relief of the poor in
them having been ordered on June 22, 1605. Plague-deaths
occur in the registers of Macclesfield and Congleton in 1603.
At Stockport 51 were buried of plague from October 9, 1605, to
August 14, 1606, most of them in the latter year[11]. Straggling
epidemics are also reported from Northamptonshire—31 burials
from plague at Merston Trussell in 1604, and 16 at Eydon in
1605[12].

One of the severest epidemics of the period occurred at York
in 1604. The markets were closed, the courts adjourned

[1] *Hist. MSS. Commis.* IX. 160.
[2] Izacke's 'Memorials of Exeter' (in *N. and Q.*, 3rd ser. VI. 217).
[3] Bailey, *Transcripts from the MS. Archives of Winchester*, 1856, p. 109.
[4] Cromwell.   [5] *Hist. MSS. Commis.* IX.   [6] *Ibid.* X. pt. 1, p. 89.
[7] Thompson's *Boston.*   [8] *Hist. MSS. Com.* IX.   [9] *Archæologia*, VI. 80.
[10] Rogers' MS. in Hemingway's *Hist. of Chester.* Harl. MS. 2177.
[11] Earwaker, *East Cheshire*, II. 471; I. 406.
[12] Bridges and Whalley, II. 53; I. 124.

to Ripon and Durham, and the Minster and Minster-yard closely shut up. The infected were housed in booths on Hobmoor and Horsefair. The number of those who died is put down at 3512[1]. Durham also had a visitation in St Giles's parish, but a minor one[2].

At Shrewsbury, however, the plague of 1604 was on the same disastrous scale as at Chester and York, the deaths in the five parishes from June 2, 1604, to April 6, 1605, having been 667. On October 11, 1604, a proclamation was issued against buying or receiving apparel, bedding, etc., as it was suspected that plague spread greatly in the town by such means[3]. A weekly tax was levied upon the inhabitants of Manchester, sometime previous to 1606, for the relief of the poor infected, or suspected of being infected, with the plague[4]. It was in Nottingham in 1604, and in at least one of the parishes in the county (Holme Pierrepont)[5].

There are few parts of England from which evidence of plague does not come in the years immediately following the great plague in London in 1603. To those already mentioned we have to add Cranborne, in Dorset, where 71 died of plague (in a total of 91) from June to December, 1604, six deaths having occurred in the family first infected and eight in another[6]. The parish register of Monkleigh in North Devon has the words "cessat pestis" opposite the entry of a burial on March 30, 1605[7]. In 1606 Peterborough was visited, the infection lasting "until the September following[8]." In 1606 Eton also was "visited," as appears from payments made[9].

In the years 1606–1610, as we have seen, the plague in London occurred as a regular product of the summer and autumn seasons. The outbreak in 1608 has left several traces in the state letters[10]. On September 12, Lord Chancellor Ellesmere writes from Ashridge (Berkhamstead) to the Secretary

---

[1] Drake's *Eboracum.* Lond. 1736, p. 121.
[2] Sykes, *Local Records of Northumberland and Durham.*
[3] Phillips, Owen and Blakeway.
[4] *Cal. State Papers.* Addenda, 1580–1625.
[5] Parish Register (in a local history).   [6] *Notes and Queries*, 6th ser. II. 390.
     [7] *Ib.*   [8] *Ib.*   [9] *Ib.*   [10] *Cal. State Papers*, 1608-9.

of State that he will remain away until he is fully sure of his London house being clear of the infection. On September 20 the City ditch was being cleaned out, and Parliament was put off until February. On November 26 a letter from the court at Newmarket states that the king is angry that my Lord Chamberlain has not sent him the bill of sickness. In 1609 there were 13 plague-deaths in Enfield parish, and in 1610 some suspicious cases near Theobalds.

In the provinces there is no record of plague again until 1608: at Chester, in that year, 14 died of it "at the Talbot[1]." In 1609 the infection was at work in a number of provincial centres. On June 1 a letter from Rochester reports it prevalent in Kent, impeding the work of the Commissioners for the Aid. On June 15 the Commissioners at Hereford request farther time on account of the plague. On August 22 the king's tenants of Long Bennington, near Grantham, are brought to great poverty by the plague[2]. These accounts relate to the counties of Hereford, Lincoln and Kent, and with the last may be taken the brief reference to plague at Sandwich[3]. Other counties affected in 1609, perhaps only at a few spots, are Derbyshire, Norfolk, Northumberland, and Leicestershire. In the first, there died at Chesterfield a few persons of the plague from March 18 until May; at Belper, 51 between May 1 and September 30; and at Holmesfield, the curate on March 12[4]. At Norwich the outbreak of 1609 was slight compared with other experiences of that city[5]. Its existence at Newcastle the same year is known only from the register of St Nicholas parish[6].

The plague in Loughborough was one of the severer kind. The first case of it appears to have been on the 24th August, 1609, in a woman who had given birth to a child on the 19th. The last plague entry in the parish register is on February 19, 1611; so that the epidemic went on for about eighteen months. During that time the whole mortality was 452, of which by far the most were plague-burials. Within a mile of Loughborough is a spot of ground, long after known as the Cabbin Lees,

---

[1] Hemingway.   [2] *Cal. S. P.*   [3] *Hist. MSS. Com.* v. 570.
[4] *Archæologia*, vi. 80.   [5] Blomefield.   [6] Sykes.

whereon many of the inhabitants "prudently built themselves huts and encamped to avoid the infection[1]."

In Leicester there was a slight amount of plague in 1607, and it reappeared in 1608 (payments on account of it in the former year, and an item of "30 hurdells used at the visited houses" in the accounts of 1608). A more severe outbreak occurred in 1610 and 1611, during and after the great plague at Loughborough. The streets lying towards the Castle were exempt; a pest-house was built in Belgrave Gate; the burials for 1610 were 82 in St Martin's parish alone (more than half being from plague), and in 1611 the same parish had 128 burials[2].

In 1610 the infection was at work in one or more villages of the county of Durham; 78 deaths "of the pestilence" occur in the register of Lamesley parish, and the same year was probably one of the numerous plague seasons down to 1647 in Whickham parish, where it is said that the people, perhaps the plague-stricken, lived in huts upon Whickham Fell[3]. At Chester in 1610 "many died of the plague[4]"; and at Evesham there was a visitation which caused the wealthier inhabitants to leave the town and the authorities to effect a much-needed improvement in the cleanliness of the streets (swine found at large to be impounded, stones, timber, dunghills and carrion to be removed from the streets, and the paving in front of each house to be repaired and cleansed once a week)[5].

Between 1610 and 1625, which was an almost absolutely clear interval for London, there are few accounts of plague from the provinces. In 1611, moneys were levied for "the visited" at Sherborne[6], and there was a local rate for the same class at Canterbury in 1614–15[7]. Accounts of the same kind for Coventry probably belong to the year 1613[8]. Then, as we come near the next great plague-period, which began with the new reign in 1625, we find an entry of 26 plague-deaths at Banbury in 1623, "recorded in a part of the original register

[1] Nichols, III. 892–3.

[2] Nichols (parish registers); Kelly, *Trans. Roy. Hist. Soc.*, 1877, VI. 395.

[3] Sykes.   [4] Hemingway.   [5] May, *Hist. of Evesham*, 1845, p. 371.

[6] Add. MS. 29,975. f. 25.   [7] *Hist. MSS. Com.* IX. 162.   [8] *Ib.* I. 101.

which has not been transcribed into the parchment copy[1]:" if the date be correct, Banbury was the first town to break the somewhat prolonged truce with the plague, which became broken all over the country in 1625. There appears also to have been distress in Grantham from sickness of some kind in 1623; in September of that year the corporation of Stamford made a collection "in this dangerous time of visitation," and sent £10 of it to Grantham, the rest to go "to London or some other town as occasion offered." But the years 1623 and 1624 were so much afflicted with fevers that the "dangerous time of visitation" may not have meant plague.

Ireland.

The accounts for Ireland are so casual that one suspects there may have been more plague in that country than the records show. Thus, on January 25, 1604, there is a municipal order at Kilkenny, for men to stand at every gate to keep out all strangers or suspected persons that might come from any infected place within the kingdom; and on October 24 there is another order, from which it appears that the plague was then in the town, that it was needful to have the sick persons removed to remote places, that no dung should be in the open streets before the doors, and that no hogs should go or lie in the streets[2]. Towards the end of 1607 and beginning of 1608 there was a "most dreadful pestilence" in the city of Cork, which "by degrees ceased of itself[3]."

Plague in Scotland, 1603-24.

The history of the plague in Scotland, which we left in a former chapter at the year 1603, begins again in that year and goes on at one place or another continuously until 1609. From June, 1603, until February, 1604, it continued in the south of Scotland. At Edinburgh, in April, 1604, the house of Mr

---

[1] Beesley, *Hist. of Banbury.*
[2] Dean Butler's notes to Clyn's and Dowling's *Annals.*
[3] Smith's *Cork,* from MS. Annals.

John Hall was "clengit," because a servant woman's death was suspected of the plague: which infection certainly spread in May and became so severe in July that people fled the city[1]. A letter of July 18 from Codrus Cottage, relating to gold-mining, and making mention of Closeburn, says that the plague is amongst the men[2].

In 1605, towards the end of July, the infection reappeared at Edinburgh, Leith, and St Andrews[3]. On October 7, the chancellor of Scotland, Lord Dunfermline, wrote to the earl of Salisbury that the plague was rife in the small towns about Edinburgh, probably its old favourite seats along the Firth and on the Fife coast[4]. The chancellor himself, as we know from another source, had had a sad experience of it in his own house; his son and niece had died of the plague, and his daughter "had the boils" but recovered[5]. The next year, 1606, was the worst of this plague-period in Scotland: "It raged so extremely in all the corners of the kingdoms that neither burgh nor land in any part was free. The burghs of Ayr and Stirling were almost desolate, and all the judicatures of the land were deserted[6]." It is to this epidemic that a curious transaction, discovered by Chambers, seems to belong. Two houses, on the line of the great road from the south towards Aberdeen, situated on opposite sides of the Dee, the one being the house of a proprietor and the other of a minister, were suspected of having received the infection. The gentlemen of the county met and resolved to send to Dundee for two professional "clengers" or disinfectors, giving a bond to the borough of Dundee for 500 merks for the services of its "clengers[7]."

In April of the year following, 1607, we hear of the plague in Dundee itself, despite the experts, as well as in Perth and other places[8]. In July, 1608, many houses in Dundee were infected, and so many magistrates dead that new appointments were made by the Privy Council[9]. It broke out again at Perth

[1] Chambers, *Domestic Annals.*   [2] *Cal. State Papers.*
[3] Chambers.   [4] *Cal. State Papers.*
[5] Balfour's *Annals of Scotland* (in Chambers, I. 399).
[6] *Ibid.*   [7] Chambers.
[8] *Aberdeen Burgh Records.*   [9] Chambers.

on August 29, and continued till May, 1609, "wherein deit young and auld 500 persons[1]."

Until 1624 there is no other Scottish reference to plague except an entry, November 7, 1609, touching the arrival at Leith of a vessel from the Thames, with some of her crew dead of the plague, and the quarantining of her at Inchkeith[2]. Edinburgh had a small outbreak the year before the next great English plague that we come to. On November 23, 1624, the infection was discovered to be in several houses, and the session of the law courts was adjourned to January 8[3]; but Scotland appears to have had no part in the great infection of English soil which immediately followed.

Malignant Fever preceding the Plague of 1625.

The period of immunity from plague both in London and in the provinces, which began about 1611, was at length broken in 1625. The health of London, and of country districts as well, had not been good for two years before, but plague was not the reigning type of disease. Thus, in London, the burials rose from 8959 in 1622, to 11,102 in 1623 and to 12,210 in 1624. The letters of the time enable us to see what it was that disturbed the public health. On August 21, 1624, Chamberlain writes from London to Dudley Carleton[4]:

"We had 328 died this week, a greater number than hath been these fifteen or sixteen years, and yet no mention of plague. God keep it from among us, for we are in danger. But this spotted fever is cousin-german to it at least, and makes as quick riddance almost. The Lady Hatton hath two or three of her children sick of it at her brother Fanshaw's, in Essex, and hath lost her younger daughter, that was buried at Westminster on Wednesday night by her father; a pretty gentlewoman, much lamented." Again, on September 4: "We have here but a sickly season, which is easily seen by the weekly mounting of our bill, which is come this last week to 407, and yet we will acknowledge no infection [i.e., of plague]. Indeed, by

---

[1] *Chron. of Perth.*   [2] Chambers.   [3] *Ibid.*

[4] The invaluable letters of Chamberlain, as well as those of Mead (of Cambridge) and others, were collected by Dr Thomas Birch in the last century, and printed in 1848 under the titles *The Court and Times of James I.*, and *C. and T. Charles I.*, without an index but with some useful notes.

the particulars we find about 250 of them to be children, most of the rest carried away by this spotted fever, which reigns almost everywhere, in the country as ill as here...The mortality is spread far and near, and takes hold of whole households in many places." On October 9: "The town continues sickly still, for this week there died 347." On October 23 we hear of the Lord Keeper being "troubled with the fluent disease of the time"—the flux, or flix. On December 18 (as well as previously on August 21) a cure of smallpox is mentioned in a person of quality.

These, then, were the prevalent types of epidemic sickness, in the houses of the great as well as among the poor—spotted fever or typhus, dysentery or flux, and smallpox. Two of these continued into the plague-year, 1625, as Taylor, the Water-poet, says of that occasion:

"Thou see'st the fearful plague, the flix and fever,
Which many a soul doth from the body sever."

An eminent victim of the "pestilent fever" was the marquis of Hamilton, who died of it while at Moor Park, Rickmansworth, on Ash-Wednesday, 1625[1]. His residence in London was the house called Fisher's Folly (mentioned by Stow) outside Bishopsgate in a parish which was now "pestered" with tenements of the poor.

The fever was not always called the spotted fever. It may have been the same disease that is often spoken of under the name of ague—"the ague with a hundred names," as Abraham Holland says (1625). Thus, Mead, of Christ's College, Cambridge, writes on September 4, 1625: "Agues grow wonderfully rife both here and everywhere; so that one told me yesterday that about Royston and Barkway they wanted help to gather their harvest out of the fields"—perhaps the same sort of "burning fever" which we shall have to trace a few pages later, both in town and country, in time of peace as well as in the Civil Wars, the type of sickness which became the common one in England when the plague had ceased, reaching its highest point in the 18th century. But here again we meet the old difficulty of "influenza."

These historical glimpses of spotted fevers, or pestilent fevers, in the houses of the great, as well as among the common

---

[1] Chamberlain to Carleton, *C. and T. James I.,* II. 504.

people, are in accordance not only with the London bills of mortality for the respective years, but also with the registers of country parishes and market towns as abstracted by the laborious Dr Short. Repeating the form of table used in a former chapter, which dealt with the epidemic years 1557–8 and 1580–82, we find the years 1623–25 distinguished as follows:

Country Parishes.

Year.	No. of registers examined	No. of unhealthy parishes	Baptised in same	Buried in same
1622	85	11	177	223
1623	84	30	601	836
1624	87	19	362	511
1625	88	13	246	327

Market Towns.

Year	No. of registers examined	No. of unhealthy towns	Baptised in same	Buried in same
1622	25	4	345	442
1623	25	16	439	2254
1624	25	9	714	978
1625	25	9	563	666

The incidence upon the year 1623 is the more noteworthy as there appears to be no record of plague in England that year in its more usual seats, except an entry in a parish register at Banbury. Fever, we may take it, was the prevalent epidemic types both in London and provincial places, urban and rural. In his other treatise Short calls it "malignant spotted fever," and refers specially to the parish registers of Keswick, Penrith, and Wigton for its prevalence in 1623[1].

Chamberlain, in the letter of August 21, 1624, says the spotted fever was cousin-german at least to the plague; and therein he expressed as a layman an opinion which was afterwards formally expounded by Willis Sydenham and Morton. Along with the flux and the smallpox it stood for the unhealthiness of London in 1623 and 1624 and the first months of

---

[1] *Chronological History of the Air, Weather, Seasons, Meteors, etc.* 2 vols. Lond. 1749, I. 306:—"This fever began, and raged terribly in England in 1623; was little, if at all, short of the plague."

1625, just as the trio were the chief causes of epidemic mortality in the capital in the latter part of the seventeenth century and throughout the whole of the eighteenth. But in 1625 London was not yet done with plague. As the year passed from spring into summer, the spotted fever did not, indeed, cease (as we may infer from casual references and from the known facts of the analogous plague-years, 1636 and 1665); but it was soon overtaken, surpassed, and eclipsed by the greater infection, the old "common infection" of the sixteenth century, the bubo-plague itself. To explain the existence of typhus in the Liberties and out-parishes of London in 1623 and 1624, we find ready to hand the evidence of overcrowding while the plague was quiet from 1611; the births in 1624 were about half as many again as immediately before the last great plague of 1603, and the deaths were twice as many. The fringe of poverty had grown once more, despite the epidemic checks of flux, fever and smallpox: the harvest was ready for the sickle, and the reaping took place in the summer and autumn of 1625. The infection of plague was lurking in London, as it had been for nearly three centuries; but it depended for its activity upon the times and seasons, and the season of 1625 was a favourable one.

The London Plague of 1625.

The previous summer of 1624 had been unusually hot and dry. The weather in October was exceptionally fine, and the fruit crop was abundant. In January the weather was warm and mild. On February 25 there occurred one of those very high tides that come perhaps once in a generation. Thames Street was wrecked, Westminster Hall was "full three feet in water all over. But the greater loss we hear of in the drowning of marshes, and overthrowing the walls in Kent, Essex, Lincoln-shire, Yorkshire, and other places near the sea[1]." For the first three months of 1625 the deaths from plague were two or three in a week, some weeks being clear. In the last week of March they were 11, and in the week after, 10. In the last week of

---

[1] Chamberlain to Carleton, in *Court and Times of Charles I.*, 1. 28.

May they were 69, reported from twenty parishes. The spring is described by the Water-poet as "wholesome;" but the early summer was unusually cold. On June 12 Chamberlain writes: "We have had for a month together the extremest cold weather ever I knew in this season." The whole month of June was a time of "ceaseless rain in London[1]." In the country, the hay-harvest was spoilt, and the corn-harvest was only a half crop[2]. Another says (in verse), that the summer sun wore sallow hair and a languishing complexion; the air was full of black mists and damp, with no dewdrops at night, but a vaporous smoke[3]. The following table of the weekly burials (with christenings) in London will show how the plague increased after the rains of June. The mortality of May and June had been a good deal higher for the season than in the moderate endemic years of plague, such as the last series from 1606 to 1611; but it was not until July that a plague of the first degree declared itself.

A Table of the Christenings and Mortality in London for the year 1625[4].

Week ending	Christened	Buried	Of Plague	Parishes Infected
Dec. 23	165	183	0	0
30	176	211	0	0
Jan. 6	199	220	1	1
13	194	196	1	1
20	160	240	0	0
27	178	226	0	0
Feb. 3	178	174	3	1
10	161	204	5	2
17	181	211	3	1
24	190	252	1	1
Mar. 3	185	207	0	0
10	196	210	0	0
17	175	262	4	3
24	187	226	8	2
31	133	243	11	4
Apr. 7	184	239	10	4
14	154	256	24	10
21	160	230	25	11
28	134	305	26	9

[1] Salvetti's Diary, in *Hist. MSS. Com.* XI. pt. 1, p. 26.
[2] *Cal. S. P.* 15 Sept.　　　　　　　　　　[3] Holland.
[4] Bell, *London's Remembrancer.*

Week ending	Christened	Buried	Of Plague	Parishes Infected
May 5	158	292	30	10
12	140	332	45	13
19	182	379	71	17
26	145	401	78	16
June 2	123	395	69	20
9	125	434	91	25
16	110	510	165	31
23	110	640	239	32
30	125	942	390	50
July 7	114	1222	593	57
14	115	1741	1004	82
21	137	2850	1819	96
28	155	3583	2471	103
Aug. 4	128	4517	3659	114
11	125	4855	4115	112
18	134	5205	4463	114
25	135	4841	4218	114
Sept. 1	117	3897	3344	117
8	112	3157	2550	116
15	100	2148	1674	107
22	75	1994	1551	111
29	78	1236	852	103
Oct. 6	77	838	538	99
13	85	815	511	91
20	91	651	331	76
27	77	375	134	47
Nov. 3	82	357	89	41
10	85	319	92	35
17	88	274	48	22
24	88	231	27	16
Dec. 1	93	190	15	12
8	90	181	15	7
15	94	168	6	5
	6983	54265	35417	

The deaths from all causes in May and June were so many more than the reported plague-deaths could account for that those who watched the bills of mortality (Mead at Cambridge, Salvetti in London) suspected that plague was being concealed. " It is a strange reckoning," says Mead of the bill for the week ending June 30: " Are there some other diseases as bad and spreading as the plague, or is there untrue dealing in the account[1]?" Probably there were both; at the end of the year the deaths from all causes were some 20,000 more than the plague accounted for; and at least half of that excess was extra to the ordinary mortality. The spotted fever and the flux

[1] *C. and T. Charles I.,* letter of 2 July, 1625.

doubtless continued side by side with the plague, having been its forerunners. The parishes most affected were, as in 1603, St Giles's, Cripplegate, St Olave's, Southwark, St Sepulchre's, without Newgate, and St Mary's, Whitechapel, corresponding to the mazes of lanes and twisting passages, "pestered" with the tenements of the poorer class, of which only a few examples now remain from 18th century London. The following are the parishes with greatest mortality, in their order (Bell):

	Total deaths	Plague deaths
St Giles's, Cripplegate	3988	2338
St Olave's, Southwark	3689	2609
St Sepulchre's, Newgate	3425	2420
St Mary's, Whitechapel	3305	2272
St Saviour's, Southwark	2746	1671
St Botolph's, Aldgate	2573	1653
St Botolph's, Bishopsgate	2334	714
St Andrew's, Holborn	2190	1636
St Leonard's, Shoreditch	1995	1407
St George's, Southwark	1608	912
St Bride's, Fleet St.	1481	1031
St Martin's in the Fields	1470	973
St Giles's in the Fields	1333	947
St Clement's Danes	1284	755
St James's, Clerkenwell	1191	903
St Magdalen's, Bermondsey	1127	889
St Katharine's, Tower	998	744
St Dunstan's in the West	860	642
97 parishes within the walls	14342	9197

The original printed bill of the Parish Clerks is extant for the worst week but one, August 4th to 11th[1]. Its mortalities for the week in each of the 122 parishes are almost exactly in the order of the final summation for the year, so that the details throw no light upon the question, in what direction the infection spread, or what parishes felt its incidence most as the season advanced. The total mortalities for the week within the walls, in the Liberties, and in the nine out-parishes (within the Bills) are respectively 1144, 2717 and 994. The infection is said[2] to have begun in Whitechapel, as we conclude that it did also in 1603; but the City had its due share at length, the parishes of St Stephen, Coleman Street (full of tortuous passages), of

[1] In a volume of Topographical Papers in the British Museum, 1298, m (18).

[2] W. Heberden, Junr., *Increase and Decrease of Diseases*. Lond. 1801, p. 66. He gives no authority; "1626" is clearly a misprint.

Allhallows the Great, and of Christ Church having the largest mortalities.

In the 97 parishes of the City, the 16 parishes of the Liberties, and 9 out-parishes, the deaths at the end of the year were 54,265 from all causes, whereof of the plague 35,417. But that was by no means the whole mortality. A separate account was kept for the parishes of Stepney, Newington, Lambeth, Islington, and Hackney, and for the Westminster parishes, in all of which the deaths from December 30, 1624, to December 22, 1625, were from all causes 8,736, whereof of the plague 5,896[1]. The grand total of deaths in 1625 was, accordingly, 63,001, whereof of the plague 41,313.

The large parish of Stepney, extending from Shoreditch to Blackwall, was one of the worst plague-districts in London. It is mentioned as such by Dekker in 1603; and in the plague of 1665 it headed the list, with 8,598 deaths, whereof of the plague 6,583. We have some particulars of it for 1625: in the week July 18 to 24, there died in it 184, whereof of the plague, 144; and from July 25 to 31, 259, of which 241 were plague-deaths[2]; and those figures would have been nearly doubled in the weeks of August. Stepney alone would have had about half the deaths in the additional bill for the year; the parish register of Lambeth gives 623 burials, of Islington 213, and of Hackney 170[3], while Westminster with St Mary Newington (or Newington Butts, between Lambeth and Southwark) and Rotherhithe would account for most of the remainder. The parishes farthest out, and on higher ground, such as Hackney, Islington and Stoke Newington had fewer burials than in 1603.

The plague of 1625 was a great national event, although historians, as usual, do no more than mention it. Coinciding exactly with the accession of Charles I., it stopped all trade in the City for a season and left great confusion and impoverishment behind it; in many provincial towns and in whole counties the plague of that or the following years made the people unable, supposing that they had been willing, to take up the

---

[1] *Calendar of State Papers*, 1625—26, p. 184.
[2] *The Red Crosse* (broadside). London, 1625.
[3] Parish Histories, and in Lysons' *Environs of London*.

forced loan, and to furnish ships or the money for them.   The
history might have proceeded just the same without the plague ;
but historians would doubtless admit that all causes, moral and
physical, should be taken into the account ; and it will not be
thought beyond the scope of this history to enter as fully
as possible into these events of sickness.   First as to the sources,
other than statistical.   Four or more poems were written on the
plague of 1625—an interminable one by George Wither (with
other topics brought in) in eight cantos and about thirty
thousand lines[1], a piece by John Taylor, the water-poet and
Queen's bargeman, not wanting in graphic touches[2], a short
piece by Abraham Holland[3], the son of Philemon Holland, doctor
of physic, and another short poem by one Brewer[4].   Besides
the poems, there were sermons, mostly when the epidemic was
over, and various other moral pieces to improve the occasion.
A broadside called *The Red Crosse* gives a few details of
former plagues.   The letters of Chamberlain to Carleton, those
of Mead, at Christ's College, Cambridge (whose relation Dr
Meddus, rector of St Gabriel's, Fenchurch Street, was in the
City during the epidemic), and the diary of Salvetti, the envoy
of the Grand Duke of Tuscany[5], supply many particulars ; while
the *Calendar of State Papers* brings together other information
both for London and the provinces.   I know of no account of
the plague of 1625 from the medical side[6].

James I., prematurely worn out at fifty-seven, died at

[1] *Britain's Remembrancer, containing a Narrative of the Plague lately past.*
London, 1628.

[2] *The Fearfull Summer, or London's Calamitie.*   Printed at Oxford, 1625 (reprinted with additions, Lond. 1636).

[3] Holland's *Posthuma.*   Cantab. 1626.

[4] *The Weeping Lady, or London like Ninivie in Sackcloth.*   By T. B.   London,
1625.

[5] *Hist. MSS. Commission,* XI. pt. 1, p. 6.

[6] Bradwell's book, to be mentioned in the sequel, was written for practice during
the plague.   There is a reference to something of Sir Theodore Mayerne's on the
plague of 1625, which I have not succeeded in finding.   His *Opera Medica* contain
ordinary cases treated by him in London in December, 1625, but there is no mention
of plague-cases.   Woodall's essay on plague, published in 1639, thus refers to his
experience in the epidemic of 1625 : "In anno 1625 we had many signes contrarie to
the plagues in other times ; yea, and many did dye dayly without any signes or markes
on their bodies at all."

Theobalds on March 27, from the effects of a tertian ague, for which he preferred to be treated by the plasters and possets of an obscure ague-curer from Dunmow, setting aside his physicians, who would have succeeded no better. A great funeral, for which 14,000 " blacks" were given out, followed on May 7. Meanwhile the marriage of Charles I. to the princess Henrietta of France was being arranged. The king met his bride at Dover on June 13, and entered London with her on the 18th, passing up the river in a state barge to Denmark House, amidst an immense concourse of people on the houses and shipping, and in wherries on the water, with salvoes of artillery and demonstrations of welcome to the Catholic princess. On the 13th the Lord Keeper had written to Conway, Secretary of State, that cases of plague had occurred in Westminster, and that he could have wished that his majesty had determined to come no nearer than Greenwich. The nobility were kept in town to await the coming of the new queen, and some of them by the summons to Parliament. The Houses met on June 18, and were advised in the king's speech to expedite their business on account of the plague. However, those who were disposed to refuse supplies until grievances were redressed could make use of the plague as well as the king, and it was proposed by Mallory and Wentworth to adjourn on that plea until Michaelmas. The Houses sat for three weeks, until July 11, when they were adjourned to meet at Oxford on August 1. On a day in June Francis, Lord Russell (afterwards earl of Bedford), " being to go to Parliament, had his shoemaker to pull on his boots, who fell down dead of the plague in his presence," so that his lordship avoided the House. In the first week of July, the court removed to Hampton Court, and thence to Woodstock and to Beaulieu in the New Forest. The Coronation was put off until October, for reasons connected with the queen's religion as well as for the infection, and eventually until February 2, 1626.

Before Parliament rose, it obtained the king's sanction to a solemn fast. " This," says the Tuscan, Salvetti, " is a ceremony which is performed in all the parishes, and consists in staying in church all day singing psalms, hearing sermons, the one shortly

C.   33

after the other, and making I know not how many prayers, imploring God for stoppage of the plague, and of the ceaseless rain which for a month past has fallen to the detriment of all kinds of crops." At that date, July 1, he says that plague is now spread through all the streets and has reached other parts of the kingdom. A general exodus took place to the country, of all who had the means to remove. As in 1603, the magistrates, the ministers, the doctors, and the rich men seem to have left the city to take care of itself. On August 9, Salvetti, who had himself escaped to Richmond, writes: "The magistrates in desperation have abandoned every care; everyone does what he pleases, and the houses of merchants who have left London are broken into and robbed." On September 1, Dr Meddus, rector of St Gabriel's, Fenchurch Street, wrote: "The want and misery is the greatest here that ever any man living knew; no trading at all; the rich all gone; housekeepers and apprentices of manual trades begging in the streets, and that in such a lamentable manner as will make the strongest heart to yearn." The city an hour after noon was the same as at three in the morning in the month of June, no more people stirring, no more shops open[1]. This is re-echoed in verse by Abraham Holland:

> "A noon in Fleet Street now can hardly show
> That press which midnight could, not long ago.
> Walk through the woeful streets (whoever dare
> Still venture on the sad infected air)
> So many marked houses you shall meet
> As if the city were one Red-Cross Street."

And by the Water-poet:

> "In some whole street, perhaps, a shop or twain
> Stands open for small takings and less gain.
> And every closed window, door and stall
> Makes every day seem a solemn festival.
> All trades are dead, or almost out of breath,
> But such as live by sickness and by death."

The circumstances are so exactly the same as in 1603 that it is needless to repeat much: the sextons, coffin-makers,

---

[1] *C. and T. Charles I.* 1. 48.

bearers, searchers, apothecaries and quacks are all profitably employed ;

> " And last to dog-killers great gain abounds,
> For braining brawling curs and foisting hounds."

The clocks striking the hours are not heard for the constant tolling of bells. " Strange," says Holland,

> " Strange that the hours should fail to tell the day
> When Time to thousands ran so fast away."

Of the sick, Taylor says there were

> " Some franticke raving, some with anguish crying."

—delirious ravings and cries of pain (from the buboes) which we know from the accounts for 1665 to have been no rhetorical exaggeration. There were the same crowded common graves as in 1603, probably in the same graveyards :

> " My multitude of graves that gaping wide
> Are hourly fed with carcases of men.
> Those hardly swallowed, they be fed again."

Or as Taylor says,

> " Dead coarses carried and recarried still
> Whilst fifty corpses scarce one grave doth fill."

The treatment seems to have been mostly in the hands of quacks. Taylor says :

> " On many a post I see Quacksalvers' bills
> Like fencers' challenges to show their skill."

The Water-poet, being Queen's bargeman, appears to have had a proper feeling for all constituted authorities. After denouncing the quacks, as men who " pick their living out of others' dying," he proceeds to eulogise the regular practitioners, forgetting to add that they were now conspicuous by their absence :

> " This sharp invective no way seems to touch
> The learned physicians whom I honour much.
> The Paracelsists and the Galenists,
> The philosophical grave Herbalists,—
> These I admire and reverence, for in those
> God doth dame nature's secrets fast inclose,
> Which they distribute as occasions serve."

33—2

—the prevalence of plague not being one of the occasions for revealing the secrets entrusted to them.

The medical faculty is hardly at all in evidence the whole time. Thayre's surgical treatise of 1603 was reprinted; while a semi-empiric, one Stephen Bradwell, the grandson of Banister, a well-known Elizabethan practitioner, published a poor essay on plague, patched up from the usual stale sources and plagiarised even from the lay dialogue of the rector of St Olave's in 1603[1]. Bradwell addressed the reader, on July 15 "from my study in Mugwell-street, ready to my power to do thee any pleasure."

"I have two powders. I have also an excellent electuary. I have likewise lozenges, and rich pomanders to smell of. These are all of my grandfather's invention, and have been proved to be admirably effectual both by his and my father's experience. I confess they are costly; but slight means and cheap medicines (however they promise) prove as dear as death. The first powder is 12 pence a dram. The second is 3 pence a grain (the quantity is 10 or 12 grains). The electuary is 2 shillings and 6 pence an ounce, the quantity is one or two drams. There is a fellow in Distaff-lane that disperseth his bills abroad, bragging of a medicine that was my grandfather Bannister's. My grandfather was very scrupulous of giving any special receipts to others. But if any man can say he hath any receipt of his, I am sure, if it were of any value, I have the copy of it. Because many men know that I have a whole volume of excellent receipts left me both by my grandfather and my father, and lest they should conceive me as too strict and covetous in keeping all secret to myself, I have thought fit for the common good to divulge this excellent antidote following:"—the ingredients occupying a whole page.

This enterprising tradesman had been at Oxford, where he failed to take a degree in medicine, but he was a licentiate of the College of Physicians. He is the single literary representative of the faculty, so far as appears, in 1625; and there is nothing in his essay that concerns us, except the following corroboration of a well-known character of the epidemic:

"Poor people, by reason of their great want, living sluttishly, feeding nastily on offals, or the worst and unwholesomest meats, and many times, too, lacking food altogether, have both their bodies much corrupted, and

---

[1] *A Watchman for the Pest, teaching the true Rules of Preservation from the Pestilent Contagion, at this time fearfully overflowing this famous Cittie of London. Collected out of the best authors, mixed with auncient experience, and moulded into a new and most plaine method.* By Steven Bradwell, of London, Physition. 1625.

their spirits exceedingly weakened ; whereby they become (of all others) most subject to this sickness. And therefore we see the plague sweeps up such people in greatest heaps."

It is impossible to know whether any considerable proportion recovered. It appears that, as in 1603, the buboes and boils might come out in the same person more than once, and that the best chance was from their suppuration :

> "Some with their carbuncles and sores new burst
> Are fed with hope they have escaped the worst."

But the best hope was in flight, as Bradwell was candid enough to say, although he remained behind with his shilling powders and half-crown electuaries. *Cito cede, longé recede, tardé redi*—is the proverbial advice which he quotes.

However, the people in their flight, unless they were nobles or squires with country houses, fared but ill in the provinces. The story of their reception in country towns and villages is so like that of 1603 that one might suppose in this, as in other things, that the writers of 1625 were copying from Dekker. One of the versifiers, Brewer, has a section specially devoted to a "Relation of the many miseries that many of those that fly the City do fall into in the country." They are driven back by men with bills and halberds, passing through village after village in disgrace until they end their journey ; they sleep in stables, barns and outhouses, or even by the roadside in ditches and in the open fields. And that was the lot of comparatively wealthy men. Taylor says that when he was with the queen's barge at Hampton Court and up the river almost to Oxford, he had much grief and remorse to see and hear of the miserable and cold entertainment of many Londoners :

> "The name of London now both far and near
> Strikes all the towns and villages with fear.
> And to be thought a Londoner is worse
> Than one that breaks a house, or takes a purse....
> Whilst hay-cock lodging with hard slender fare,
> Welcome, like dogs into a church, they are.
> For why the hob-nailed boors, inhuman blocks,
> Uncharitable hounds, hearts hard as rocks,
> Did suffer people in the field to sink
> Rather than give or sell a draught of drink.

> Milkmaids and farmers' wives are grown so nice
> They think a Citizen a cockatrice,
> And country dames are waxed so coy and brisk
> They shun him as they shun a basilisk."

Taylor gives various instances in prose :

> "A man sick of an ague lying on the ground at Maidenhead in Berkshire, with his fit violently on him, had stones cast at him by two men of the towne (whom I could name), and when they could not cause him to rise, one of them tooke a hitcher, or long boat-hook, and hitched in the sick man's breeches, drawing him backward with his face grovelling on the ground, drawing him so under the bridge in a dry place, where he lay till his fit was gone, and having lost a new hat, went his way."

One at Richmond was drawn naked in the night by his own wife and boy, and cast into the Thames, where the next day the corpse was found. The village of Hendon distinguished itself by relieving the sick, burying the dead, and collecting eight pounds, at the least (being but a small village) for the poor of St Andrew's, Holborn, besides allowing good weekly wages to two men to attend and bury such as died. The village of Tottenham appears to have been equally hospitable ; but as it was on the road to Theobalds, and some of his majesty's servants dwelt there, the Privy Council on July 19, wrote to the justices of Middlesex to order the inhabitants of Tottenham, who had received into their houses "multitudes of inmates," to remove the new-comers and not to receive any in future[1]. Although the king was not at Richmond, yet as there was a royal residence there, the inhabitants sought to drive away citizens on the ground of the warrant forbidding them to approach any of his majesty's houses[2]. At Woodstock, where the Court was in August, no one was allowed to go from thence to London, nor any to come thither, and for contraveners a gibbet was set up at the Court gate[3]. It was hardly possible to get a letter smuggled into London[4]; in the provinces "no one comes into a town without a ticket, yet there are few free places." At Southampton on August 27, a stranger died in the fields : "He came from London. He had good store of money

---

[1] *Cal. State Papers.*   [2] *Ib.*
[3] Th. Locke to Carleton, *Cal. S. P.*, 14 Aug.   [4] Salvetti.

about him, which was taken before he was cold[1]." Dr Donne, the dean of St Paul's, confirms these experiences in a letter of November 25, from Chelsea[2]:

"The citizens fled away as out of a house on fire, and stuffed their pockets with their best ware, and threw themselves into the highways, and were not received so much as into barns, and perished so : some of them with more money about them than would have bought the village where they died. A justice of the peace told me of one that died so with £1400 about him."

Meddus, rector of St Gabriel's, heard of one sad case of a citizen in Leadenhall-street who removed to the country with his seven children, "but having buried all there is come again hither," in July[3]. In October, the people began to come back, although the infection was by no means over ; Salvetti, who was himself near Huntingdon, says that many of the returning artisans caught the infection in the city, which is probable enough, as it happened also in 1665. On October 15, a correspondent of Mead's wrote that in his passing through London he found the streets full of people, and the highways full of passengers, horse and foot. On October 24, we hear of great distress among tradesmen, artificers and farmers round London, and of discontent at the forced loan[4]; although the Court itself was in as great extremity during the plague for want of money as any private house could have been. On November 22, the lord mayor and aldermen wrote to the Privy Council that the great mortality, although it had taken many poor people away, yet had made more poverty by decay of tradesmen, the want and misery being still very great[5]. Still, the effect of this great plague on London, cutting off some fifty thousand in a year, or more than a fifth part of the population, must have been, like that of all other great plagues in London, to cut off the fringe of poverty and broken fortunes, and to raise the general average of well-being of those that remained. Trade would come back ; but the submerged tenth, or sixth, or fourth, or whatever fraction they made, were drowned for good.

[1] Locke to Carleton, 27 Aug. [2] *Cal. S. P.*
[3] Mead, letter in *C. and T. Ch. I.* i. 43.
[4] *Cal. S. P.* [5] *Ibid.*

London soon filled up the gaps made by the plague, doubtless by fresh blood from the country. In 1627, the christenings were again at 8,408, having been at a maximum of 8,299 the year before the plague. In 1629 they actually exceeded the burials by more than a thousand (9,901 to 8,771), and continued to be slightly in excess until the next plague of 1636.

The Plague of 1625 near London.

In the immediate neighbourhood of the capital the parishes on the Kentish chalk below London, such as Deptford, Greenwich, Lewisham, Eltham and Bromley had more plague in 1625 than in 1603. Kensington, for some unknown reason, has 80 deaths from all causes in the register, as against 32 in 1603 and 62 (of plague 25) in 1665. The group of parishes in Middlesex, such as Enfield, Edmonton and Finchley, had each a large number of deaths, but somewhat less than in 1603 and 1665, and the same holds for Hackney and Stoke Newington, Islington and Hampstead. Places up the Thames all the way from Battersea to Windsor were infected, including Wandsworth, Putney, Isleworth, Richmond, Kingston and Hampton Court. Eton was "visited;" even the sequestered village of Stoke Pogis had houses shut up "by reason of the contagion" and a collection made for their impoverished inmates. Among the Hertfordshire towns to which Londoners resorted in plague-times, Watford is known to have had plague-deaths in 1625. In Essex,—Stratford, Tottenham, Romford and Barking had each a large number of plague-deaths, and, in Surrey, Croydon and Streatham. At Carshalton, oddly enough, the heavy mortality was the year after (1626) "not from plague, but from a disease somewhat akin to it[1]."

Plague in the Provinces in 1625 and following years.

It is stated by Salvetti and other gossips of the time that the infection of plague in 1625 was carried all over the country from London by the fleeing citizens, and that few places

---

[1] Mostly from parish registers in Lysons' *Environs of London.*

remained free from it, just as it was said afterwards for the
plague of 1665. So far as records show, one would not be
warranted in inferring a great provincial prevalence of plague
either in 1625 or in 1665. There was plague at Plymouth, and
in the south-western counties, under very special circumstances,
as we shall see. There was plague also at Norwich, said to
have been brought from Yarmouth, and at Colchester the year
after. Newcastle, also, which hardly ever escaped the infection
when it was afoot, had one of its minor visitations. But, on
the whole, it is impossible to show by local evidences that
the plague of 1625 was diffused universally over England, either
in that or in the following year, or that it grew to a great
epidemic in but a few provincial centres[1]. Probably all the
plague-deaths in the provinces together, in 1625 and 1626,
would not have made a fifth part of the mortality in London.

The interest centres in the plague at Plymouth, with which
the outbreaks at Ashburton, Exeter, Dartmouth, Bridport, and
perhaps Portsmouth, Rye and other places, may be connected,
if not causally, yet in neighbourhood. The first that we hear of
sickness at Plymouth is under date July 26, 1625; some of the
ships arrived there had been visited with sickness, and the sick
had been landed and lodged under sails[2]. It is not called "the
sickness," and it is not clear that it was bubo-plague. There
may, indeed, have been real plague on board ships of war: Stow
says that it was in the fleet in 1603, and there is evidence of its
existence now and again in the Venetian galleys of an earlier
day. But we are now come to the period of the beginnings of
ship-fever, as we shall see in the next chapter; and, for the
present, we must not assume that the sickness on board ship
in 1625 was all plague, or chiefly plague.

---

[1] Winchester was probably a fair sample. In the city archives under the year
1625 there is this entry: "Item, it is also agreed that the decayed cottage where
Lenord Andrews did dwell, he lately dying of the plague, shall be burned to the
grounde for fear of the daunger of infection that might ensue if it should stande."
(Bailey, *Transcripts*, etc. Winchester, 1856, p. 110.) In a petition relating to
Farnham, Jan. 1628, the town is described as being "impoverished through the
plague and many charges," which may mean that plague had been diffused in Surrey
and Hampshire.

[2] *Cal. State Papers*.

The ships at Plymouth in July were doubtless a part of the squadron of ninety sail, which sailed thence in autumn, carrying ten thousand men to make war on Spain, in accordance with the anti-Catholic policy which had been forced upon James I. in the last years of his reign, and was now being carried out by Charles I. and Buckingham. This was not the first fruit of that policy. The immediate result of it was Mansfeld's English troops for the recovery of the Palatinate to Protestant rule. That expedition failing to effect a landing was speedily broken with disease, and before it had been many days on shore in Holland was burying 40 or 50 men a day. The fleet eight months later had a similar experience. The ships were victualled with rotten food, and the men were supplied with worthless clothing. As the facts were never investigated, the king having interfered to shield the duke of Buckingham from the attack on him by Sir John Eliot, peculation and jobbery were never proved, although it was known to everyone that honesty was the last quality to be looked for in those about the king and the favourite. The fleet reached the Bay of Cadiz and made a futile demonstration there. It is in the month of November that we begin to hear of sickness. On the 9th Viscount Wimbledon writes from on board the 'Anne Royal' to Secretary Conway that there are not men enough to keep the watches owing to sickness. On December 22, the Commissioners at Plymouth write to the Council that about thirty sail had arrived there with 4,000 soldiers "in such miserable condition as for the most part to be incapable of such comforts as the country would afford them." Captain Bolles, who died since their coming in, declared the occasion of his sickness to be scarcity and corruption of the provisions. Great numbers of the soldiers are continually thrown overboard. Yesterday seven fell down in the streets. The rest are weak, and want clothes, for the supply of which some thousands of pounds were needed. The despatch of December 29, says, "They stink as they go, and the poor rags they have are rotten and ready to fall off if they be touched"[1].

So far there is no word of plague; on the other hand there

[1] *Cal. State Papers.*

is a strong probability that the sickness was ship-fever, or typhus. It is not until the spring of 1626 that the plague is mentioned at Plymouth. On March 18, sickness increases at Plymouth and the plague is wondrous rife. On March 28, the plague is dispersed about the town. On April 5, the sickness increases very much. On the 11th, 40 died last week and twenty houses are shut up; some of the sick died and were buried in less than twenty-four hours. On 8th June, the plague is very bad in Plymouth, and the town is destitute of its best inhabitants. The town-council records bear witness to a rate having been levied for the relief of the plague-stricken, and to attempts as late as 1628 to collect their share of it from those who had fled the town in 1626. The deaths at Plymouth are stated in a manuscript book of the municipal annals to have been 2,000[1].

Meanwhile plague appeared in other parts of Devonshire. In Exeter it had been prevalent sooner than in Plymouth itself; a letter of November 17, 1625, speaks of the afflicted state of the city, and of the weekly contributions for the plague-stricken. Some particulars of the state of Exeter at this time are given in a memorial to the Privy Council by the mayor and bailiffs of the city, dated October 15, 1627. During the great sickness which fell on their city, and was not cleared in sixteen months, all trading was stopped and the inhabitants generally left the town. To appease a mutiny of the more disordered people, who threatened to burn the city, a rate was assessed generally on the city, but most of the inhabitants being absent, the corporation took up the amount at interest on their own credit. The persons whose names are inclosed, being inhabitants who have returned to the city, now refuse to pay the rate assessed in their absence; and the Council is petitioned to summon them before it[2].

---

[1] MSS. of the Corporation of Plymouth. *Hist. MSS. Commis.* IX. 278. Accounts are given (p. 280) of the monies collected for the relief of the poor and sick people of Plymouth "in the time of the infection of the pestilence from Sept. 29, 1625, to that day A.D. 1627." But that does not imply that the infection lasted all that time. The civic year began with September 29, and the accounts are those that fall within two complete financial years.

[2] *Cal. State Papers.*

On May 17, 1626, the plague is reported to be rife "in Devonshire," and specifically, on July 28, at Okehampton and Ashburton. The epidemic at Ashburton was on the same severe scale as at Plymouth. It began in the end of 1625, but was most fatal in April and May, 1626. The deaths in a twelvemonth were 365, "probably a fourth of the inhabitants[1]." (In 1627 there were only 27 deaths, doubtless from the empty state of the town.) The same summer it is heard of in Dorsetshire. On September 2, the deputy lieutenants and justices of the county petition the Privy Council that the 1000 soldiers who were to be removed from Devon and Cornwall, should not be quartered in Dorset, but in Somerset, as the former was visited with the plague[2]. Perhaps Bridport was the centre of plague referred to. Sometime later in the year, perhaps in November, the bailiffs and burgesses of that town explain to the Council that, although they had subscribed to the loan, yet they were unable to pay the amount subscribed as the town was destitute by reason of a twenty weeks' visitation of plague[3].

The last of this series of outbreaks in the south-west appears to have been at Dartmouth in the summer of 1627. On June 29, it was reported that the plague was so hot there that the inhabitants had left. The mayor wrote on July 19 to the Privy Council that it was true the inhabitants were still away, but the plague had ceased; only 15 houses had been infected, the inhabitants of which had all been removed to the pest-houses remote from the town[4].

Farther east on the Channel coast, Portsmouth had a visitation of plague previous to September 28, 1625, perhaps in connexion with the Cadiz fleet; the mayor and bailiffs, being at the end of their year's office, had refused to take steps to sever the infected[5]. At Southampton, only one house was infected on August 27. The infection is reported also from Rye in 1625, and from Canterbury, where the famous composer, Orlando Gibbons, died in the beginning of June, 1625, "not without suspicion of the sickness," says Chamberlain, but, according to Anthony Wood, of the smallpox. The king and queen lodged

---

[1] *Notes and Queries,* 6 ser. III. 477.   [2] *Cal. S. P.*   [3] *Ib.*
[4] *Cal. S. P.*   [5] *Ib.*

at Canterbury on June 14; but on July 23 the place had to be avoided "for the great infection."

From Oxford, where the Parliament met on August 1, the vice-chancellor wrote on July 27, that Sir John Hussey came thither infected from London, and died, that Dr Chaloner, being in the same house, was since dead, that the infection was in other parts of Oxford, and that All Souls College was shut up. There was a slight revival of it in January, 1626, which caused the exercises and the sermons at St Mary's to be put off[1]. Anthony Wood gives much the same account as for 1603, and blames the great increase of "cottages" erected by townsmen, to which scholars were enticed.

Cambridge kept free in 1625; but on October 3, three deaths are reported at Trumpington—one Peck, his wife, and maid. On the same date three houses were shut up at Royston, and the infected "translated into the fields[2]."

The outbreak at Norwich was one of the severer degree[3]. It was said to have been brought in the end of June, 1625, from Yarmouth, where nothing is recorded of it. A king's order to the mayor imposed extensive cleansings, &c, but the plague increased from 26 deaths in a week in July, to 40 in September, reaching a maximum of 73 from plague in a week, besides 18 from other causes. On August 27, Mead, the Cambridge don, writes that he had met the Norwich carrier, who told him that the number of burials there the last week was 77, whereof of the plague 67, and but 14 the week before. The infection lingered on until December of the year after (1626), the total deaths from plague having been 1431. The plague at Norwich was made the excuse, by the mayor and aldermen writing to the Privy Council on January 30, 1627, for not contributing towards shipping for the king's service; the city was distressed from inundations and the plague, "many hundreds of houses" standing empty. There appears to have been some plague at Lynn in the end of 1625, a Privy Council order of January, 1626, authorising the fair to be held there, the disease having ceased.

In April, 1627, the bailiffs and aldermen of Colchester offer

---

[1] *Cal. S. P.*   [2] Letter from Mead in *C. and T. Charles I.* 1. 51.
[3] Blomefield.

the same excuse as Norwich; they are unable to set forth any ships as directed on account of the heavy visitation of their town by the plague, the decay of their trade in the new draperies and baize, and the loss of their ships at sea.

Leicestershire, also, would appear to have had another visitation in 1626. On July 28, the muster in that county was respited on account of the shire town and nine or ten other towns being visited with the plague. Of that there is no trace in the excellent county history by Nichols. Leicester, like Bristol and other places, is known to have imposed quarantine against Londoners in the summer of 1625. It is probable that plague was also in Warwickshire in 1626[1].

Among other outbreaks in 1625 was one at Newcastle, but it does not compare in extent with some earlier and later plagues there. On September 10, Lord Clifford writes from Appleby Castle to Secretary Conway that Newcastle is so infected with plague, so ill fortified, and ill neighboured, that 500 men would disarm it. In his own county of Cumberland there was plague in Lord William Howard's house. Sir Francis Howard's lady took the infection from a new gown she had from London, so as she died the same day she took it; they are all dispersed most miserably, with the greatest terror in the world. Cheshire also had the infection in 1625[2].

---

[1] At Coventry in 1626, £20 was paid to the poor in lieu of a feast at Lammas, by reason of the infection. (Dugdale, *Warwickshire.*)

[2] The following curious extract was sent by J. A. Picton to *Notes and Queries,* 6th ser. I. 314 from the parish register of Malpas, Cheshire, 1625:

"Richard Dawson (brother of the above-named Thomas Dawson of Bradley) being sick of the plague and perceiving he must die, at that time arose out of his bed and made his grave, and caused his nephew John Dawson to cast straw into the grave, which was not far from the house, and went and laid him down in the said grave and caused clothes to be laid upon, and so departed out of this world. This he did because he was a strong man and heavier than his said nephew and another wench were able to bury. He died about the 24th of August. Thus much was I credibly tould. He died 1625.

"John Dawson, son of the above-mentioned Thomas, came unto his father when his father sent for him being sick, and having laid him down in a ditch died in it the 29th day of August, 1625, in the night.

"Rose Smyth, servant of the above-named Thomas Dawson, and last of that household, died of the plague and was buried by Wm. Cooke the 5th day of September, 1625, near unto the said house."

After a clear interval of two or three years, the history of plague begins again in London, and in the provinces. The London plague of 1630 was a small affair (1317 deaths), the city being otherwise so healthy that the christenings exceeded the total burials (9315 to 9237). In 1630, at the same time as the small London outbreak, Cambridge had what appears to have been its most considerable plague, but a very small one at the worst. It began about February 28, caused the colleges to break up and the midsummer assizes to be transferred to Royston, and from first to last produced 214 deaths, known or suspected from plague [1].

Along with it there were a good many cases at Wymondham (Windham), and some straggling cases at Norwich and Colchester, continuing into 1631, some 20 or 30 dying at Norwich of plague in the latter year [2]. The other centre in 1630 was in the north-west. Shrewsbury, an old-world town which seldom escaped, had a localised epidemic in St Chad's parish. It began on May 24 in Frankwell, but was confined to that street by cutting off the residents therein from the rest of the town, and by removing the infected to pest-houses in Kingsland [3]. It continued at Shrewsbury into 1631, and is heard of also at Preston, Wrexham, and Manchester, collections having been made in neighbouring places for the infected [4]. But the one great outbreak of those years fell upon the town of Louth, in Lincolnshire, of which the sole particulars are that the plague from April to the end of November, 1631, swept away 754 persons of whom nearly 500 in July and August [5].

After four years clear in London and in all parts of England (years occupied with the growing quarrel between the king and the Parliament), plague broke out again not far from Louth, where we saw it last, namely at Hull. A century and a half had passed since Hull's last great devastation by plague year after year from 1472 to 1478. It was then

---

[1] Memoranda of Rev. Thomas Archer, of Houghton Conquest. MSS. Addit. Brit. Museum.

[2] Blomefield.   [3] Phillips' *Hist. of Shrewsbury. Hist. MSS. Com.* x. pt. 4. p. 498.

[4] *Hist. MSS. Com.* II. 258.

[5] *Hist. of County of Lincoln,* II. 187. *Notitiae Ludae,* p. 41.

a medieval town, with a chain drawn across the mouth of its creek of the Humber, surrounded by great abbeys, and owing its importance to its trade in stock fish from Iceland and the North Sea. In the Tudor times it had experienced one small epidemic about the Blackfriars Gate in 1576, causing about a hundred deaths. The date of the outbreak in 1635 is not given exactly; but, as in the 15th century, it was the peculiarity of Hull among provincial towns that it kept the infection for several years,—down to June, 1638. Business was paralysed, schools shut up, and the town deserted by the wealthier classes. The deaths from plague from first to last are counted at 2730, besides those which occurred in flight to other places. Upwards of 2,500 persons, once in easy circumstances, are said to have been reduced to seek relief, to which the county of York contributed [1]. In 1643 Hull stood a siege, but there is no farther mention of plague ; nor did the town suffer in 1665.

The year 1635, which saw the beginning of the Hull plague, at a time when the infection was absolutely quiet in the capital, saw also the beginning of an outbreak at Sandwich, with accompanying cases at Canterbury, and a beginning at Yarmouth, Lynn and Norwich [2], in all which places the infections lingered at a low endemic level for a year or more. The dates are important only as showing that these provincial infections were looking up some months before the sharp outburst in London in the late autumn of 1636 made any sign. In Sandwich, on the 12th of March, 1637, there were 78 houses "visited," and 188 persons infected ; on June 30, 24 houses shut up, with 103 persons, some of them lodged in tents; from July 6 to October 5, there were buried of the plague about ten every week in St Clement's parish. Considerable expenses were incurred (more than £40 a week), to which the county of Kent and the other Cinque Ports contributed [3].

Besides these lingering endemics in Kent and Norfolk, the great plague epidemics of 1636 were in Newcastle and London.

---

[1] Tickell's *Hist. of Kingston-upon-Hull.* Hull, 1798.

[2] Gawdy MSS. (*Hist. MSS. Com.* x. pt. 2), various letters from Sept. 14, 1636, to Nov. 26, 1638, relating chiefly to Norwich.

[3] Boys, *Hist. of Sandwich*, pp. 707—8.

The Newcastle epidemic was both earlier and relatively far more severe than that of the capital. For a town of some 20,000 inhabitants, the following weekly figures[1] indicate a plague of the first degree, comparable to the London death-rates of 1625 and 1665:

Died of plague at Newcastle, within the liberties, from May 7 to December 31, 1636:

Week ending	Plague deaths	Week ending	Plague deaths
May 14	59	July 23	270
21	55	30	366
28	99	Aug. 7	337
June 4	122	14	422
11	99	21	346
18	162	28	246
25	133	Sept. 4	520
July 2	172	11	325
9	184	To end of Dec.	908
16	212		
		Total to 31st Dec.	5027

Besides in Garthside, from May 30 to October 17, 515, making a total of 5542.

This tremendous visitation of Tyneside is said to have begun in October, 1635, at North Shields, where the infection rested during the winter cold, to begin again at Newcastle in spring. During the height of the epidemic in summer and autumn all trade was suspended, no one being about in the streets or in the neighbouring highways. The means tried to check the infection were fumigations with pitch, rosin, and frankincense. Newcastle had one other visit from the plague, as we shall see, in 1644 and 1645, during and after the siege by the Scots Presbyterian army; but in 1665 it is said to have escaped, although Defoe says that the infection was introduced by colliers returning from the Thames.

The London Plague of 1636.

The London plague of 1636 was one of the second degree, for the capital, and was otherwise peculiar as being rather later

[1] R. Jenison, D.D., *Newcastle's Call to her Neighbor and Sister Towns.* London, 1637.

in the autumnal season than usual. The following table of the weekly mortalities shows how it increased, reached a height, and declined.

	Christ-ened	Buried in all	Buried of plague			Christ-ened	Buried in all	Buried of plague
Dec. 24	231	170	0	**1636**				
31	195	174	0	June 23		149	257	65
1636				30		141	273	82
Jan. 7	217	189	0	July 7		152	265	64
14	242	174	0	14		142	298	86
21	220	190	0	21		146	350	108
28	214	171	0	28		183	365	136
Feb. 4	227	183	0	Aug. 4		152	394	181
11	234	160	0	11		166	465	244
18	207	203	0	18		167	546	284
25	198	238	0	25		161	690	380
Mar. 3	221	198	0	Sept. 1		163	835	536
10	231	194	0	8		153	921	567
17	244	187	0	15		166	1106	728
24	215	177	0	22		172	1018	645
31	193	196	0	29		168	1211	796
Apr. 7	202	199	2	Oct. 6		170	1195	790
14	221	205	4	13		164	1117	682
21	202	205	7	20		174	855	476
28	271	210	4	27		133	779	404
May 5	197	206	4	Nov. 3		153	1156	755
12	199	254	41	10		164	966	635
19	171	244	22	17		143	827	512
26	160	263	38	24		162	747	408
June 2	189	276	51	Dec. 1		168	550	290
9	153	275	64	8		175	385	143
16	145	325	86	15		134	324	79
						9,522	23,359	10,400

The parishes chiefly affected were the same as in 1625 and 1603. Stepney is still wanting from the general bill; but after 1636 it was included therein, along with Newington, Lambeth, Westminster, Islington and Hackney. These omitted parishes doubtless contributed largely, Stepney in particular, so that the total of plague-deaths would have to be increased by perhaps two thousand. The following parishes had the severest mortalities:

	Total deaths	Plague-deaths
St Giles's, Cripplegate	2374	870
St Mary's, Whitechapel	1766	1060
St Olave's, Southwark	1537	847
St Botolph's, Aldgate	1506	735

	Total deaths	Plague-deaths
St Sepulchre's, Newgate	1327	566
St Saviour's, Southwark	1269	742
St Botolph's, Bishopsgate	1239	515
St George's, Southwark	1044	514
St Andrew's, Holborn	922	419
St Giles's in the Fields	863	428

Like the greater plagues of 1603 and 1625, that of 1636 appears to have begun in the suburbs[1]. Taylor, the Water-poet, in reprinting his poem on the plague of 1625, with some notes for 1636, says that of 1076 plague-deaths from April 7 to July 28 (the summation in the annual bill comes to 864), only 40 had occurred within the walls, so that the general infection of the City must have followed that of the Liberties and out-parishes. As early in the epidemic as 31 May, according to a record of the Middlesex Sessions, "the plague increases most at Stepney," wherefore the Greengoose Fair at Stratford was prohibited, (the parish of Stepney extending as far as Shoreditch)[2]. From Taylor we learn that Gravesend and Faversham had calamitous visitations, and that the infection was in many other towns and villages.

The epidemic of 1636 was like the plague of 1625 in having been preceded by much typhus fever in London, and accompanied by the same, as many as 2360 deaths being put down to fever in the plague-year in the classified causes of death now issued regularly (since 1629) in their printed bills by the Parish Clerks' Hall. The letters and state papers of the time bear witness to the usual exodus from the City, the movements of the Court, and personal incidents, which have no farther interest after the samples given for 1625. One incident relating to the worst week of the plague in London in 1636 is preserved: eleven persons were committed to Newgate on 5 October for going with one Samuel Underhill, a trumpeter, who died of the plague, to his grave with trumpets and swords drawn in the night time in Shoreditch[3]. The profession still

[1] Heberden says that it began in Whitechapel, but does not say where he got the information.
[2] *Middlesex County Records*, III. 62.   [3] *Ibid.*

makes no appearance in the way of epidemiological writing; but some "necessary directions" were drawn up by the College of Physicians, in substance the same as certain statutes issued on the alarm of plague in 1630[1].

Next year, 1637, the plague continued in London, causing 3082 deaths out of a total of 11,763 in the bills. In 1638 there were only 363 plague-deaths, but the total mortality was 13,624, or nearly 2000 more than in the previous year, when plague alone had claimed its 3000. What were the epidemic types of disease that caused the high mortality in 1638?

Fever in London.

There ought to have been no difficulty in answering the question. The causes of death in the metropolis had been assigned in the books kept at Parish Clerks' Hall since 1604, and had been printed since 1629. The printed series was in the hands of Graunt, from 1629 down to the date of his writing, January 1662; and he did abstract the deaths under each head of disease and casualty from 1629 to 1636 inclusive, and again from 1647 to 1661; but the ten years from 1637 to 1646 inclusive, he omitted as presenting nothing of importance and as being "inconsistent with the capacity" of his sheet of paper[2]. All the original documents prior to 1658 appear to have been lost in the fire of 1666, so that Graunt's omission cannot now be made good. One could wish that the worthy citizen had made no difficulty about the size of his paper. The omitted years are not only those of great political revolution, which may have had an effect upon the public health, but they are of special interest for the beginning of that great period of fever and smallpox in London which continued all through the 18th century.

---

[1] The College of Physicians reported also in May, 1637, on the causes of plague—overcrowding, nuisances, &c.; among the causes assigned the following is noteworthy: Those who died of the plague were buried within the City, and some of the graveyards were so full that partially decomposed bodies were taken up to make room for fresh interments. (Cited by S. R. Gardiner, *History, &c.*, VIII. 237–9, from the State Papers.)

[2] *Natural and Political Reflections on the Bills of Mortality.* London, 1662.

The following section of London mortality, down to the end of our present period, will show, by reference to the total deaths, how important the omitted years are for the epidemiological history.

Year	Plague	Fever	Small-pox	Total deaths
1629	0	956	72	8771
1630	1317	1091	40	10554
31	274	1115	58	8562
32	8	1108	531	9535
33	0	953	72	8393
34	1	1279	1354	10400
35	0	1622	293	10651
36	10400	2360	127	23359
37	3082	—	—	11763
38	363	—	—	13624
39	314	—	—	9862
1640	1450	—	—	12771
41	1375	—	—	13142
42	1274	—	—	13273
43	996	—	—	13212
44	1492	—	—	10933
45	1871	—	—	11479
46	2365	—	—	12780
47	3597	1260	139	14059
48	611	884	401	9894
49	67	751	1190	10566
1650	15	970	184	8754
51	23	1038	525	10827
52	16	1212	1279	12569
53	6	282	139	10087
54	16	1371	832	13247
55	9	689	1294	11357
56	6	875	823	13921
57	4	999	835	12434
58	14	1800	409	14993
59	36	2303	1523	14756
1660	13	2148	354	12681
61	20	3490	1246	16665
62	12	2601	768	13664
63	9	2107	411	12741
64	5	2258	1233	15453
65	68596	5257	655	97306
1666	1998	741	38	12738

The year 1638, and the four successive years 1640–43, have exceptional mortalities, which plague alone can by no means account for. In one of those years, 1641, we know that smallpox was rife, along with plague, in the autumn; in the third week of August there were 118 deaths from smallpox (133 from plague), and in the second week of September 101 from smallpox (185 from plague), the plague continuing at even higher figures all through September and October, while smallpox ceases to be mentioned in the letters of the time[1]. According to earlier and later experience, the epidemic of smallpox would have been followed by a quiet interval of that disease; so that the high mortality, beyond what plague could account for, would have been due to some other epidemic type. There is little doubt that that type was fever, less heard of in letters of the society people because it was, in its steady prevalence from year to year, an infection of the crowded quarters of the poor.

We begin about this period to find fever, or typhus fever, taking that place in the medical history of England which it continued to hold down to the generation before our own. What remains of the history of plague until its extinction in 1665–66, is so closely interwoven with the history of malignant fever, that it will be more convenient to carry the latter on side by side with it instead of in a separate chapter.

The first medical essay upon the malignant fever which got the name of typhus at the beginning of the 19th century, was that of a physician, Sir Edward Greaves, published at Oxford in 1643 in connexion with the sickness in that city while the king and the Royalist army lay there, and with the sickness in the Parliamentary army of the earl of Essex which lay at Reading. Greaves describes the unmistakable characters of spotted fever or typhus, and calls it, in his title "*Morbus Epidemicus Anni* 1643, or the New Disease." In his text he speaks of "this so frequently termed the New Disease." The name of "New Disease" was used also for influenza; but there can be no doubt that typhus did become common in England during the Civil Wars, between the Royalists and the Parliamentarians, which were the first and also the only sieges and campaigns on English soil that really touched the life of the nation.

The continent of Europe had been familiar with the same type of fever ever since the beginning of the 16th century, now in Italy, now in Spain, another time in the Low Countries,

---

[1] *Cal. State Papers.*

or in Hungary, or in Germany in the Thirty Years' War. Greaves, our first writer on epidemic typhus, had been preceded a whole century by Fracastori, whose description of the fever at Verona in 1505 is perhaps the first account of epidemic sickness free from subservience to ancient or medieval authority, and based upon direct observations made in modern Europe. At the same time typhus or spotted fever was not new to England in 1643. There is always the difficulty whether some epidemics of fever should be called influenza or typhus; but the fever of the Black Assizes, as well as the standing "sickness of the house," was certainly typhus, and so probably was the "new disease" in 1612.

The history of fever in England has been partly traced in the chapter on gaol-fevers in the Tudor period and on the Protean "hot agues," "new sickness," "strange fevers" or influenzas of 1540, 1557–8 and 1580. At a much earlier period, fevers of the same type (with dysenteries, lienteries, and pestilent sore throats) have been described, with whatever details there are, in connexion with the periodic famines, especially since the Conquest. But we are now come to a time in the history when typhus fevers appeared in the country unconnected with gaols or with famines. We are come, indeed, to the new era of epidemics, which is revealed more clearly after the plague was extinguished for good, but was really concurrent with the last half-century of plague, preparing, as it were, to succeed the long reign of that infection. The Civil Wars may be admitted to have given the new types of sickness an impulse, but the wars did not originate them, nor did they serve in any way to establish them as the predominant forms of epidemic sickness for nearly two centuries. Whatever it was in the condition of England that favoured the prevalence of fevers, fluxes, and smallpox, that factor was beginning to make itself felt shortly after the Tudor period ended : it continued in operation through all political changes of Restoration, Revolution, and Georgian rule ; and if the conditions at length changed, largely for the better so far as the adult population is concerned, and for the better even as regards infancy, there has followed the "*nova cohors febrium*" of our own time, appropriate to its own state of society, as was the old troop before it. This theme is really the subject with which a new volume should open; but as the plague-period overlaps its successor the fever-period by half a century, and as one must pay heed to the chronology, it remains to insert some facts about fevers in this place.

Review of Fever in England to 1643.

Of the prevalence of malignant fevers in England in the earlier years of the 17th century we have only occasional glimpses. Thus, in London in November, 1612, there were several deaths of prominent personages. Prince Henry, eldest son of James I., died of a fever in the course of that month, the illness being thus referred to by Chamberlain in one of his letters to Carleton, written on November 12 from London:

"It is verily thought that the disease was no other than the ordinary ague that hath reigned and raged almost all over England since the latter end of summer, which, by observation, is found must have its ordinary course, and the less physic the better, but only sweating and an orderly course of keeping and government. The extremity of the disease seemed to lie in his head [a sure sign of typhus], for remedy whereof they shaved him and applied warm cocks and pigeons newly killed, but with no success."

Sir Theodore Mayerne, the king's physician (who had been driven from Paris by the intolerance of the Galenists towards those who used antimony and other Paracelsist remedies), was a good deal blamed because he had purged the patient instead of bleeding him.

Writing again on the 19th November, Chamberlain says: "On Friday Sir Harry Row, our alderman died, and, same morning, Sir George Carey, master of the wards, of this new disease." Chamberlain's statement that an epidemic fever, which he calls "the ordinary ague," had raged all over England from the end of summer, 1612, is supported by Short's abstracts of the parish registers for that year, while the following year, 1613, stands out as still more unhealthy. The next unwholesome year in Short's tables is 1616; and of that sickly time we have one great personal illustration. Shakespeare died on April 23 at Stratford-on-Avon, after three days' illness of a fever (but possibly of a chill) having just completed his 52nd year.   So far as is known, he was not in failing health.   It is a singular coincidence that he made his will on March 25 preceding, the first day of the year, old style; but the customary phrase, "in perfect health and memory (God be praised!)," would have been perhaps varied a little if illness had been creeping upon him. Now the year 1616 is the most unhealthy in Short's tables from the beginning of the century; the parish registers do not bear witness again to so much sickness until 1623, which, as we have seen, was a year of typhus.   The winter of 1615–16 was altogether exceptional: warm and tempestuous south-westerly and westerly winds prevailed from November until February; on the 8th February, there were East Indiamen lying in the Downs, which had been at anchor there for ten weeks waiting for a change of wind to take them down the Channel.   The warm winds brought "perpetual weeping weather, foul ways and great floods," and brought also an early spring.   In the last week of January the archbishop found a nest of young blackbirds in his garden at Lambeth, and had " another sent to him from Croydon about four days after."   That was proverbially the kind of Christmas to make a fat churchyard; but it is impossible to say whether one type of sickness, such as fever, predominated, as in the preceding sickly years, 1612–13, and in the next following 1616, namely 1623–24.   The following figures from Short's tables will prove, at least, that there was excessive mortality:

In the year 1616, twenty-one parish registers out of eighty-eight examined, showed excessive mortality, the burials being 601 and the baptisms 417, the year 1617 showing a somewhat improved state of health.   In the market towns for the same two years, the excessive proportion of burials to christenings is equally striking: of sixteen town registers examined, ten showed a bad state of health in 1616 (714 burials to 568 baptisms), and in 1617, nine towns had 786 burials to 652 baptisms.   But neither in town nor country do the years 1616–17 stand out so unhealthy as the years 1623–24.   Those two biennial periods are the only very conspicuous ones in Short's list for the first quarter of the 17th century, the year 1613 coming next in unhealthiness.

Let us now seek for any causes such as unwholesome conditions of living upon which these epidemic fevers might have depended. One of the most notorious forms of typhus in the 18th century was the ship-fever. The problem how to destroy its infection in the hulls of transports and ships of war occupied the attention of the men of science, Stephen Hales among the rest. Parliament, eager for any cure of so disastrous a pest, voted some thousands of pounds to a projector whose method, when tried, resulted in nothing but the burning of three ships to the water's edge. This ship-fever became notorious early in the 17th century, having occurred before in 1588. If the Elizabethan naval annals in Hakluyt's collection were less engrossed than they are with adventures and doughty deeds, we should probably have had more glimpses of an unwholesome state of things in the 'tween-decks. At all events there is no doubt that fever infested the shipping of England as well as of France about the year 1625. The conditions on board ship are, of course, special; there might have been ship-fever, when there was no gaol-fever, workhouse-fever, or domestic typhus in general. But what happened on board ship was no bad index of what was happening on shore. The nation, both on sea and on land, was expanding far beyond its old medieval limits, with very crude notions of the elbow-room that it needed. The ideas of cubic space, ventilation, and the like, with which we are now so familiar, had then no existence. A few facts about the shipping, gaols and houses will serve to illustrate this statement.

The fleet which sailed from Plymouth to make war on Spain in the autumn of 1625 consisted of 90 sail, and carried 10,000 men. Whether there was overcrowding would depend, of course, on the size of the ships; and it may be safely said that the largest ship of the fleet was not a fourth part the size of a transport that would be allowed to carry five hundred men today. The expedition came back in a few weeks broken by sickness and mutiny, just as the expedition of Mansfeld for the relief of the Palatinate had fared. The wretched state of the thirty ships which arrived at Plymouth in November, 1625, has been mentioned already. At the same date we read of French ships of war also throwing overboard two or three dead men every day.

There are some more precise figures for French ships in 1627, to be given in the next chapter, which will enable us to measure the provocation to ship-fever afforded by the conditions of a transport service in those years.

Besides ship-fever, in the great typhus period of the 18th century, there used to be named gaol-fever, and workhouse-fever. Of the gaol-fever one hears little in these years. It was severe in the Queen's Bench prison in Southwark in March, 1579; a petition of that date complains that the prison held double the usual number, that "the sickness of the house" was rife, and that near a hundred had died of it there during the previous six years, many more having been sick[1]. "The sickness of the house" is a name suggestive of what was usual. These events of prison life made little stir unless they involved the health of classes far removed from the prison-class, as in the three memorable instances of the Black Assizes at Cambridge, Oxford and Exeter. But it is not certain that even such cases have been all recorded, or that instances of gaol-fever spreading to those outside may not have been more frequent than appears. Whitmore in his book of 1659 on fevers in London and the country, quotes Bacon's remarks upon the Black Assizes of the Tudor period and adds: "and within this eight or nine years there happened the like at Southwark, as I am credibly informed." That would have been in the King's Bench prison some time about 1650, which is not far from the date we have brought the history down to[2].

The overcrowding of the ships and of the gaols had its counterpart in the dwelling-houses of London and other towns such as Portsmouth. The proclamations against the erection of houses on new sites within three miles of the city gates continued to be issued to the time of Cromwell. The effect of them was merely to call into existence a class of poor tenements in odd corners or to overcrowd the existing houses. Thus, on

---

[1] Strype's ed. of Stow's *Survey of London.*

[2] Rendle (*Old Southwark*, 1878, p. 96) quotes the following from a letter written in 1618 by Geoffrey Mynshall from the King's Bench prison: "As to health, it hath more diseases predominant in it than the pest-house in the plague time...stinks more than the Lord Mayor's dog-house or Paris Garden in August...three men in one bed."

June 27, 1602: "The council have spied an inconvenient increase of housing in and about London by building in odd corners, in gardens and over stables. They have begun to pull down one here and there, lighting in almost every parish on the un-luckiest, which is far from removing the mischief[1]." Again, on February 24, 1623, certain inhabitants of Chancery Lane were indicted at the Middlesex Sessions for subletting, "to the great danger of infectious disease with plague and other diseases[2]." Again, in May, 1637, there were found in one house eleven married couples and fifteen single persons; in another the householder had taken in eighteen lodgers[3]. The monstrous window-tax, which did more than anything else to breed typhus and perpetuate smallpox, was not imposed until after the Revolution; but there was enough in the London of the Stuarts to explain the great increase of those diseases.

We have already had evidence of the wide prevalence of spotted fever in 1624, even in the houses of the rich. In the harvest of 1625, Mead, of Cambridge, heard of much sickness which he calls "ague," about Royston and Barkway, localities by no means malarious; so many were ill that the people wanted help to gather the harvest out of the fields. The nature of these "agues" is a question of great difficulty. The intermissions or remissions of the country fevers are clearly enough asserted by Willis and others, whatever they were; at the same time the general characters of the disease, or diseases, are not those of intermittent malarial fever; and "influenza" does not help us. Chamberlain calls the fever of 1624 "the spotted fever," and Sir Theodore Mayerne, physician to James I., in a long opinion upon the king's state of health and the treatment, dated Aug. 20, 1624, introduces a paragraph "Ad Febrem Purpuream," which, he says, was prevalent that year, "not so much conta-gious as common through a universal disposing cause," seizing upon many in the same house, and destroying numbers, being most full of malignity etc. These various accounts for town and country point to a form of typhus; and we find that

[1] *Cal. S. P.* 1601-3, p. 209.
[2] *Middlesex County Records*, II.
[3] Cited by Gardiner, *History*, VIII. 289.

diagnosis confirmed for the country fevers which were again widely prevalent a few years later, about 1638.

Among other statistics in Graunt's essay of 1662 we find the figures from the register of " a parish in Hampshire " from 1569 to 1658. There were several years of excessive mortality in that period just as in Short's tables, but the worst were 1638 and 1639—the years of high mortality (not plague) in London also. Of that mortality in the Hampshire parish Graunt has given a brief account, which he seems to have based on first-hand information. The parish contained about 2700 inhabitants, and enjoyed average good health during the period of 90 years covered by the figures, the births exceeding the deaths by twelve on an average in the year. In the year 1638 the deaths were 156 and the births 66 (about the average); in 1639 the deaths were 114 and the births 55. The cause of this great excess of mortality in a country parish was, says Graunt, not plague, " but a malignant fever raging so fiercely about harvest that there appeared scarce hands enough to take in the corn ; which argues, considering there were 2700 parishioners, that 7 might be sick for one that died ; whereas of the plague more die than recover. They lay longer sick than is usual in plague," and there were no plague-tokens.

This considerable epidemic of fever, which must have affected some hundreds of people, occurred in a Hampshire parish. In the very same season (autumn and winter of 1638) we hear of what is obviously the same sickness being epidemic all over the county of Monmouth. On April 23, 1639, the sheriff of Monmouthshire thus explained his delay in executing the king's writ for an assessment : " In January last I sent forth my warrants for the gathering and levying thereof, but there has been such a general sickness over all this country, called 'the new disease,' that they could not possibly be expedited.... Besides, the plague was very hot in divers parts of the county, as Caerleon, Abergavenny, Bedwelty, and many other places[1]." Here the sheriff uses the same name as Greaves put on his title-page five years after, and he distinguishes clearly between the fever and the plague. The mayor and others of Northamp-

---

[1] *Calendar of State Papers.*

ton, in a memorial to the Recorder, dated May 1, 1638, touching the exclusion of Northampton tradesmen from fairs in the vicinity owing to suspicions of the plague in their town, had been informed by the physicians that some cases were of the plague, and some of "the spotted fever[1]." The same distinction had been made at Norwich, in 1636: in October there was a suspicion of the plague, "but the physicians say it is some other contagious disease which die with the spots[2]." At Northampton, the coexistence of plague and some other sickness is asserted also by the sheriff (Sept. 18, 1638), who had to excuse himself, like so many other sheriffs, for his failure to remit the ship-money: he himself and his servants had had sickness, and the plague was so great and so long in Northampton that the county still allowed £148 a week for relief of the sick. The deaths in that epidemic from March to September were 533[3]. The sheriff of Montgomery, making a like excuse on October 25, 1638, speaks of the plague only: "It pleased God to visit a great part of the county with the plague, and three of the greatest towns, Machynlleth, Llanidloes and Newton[4]." The sheriff of Radnorshire, in his excuse to the Privy Council, on November 14, says he could not collect the ship-money at Presteign "by reason of the plague, which continued there for two years together, and did not cease until the latter end of April last[5]." We may take it, then, that there was a great deal of plague in Wales about 1637 and 1638, that there was also "the new disease," or spotted fever, all over Monmouth and probably other Welsh counties, that the same two forms coexisted at Norwich and Northampton, just as they coexisted in London, and that Graunt's parish in Hampshire in 1638 had probably the fever only.

Short's statistical tables again bear out the concrete history. In 1638, nineteen country parishes, out of ninety-four examined, had 699 burials to 542 baptisms, and in 1639, eighteen parishes

---

[1] *Cal. S. P.*   [2] *Ibid.*

[3] *Ibid.* The coexistence of malignant fever with plague at Northampton in 1638 is decisively shown by particulars of cases published by Woodall, *Op. cit.* 1639. See also Freeman, *Hist. of Northampton*, p. 75 (but under the year 1637).

[4] *Ibid.*   [5] *Ibid.*

had 585 burials to 386 baptisms. In the market towns the unhealthy period (which may have been due to plague in great part) is a year earlier. In 1637, ten towns out of twenty-four whose registers were added up, show 1474 burials to 1008 baptisms, the proportion in 1638 for the same number of unhealthy towns being 1438 to 1025.

It would have been one of the country epidemics of those years that Boghurst brings into his account of the plague of London in 1665: "I was told by an ancient woman that in Somersetshire the spotted fever was very epidemical, so that whole families died; but being told that plantan [plantain] was very good, all of them almost took it, which wrought an admirable change, for very few died that took it, whereas before they died very fast." He thinks plantain was as likely to have effected a cure as "higher priced medicines." We shall find a corresponding prevalence of fever described by a competent physician, Whitmore, for rural parts of Cheshire and Shropshire in 1651 and 1658. Thus we have a remarkable epidemiological phenomenon, somewhat new to England unless, indeed, we bring all those spotted fevers and the like under the generic name of influenza. It was in country districts in 1612–13 and from 1623 to 1625, it was extensively prevalent in 1638 in places as far apart as Hampshire, Monmouth and Northampton, it appeared in Berkshire and Oxfordshire in 1643 in connexion with the military movements of the Royalist and Parliamentary armies, it caused a disastrous loss of life in Tiverton within a few weeks of Essex's army passing through the town in 1644; it is heard of again in Shropshire and Cumberland in 1651–52, and in the same parts in 1658, as well as in Somerset, and in London steadily from year to year.

It was in its steadiness from year to year in the poor quarters of towns, as well as in its more frequent recurrences as a country epidemic, that the spotted fever deserved the name of "new disease" in the reign of Charles I. But more than one epidemic fever had been called a "new disease" in England before; and no fewer than five epidemics were so called from 1643 to 1685, of which only one or two can be classed among the influenzas.

If it had been possible to keep in mind the history of

sicknesses from century to century or even from generation to generation, the "new disease" might have been recognised as not unlike the type that overran England in 1087, that was described by William of Newburgh in 1196, by Matthew Paris in 1258, and by Trokelowe in 1315–16.   The conditions producing it or favouring it were not, indeed, the same in all particulars in the medieval period, in the Tudor period, and in the Stuart period.   In the medieval period, the extreme want and misery which brought epidemic sickness were due to occasional sharp famines at long intervals, from failure of the crops.   In the Tudor period epidemics were still so occasional (so far as is known) that something more special will have to be blamed for them than the swarms of vagrants and criminals all over England, which made the reign of Henry VIII. notorious, and were still a source of trouble until late in the reign of Elizabeth ; the four chief periods were in 1540, 1557–8, 1580–82, and 1596–97 so that some special cause would have to be assumed in those years to account for their peculiar "epidemic constitution." Almost from the beginning of the Stuart period, the seasons of fever (to say nothing of flux and smallpox), seem to come in quicker succession ; they are heard of in 1612–13, 1623–25, 1638, 1643–44, 1651, 1658–9, and 1661–65, and heard of in those years over wide tracts of rural England as well as in London and other towns.   It was from such experiences that the doctrine arose, so unintelligible to us now, of an "epidemic constitution of the air," which may be traced, indeed, to much earlier writings than those of the 17th century, but finds its most frequent applications in the latter.   The fevers were in part contagious and not contagious ; contagion could not explain them all, and yet there was an undoubted infective element in them.   The universality or generality of their incidence was accounted for by assuming, on the one hand, something common in the state of the air and, on the other hand, some common predisposition in the bodies of men, which might itself have had seasonal causes. We have now only one name for such common infection of the air, namely influenza; and it is significant that the catarrhal influenzas of 1658 and 1659 were regarded by some at the time as only the appropriate vernal form of the fever which in the hot weather of 1657 and 1658 had prevailed almost in the same general way as influenza, but with the symptoms of typhus. One thing which should not be overlooked, is that plague was still in the country, not always at the same time as the fever, and perhaps not usually coincident with it. Another thing, which will come out in its due order at a later part of the history, is that after the extinction of plague, fever became far more steady in the towns from year to year, and in certain years was not less prevalent in influenza-like epidemics all over the country. One might offer some suggestions as to the meaning of these epidemiological phenomena; but it will perhaps be more convenient that critics who have a speculative turn or a craving for generalities should exercise the one or gratify the other at their own risk.

Along with the prevalence of plague in 1637–38 in many towns of Wales, we may associate the outbreak of 1638 in Gloucester on the one side and in the small Salopian town of Clun on the other. From a letter of the Privy Council to the justices of Gloucestershire, it appears that a rate in aid of the plague-stricken in the city had been imposed upon the county in December, 1637, and that the infection still continued in Gloucester in September, 1638. Contributions made in Bridgenorth for the relief of the visited in Clun appear to belong to the same year. At Reading a tax for the "visited" had been collected once or oftener between 1638 and 1641. In 1641 the town of Leicester was put to some expense (£46. 8s. 7d.) in watching to keep out the sickness which prevailed in Thurmaston, Birstal, Whetstone and Oakham. The very severe plague in Stamford the same year would have been the most intense part of the epidemic in that corner of England; "Camden," quoting from bishop Sanderson's manuscript, says that it began at St James's tide, 1641, and ended in March following, whereof are said to have died between 500 and 600 persons[1].

Another centre of plague in 1641 was Congleton, in Cheshire, if we may trust the accuracy of the date given in a manuscript written some time after and seemingly based upon tradition[2].

---

[1] Camden's *Britannia*, ed. Gough, II. 244.
[2] *Notes and Queries*, 6th series, IV. 199.

The infection was traced to a box of clothes which had belonged to one dead of the plague in London and were sent to the dead man's relations at North Rede Hall. The family who received the box "caught the infection and died." It spread "all over the country," and came to Congleton, where it made dreadful ravages. The traditions which the anonymous narrator has put on record are, indeed, those of a plague of the greater degree—stories of corpses that no one would bury, of the sick left to their fate, of money dropped into water before it changed hands. This somewhat doubtful narrative ends with the statement that "the greatest part of the inhabitants died."

The period from 1643 to 1650 contains all the outbreaks of plague that remain, whether in London or the provinces, until we come to the final explosion of 1665. In London the plague continued at a low endemic level from the outburst of 1636 until 1648, the deaths in 1647 reaching the considerable figure of 3597. This series of plague-years has no other interest than as showing how regularly every season the infection increased from a few cases in May or June to a maximum in September or October. One incident, out of many, may find a place. In August, 1647, Sir Philip Stapleton, one of the Eleven Members, leaders of the Presbyterian party, who were accused of treason by the Army, went over to Calais with five more of the accused, and died of the plague almost as soon as he landed. The people of the house where he died made the rest of the party pay them £80 before they would let them come forth, for bringing the sickness into their house[1].

The plagues in provincial towns were in those years much more serious relatively than those in London. All of them occurred in towns that were besieged, or had been besieged, or had been occupied by bodies of troops or by garrisons. At the same time most of them were towns which had suffered plagues before. But the first effects of the war in the way of epidemic sickness were not of the type of plague.

[1] *Hist. MSS. Com.* v. 173.

War-typhus in Oxfordshire and Berkshire.

It was in the spring and summer of 1643 that England had a first experience of the war-typhus which had been familiar to the continent of Europe for a century and a half, having reached perhaps its greatest prevalence in the Thirty Years' War. It is only in the sense of war-typhus that Shakespeare's boast, put into the mouth of John of Gaunt, holds good :

> "This fortress, built by nature for herself,
> Against infection and the hand of war."

The medieval civil wars in England do not seem to have bred infection among the people, unless, perhaps, during the anarchy of Stephen's reign : there is reason to think that the faction-fights of York and Lancaster had no such result. But the wars of the Parliament against the Royalists produced war-sickness in its most characteristic form, and that too, at the very beginning of the struggle.

The existence of sickness in 1643 among the troops of the Parliament in Berkshire and Oxfordshire, under the earl of Essex, is briefly stated by Rushworth. But, for the first time in the history, we find a medical account of the type of sickness, of its circumstances, and of the extent of its prevalence, which is not without interest even for the military history. It happened that the afterwards celebrated Dr Thomas Willis, chemist, anatomist, physiologist and physician, was at Christ Church, Oxford, in 1643, being then aged twenty-one, and intending to enter the Church. In 1659 he published at the Hague his first medical essays, one on Fermentation and the other on Fevers[1]; and in the latter he recalls many particulars of what he had seen in his earlier years in and around Oxford. The sickness of 1643 was also the subject of a tract published that year in Oxford, by his majesty's command, by Sir Edward Greaves, physician to the king, which appears to have been in sufficient request in the town to be reprinted within the year[2].

---

[1] *Diatribae duae de Fermentatione et de Febribus.* Hagae, 1659.

[2] *Morbus Epidemicus anni* 1643; *or the New Disease.* Published by command of his Majesty. Oxford, 1643.

The preceding events may be briefly summarized[1]. In November, 1642, the king moved from Oxford with his army towards London and seized Brentford. The forces of the Parliament, under Essex, concentrated round the capital, where they were joined by the trainbands of the City, so that the king recrossed the Thames at Kingston and retired upon Reading and Oxford. All through the months from January to April 1643, tedious negociations went on for a treaty, the details largely relating to the places to be occupied by the Parliamentary troops on the one hand (around Windsor) and by the Royalist troops on the other (in Oxfordshire and Bucks). In April the negociations fell through, and Essex came before Reading on the 15th, with an army of 15,000 foot and 3000 horse. The king and prince Rupert attempted to raise the siege by a march from Oxford, but were stopped at Caversham bridge, and on the 26th April, Reading was surrendered to the Lord General, the garrison marching out the day after.

The siege had lasted only eleven days; the Royalist commandant was sentenced to death at Oxford for betraying the town, but was pardoned. When Essex entered Reading he found the place "infected," and a great mortality ensued among his men, who were discontented at the want of plunder and of pay. In June he moved his troops across the chalk downs to Thame, on the borders of Bucks; but the weather being wet and unseasonable in the early summer, and afterwards hot, the sickness so increased among them that "he judged the design upon Oxford impracticable" (Rushworth), and on July 9, wrote to the Parliament advising a peace. In his letter, Essex explained that it was impossible to keep the counties from being plundered, "so that they must suffer much wrong, and the cries of the people are infinite." Eventually he brought what remained of his army to the neighbourhood of London, and having received 2000 recruits from the City, he held a muster on Hounslow Heath, when his whole force amounted to 10,000 men. With his recruited army he marched to the relief of

---

[1] From Rushworth.

Gloucester[1], raised the siege, and on September 20 won the (first) battle of Newbury.

The realities of that inactive summer at Reading and Thame may be conceived from what Willis tells us of the state of things within the Royalist lines in Oxfordshire. These things, he says, " fell under our own observation," he being then at Christ Church and not yet entered on the physic line.

In the spring of 1643, Reading being held for the king,

" In both armies there began a disease to arise very epidemical ; however they persisting in that work till the besieged were forced to a surrender, this disease grew so grievous that in a short time after, either side left off and from that time for many months fought not with the enemy, but with the disease ; as if there had not been leisure to turn aside to another kind of death....

Essex's camp moving to Thame, pitched in the places adjacent, where he shortly lost a great part of his men.

But the king returned to Oxford, where at first the soldiers, being disposed in the open fields, then afterwards among the towns and villages, suffered not much less. For his foot (which it chiefly invaded) being pact together in close houses, when they had filled all things with filthiness and unwholesome nastiness and stinking odours (that the very air seemed to be infected) they fell sick by troops, and as it were by squadrons. At length the fever, now more than a camp fever, invaded the unarmed and peaceable troops, to wit, the entertainers of the soldiers, and, generally, all others : yet at first (the disease being but yet lightly inflicted) though beset with a heavy and long languishment, however, many escaped. About the summer solstice this fever began also to increase with worse provision of symptoms, and to lay hold on the husbandmen and others inhabiting the country, then afterwards spread through our city and all the country round for at least ten miles about. In the mean time they who dwelt far from us in other counties remained free from hurt, being as it were without the sphere of the contagion. But here this disease became so epidemical that a great

1 "The City, with much emotion, ranks its trained bands under Essex : making up an Army for him, despatches him to relieve Gloucester. He marches on the 26th [August]; steadily along, in spite of rainy weather and Prince Rupert; westward, westward; on the night of the tenth day, September 5th, the Gloucester people see his signal-fire flame up, amid the dark rain, 'on the top of Presbury Hill;'—and understand that they shall live and not die. The King 'fired his huts,' and marched off without delay. He never again had any real chance of prevailing in this war...The steady march to Gloucester and back again, by Essex, was the chief feat he did during the war; a considerable feat, and very characteristic of him, the slow-going inarticulate, indignant, somewhat elephantine man." Carlyle, *Letters and Speeches of Cromwell.*

part of the people was killed by it ; and as soon as it had entered a house it ran through the same, that there was scarce one left well to administer to the sick.   Strangers, or such as were sent to help the sick, were presently taken with the disease ; that at length for fear of the contagion, those who were sick of this fever were avoided by those who were well, almost as much as if they had been sick of the plague.

Nor indeed did there a less mortality or slaughter of men accompany this disease ; because cachectic and phthisical old men, or other ways unhealthful, were killed by it ; also not a few children, young men, and those of a more mature and robust age.   I remember in some villages that almost all the old men died this year, that there were scarce any left who were able to defend the manners and privileges of the parish by the more anciently received traditions[1]."

Willis recalls how this epidemic disease changed its type as the season wore on.   At first it was a " putrid synochus," which seemed to be helped by a sweat or a looseness; a relapse or renewal followed the crisis.   Later, it became a continual fever of six or seven days, with no crisis ; when the fever ceased the sick kept their beds, sometimes raging, more often in a stupor, great weakness continuing, and sometimes convulsions ensuing. About midsummer "the disease betrayed its malignancy by the eruption of whelks and spots."   It would often begin with an insidious languishing, the strength being totally withdrawn.   At length buboes appeared in many, as in the plague.   At this time, during the dog-days, the disease began to be handled, not as a fever, but as a lesser plague—by vomits, purges, and sudorifics.   The autumn coming on, the disease by degrees remitted its wonted fierceness, so that fewer grew sick of it, and of them many grew well.   At the approach of winter the fever almost wholly vanished, and health was fully restored to Oxford and the country round about.   Among the victims are mentioned "some belonging to the king's and queen's Court, with a few scholars[2]."

Of the causes, Willis says that, so far as concerned the army, the evident causes were "errors in the six non-naturals."   The spring was very moist and "flabbery," with almost continual showers, to which a hot summer succeeded.   The tract upon

---

[1] From the translation by S. Pordage.   London, 1681.
[2] Anthony Wood, II. pt 1. p. 469.

the Oxford fever by Greaves, a short piece of some 25 pages, which was written for use in the city during the epidemic, bears out the account by Willis, without developing the doctrine of increasing malignancy. He is concerned to prove that it was not the plague "as the relations and hopes of your enemies, and the fears of others, have suggested." One of his proofs is the insidious mode of invasion, which Willis ascribes to the sickness in its later type—great weakness without any manifest cause appearing, such as sweating or looseness, so that even strong men were prostrated, with a quick, weak and creeping pulse, sometimes intermittent, with pains in the head, vertigo &c. The most distinctive thing was the spots; "But what need we any farther signs than the spots, which appear upon half the number, at least, of those that fall sick?" Greaves seems to claim that Oxford had some immunity for a time: "God hath been most merciful to this city in sparing us heretofore, when our neighbours round about us were visited."

Among the causes, he mentions putrid exhalations from stinking matters, dung, carcasses of dead horses and other carrion; "and were there care taken for the removing of these noisome inconveniences, and keeping the streets sweet and clean, it would doubtless tend much to the abatement of the disease." The diet, also, may have had something to do with it; more particularly the brewers should dry their malt better, boil their beer longer, and put in a sufficiency of hops. But the great cause was the presence of the army.

"We need not look far for a cause where there is an army residing, which the Athenians called to mind in their calamity, or as Homer speaks of his Greeks :

εἰ δὴ ὁμοῦ πόλεμός τε δαμᾷ καὶ λοιμὸς Ἀχαιούς.

—it being seldom or never known that an army, where there is much filth and nastiness in diet, worse lodging, unshifted apparel, etc., should continue long without contagious disease." Whole families were infected, "and seldom in any house where sick soldiers of either side are quartered, but the inhabitants likewise fall sick of the same disease."

There appears to have been the almost inevitable doubt in some minds, whether the disease were contagious: "But if anyone be yet obstinate, and will not believe it contagious, let him go near and try." Among the remedies, he mentions a favourite one of the empiric sort, " Lady Kent's powder," which Willis also refers to; but Greaves, as became an academical physician, would not admit that it had any advantage over medicines of known ingredients.

This widespread epidemic of typhus, perhaps not without some relapsing fever, and, according to what Willis says in one of his general chapters, complicated, in its diffusive form in the villages around, "with squinancy [sore throat], dysentery, or deadly sweat," is the only one medically recorded of the Civil Wars. But there was certainly a renewal of it, in the same circumstances, next year at Tiverton; and it seems probable, from the heavy mortality which the parish registers witness to in that year (1644) that some kind of epidemic sickness had spread far and near. Thus, in Short's abstracts of the burials and christenings in country parishes and market towns, the years 1643 and 1644, and especially the latter, stand out as the most unhealthy for a long time before and after, the next sickly period, as we shall see, being the years 1657–1659. In the year 1643, out of eighty-eight country registers examined, twenty-nine showed a sickly death-rate, although the disproportion of births to deaths does not appear great (821 to 847). That was the year of the epidemic fever in Berkshire, Oxfordshire and Bucks. Next year, which was the year of the Tiverton epidemic, there are again twenty-nine country registers indicating unusual sickness (715 baptisms to 938 burials). In nineteen out of twenty-four market towns, the same two years come out still more unhealthy (844 births to 1193 deaths in 1643 and 1008 births to 1647 deaths in 1644). The registers examined by Short were mostly from Northern and Midland parishes; but they included two or three from Devonshire, and among his market towns was Tiverton. We shall now see what these bald figures mean in that concrete instance.

War-typhus at Tiverton in 1644.

Tiverton was then a town of some 8000 inhabitants, mostly occupied in the weaving industry. On July 5, 1644, Essex arrived with his army on his way to Cornwall to subdue prince Maurice, and lay there till the 18th.   The diary of one farmer Roberts has an entry that Mr Thomas Lawrence, who came from Tiverton, reported to him that the earl had 350 and odd carriages, and of horse belonging thereto for draught 2000[1]. This would have been his large artillery train, baggage and ammunition waggons, etc.   His infantry would be some 6000, and his cavalry perhaps 1000.   The king's force meanwhile advanced after Essex, and on July 25 lay in the great meadow at Crediton.   They had advanced by Yeovil and may or may not have passed through Tiverton.   The two armies came to blows in Cornwall, a prolonged series of encounters in the country around Lostwithiel in wet August weather ending in the escape of Essex to the coast, the retreat of his cavalry through the Royalist lines, and the surrender of the infantry on 1st September. The disarmed foot-soldiers were convoyed back to Poole and Wareham, and did not trouble Tiverton again.   The retreating cavalry passed that way, but did not enter the town, which was now held by the Royalists.   But the king's army came back by the way of Tiverton, which they reached on Saturday, the 21st September.   They had got no farther than Chard on the 30th, and may have halted in Tiverton some days.   A Royalist garrison of 200 men was left in it, and held the place until October 1645, when it was taken by Fairfax after a short siege[2].

Tiverton was thus occupied by both armies in the summer and autumn of 1644, that of Essex having been quartered in and around the town for a fortnight in July.   A serious epidemic followed, especially in the suburb on the western side of the Exe.   The particulars of it are in the parish register, from which it would appear that the sickness began in August and lasted until November.   The greatest mortality was in October, when 105 were buried, the whole mortality of the year having been 443. The ordinary monthly burials would hardly have exceeded a dozen or fifteen ; and as the 105 burials in October would have meant some eight or ten times as many sick, it is not

---

[1] Dunsford's *Histor. Mem. of Tiverton*, p. 184.
[2] The military events from Rushworth.

surprising to read that the town was desolate, and that grass grew in the streets[1]. Of this epidemic there are no medical particulars; but it appears from the parish register that it was known as "the sweating sickness." It would hardly have been so called if sweating had not been a prominent symptom. Besides the English sweat proper, with its five epidemics from 1485 to 1551, we have had occasion to notice a sweating type in several epidemics of fever. That symptom was so marked in the epidemic of 1558 at Southampton, Portsmouth, and Isle of Wight when they were full of troops, that Dr John Jones, who had personal experience of it, compares it to the sweat proper. It was a sufficiently prominent symptom in the Oxford gaol-fever of 1577 for the *sudor Anglicus* to be called to mind. In the English fevers and influenzas of 1580–82, a sweat or a lask is mentioned by Cogan as a least occasional; but the fevers of the same years on the Continent had so often the sweating character that it was sometimes said the English sweat had come back. Lastly for the war-fevers of 1643 around Reading and Oxford, Willis asserts in more than one place the occurrence of sweats, critical or giving relief for a time in the milder form, "deadly sweats" in fevers of an aggravated type. To anticipate somewhat, it may be mentioned also that a sweating character is recorded of some cases of the perennial London typhus at its worst period in the middle of the 18th century.

Admitting all these facts, we must still hold to the opinion expressed in the chapter on the Sweating Sickness, that sweating was never again the *signum pathognomicum* of a whole epidemic, as it had been of the sudor Anglicus in its five outbursts. But if there be gradations of type, or approximations of typhus to sweating sickness (as well as to influenza), then we may perhaps take the Tiverton epidemic as coming nearer than any other to the sweating sickness, on the strength of the name given to it in the parish register.

Nothing is known of sickness in the army of Essex, which lay at Tiverton from 5th to 18th July, 1644. It suffered much in the fighting in Cornwall, and the Parliament on 7 September sent to Portsmouth arms for 6000 foot and 6000 suits of clothes

---

[1] Dunsford, *Histor. Memoirs of Tiverton.* Harding, *Hist. of Tiverton.*

and shirts for the infantry who had surrendered and been convoyed back along the coast. The king's troops which occupied Tiverton on 21 September on their way back, had doubtless suffered also, from the campaigning in wet fields and miry ways, and are known to have been discontented for want of pay. Probably the epidemic at Tiverton was due to aggravation of the usual circumstances of war. It must be classed as a form of typhus; while its distinctive character of sweating might find an explanation, on the analogy of the sweat of 1485 in London after the arrival of Henry VII. from Bosworth Field, if we had sufficient reason to suppose that the soldiers who successively occupied Tiverton were not themselves suffering from fever. Contact alone, especially the contact *en masse* of men reduced by hardships and disorderly in their habits, will sometimes serve to breed contagion among a population unlike them in these respects. The converse of that principle, namely that contagion need not follow from the introduction of developed sickness *en masse*, finds an illustration in the case of Tiverton itself within little more than a year after the epidemic of 1644. In November, 1645, Fairfax lay at Ottery St Mary with his army, pending the investment of Exeter. On account of much sickness and heavy mortality among his infantry (not medically described) he removed them on December 2, to Crediton and ultimately to Tiverton, which was supposed to be a healthier situation and became his head-quarters until January 8, 1646[1]. But no outbreak in the town is mentioned, and almost certainly none occurred; the health of the place continued to be good every year of the time that it was under the rule of the Parliament, as the parish register proves. On the other hand Totness, which was occupied by the same convalescent force after it left Tiverton, had a severe epidemic of plague in the end of the year, 1646.

Plague in the Provinces during the Civil Wars.

The type of sickness, after the first two years of the war, does not appear to have been typhus-fever, but always the old

---

[1] Rushworth. Moore, *Hist. of Devonshire,* I. 149.

bubo-plague of the towns.   So far as the history is known, the experience of war-sicknesses upon English soil began in 1643 and ended in 1644, except in the instance of Fairfax's troops at Ottery St Mary in November, 1645.

Perhaps the "new model" of the Parliamentary forces, after the pattern of Cromwell's Ironsides, may have had something to do with the immunity of England from war-typhus in all the marchings and counter-marchings, battles, occupations and sieges, from 1645 to the end of the Civil Wars.   Cromwell pointed out to Hampden that the army of Essex was composed of "a set of poor tapsters and town-apprentices," and gave it as his opinion that these were not the men to win with.   When the original commanders, Essex, Manchester, Sir W. Waller, and others, had retired in 1645, in terms of the self-denying ordinance, the army of the Parliament acquired a new character under Fairfax and Cromwell: it contained a large proportion of "men of religion," especially among the officers ; and there is sufficient evidence that the war was in future carried on so as to produce as few as possible of those effects of campaigning among the people at large which had marked the Thirty Years' War in Germany and had attended the operations of Essex and the Royalists in 1643 and 1644.

What remains to be said of the epidemics of the Civil Wars relates almost exclusively to plague, with an occasional reference to the spotted fever which was widely prevalent in the autumn of 1644.   These epidemics of plague in the English provinces, during the political troubles, more numerous than usual from 1644 to 1650, are the last on English soil until we come to the final grand explosion of 1665–66.

In 1644 there were two principal centres of plague (besides London), namely Banbury, and the valley of the Tyne.   Banbury was near enough to the Royalist head-quarters to have shared in the fever-epidemic of 1643 ; in that year the burials of 58 soldiers are entered in the parish register, besides a large excess of burials among the civil population (total of 225 deaths in the year as against an annual mortality in former years ranging from 30 to 98).   The siege by the Parliamentary forces did not begin until July 19, 1644, and ended in the surrender of the castle in October. The epidemic of plague may have begun as early as January, a soldier having "died in the street" on the 16th; but it is not until March 1644, that plague-deaths appear in the register. In that month there were 10 deaths from plague, in April 34, and so until November, when there were 2, the total mortality from plague having been 161. After the plague ceased, the town remained otherwise unhealthy until 1647[1].

The information as to Newcastle and Tyneside comes from the observant Scotsman, William Lithgow, who was with the Presbyterian army when Newcastle was stormed on October 20, 1644[2]. The town had suffered heavily from plague, as we have seen, in 1636, and there had been a slighter outbreak in 1642. Although the state of things during the siege in 1644 was wretched in the extreme, there does not appear to have been plague until after the surrender. The infection was already at work, however, in places near. Thus Tynemouth Castle was surrendered by the Royalist commander, Sir Thomas Riddell on October 27: "The pestilence having been five weeks amongst them, with a great mortality, they were glad to yield, and to scatter themselves abroad; but to the great undoing and infecting of the country about, as it hath contagiously begun" (Lithgow). Among the places infected were Gateshead, Sandgate, Sunderland, and many country villages, the plague being reported in Newcastle itself in 1645 as well as in Darlington[3].

The year 1645 was one of severe plague in several towns at the same time, some of them in a state of siege and all of them occupied by troops. The largest mortality was at Bristol, being proportionate to its size. The town was taken by prince Rupert on July 22, 1643, and was held by a strong garrison for two years and some weeks. It was towards the end of the Royalist occupation that the plague broke out, probably in the spring of 1645[4]. On the 16th May, Sir John Culpepper wrote to Lord Digby: "The sickness increases fearfully in this city. There died this week according to the proportion of 1500 in

---

[1] Beesley's *Hist. of Banbury*, p. 387.
[2] In Somers's *Tracts.* Scott's ed. v. 294.   [3] Sykes.
[4] Clarendon, referring to a proposed Royal visit to Bristol in April says: "The plague began to break out there very much for the time of the year."

London[1]." When it had been stormed by Fairfax and Cromwell in September 1645, it was found that prince Rupert's garrison consisted of 2500 foot, and about 1000 horse. The auxiliaries and the trained bands of the town were reduced in June to about 800, and of the 2500 families then remaining in the town, 1500 were in a state of indigence and want[2]. In Cromwell's despatch of September 14 to Mr Speaker Lenthall he says: " I hear but of one man that hath died of the plague in all our army, although we have quartered amongst and in the midst of infected persons and places[3]." The deaths from plague in the whole epidemic approached 3000, according to the MS. calendars[4].

While this was going on within the walls of Bristol, an epidemic of plague more severe for the size of the town was progressing at Leeds. The town had been taken by Fairfax on January 23, 1643, and had remained in the quiet possession of the Parliament, under a military governor. In August, 1644, there were buried 131 persons, "before the plague was perceived," says the parish register; which means that the excessive mortality was not from plague, but probably from the spotted fever which reigned that autumn in other places in the North. The plague proper began with a death in Vicar-lane on March 11, 1645. The weekly bills of mortality which were ordered by the military governor showed a total mortality, from March 11 to December 25, of 1325. It raged most in Vicar-lane and the close yards adjoining; it was also very prevalent in March-lane, the Calls, Call-lane, Lower Briggate, and Mill-hill. The largest number of burials in a week (126) was from July 24 to 31; the mortality kept high all through August and September (60 to 80 weekly), and declined gradually to 3 in the week ending Christmas-day. Whitaker estimates that probably the fifth part of the population died, and he cannot discover any person of name among the victims. The air was so warm and infectious that dogs, cats, mice and rats are said to have died (of rats and mice it can well be believed), and that several birds dropped

---

[1] *Cal. State Papers.*   [2] Rushworth.
[3] *Letters and Speeches,* I.
[4] Seyer's *Memorials of Bristol,* II. 466.

down dead in their flight over the town[1]. This appears to have been the only visitation of plague in Leeds, at least since the medieval period.

The plague of Lichfield in 1645–46, like that of Bristol, went on during a constant state of military turmoil. On April 21, 1643, the Close was taken by prince Rupert and was held as a Royalist stronghold until July 26, 1646, the king having repaired thither after his defeat at Naseby in June, 1645, and again in September. The plague is said to have been active both in 1645 and 1646; in twelve streets there occurred 821 deaths, the largest share (121) falling to Green Hill[2]. In what way the state of siege may have contributed to the plague is uncertain. The fosse was drained dry at one stage, and was choked with rubbish at another. Many of the inhabitants of the town would appear, from the 4th article of the capitulation, to have taken refuge with their effects within the fortified Cathedral Close, which was almost enclosed by water. This was one of several outbreaks of plague that Lichfield had suffered since early Tudor times.

Minor plague outbreaks of 1645 were at Derby and Oxford. Of the latter we have a glimpse from Willis of Christ Church.

"Sometime past in this city [Oxford] *viz.*, 1645, the plague (tho' not great) had spread. Doctor Henry Sayer, a very learned physician, and happy in his practice, many others refusing this province, boldly visited all the sick, poor as well as rich, daily administered to them physic, and handled with his own hands their buboes and virulent ulcers, and so cured very many sick by his sedulous though dangerous labour. That he might fortifie himself against the contagion, before he went into the infected houses, he was wont only to drink a large draught of sack, and then his perambulation about the borders of death and the very jaws of the grave being finished, to repeat the same antidote.

After he had in this city, as if inviolable as to the plague, a long while taken care of the affairs of the sick without any hurt, he was sent for to Wallingford Castle, where this disease cruelly raged, as another Æsculapius, by the governor of the place. But there, being so bold as to lie in the same bed with a certain captain (his intimate companion), who was taken with the plague, he quickly received the contagion of the same disease ; nor were the arts then profitable to the master which had been helpful to so many others, but there with great sorrow of the inhabitants, nor without great loss to the

---

[1] Whitaker, *History of Leeds,* p. 75.   [2] Harwood, *Hist. of Lichfield,* p. 306.

medical science, he died of that disease." He treated the sick, in the pre-bubonic stages, by a vomit of Crocus Metallorum, and then by diaphoretics[1].

None of the other localized epidemics of plague in those years would appear to have been of the first magnitude. Thus, the 22 deaths from plague at Loughborough from 1645 to May 14, 1646, and the renewed prevalence, after a year's interval, (83 plague-deaths from July 20, 1647 to March 25, 1648)[2], are samples of local mortalities from plague that other parish registers might bear witness to if they had been examined by antiquaries as closely as Nichols examined those of Leicestershire.

Newark was one of the towns which suffered much during the Civil War. Besieged time after time, it was at length surrendered to the Parliament on May 6, 1646. A letter written shortly after the surrender says[3]:

"Truly it is become a miserable, stinking, infected town. I pray God they do not infect the counties and towns adjacent....By reason of the sickness in divers places, the officers dare not yet venture to fetch out the arms...Tradesmen are preparing to furnish their shops...but the market cannot be expected to be much whilst the sickness is in the town."

The parish register of Newark bears no witness to deaths from plague ; but that of the adjacent parish of Stoke, in which stood the Castle and the suburb of Newark surrounding it, has numerous entries of plague-deaths, beginning with one some three weeks after the surrender, on May 28, 1646, and continuing through July, August, and September. Several of the same household are buried in one day, one is "buried in the field," another "in his croft." The vicar sums up the mortality thus : "There dyed in the towne of Stoke, 1646, eight score and one, whereof of the plage seven score and nineteen." · The whole deaths in Stoke parish the year before had been nine, and the year after they were six[4]. If the plague had been at all proportionate in Newark town itself, the deaths would have far exceeded 159 ; but, as the parish register does not record plague-

[1] Pordage's translation of Willis's *Remaining Works*, p. 131.
[2] Nichols, III. 893.
[3] Cornelius Brown, *Annals of Newark*. London, 1879, p. 164.
[4] *Ibid.*

deaths at all, it may be inferred that the infection lay mostly around the Castle.

Whitmore speaks of having practised in the plague in Staffordshire in 1647–8, and there is some other evidence, without particulars, of an epidemic in the town of Stafford.

One more epidemic of plague is reported from the theatre of Civil War in the south-west, the outbreak at Totness in 1646–7. In the parish register there is a burial entered on July 30, 1646, " suspected she died of the plague." A leaf of the register has the following : " From December 6, 1646, till the 19th October, 1647, there died in Totness of the plague 262 persons "—a number greater than the register shows in detail. The stereo-typed remark is added, that the town was deserted and that grass grew in the streets[1]. For months before the first suspected case of plague in 1646, Totness had been occupied by one body of troops after another. In November or December, 1645, Goring's Royalist cavalry, to the number of nearly 5000, were quartered at Totness and two or three other places near. On January 11, 1646, Fairfax came with his army to Totness for the siege of Dartmouth, which was carried by storm on the 20th. The Lord General then withdrew to resume the investment of Exeter. Before doing so he issued warrants to four Hundreds to assemble their men at Totness on the 24th January. The men came in to the number of about 3000, and a regiment was formed from them[2]. What connexion with the plague in the end of the year all this military stir at Totness may have had, it would not be easy to determine. There had been a great deal of sickness in the army of Fairfax while it lay at Ottery St Mary in the latter half of November, 1645. " By reason of the season," says Rushworth, " and want of accommodation, abundance of his army, especially the foot, were sick, and many died, seldom less than seven, eight or nine in a day in the town of Autree, and amongst the rest Colonel Pickering died and some other officers. The Royal party had notice of this consumption of Fairfax's army," and took heart to make a new effort. The type of sickness is unknown ; but it was such as to cause the removal of the head-quarters on December 2 to Tiverton, for better air.

[1] *Notes and Queries*, 6th ser., III. 477.   [2] Rushworth.

The army lay there until January 8, and came to Totness, for the siege of Dartmouth, on the 11th. Thus Totness had not only been occupied by an army some months before the plague, but by an army which had lately had a fatal form of sickness in it. The troops march away, and the historical interest goes with them; what they may have left behind them concerns only the domestic history. Fifty-six years had passed since Totness had the plague before; and on that occasion the epidemic was equally disastrous.

Two other centres of plague in 1646-7 are casually mentioned, one at Reading[1], which affected " a great number of poor people," and the other at Carlisle[2]. Of the latter there are no particulars; but the circumstances of the town for several years were such as to make an outbreak of plague in 1646 credible.

Carlisle suffered much from the war for a series of years. In July, 1644, it was seized for the Royalists, and was besieged by Lesley in October, the siege lasting many months. It had a garrison of about 700, including some of the townsfolk armed. About the end of February, 1645, all the corn in the town was seized to be served out on short allowance; on June 5, "hempseed, dogs and rats were eaten." The surrender was on June 25, and the place was held by a Scots garrison until December, 1646. It was again seized for the Royalists in April, 1648, was recaptured by Cromwell in October, and held by a strong garrison of 800 foot and a regiment of horse, besides dragoons to keep the borders. All Cumberland was in such a state of destitution that the Parliament ordered a collection for its relief; numbers of the poor are said to have died in the highways, and 30,000 families were in want of bread[3].

Plague in Scotland during the Civil Wars.

Connecting with plagues in the north of England, there was a great prevalence of the infection in Scotland. After the storming of Newcastle by the Scots Covenanters in October, 1644, the plague appeared in Edinburgh, Kelso, Borrowstownness, Perth

---

[1] *Histor. MSS. Com.* XI. 7, p. 190.   [2] *Ibid.* IX. 1, p. 201.
[3] *Hist. of Carlisle,* 1838.

and other places.   On April 1, 1645, Kelso was burned down, the fire having originated in a house that was being "clengit" or disinfected after plague in it.   At Edinburgh the plague-stricken were housed in huts in the King's park below Salisbury Crags. Collections were made for the relief of people in Leith impoverished by the plague.   The epidemic in and around Perth is said to have given rise to the story of Bessie Bell and Mary Gray, who fled from the plague-tainted ground and built themselves a bower by a burn side[1].   At Glasgow the infection was severe in the end of 1646, and did not cease entirely until the autumn of 1648.   There are numerous references to it in the letters of principal Baillie of Glasgow University, of which the following are the most important[2].

On September 5, 1645, he writes that the pest has laid Leith and Edinburgh desolate, and rages in many more places : never such a pest seen in Scotland (in his time, perhaps).   About January, 1646, he writes of "the crushing of our nation by pestilence and Montrose's victories."   At the end of that year, the plague was in Glasgow : on January 26, 1647, during winter cold, "all that may are fled out of it."   On June 2, the plague had scattered the St Andrews' students, the principal of St Leonard's College was dead of it, and it was killing many in the north.   The same summer, principal Baillie was shut up in the town of Kilwinning, cut off, with all the inhabitants, from communication with the outer world owing to a suspicion of plague in the place.   Edinburgh and Leith, which had suffered earliest, were almost free in the autumn of 1647, but "Aberdeen, Brechin and other parts of the north are miserably wasted ; the schools and colleges now in all Scotland, but Edinburgh, are scattered."   Glasgow had its worst experience of plague in the summer and autumn of 1648, which were wet seasons : on August 23, "our condition for the time is sad ; the plague is also in Edinburgh and Aberdeen.... At this time I grieved for the state of Glasgow.... My brother's son's house was infected ; my brother's house enclosed many in danger ; one night near a dozen died of the sickness.... The long great rains for many

[1] Chambers, *Domestic Annals of Scotland.*
[2] Baillie's *Letters.* 3 vols. Edited by D. Laing for the Bannatyne Club.

36—2

weeks did prognosticate famine ; but these three days past there is also a great change of weather ; the Lord continue it." The infection which began at Glasgow in January, 1647, reached Aberdeen in April, having been carried, it was said, by a woman from Brechin. It was still raging at Aberdeen in September, and there were straggling cases as late as November of the following year (1648). The deaths from plague are put down at 1600, besides 140 in the adjacent fishing villages of Futtie and Torrie on either side of the Dee mouth. This enormous mortality ensued despite the usual rigorous measures—the removal of the infected to huts on the Links and Woolmanhill, a cordon of soldiers to shut them in, a gibbet for the disobedient, and "clengers" for the infected houses[1]. This disastrous epidemic of 1647–1648 is the last that is heard of plague in Scotland.

Plague in Chester &c. and in Ireland, 1647–1650.

The two remaining English plagues of those years were both in cities that had suffered much from plague before, and were in a constant state of turmoil during the war, namely Chester and Shrewsbury. Chester was held for the king, and surrendered to the Parliament on February 3, 1646, after a siege of twenty weeks, during the latter part of which there was famine within the walls. It was not until 1647 that plague broke out. From June 22 until April 20, 1648, the numbers that died of plague are stated in the MS. of Dr Cowper to have been 2099 ; all business was suspended, and cabins for the plague-stricken were built outside the town[2].

The Shrewsbury plague of 1650, like that of Chester, is described as having been dreadful in its effects upon the town. It broke out during the occupation by the Parliament's troops, on June 12, 1650, in a house in Frankwell, and continued until

---

[1] Kennedy, *Annals of Aberdeen*, I. 270 (expenses of the epidemic from the Council Register, vol. LIII. p. 130).

[2] Hemingway, Ormerod. *The Report of the Hist. MSS. Commission* (v. 339) notes that Dr Cowper's MS. contains details of 2,099 deaths, but reproduces none of them.

January, 1651. Only one parish, St Chad's, appears to have
kept account of the plague-deaths: in that register from
June 12 to January 16, there are entered 277 burials, whereof
of the plague 250, the highest monthly mortality (76) being in
August, 1650. Of these 250 deaths, 123 took place in the
pest-houses. A letter of August 21 says that 153 died in two
months, and that there were near 3000 people in the town
dependent upon common charity[1]. On November 21, there
were still 200 cases in the pest-houses, most of them being in
the way to recover, as usually happened towards the end of
an epidemic through the greater readiness of the buboes to
suppurate.

From the small number of burials due to ordinary causes in
the St Chad's register, it would appear that many citizens had
fled. The severity of incidence upon certain houses appears
from the fact that five servants in Mr Rowley's house died of it;
and that 15 out of 21 burials in St Julian's parish came from
four families[2]. These are incidents like those of the great
plague of London in 1665, which is the next in time in the
English annals after Shrewsbury's visitation in 1650.

The plague in Ireland in 1649–50 was connected, directly
and indirectly, with the military operations under Ireton and
Cromwell. The previous year, 1648, had been one of famine:
at the attack on Kildare by the rebels in the spring, both the
English garrison in the town and the attacking Irish were
half-starved, and there was a great mortality on both sides,
as well as a murrain of cattle. On May 4, corn in all the
rebel quarters is said to be at the incredible price of £8 the
quarter, both men and cattle dying in large numbers[3]. In 1649
the plague broke out in Kilkenny, obliging the supreme council
of Confederate Catholics to remove to Ennis. Ireton, "thinking
he ought not to meddle with what the Lord had so visibly
taken into his hands, has declined taking Kilkenny into his
own." But Cromwell besieged it on March 23, 1650, by which
time the garrison of 200 horse and 1,000 foot had been reduced

[1] *Hist. MSS. Commiss.* v. 342.
[2] Owen and Blakeway.
[3] Rushworth, Pt. 4, vol. II., pp. 1100, 1109.

to 300 men through the ravages of the plague, the inhabitants having also suffered heavily[1].

The Royalist letters from the Hague speak of the plague in the summer of 1650 as disastrous in Ireland, particularly in Dublin[2]. On August $\frac{5}{15}$: "Lady Inchiquin came hither last night; those with her report that the plague will devour what the sword has not in Ireland." On September $\frac{2}{12}$: "All I hear out of Ireland is that the plague has made a horrid devastation there; 1100 in a week died in Dublin"—an improbable estimate[3]. The ranks of the rebels were so thinned by the sword and pestilence that "not above 200 suffered by the hands of the executioner," after trial at the high court of justice held in County Cork in 1651[4]. The epidemic appears to have ceased in the autumn of 1650, when the Council of State, in a despatch to the Lord Deputy, take notice of the goodness of God in stopping the plague[5].

Fever in England, 1651-2.

Between those plagues of the years 1644–1650 and the final re-appearance of the infection on English soil from 1665 to 1666, the interval is occupied with a good deal of fever both in town and country. The sicknesses of those years are of interest as having been described by two competent physicians, Willis and Whitmore.

There were two principal periods of the epidemics, the years 1651–2 and 1657–9. In the former period the sickness appears to have been mostly in the north-west. Whitmore, who had seen practice in the Civil War, in Staffordshire and Shropshire, appears to have been in Chester in 1651, and was settled in

---

[1] *Annals of Ireland* by Clyn and Dowling, Dean Butler's notes pp. 64, 65 (ref. to Carte's *Life of the Duke of Ormonde*).

[2] *Cal. State Papers.*

[3] The weekly bills of mortality for Dublin, July 20—Aug. 2, 1662, showed only 14 baptisms and 20 burials in ten parishes; but these can hardly have been all the births and deaths in the city.

[4] Smith's *Cork*, vol. II. from Cox MSS.

[5] *Cal. S. P.* Sept. 21, 1650.

London in 1657. It is from him that our information mostly comes[1].

"It is well known," he says, "that this disease in the year 1651 [the same fever that he describes more fully for the years 1658 and 1659] first broke out by the seaside in Cheshire, Lancashire, and North Wales....In Cheshire in the year 1651 this disease seized most upon the country people who were laborious, the seeds being sooner dispersed in them through the agitation of the humours and spirits in their harvest labours, than on those who lead a more sedentary life ; and that might be one reason why we were so free in the city of Chester, when within three or four miles of us round about, whole towns were infected with it, there being 80 and 100 sick at a time in small villages, as at Stanney, Dunham-on-the-hill, Norton and all there abouts by the water side it extremely raged."

Whitmore refers to something that he had written, "for my private use," on the subject of this fever as far back as 1642 ; he remarks also that it raged every autumn in some place or other of the kingdom, and mentions his own experience in Staffordshire and Shropshire during the late war. But it is the epidemic in Cheshire, Lancashire and North Wales, in 1651 that he specially describes, side by side with those of 1658 and 1659 ; and it is of interest to note his suggestion as to the origin of the fever on both shores of the Mersey. It was well known that the fever in 1651 first broke out by the seaside in Cheshire, Lancashire and North Wales :

"And if it were observed in Holland that on a misty day, that infectious disease the Sudor Anglicus came into Amsterdam in an afternoon, five hundred or more dying that night of it, as Lemnius reports, I know not why we may not as well suppose their opposite neighbour, Dublin, then visited for two years with the plague, should not have communicated the same to them though in a more remiss degree."

Here the suggestion is that the prevalence of plague on the opposite coast of Ireland had given rise to a minor and "more remiss" contagion along the coasts of North Wales, Cheshire and Lancashire. But the plague had been most severe in Chester itself before it broke out in Ireland, and had been severe in Shrewsbury at the same time as in Ireland.

[1] H. Whitmore, M.D. *Febris Anomala ; or the New Disease that now rageth throughout England, with a brief description of the Disease which this Spring most infested London.* London, 1659 (4 November).

Whatever the theory, it is significant that the corner of England
which was the worst and perhaps only seat of plague in 1648
and 1650, was the seat of a malignant fever in 1651, the former
having been in the towns, and the latter in the country villages.

We get a glimpse of a heavy mortality among the country
people the year after at Bootle, in Cumberland, just across the
border from Lancashire[1]. On July 8, 1652, Thomas Wharton
writes from Kirkdale to Edward Moore :

"There was a boy at widow Robinson's died upon Saturday in Whitsun
week, and upon the Wednesday before he was sawying at the steward
Worsley's house with his wrights. The boy and the steward's man slept
together in Worsley's barn ; towards night the boy was not well, and could
work no longer. All this John Wiggan of Kirkdale did see. Next, John
Birch died, and four of his children—all are dead but his wife. At John
Robinson's, one child and his wife died last week, and upon Wednesday last
two children more died ; and it was thought by the constable of Bootle that
he would be dead before this day at night. Upon Wednesday at night last,
at James Pye's, there died two, his son and daughter ; and a servant of
Thomas Doubie's is dead ; and it is this day broken forth in Bridge's, as we
hear."

On what evidence this country epidemic is called "the
plague" by the antiquary who prints the document does not
appear. The fatality of the disease would suggest plague,
rather than fever ; but the fever itself would seem to have been
more malignant at one place than another, and at one time
than another, and there may have been at Bootle cases unmentioned which recovered. If it had been true bubo-plague, it
is a solitary instance, so far as records go, in the fifteen years
between the extinction of plague at Shrewsbury in 1650, and
its revival in London and elsewhere in 1665. The epidemic
disease that we ordinarily hear of in that interval is fever ; and
of the fever our best accounts, after Whitmore's reference to
1651, are of the epidemics in 1657, 1658 and 1659.

Fever and Influenza, 1657–9.

The account by Willis of three consecutive epidemics in
the autumn of 1657, the spring of 1658, and the autumn of 1658,

---

[1] *Hist. MSS. Commission,* x. pt. 4, p. 106.

is of peculiar interest for the reason that it is the first systematic piece of epidemiology written in England, and that the middle epidemic of the three was one of influenza[1]. On reading the narrative of events by Willis, we can understand how it was that the physicians of that period were so impressed by the doctrine of an epidemic constitution of the season, and by its counterpart doctrine of a seasonal predisposition in the human constitution. That teaching was afterwards expounded in successive essays by Sydenham ; but it was held generally in those times, and Willis found apt illustrations of it in the three epidemics one after the other in 1657–58. Let us follow his narrative, and add to it some particulars from Whitmore.

The spring and summer of 1657 were extremely dry and hot; but especially after the summer solstice the heats were so intense for many weeks following that, day and night, there was none that did not complain of the heat of the air, and were almost in a continual sweat and were not able to breathe freely. About the calends of July, the fever which was at first sporadic and particular, began to break forth in some places, perhaps two or three cases in the same city or village. The fever fits at this period occurred every other day, but there was no cold fit or rigor preceding, as in an ordinary ague, the heat being intense from the outset. Vomiting and bilious stools occurred plentifully to most, with sweat succeeding, not however an easy, uninterrupted and critical sweat. The remission of the fever fit was rarely complete in the intermediate day, weakness, languor, thirst and restlessness always remaining. In some the type improved after three or four of these quasi-tertian paroxysms; the later fits were ushered in with a rigor and a cold stage, so that the fever became an exact tertian intermittent. But in most the type became worse, which may have been due to errors of regimen and physicking. The fever became, indeed, a continued one, and might end in nervous symptoms—lethargy, delirium, cramps or convulsions.

In August it was spreading far and near, so that in every region or village round Oxford, many were sick of it; but it was much more frequent in the country cottages and in the

[1] Willis, *Diatribae duae.* Hagae, 1659.

smaller villages than in cities or towns. It was called "the new disease," as the war-typhus of 1643 had been called, and other epidemics both earlier and later.

Willis continues: It crept from house to house, infecting most of the same family, and especially those in familiar converse with the sick. "Yea old men, and men of ripe age, it ordinarily took away." It lasted many days in an individual, nay even months, attended with much evacuation and almost daily vomits and sweats. "Scarce one in a thousand died of it, which I never knew in an epidemical synochus." This singular malady, which differed from ague not only in its want of clear intervals between the fits of fever, but also in being propagated by contagion, raged throughout all England in the autumn of 1657. Only in some few limited localities, and in these only in some cases, was it accompanied by true dysentery. Willis is not satisfied with the facile explanation of an infection of the air, "the little bodies of which infections, being admitted within, did ferment with the blood and humours." There must have been something equally general in the human body, a predisposition to be so acted upon ; and of that proneness to fever he finds the cause in the intemperance of the year, namely the great heat of the summer and autumn.

But the most remarkable illustration of these doctrines was the epidemic of the following spring, which was a pure and unmistakeable epidemic of influenza-cold. After the very hot summer and autumn, there was a long winter of intense frost. From the ides of December to the vernal equinox the earth was covered with snow, the wind blowing steadily from the north. The state of health through the winter was fairly good. The north wind continued until June. "About the middle of April, suddenly a distemper arose as if sent by some blast of the stars, which laid hold of very many together; and in some towns in the space of a week above a thousand fell sick together." They had a troublesome cough, great spitting, and catarrh "falling down on the palate, throat, and nostrils." The illness approached with fever, thirst, want of appetite, weariness, grievous pains in the head, back, loins and limbs, and heat in the praecordia. Some were very ill in bed, with hoarseness and almost continual coughing; others had bleeding at the nose, bloody spittle or bloody flux. Not a few old and infirm died, but the more strong, and almost all the healthy constitutions recovered. Those that died "wasted leisurely," like persons sick of a hectic fever. About the third part of mankind was distempered in a month. Willis's explanation of it is that the constant north wind checked the natural action of the blood in spring. The spring blood is more lively, like the juices of vegetables. The catarrhal fever was a disorder of the spring blood, like new wine close shut up in bottles.

This outbreak about the middle of April is evidently described for Oxford and the country around. Willis then describes his third epidemic, that of the summer and autumn of 1658, which was the same type of fever as in the summer and autumn of 1657. The vernal fever of 1658 did not last longer than six weeks. The wind continued still north, until the summer solstice; a little before the beginning of July there was a most fierce heat for a few days, and when the dog-days were begun, the air grew most cruelly hot, so that one could scarce endure it in the open. The new fever arose mostly about the end of August, and began to spread through whole regions about us (at Oxford), and chiefly, like that of 1657, in country houses and villages; but in the meantime few of the inhabitants of the greater towns and cities fell sick. The symptoms were much the same as in the previous autumn. The fever was continual in some; in others it was of an intermitting type at first; but very many were ill "in their brain and nervous stock," with cruel headache, noises in the ears, dullness of hearing, stupor, vertigo, waking, and delirium. In some, on the first or second day, "little broad and red spots like to the measles have leisurely broken forth in the whole body, which being shortly vanished, the fever and headache became worse." The patients lay for a few days as if dying, without speaking or knowing their friends, after which came lethargy and delirium. The young men mostly recovered, the old men died. In the fits of old men, the heat was not very sharp, but there were restlessness, tossing about, idle and random talking, with dryness of the mouth, surfiness of the tongue, and viscous sordes. Usually the pulse was strong and equal; a weak, unequal and intermittent pulse, with contractures of the tendons and convulsive motions in the wrists, was an omen of death. Those who died passed away in a stupor, without consciousness to dispose of their goods; the recovery of others was long and doubtful. One notable thing in this fever was the exanthem, which reminds one more of the rash of sweating sickness or dengue (break-bone fever), than of the spots of typhus.

Willis ends his book on fevers with that account of the autumnal epidemic of 1658, "taken the 13th of September," his work having been published at the Hague in 1659. Whitmore, whose short essay is dated from London, November, 1659, begins with the autumnal epidemic of 1658, which is the last of Willis's three; and, strangely enough, he also has a vernal epidemic of influenza to describe—an epidemic clearly belonging to the spring of 1659. Unless there be some error in Whitmore's dates, it is impossible to avoid the conclusion that the second autumnal fever, that of 1658, was followed by a spring influenza, just as the first, of 1657, had been.

Whitmore's account of the autumnal fever of 1658 agrees in the main with that given by Willis. He defines it as "a putrid continued and malignant fever containing in it the seeds of contagion." It raged in the last autumn through all England, "and now begins again," (his preface being dated November, 1659), seizing on all sorts of people of different nature, which shows that it is epidemic. The part affected is chiefly the heart, and therefore some call it *cordis morbus.*

"In this, as in the plague at the first catching of it, some seem to be very pleasant, so far are they from perceiving themselves to be amiss, when indeed death itself hath set his foot within the threshold of their earthly houses." There were pains in the head, inclination to vomit, sudden fainting of spirits, and weakness without any manifest cause, the pulse feeble and sometimes intermittent, so as very lusty and strong men in Cheshire (in the year 1651 where this disease then raged) in a very short space so lost their strength that they were not able to stand or turn themselves in their beds. Some also are taken with bleeding, purging, and sweating, and many have the spots. But for the most part it appears in the livery of some other kind of ague. It begins to show its malignity after the 5th, 7th, or 9th day, with loss of appetite, thirst, and a dry black tongue.

Letters of 1658 from London bear out the prevalence of autumnal sickness. On August 3, one writes that the weather is hot and dry, the town extremely empty, and the flux beginning. On January 4, 1659, there is much sickness, especially fevers, agues and the smallpox.

A good deal of the interest of Whitmore's essay lies in his arguments against blood letting in this fever; but that is part of a history which will have to be dealt with as a whole at a later stage.

Whitmore then proceeds to the vernal epidemic of 1659, just as Willis had done to that of 1658. His words are (4 Nov. 1659):

"Having given an account of the nature and cure of this disease which now rageth throughout England, I shall briefly describe that which this spring universally infested London ; and show how it agreed and how it differed from that disease which last fall invaded the whole nation." He then describes the typical influenza, just as Willis had done under a date a year earlier—pains in the limbs of some, coughs, and aguish distempers in others ; "so that in a week or a fortnight's time, when it had fermented and caused a putrefaction of humours, it quickly tended to a height, and struck many thousands in London down, scarce leaving a family where any store were, without some being ill of this distemper, suddenly sweeping very many away, being the same, in the judgment of no mean physician, with that in autumn last, though in a new skin." Whitmore then gives a reason "why this should hold them all with coughs, which it did not in the fall."

Assuming an affinity to the autumnal epidemic of 1658, he proceeds to state the circumstance of a reappearance in the spring of 1659: "Upon this hush it lay all the winter, until the Easter week, and then in two or three warm days broke loose, having had no warm weather all before, but a rainy and black week, the sun not appearing for five or six days together just before the holiday; when on a sudden that warm weather breaking forth, the citizens in their summer pomp, being thinner clothed many of them than before (like bees on a glorious day) swarmed abroad, and the pores etc."

Both Willis and Whitmore incline to the view that the catarrhal fever of the spring was akin to the strange fever of the autumn, the differentia of each being appropriate to the season. Willis, however, keeps the two types more apart than Whitmore. The latter speaks of both fevers as "this Protean-like distemper," whose various shapes "render it such a hocus pocus to the amazed and perplexed people, they being held after most strange and diverse ways with it." It is "so prodigious in its alterations that it seems to outvie even Proteus himself." Thus the strangest part of these narratives is not the catarrhal influenza, which has so often reappeared as to be familiar, but the prevalence of anomalous fevers, in some respects like intermittents without the clear interval between the fits, but in respect of contagion, spots, pains and other symptoms, like typhus—a volatile typhus of the country and of the towns. Although this epidemiological phenomenon be a strange one, there is no reason to question the correctness of Willis's observations, corroborated as they are by those of Whitmore. But there are, indeed, many more experiences of the like kind in the years to follow, which fall without the limits of the present volume. One only of these later observers need be mentioned here. The third of the famous trio with Sydenham and Willis was Morton. He had a long experience in London of fever and smallpox, which he made the subject of a book in 1692–4[1]. His history goes as far back as 1658—"*historia febris* συνεχὴς *ab anno* 1658 *ad annum* 1691." Of the year 1658 he says the fever was everywhere through England and refers to Willis; the only facts of his own being that Oliver Cromwell and his (Morton's) father were carried off by it in September of that year, that he had it himself (aged 20) and was three months in recovering, and that the whole household (in Suffolk) were infected. Cromwell's attack came upon him at Hampton Court on August 21; but it was not the first sickness of the kind that he had suffered. He was only fifty-nine, but worn out with many cares, and at that time distressed by the death of his favourite daughter, Lady Claypole, under his roof on August 6, from some painful internal female trouble. The Lord Protector's fever was called a "bastard tertian," which might have been a name for the fever described by Willis. He was removed on the 24th August to Whitehall, where the air was thought to be more wholesome; and died between three and four in the afternoon of September 3, the

[1] *Pyretologia.* 2 vols. London, 1692–4. Appendix to 1st volume, p. 415.

anniversary at once of "Dunbar field and Worcester's laureat wreath."

This prevalence of fevers, Protean in their varying types, all over England in 1657–59 corresponds to the fever period of 1623–24. In each case the fever was a minor plague, and in each case it was followed by a revival of the plague proper, which had been dormant all over the country for a dozen or fifteen years. The principal difference is that the fever-period of 1623–24 was followed by the plague in 1625, whereas the fever-period of 1657–59 was followed by several years not free from fever and then by the plague in 1665. It is clear that the fevers of 1657–59 made a great impression all over England, and were afterwards popularly spoken of as a warning of the Great Plague itself. In the parish register of Aldenham, Hertfordshire, there is inserted a poem on the Great Plague of 1665, which has the following verses[1] :

> "Seven years since a little plague God sent,
> He shook his rod to move us to repent.
> Not long before that time a dearth of corn
> Was sent to us to see if we would turn."

In Short's abstracts of parish registers, the years preceding 1665 stand out as sickly in country districts, according to the following figures :

	No. of registers examined	No. with sickness	Baptisms in same	Burials in same
1657	98	36	991	1305
1658	96	33	704	1159
1659	101	29	553	825
1660	107	17	342	489
1661	182 (?)	25	448	685
1662	105	20	376	504
1663	119	15	325	443
1664	118	12	328	364
1665	117	14	229	446

Periods as unhealthy as 1657–59 do not occur again until 1667–71, and 1679–84.

Willis says, of the autumnal epidemic of 1658 : "But in the meantime few of the inhabitants of the greater towns and cities

---

[1] Sent to *Notes and Queries*, 1st ser. XII. 281, by Mr H. Hucks Gibbs.

fell sick." That is confirmed for London, in a letter of October 26, 1658 : " A world of sickness in all countries round about London. London is now held the wholesomest place;" but on January 4, 1659: " There is much sickness in the town, especially feavers, agues, and smallpox[1]." In Short's tables, the registers of market towns bear the same traces of much sickness in 1657 and 1658 as those of country parishes.

A high mortality from fever and spotted fever continued in London every year from 1658 to the year of the great plague. The largest number of deaths from fever was in the year of the plague itself, when the bills of mortality returned them as 5257 (without much certainty, however, owing to the confusion of the plague). The next highest figures had been in 1661, when the fever deaths were 3490. We get a glimpse of that epidemic from Pepys ; on August 16, 1661, he writes: " But it is such a sickly time both in the city and country everywhere (of a sort of fever) that never was heard of almost, unless it was in plague-time. Among others, the famous Tom Fuller is dead of it, and Dr Nicholls [Nicholas], dean of St Paul's, and my Lord General Monk is very dangerously ill." On August 31 he enters in his diary : " The season very sickly everywhere of strange and fatal fevers." The same diarist, on October 20, 1663, has an entry that the queen is ill of a spotted fever and that " she is as full of spots as a leopard ;" on the 24th the queen was in a good way to recovery.

It is at this period that Sydenham's famous observations of the seasons and the public health in London begin. The autumnal intermittents, he says, which had been prevalent some years before, came back in 1661 with new strength, about the beginning of July, being mostly tertians of a bad type : they increased so much in August as to sweep away families almost entirely, but declined with the winter cold coming on. He then draws the distinction between them and ordinary tertians. In the same years, 1661–2–3–4, a continued fever is described at great length, and then he comes to the " pestilential fever " and the plague itself of 1665 and 1666[2]. Taking from Sydenham

---

[1] *Hist. MSS. Commiss.* v. 146 (Sutherland letters).
[2] Greenhill's edition (Sydenham Society, 1844), pp. 37, 93, 95–98.

the single fact, for the present, that an unusual amount of pestilential fever led up to the plague of 1665 (which he did not stay in London to witness), we shall proceed in the next chapter but one to that crowning epidemic of the present section of our history. Something more remains to be said of the fevers of 1661 (specially described by Willis as a fever of the brain and nervous stock, but called "the new disease" in its turn); but as it is the first of Sydenham's "epidemic constitutions," and as these are recorded continuously to 1685, when there was another "new fever," it will be convenient to end the detailed history of fevers for the present with the remarkable epidemics of 1657–59.

CHAPTER XI.

SICKNESSES OF VOYAGES AND COLONIES.

(Sea Scurvy, Flux, Fever, and Yellow Fever.)

THE sicknesses of the first voyages and foreign settlements come into the history of national maladies, both as concerning Britain on the sea and beyond sea, and as showing forth the disease-producing conditions of those early times. In the latter respect there is more to be learned from voyages and colonial experience than the records of domestic life at home are likely to inform us of otherwise than vaguely. The Englishman of the time carried his habits with him to sea and to foreign parts, where the circumstances were more trying and the consequences more obvious.

This history divides itself at once into several branches. There are the disease-incidents of ocean voyages, irregular at first but becoming somewhat uniform after the East India Company's start in 1601, chief among them being scurvy. There are next the early discouragements from sickness, both on the voyage and after landing, in the planting of colonies in Virginia, New England and the West Indies, among which the troubles of Jamaica were on a sufficiently great scale to deserve minute study. Lastly, among the larger sections of this chapter, we have to notice the beginnings and circumstances of the terrible and long-enduring scourge of West Indian colonies—yellow fever. While we are mainly, in this record of the sicknesses of voyages and of new colonies, concerned with British enterprise, we shall have occasion to glance at the similar experiences of other nations.

The first accounts of Sea Scurvy.

The malady that figures most in the narratives of the long ocean voyages which began with the modern period is scurvy. In the very first of the great voyages, that of Vasco de Gama to the Indies by the Cape of Good Hope in 1498, scurvy appeared when the ships were on the West African coast, fifty-five deaths occurring within a short period. Of all the known subsequent occurrences of the kind, there are accounts more or less full in the collections of Hakluyt and Purchas, from which the facts in the sequel have been taken.

In the voyage of Ferdinand Magellan to the Pacific, scurvy is mentioned first at a late stage; in the year 1520 the ships had passed the straits called by his name and had been three months and twelve days sailing westwards from the last land; their provisions had run short, and, "by reason of this famine and unclean feeding, some of their gums grew so over their teeth that they died miserably for hunger." Nineteen men, as well as a giant from Patagonia and an Indian from Brazil, were dead, and some twenty-five or thirty others were sick, "so that there was in a manner none without some disease[1]."

There were no voyages of the same length by English ships until many years after: and then we find the same troubles in them from scurvy and other sickness. While the Portuguese and Spaniards were navigating in tropical waters, the English and French were sending most of their expeditions to the North. The French attempted to found a colony on the shores of the Gulf of St Lawrence, while the English sought to establish a trade with Muscovy by way of the White Sea, and to open a nearer route to the far East by way of the polar regions. The voyages in all these enterprises were short, the ships for the most part returning after an absence of four or five months, and without any notable experience of sickness: it was only

[1] Purchas, *His Pilgrimes.* 4 vols., folio. London, 1625, vol. I. Book II. p. 36.

when the French wintered in Canada that scurvy broke out. Thus the English voyages for the Muscovy Company have little or no interest for our subject; while the three voyages of Frobisher in search of the North-West passage in 1576, 1577 and 1578, and the three of Davis in 1585, 1586, and 1587 (in which last he got to 73° N.) are as nearly as possible free from records of sickness.

Jacques Cartier's second expedition to the St Lawrence in 1535 had a disastrous experience of scurvy. In his first voyage in 1534, with two ships of sixty tons each and each carrying sixty-one men, he appears to have had no sickness, having left St Malo on April 20, traded with the Indians on the Gulf of St Lawrence, and returned on September 5 of the same year. The expedition of the following year, with three ships, wintered on the coast, amidst heavy ice, and about mid-winter began to suffer from scurvy[1]. The crews appear to have had no lack of stores, both meat and drink, and the outbreak of scurvy, described as an unknown disease, was so surprising that it was traced to infection from the Indians, who are said to have admitted the deaths of some fifty of their number from "pestilence."

"The said unknown sickness began to spread itself amongst us after the strangest sort that ever was either heard of or seen, insomuch as some did lose all their strength, and could not stand on their feet; then did their legs swell, their sinewes shrink as black as any coal. Others also had their skins spotted with spots of blood of a purple colour; then did it ascend to their ankles, knees, thighs, shoulders, arms, and neck; their mouth became stinking, their gums so rotten that all the flesh did fall off even to the roots of the teeth, which did also almost all fall out. With such infection did this sickness spread itself in our three ships that about the middle of February, of a hundred and ten persons that we were, there were not ten whole; so that one could not help the other...There were already 8 dead and more than 50 sick, and, as we thought, past all recovery." The body of one dead, aged 22, was opened to see what the disease was; he was found to have his heart white, but rotten, and more than a quart of red water about it[2]; his liver was indifferent fair; but his lungs black and mortified...his milt toward

---

[1] Hakluyt, *The Principal Navigations*, &c.   3 vols.   London, 1599, III. 225–6.

[2] Pericarditis scorbutica—a condition which has been observed mostly in Russia in recent times. The whiteness of the heart would have been due to the fibrinous layer of lymph on its surface, from the pericarditis.

the back was somewhat perished, rough as if it had been rubbed against a stone.

"From the midst of November to the midst of March there died 25 of our best and chiefest men, and all the rest sick except three or four; then it pleased God to cast his pitiful eye upon us, and sent us the knowledge of remedie of our healths, and recovery....The Captain, walking upon the ice, asken of Domagaia [an Indian] how he had done to heal himself; he answered that he had taken the juice and sap of the leaves of a certain tree, and therewith had healed himself! for it was a singular remedy against that disease." The Indian's advice was "to take the bark and leaves and boil them together and to drink of the said decoction every other day, and to put the dregs of it upon the legs that is sick."...

"It is thought to be the sassafras tree. After this medicine was found and proved to be true there was such strife about it, who should be first to take of it, that they were ready to kill one another, so that a tree as big as any oak in France was spoiled and lopped bare, and occupied all in five or six days, and it wrought so well that if all the physicians of Montpelier and Lovaine had been there with all the drugs of Alexandria, they would not have done so much in one year as that tree did in six days, for it did so prevail that as many as used of it, by the grace of God recovered their health."

In 1542, while Cartier was still trading on his own account to the St Lawrence from Brittany, a more ambitious project, under a Crown patent, issued from La Rochelle[1]. With De la Roche, count of Roberval, as governor, a number of adventurous nobles and gentry, with men, women and children to the number of two hundred in all, sailed in three ships, and established themselves in Lower Canada with all the formalities of occupation. Two of the three ships were sent home in September, the colonists proper being left to taste the rigours of a Canadian winter: "In the end many of our people fell sick of a certain disease in their legges, reynes and stomacke, so that they seemed to bee deprived of all their lymmes: and there died about fiftie."

The first English records of scurvy at sea are in connexion with the early voyages to Guinea for gold-dust[2]. Mr John Lok sailed on the second voyage to Guinea, on October 11, 1554, his ships being the 'Trinitie,' 140 tons, the 'Bartholomew,' 90 tons, and the 'John Evangelist,' 140 tons. After trading some months on the African coast the ships sailed for home:

---

[1] Hakluyt, III. 241.   [2] Hakluyt, II. Part II., pp. 22, 36, 48.

"There died of our men at this last voyage about twenty and four, whereof many died at their return into the clime of the cold regions, as between the islands of Azores and England." The disease is not named; but it is probable from what follows that it was scurvy.

The next voyage to Guinea was Towrson's first, in October 1555, from Newport, Isle of Wight, in the 'Hart' and the 'Hind;' the death of only one man is mentioned; he died "in his sleep" on March 29; by the 7th May, the provisions were so reduced that the ships put in on the coast of Ireland to purchase milk and two sheep from the wild kernes, paying in gold-dust.

In Towrson's second voyage there is no word of sickness; but in his third voyage in 1577, it is a prominent topic of the narrative. The vessels 'Minion,' 'Christopher' and 'Tiger' left Plymouth on January 30, 1577. On the 8th of May, "all our cloth in the 'Minion' being sold, I called the company together to know whether they would tarry the sale of the cloth taken in the prize at this place or no: they answered that in respect of the death of some of their men, and the present sickness of 20 more, they would not tarry, but repair to the other ships, of whom they had heard nothing since April 27." Having at length bartered for gold until the natives would barter no longer, the three ships bore up for home. On July 24 the master of the 'Tiger' came aboard the 'Minion' and reported that "his men were so weak and the ship so leak that he was not able to keep her above the water." A muster held of all the three crews the same day showed that there were not above 30 sound men in them. On September 3, there being only six men in the 'Tiger' who could work, the gold and stores were taken out of her, and she was abandoned. On October 6, when off the coast of Portugal, the 'Christopher' reported herself so weak that she was not able to keep the sea. The 'Minion' promised to attend her into Vigo; but a fair wind springing up, she signalled that she was off for home, whereupon the 'Christopher' followed. On October 16, a great south-westerly storm arose; the men in the 'Minion' were not able, from weakness, to handle the sails, which were blown away: however, they made shift to reach the Isle of Wight on October 20, nothing more being said of the 'Christopher.'

The English voyages to Guinea for gold-dust were shortly followed by the three expeditions of John Hawkins in 1562, 1564 and 1567 to the West coast of Africa for negro slaves to be sold to the Spaniards in Hispaniola and Cuba and on the Spanish Main[1]. Only a brief summary remains of the first voyage, in which nothing is said of sickness; in the second, the negroes, at least, appear to have suffered on the somewhat long passage across the tropical belt, especially from want of water; and the third was so calamitous in various ways that Hawkins himself wrote of it : " If all the miseries and troublesome affairs of this sorrowful voyage should be perfectly and thoroughly written, there should need a painful man with his pen, and as great a time as he had that wrote the lives and deaths of the martyrs." Little or nothing is said of one class of martyrs in the business —the negroes, of whom the ships carried four to five hundred. English lives were lost in the kidnapping raids, from poisoned arrows, it was thought, the wounded dying " in strange sort with their mouths shut some ten days before they died, and after their wounds were whole." It was on the return from the Gulf of Mexico, more than a year out from England, that the sickness on board was worst. They cleared the Bahamas channel on November 16, 1568, after which, " growing near to the cold country, our men being oppressed with famine, died continually, and they that were left grew into such weakness that we were scarcely able to manage our ship " (the ' Jesus ' of Lubeck, 700 tons). They put in at Ponte Vedra, near Vigo, on December 31, but the fresh provisions that they got turned to their hurt: " our men with excess of fresh meat grew into miserable diseases and died a great part of them." Twelve fresh hands shipped at Vigo enabled the vessels to reach the nearest English haven at Mount's Bay in Cornwall.

Meanwhile we obtain some glimpses of seafaring among the Portuguese, who had now in the middle of the 16th century a regular trade to the Indies, established by Vasco de Gama's route round the Cape of Good Hope. Perhaps the most famous

[1] Hakluyt, III. 501.

of these records is that of the voyage of St Francis Xavier from Lisbon to Goa in the spring of 1540. The expedition with which he took passage carried, it is said, a regiment of a thousand men to reinforce the garrison of Goa ; during the voyage the Jesuit apostle " rendered to the diseased services too revolting to be described, and lived among the dying and the profligate, the unwearied minister of consolation and of peace[1]." After five months the ships arrived at Mozambique, by which time Xavier and many more were suffering from fever. Goa was not reached until thirteen months out from the Tagus. A more familiar narrative of the same voyage of the Portuguese ships a generation later is given by an English youth, Thomas Stevens, in a letter written home to his father, a citizen of London, shortly after arriving at Goa. Both in its generalities and in its particulars this excellent letter will serve to measure the prevalence of scurvy, flux, and fever in the earlier period of the East Indian trade by the Cape[2].

The five ships left Lisbon on April 5, 1579, the solemnity being marked by the firing of ordnance and the braying of trumpets. In the ships, " besides shipmen and soldiers, there were a great number of children, which in the seas bear out better than men ; and no marvel, when that many women also pass very well." After a passage along the Guinea coast, made tedious by calms and head winds, they rounded the Cape of Good Hope on July 29. From that point in the voyage the Portugal ships were wont to follow one or other of two routes according to the lateness of the season— either the route by the Mozambique Channel, in which case they were able to get fruits and fresh provisions, or the route along more southern parallels for a time, and passing to the east of Madagascar[3]. In the latter case, " by reason of the long navigation and want of food and water, they fall into sundry diseases, their gums wax great and swell, and they are fain to cut

---

[1] Sir James Stephen's *Essays in Ecclesiastical Biography*, pop. ed. p. 125.

[2] Hakluyt, II. pt. 2, p. 99.

[3] The famous figure in *Paradise Lost* (IV. 159) is taken from the route to India passing within Madagascar—a poetic colouring of dreary and painful realities :—

> As when to them who sail
> Beyond the Cape of Hope, and now are past
> Mozambik, off at sea north-east winds blow
> Sabean odours from the spicy shore
> Of Araby the blest ; with such delay
> Well pleas'd they slack their course, and many a league
> Cheer'd with the grateful smell old Ocean smiles :

them away, their legs swell, and all the body becometh sore and so be-
numbed that they cannot stir hand nor foot, and so they die for weakness.
Others fall into fluxes and agues, and so die thereby.

"And this way it was our chance to make ; and though we had more
than one hundred and fifty sick, there died not past seven-and-twenty, which
loss they esteemed not much in respect of other times."

The ships went greatly out of their course, having sighted the island of
Socotra at the entrance to the Gulf of Aden, and did not arrive at Goa until
October 24, 202 days from Lisbon without calling anywhere.

The first of the long English voyages beyond the Line was
Sir Francis Drake's famous circumnavigation from November
15, 1577, to September 26, 1580[1].   Drake must have lost many
of his men in those three years, but there is nothing in the
narrative to show that they perished of disease.   The expedition was by way of the Straits of Magellan, and was mainly
given up to plundering the Spaniards on the coasts of Chili and
Peru.   Drake set out for home loaded with treasure by way of
the Philippines and the Cape of Good Hope.   It is not until the
narrative brings us to a small island between Ternate and
Celebes that we hear of sickness ; they graved the ship there
and remained twenty-six days, during which the "sickly, weak
and decayed" recovered their strength, a large species of crayfish
found on the island being "very good and restoring meat,
whereof we had experience."   But even Drake, with all his
systematic care and resource, was destined in after years to
have a share of the common sickly experience at sea, and to
find disease a more potent enemy than the Spaniard.

Remarkable Epidemic in Drake's Fleet 1585-6.

Drake's next great expedition after his circumnavigation
was in 1585, with six Queen's ships and some nineteen others,
carrying 2,300 men.   A large number of private adventurers
had a money interest in the enterprise, which had for its object
to plunder Spanish towns in the West Indies and the Spanish
Main and to capture the treasure at the isthmus of Panama on

---

[1] *The World Encompassed* &c., Hakluyt Society, ed. Vaux, p. 149, and Hakluyt,
III. 740.

its way to Spain. The fleet experienced one of the most remarkable epidemics in the whole history of sickness[1].

Having left Plymouth on September 14, 1585, they arrived at the island of St Jago, in the Cape de Verde group, on November 16. More than a thousand men were landed, and were marched up the steep and broken ground to a hill overlooking the capital, which stood in a narrow valley, with high cliffs on the east and west and the Atlantic open before it at some distance on the south. The place was surrounded by a wall, and defended by fifty pieces of brass ordnance ; but no resistance was offered, and the English marched in to find the inhabitants fled farther inland. On the 17th November, the town was quartered out for the lodging of the whole army, which remained there for ten days or a fortnight (there are inconsistent dates), taking such spoils as the place yielded (wine, oil, meal and "trash" of the Portuguese trade to the Indies). After a week, when no one had come to ransom the town, Drake set out with 600 men to the village or town of St Domingo, twelve miles inland, with the hope of finding the governor and the bishop ; but, finding no one, he marched his men back again the same evening. On November 26 the whole force was re-embarked, all the houses in the capital as well as in the country round were set fire to, the port of Playa, a few miles to the westward, was also burned, and on the same night the ships weighed anchor from the latter, and stood away to the south-west. They had filled their water-casks from a pool, near the seashore, formed by the small stream which runs through the capital and descends the southern declivity. Nothing is said of sickness during the occupation of St Jago ; there seems to have been some lax discipline, (owing to the mixed character of the expedition), which Drake quickly remedied.

The ships were only eighteen days in crossing the Atlantic to Dominica, a distance of some forty meridians. In the midst of that quick sailing along the edge of the tropical belt of ocean, with the steady north-east trade wind behind them, the season the beginning of December and the climate the most delightful and most refreshing on the globe, the ships were visited suddenly with the fury of a deadly pestilential fever, of which the following is the account by a captain of the land-forces on board:

"We were not many days at sea but there began among our people such mortality as in a few days there were dead two or three hundred men. And

---

[1] *A summarie and true discourse of Sir Francis Drake's West Indian voyage begun in the year* 1585. Published by M. Thomas Cates. Shortened in Hakluyt, III. 542. The earlier part of the narrative is by Captain Bigges, and, after his death in the West Indies, by his lieutenant, Croftes.

until some seven or eight days after our coming from St Jago there had not died any one man of sickness in all the fleet. The sickness showed not his infection wherewith so many were stroken until we were departed thence ; and then seized our people with extreme hot burning and continual agues whereof very few escaped with life, and yet those for the most part not without great alteration and decay of their wits and strength for a long time after. In some that died were plainly showed the small spots which are often found upon those that be infected with the plague."

From Dominica the ships sailed to St Christopher, on which island Drake disembarked his whole force, and cleaned and aired his ships, according to an excellent practice which he had followed also in his great circumnavigation. Some days of Christmas having been thus spent ashore, "to refresh our sick people," the voyage was resumed to Hispaniola. Deaths continued to occur, from the same disease as at first, both among officers and men, and so continued for many weeks. However, they were able to land some 1000 or 1200 men on Hispaniola, and to carry the city of San Domingo by assault. The fleet then sailed southwards along the coast of the mainland to Cartagena, which was captured in turn, and in like manner held to ransom.

It is at this part of the narrative that we next hear of the infection in the fleet :

"We stayed here six weeks [from middle of January to end of February, 1586], and the sickness with mortality, before spoken of, still continued among us, though not with the same fury as at the first. And such as were touched with the said sickness, escaping death, very few or almost none could recover their strength ; yea, many of them were much decayed in their memory, insomuch that it was grown an ordinary judgment, when one was heard to speak foolishly, to say he had been sick of the *calentura*, which is the Spanish name of that burning ague ; for, as I told you before, it is a very burning and pestilent ague."

Then follows the Spanish theory of the *calentura*, which may or may not be rightly applied to the deadly epidemic that broke out suddenly in the English ships in mid ocean :

"The original cause thereof is imputed to the evening or first night air, which they term *la serena*, wherein they say, and hold very firm opinion, that whoso is then abroad in the open air shall certainly be infected to the death, not being of the Indian or natural race of those country people. By holding their watch our men were thus subjected to the infectious air, which at St Jago was most dangerous and deadly of all other places. With the inconvenience of continual mortality, we were forced to give over our intended enterprize, etc."

The land-captains having been consulted by Drake, on February 27, 1586, advised that the expedition should go home from Cartagena, instead of attempting to capture the treasure at Panama. In their memorandum they wrote : "And being further advised of the slenderness of our strength, whereunto we be now reduced, as well in respect of the small number of able bodies, as also not a little in regard of the slack disposition of the greater part of those which remain, very many of the better minds and men being either consumed by death, or weakened by sickness and hurts, etc." The voyage to England was accordingly begun ; St Augustine in Florida was captured by the way, and the struggling colony in Virginia, the first sent out by Raleigh, was taken up and brought back, and Portsmouth reached on July 28. "We lost some 750 men in the voyage, above three parts of them only by sickness." The names are given of eight captains, four lieutenants, and seven masters, who had died ; and there were some other officers dead unnamed. When the ransoms of San Domingo and Cartagena came to be divided, the venture must have been found as unprofitable to the shareholders as it had been disastrous to officers and men.

The Spanish name *calentura*, by which the fever in the fleet is described, was probably used generically for various kinds of fever in the tropics. But of this fever in particular, we have some details not without diagnostic value. It was doubtless contracted at St Jago in the Cape de Verde islands; it broke out suddenly in mid ocean after some seven or eight days sailing before the wind, in a delightful climate, which points to the regular incubation of an infective virus, received by hundreds of men when they were last ashore; the mortality was enormous; the symptoms were those of a burning fever ; and in some cases there were small spots or petechiae like those often seen in the plague. It was clearly a febrile form of pestilential infection, and, as few recovered, it must be considered to have had a death-rate such as typhus has rarely had, and such as yellow fever has commonly had. Nothing is said of the black vomit, the haemorrhages, and the saffron colour of skin and eyes, which are distinctive of yellow fever[1]. On the other hand there is a remarkable after-effect mentioned in both the passages quoted, the loss of memory, impairment of wits, and appearance of foolishness, which made "the calenture" a bye-word in the fleet. I shall not venture to say what the infection was; but it seems tolerably certain that it was contracted by the English during their occupation of the capital town of St Jago. More recent visitors to the Cape de Verde islands have remarked upon their towns and villages as fever-traps, and have pointed to the source of the fever; it is not malaria, or the mere climatic influence, but a pestilential emanation from spots of soil long inhabited by mankind, both black and white, and so situated in cups of the hills as to retain and multiply the filth-ferment in them. According to all analogy, the emanations from such a soil would be felt most by strangers not inured to them, and most of all by men of another stock and from other latitudes[2].

[1] Mr Froude (*History*, XII. 150) must be pronounced somewhat happy in his bold guess of "yellow fever." At the same time the enthymeme by which he had reached his conclusion is altogether wrong: first, in assuming that the infection "broke out" after the capture of Cartagena, ignoring the fact of its disastrous prevalence in mid-ocean two or three months before, shortly after leaving the Cape de Verde islands; and secondly in assuming that the yellow fever for which Cartagena and other harbours of the Spanish Main became notorious in later times had existed as an infection there in the 16th century.

[2] Sir Richard Hawkins, who commanded the galliot 'Duck' in Drake's expedition of 1585, thus refers to the Cape de Verde islands, on the occasion of touching there in his own expedition to the Pacific in 1593 (Purchas, IV. 1368):

These islands are "one of the most unhealthiest climates in the world. In two times that I have been in them, either cost us the one half of our people, with fevers and fluxes of sundry kinds, some shaking, some burning, some partaking of both; some possesst with frensie, others with slouth; and in one of them it cost me six months' sickness, with no small hazard of life." He then gives a reason for the great risk to health: the north-east breeze about four in the afternoon seldom faileth, "coming cold and fresh, and finding the pores of the body open and for the most part naked, penetrateth the very bones, and so causeth sudden distemperature, and sundry manners of sickness, as the subjects are divers whereupon they work. Departing out of the calmes of the Islands, and coming into the fresh breeze, it causeth the like; and I have seen within two days after that we have partaked of the fresh air, of two thousand men above an hundred and fifty have been crazed in their health." This seems to refer to the epidemic in Drake's fleet, as given in the text; but it is clearly an imperfect account of the facts, and in theory altogether improbable,

Sicknesses of Voyages, continued: Management of Scurvy.

The expedition to Virginia which returned in 1586 with Drake's ships homeward bound from the Spanish Main, was the first sent out by Raleigh with the intention of settling, an earlier voyage in 1584 having been made to explore the country. It is in connexion with Raleigh's second colony (and fourth expedition) in 1587 that we hear of disastrous sickness[1]. Having left 118 people to inhabit the country, the two larger ships sailed for home on August 27 of the same year. On board the " fly-boat," the provisions fell short, the water turned stinking, officers and men died, and the vessel was navigated with difficulty to the west coast of Ireland. When they reached Portsmouth, they found the admiral arrived there three weeks before them, but with an equally disastrous experience: " Ferdinando the master, with all his company were not only come home without any purchase, but also in such weakness by sickness of their chiefest men that they were scarce able to bring their ship into harbour, but were forced to let fall anchor without."

as a trade wind within the tropic cannot be credited with such effects, even if the forms of sickness were conceivably due at all to chill.

Darwin (*Naturalist's Voyage in the Beagle*, p. 366) says: " The island of St Jago, at the Cape de Verde, offers another strongly-marked instance of a country, which anyone would have expected to find most healthy, being very much the contrary. I have described the bare and open plains as supporting, during a few weeks after the rainy season, a thin vegetation, which directly withers away and dries up; at this period the air appears to become quite poisonous; both natives and foreigners often being affected with violent fevers. On the other hand, the Galapagos Archipelago, in the Pacific, with a similar soil, and periodically subject to the same process of vegetation, is perfectly healthy." But the Galapagos have been uninhabited, except in recent times by two or three hundred people banished from Ecuador. On the other hand the Cape de Verde islands are believed to have been at one time well wooded and not unfertile; and the Portuguese settlements in them, to say nothing of the native negro villages, had a fair population. It is not easy to understand the pernicious character of their fevers without assuming that spots of soil had become pestilential by human occupancy; but it is at the same time clear that a degree of befouling of the soil which would be innocuous in ordinary, would there engender deadly miasmata owing to the remarkable alternations of drought and wetness under a tropical sun.

[1] Hakluyt, III. 286.

The following year, 1588, was made memorable in the English annals of the sea by the defeat of the Spanish Armada. There was much sickness in both fleets. As regards the English ships, a writer who has had special access to original documents says[1]:

"We little think, when we peruse the melancholy tale of disease, starvation and shame, so needlessly undergone by the heroic champions of England's liberty against the invading might of Spain, from what obscure and insignificant causes the difficulties and hardships of the Island seamen may have chiefly arisen"—namely the peculation of officials, the mouldering rations, empty magazines, and the like. In the ships of the Spanish fleet the infection was like that of the plague itself; the main body of the expedition, fifty sail, reached Corunna, Santander and St Sebastian with such infection among the ten thousand men on board, that the inhabitants shut their houses against them.

Two of the heroes of that fight, Drake and Hawkins, met their death by sickness off the Spanish Main in 1595–6. The expedition, consisting of 2500 men in six Queen's ships and twenty-one others, left Plymouth on August 28, 1595[2]. Only the deaths of officers are mentioned in the narrative, but of these there seem to have been a good many, when the ships were in the Caribbean Sea. Hawkins died off Porto Rico on November 12. On December 7, Mr Yorke, captain of the 'Hope,' died of sickness, on January 15, captain Plat died of sickness, and then Sir Francis Drake began to keep his cabin and to complain of a scouring or flux: he died on January 28, off Porto Bello. On the 27th died captain Jonas of the 'Delight,' captain Egerton, and James Wood, chief surgeon of the fleet, out of the 'Garland.' On the 28th died Abraham Kendall out of the 'Saker.' Several of the ships were sunk so that their men might go to the Queen's ships, which were short of hands. A muster on February 6 showed in the whole fleet "two thousand sick and whole," or five hundred fewer than had sailed. There was some loss of life in encounters with the enemy, but much more from disease.

Of the filibustering cruises or expeditions to the East by the South American route, there remain to be mentioned two

[1] Mr Hubert Hall, of the Record Office, in *Society in the Elizabethan Age*. London, 1886, p. 120.

[2] Hakluyt, III. 583.

by Thomas Cavendish, and one at some length by Richard
Hawkins, before we come to the establishment of regular Eng-
lish trade to the East Indies by the Portuguese route round the
Cape of Good Hope. Cavendish's first voyage[1] by the Straits of
Magellan was from Plymouth, 25 July, 1586, with three ships
(240 tons in all) carrying 125 men.

Touching on the west coast of Africa, they went ashore and took
lemons from the trees. Off the coast of Brazil in November and December
two men died "of the disease called scorbuto, which is an infection of the
blood and the liver." Arrived at the Straits of Magellan they found twenty-
three Spaniards living on shell-fish, "which were all that remained of
four hundred which were left there [to found a colony] in these Straits of
Magellan, three years before, all the rest being dead with famine." They
were only too glad to hasten from this place, Port Famine, "for the noysome
stench and vile savour wherewith it was infected through the contagon
of the Spaniards' pined and dead carkeises." In one of Cavendish's own
ships, on February 21, 1588, when among the East Indian islands, Captain
Havers died of "a most severe and pestilent ague, which held him furiously
some seven or eight days. Moreover presently after his death, myself
[Pretty, the narrator] with divers others in the ship fell marvellously sick,
and so continued in very great pain for the space of three weeks or a month,
by reason of the extreme heat and intemperature of the climate."

One might guess that these were cases of ship-fever (or
calenture); but in Cavendish's last voyage we meet with a
strange sickness which will perhaps baffle all nosological conjecture. This voyage, like the first, was intended for the East
Indies by way of the Straits of Magellan[2]. The three tall ships
and two barks, having sailed from Plymouth on August 26,
1591, never got through the Straits; they were still within their
recesses in April, 1592, many men having "died with cursed
famine and miserable cold," and sick men having been put
ashore into the woods in the snow. The narrative (by John
Lane), then follows the fortunes of one of the ships, the 'Desire.'
Landing at Port Desire, in Patagonia, they found scurvy-grass
growing, which they ate with oil: "This herb did so purge the
blood that it took away all kind of swellings, of which many
[had] died, and restored us to perfect health of body, so that

---

[1] Hakluyt, III. 804, 820 ; and other details in the 1st ed. (1589) pp. 809, 810.
[2] Hakluyt, III. 842–52.

we were in as good case as when we came first out of England."
There also they took on board 14,000 penguins, which they had
dried on the rocks, mostly without salt; and sailed northwards
on December 22. With only 27 men surviving out of 76, they
left the coast of Brazil at Cape Frio (near Rio de Janeiro), and
then began their more singular experience of disease.

"After we came near unto the sun, our dried penguins began to corrupt,
and there bred in them a most loathsome and ugly worm of an inch long.
This worm did mightily increase, and devour our victuals;" it devoured
everything except iron,—clothes, boots, shirts, even the ship's timbers! "In
this woeful case, after we had passed the equinoctial toward the North, our
men began to fall sick of such a monstrous disease as I think the like was
never heard of: for in their ankles it began to swell, from thence in two
days it would be in their breasts, so that they could not draw their breath,
and then fell into their cods, and their cods and yardes did swell most
grievously and most dreadfully to behold, so that they could neither stand,
lie, nor goe. Whereupon our men grew mad with grief. Our captain [John
Davis] with extreme anguish of his soul was in such woeful case that he
desired only a speedy end, and though he were scarce able to speak for
sorrow, yet he persuaded them to patience.......For all this, divers grew
raging mad, and some died in most loathsome and furious pain. It were
incredible to write our misery as it was; there was no man in perfect health
but the captain, and one boy....To be short, all our men died except
sixteen [i.e., eleven died of the survivors after Cape Frio] of which there
were but five able to move." Those five worked the ship into Berehaven
(Bantry Bay) on June 11, 1593, and there ran her ashore.

The remarkable epidemic on board the 'Desire,' among men
living upon dried penguin infested with worms, was probably
not scurvy, or at least not all scurvy: the dropsy and dyspnœa
suggest one of the two forms of beri-beri, of a peculiarly severe
type. The co-existence of worms in the dried food may lead
one to think of a parasitic malady such as that caused by
Anchylostoma duodenale, which has also an anasarcous or œde-
matous character. But the diagnosis of beri-beri appears to be
far more likely. That epidemic, however we interpret it, must
rank among the curiosities of the history. But, in the next
that we come to, the sickness on board the 'Daintie,' Richard
Hawkins master, on a voyage in 1593 through the Straits of
Magellan, the disease is typical scurvy; and the observations
on sea-scurvy by Hawkins himself are among the best that we

C.   38

have for the period, and, indeed, until long after the Elizabethan period[1].

The 'Daintie,' a nearly new ship of 300 to 400 tons, weighed anchor from Blackwall on April 8, 1593. She was deeply laden with merchandise for trade and accompanied by a victualler, of 100 tons, the 'Hawk.' It was not until June 12, that they got away from Plymouth. They put in at the Cape de Verde islands, about whose climate and health Hawkins makes some observations already quoted. Sailing thence they had come within three or four degrees of the Line, when scurvy broke out :

"My company within a few days began to fall sick of a disease which seamen are wont to call the scurvie ; and seemeth to be a kind of dropsie, and raigneth most in this climate of any that I have heard or read of in the world, though [it is found] in all seas. It possesseth all those of which it takes hold with a loathsome sloathfulnesse, *that even to eate* they would be content to change *with sleepe and rest*, which is the most pernicious enemie in this sickness that is known. It bringeth with it a great desire to drink, and causeth a general swelling of all parts of the body, especially of the legs, and gums ; and many times the teeth fall out of the jaws without pain. The signs to know this disease in the beginning are divers,—by the swelling of the gums, by denting of the flesh of the legs with a man's finger, the pit remaining without filling up in a good space ; others show it with their laziness ; others complain of the crick of the back, etc., all which are for the most part certain tokens of the infection. The cause is thought to be the stomack's feebleness by change of air in intemperate climates, of diet in salt meats, boiled also in salt water, and corrupted sometimes ; the want of exercise, also, either in persons or elements, as in calms."

Hawkins then recalls the experience of the Queen's fleet in 1590, at the Azores, the ships being in calm weather for six months : "in which voyage, towards the end thereof, many of every ship (saving the 'Nonpereli' which was under my charge and had only one man sick in all the voyage) fell sick of this disease and began to die apace."

Hawkins wrote out the account of his 1593 voyage some time after, and did not print it until 1622 ; but it may be supposed that the views about scurvy therein expressed were the same

---

[1] Purchas, IV. Bk. 7, Chap. 5, (reprinted from Hawkins's own narrative of the voyage, published a few months after the author's death in 1622).

that he held and acted upon in his earlier life[1]. Thus his remarks upon the prevention and cure of scurvy, about to be given, may be taken to stand for the practical wisdom or sagacity of the Elizabethan period. The ship should be kept clean, vinegar should be sprinkled and tar burned. In hot latitudes salt meats should be shunned, and especially salt fish. Salt water should not be used to dress the meat, nor to wash shirts in; nor should the men sleep in their wet clothes. The crews should be set to various exercises, and encouraged to various pastimes. At this point he seems to feel that he is a layman giving medical advice, and interpolates:

"And I wish that some learned men would write of it, for it is the plague of the sea and the spoil of mariners. Doubtless it would be a work worthy of a worthy man, and most beneficial for our country, for in twenty years (since I have used the sea) I dare take upon me to give account of ten thousand men consumed with this disease."

The learned man was forthcoming in due course, in the person of John Woodall, surgeon-general to the East India Company; and we shall see what he made of it. Meanwhile, in default of professional guidance, we may hear Hawkins himself:

"That which I have seen most fruitful for this sickness is sour oranges and lemons, and a water called Dr Stevens his water, of which I carried but little, and it took end quickly, but gave health to those that used it. The oyle of vitry [vitriol] is beneficial—two drops in a draught of water with a little sugar. But the principal of all is the air of the land; for the sea is natural for fishes, and the land for men. And the oftener a man can have his people to land, not hindering his voyage, the better it is and the profitablest course he can take to refresh them."

Hawkins, as well as his contemporaries, as we shall see, knew what lime-juice could do for scurvy, and knew also the limit of its powers; it was useful, as he had himself found; but

[1] Mr J. K. Laughton (*Dict. of National Biography*. Art. "Hawkins, Sir Richard") points out that Hawkins's narrative of the 'Daintie's' voyage had not always been authenticated by reference to notes or documents. It seems probable also, from his remarks on the epidemic in Drake's fleet after leaving the Cape de Verde islands in 1585, that he trusted his memory too much. But that objection of writing from memory has no force as against his general observations and reflections on scurvy.

much else was needed to ward off scurvy. After experience showed clearly enough that some commanders with the same stores as others could carry their crews through a long voyage without scurvy ; Hawkins himself, in the 'Nonpareil' in 1590, had only one man sick of it, while it was general in the fleet. In the voyage of 1593, for all his knowledge and resource, he appears to have found circumstances too hard for him. His crew showed their bad habits while the ship lay at Plymouth ; as in Lancaster's experience two years before, the evil habits of sailors told upon their constitutions, so that they became an easy prey to monotonous living at sea. Scurvy broke out when they were within three or four degrees of the Line : "The sickness was fervent, every day there died more or less." The ship's course was accordingly turned westward, although they were too far south to benefit by the north-east trade wind ; and in the end of October they came to the coast of Brazil at Santos, four months and a half out from Plymouth. At Santos they obtained 200 or 300 oranges and lemons, and a few hens ; there were so many men sick that there were not above three or four oranges or lemons to a share: "Coming aboard of our ships there was great joy amongst my company, and many with the sight of the oranges and lemons seemed to recover heart." It is the great and unknown virtue of that fruit, he says, to be a certain remedy for this infirmity. The rest of the voyage possesses no special interest for us. The scurvy had "wasted more than half of my people;" so that Hawkins took the crew and provisions out of the 'Hawk,' and burned her. He left the Brazilian coast on December 18, passed the Straits of Magellan, and after some filibustering on the Chilian and Peruvian coasts, was captured by a Spanish ship, and sent home to Spain to be ransomed.

Hawkins, it will have been remarked, was no bigoted "lime-juicer ;" although he knew the virtues of anti-scorbutic acids, he had a correct apprehension of the need of cleanliness, dry clothing, exercise, amusements and discipline, and if he had understood the need of wind-sails for the ventilation of 'tween-decks, he would have had as scientific a grasp of the whole question as Blane had two centuries after. But in the end of the Tudor period, and in the Stuart period, with abounding enterprise and national expansion, there was little sense of the personal need of breathing space, whether in ships or in houses. The number of souls on board, in proportion to a ship's tonnage, was twice or thrice as great as the Board of Trade now allows. It was not only in long voyages, or in the monotony of tropical calms, that scurvy was apt to invade a crew. The following experience, on our own shores, is credible enough: In 1611 Purchas was shown a letter from Newfoundland, giving an account of a winter spent there, the writer taking credit to himself for the small amount of scurvy among the men under him: in a company of 39 persons, only four were wanting in the spring; but, by way of contrast, he recalls what happened at home in the year 1600[1]:

"One Richard Fletcher, that is master pilot here, and a director of the fishing, reported unto me that he was one of the company, consisting of forty persons, that went in a drumbler of Ipswich called the 'Amitie,' to the north of Ireland about eleven years ago from London in the late Queen's service under the charge of one Captain Fleming, and continued there the space of two years. In which time two and thirty died of the scurvie, and that only eight of them returned home, whereof the said Richard Fletcher was one.... notwithstanding that there were to be had fresh victuals and many other helps, which their country [Newfoundland] as yet hath not, but in good time may have."

We have not yet come to any deliverance of the faculty on the subject of scurvy; Hawkins appears to be giving merely his own experience and reflections. Beside these we may here place the contemporary observations and practice of the French laymen, which are expressly at variance on some points with medical teaching. Some time previous to 1609, Marc Lescarbot wrote an account of 'the voyage of M. de Monts into New France;' the expedition sailed from Havre in March, 1604. Their first winter in Canada is thus related[2]:

In the meanwhile the cold and snows came upon them....Many idle, sluggish companions drank snow-water, not willing to take the pains to cross the river. "Briefly, the unknown sicknesses like to those described unto us by James Quartier in his relation, assailed us. For remedies there was none to be found. In the meanwhile the poor sick creatures did

---

[1] Purchas, part IV. p. 1877.   [2] *Ibid.* p. 1623.

languish, pining away by little and little for want of sweet meats, as milk or spoon meat for to sustain their stomachs, which could not receive the hard meats, by reason of let, proceeding from a rotten flesh which grew and over-abounded within their mouths; and when one thought to root it out, it did grow again in one night's space more abundantly than before....There died of this sickness thirty-six; and thirty-six or forty more that were stricken with it recovered themselves by the help of the Spring, as soon as the comfortable season appeared. But the deadly season for that sickness is the end of January, the months of February and March, wherein most commonly the sick do die, every one at his turn, according to the time when they have begun to be sick; in such sort that he which began to be ill in February and March may escape, but he that shall overhaste himself, and betake him to his bed in December and January, he is in danger to die in February and March, or the beginning of April....M. de Poutrincourt made a negro to be opened that died of that sickness in our voyage, who was found to have the inward parts very sound except the stomacke, that had wrinkles as though they were ulcerated."

Then follow Lescarbot's views of the treatment and prevention of scurvy. After advising to avoid "cold" meats without juices, gross and corrupted, salted, "smoaky," musty, raw and of an evil scent, including dried fishes, he proceeds:

"I would not, for all that, be so scrupulous as the physicians, which do put in the number of gross and melancholy meats, beeve's flesh, bear's, wild boar's and hog's flesh (they might as well add unto them beaver's flesh, which notwithstanding we have found very good), as they do amongst fishes the tons [tunnies], dolphins, and all those that carry lard; among the birds the hernes, ducks and all other water-birds; for, in being an over-curious observator of these things, one might fall into the danger of starving. They place yet among the meats that are to be shunned, bisket[1], beans and pulse, the often using of milk, cheese, the gross and harsh wine and that which is too small, white wine, and the use of vinegar"

—just like our own great masters in prohibitory dietetics.

Lescarbot's advice agrees on the whole with that of Sir R. Hawkins: the men should be well shod and clothed, merriment should be encouraged, and again:

"Good wine taken according to the necessity of nature, it is a soveraigne preservative for all sickness, and particularly for this. The young buds of herbs in the Spring time be also very soveraigne....We have had some sick that have been (as it were) raised up from death to life, for having eaten twice or thrice of a coolice made of a cock."

[1] Woodall defends the use of biscuit in his *Surgeon's Mate*, published in 1617.

In the voyage of Sir Thomas Smith to Baffin's Bay in 1616, the treatment of scurvy by vegetable juices is mentioned: "Next day, going ashore on a little island we found great abundance of scurvie grass, which we boiled in beer, and so drank thereof, using it also in sallet, with sorrel and orpen, which here groweth in abundance; by means whereof, and the blessing of God, all our men within eight or nine days shall gain perfect health, and so continue till our arrival in England[1]."

On the other hand, those who appear to have had the most correct intuition of the teaching of the schools were the Red Indians. Lescarbot says that, in the treatment of scurvy, "they use sweating often." Perhaps they had some dim notion of the doctrine of peccant humours: at all events they clung to the alterative practice until long after that date, with a tenacity second only to that of the European faculty itself.

Scurvy in the East India Company's Ships: Professional Treatment.

Until the end of the Tudor period, scurvy had been only an occasional incident of English voyages. But as soon as the regular trade to the East begins, we find it a common experience.

The English voyages to the East Indies by the Cape route really began in 1591, when Captain James Lancaster sailed first in command of ships belonging to the Company of Merchant Adventurers; but it was not until 1601 that he sailed again to the East Indies in command of the first ships of the East India Company, which had been formed the year before.

The three ships in 1591, the 'Penelope,' 'Marchant Royal,' and 'Edward Bonaventure,' cleared from Plymouth on April 10[2]. They crossed the Line on June 6, by which time two men were dead and divers sick. In the tropics so much rain fell that " we could not keep our men dry three hours together, which was an occasion of the infection among them, and their eating of salt victuals, with the lack of clothes to shift them." On this first voyage,

---

[1] Purchas, III. 847.

[2] *The Voyages of Sir James Lancaster, Knight, to the East Indies.* Hakluyt Society, ed. Clements Markham, 1878; and in Hakluyt's *Principal Navigations*, II. pt. 2, p. 102.

Lancaster began the practice which was generally followed when the East India trade in English ships became established; before attempting to double the Cape of Good Hope, he refreshed his crews, who were weak and sick in all three ships, by a sojourn ashore at the Bay of Saldanha, a few leagues to the north of Table Bay. The voyage had already lasted more than three months from Plymouth, and about six weeks from the Line[1].

At a muster on August 1, in the Bay of Saldanha, Lancaster found that he had 198 men sound and whole, of whom he assigned 101 to the 'Penelope,' and 97 to the 'Edward Bonaventure,' sending home 50 more or less unfit men in the 'Royal Merchant.' Scurvy, he says, was the disease:

"Our soldiers, which have not been used to the sea, have best held out, but our mariners dropt away, which in my judgment, proceedeth of their evil diet at home." The voyage was continued to the East Indies, the next that we hear of the state of health being at Penang in the beginning of June 1592, or some fourteen months out. The men were then very sick and many fallen; the sick were landed, and twenty-six died there, but not of scurvy, we may surmise. They had now left but thirty-three men and one boy, "of which not past twenty-two were found for labour and help."

The two ships sailed for home from Point de Galle on December 8, 1592, and reached St Helena on April 3, 1593; one man was sick of the scurvy, and another had been suffering from the flux for nine months, but on the island both shortly recovered their perfect health. Instead of reaching England, the ships were carried to the West Indies, where, after an attempt to navigate them northwards, they were wrecked, and the small remnants of their crews dispersed.

Lancaster's first voyage for the East India Company in 1601[2] was "with foure tall shippes, to wit, the Dragon, the Hector, the Ascension, and Susan, and a victualler called the Guest." The Company, founded in 1600, began with a capital of £72,000,

---

[1] The slowness of the passage round the Cape of Good Hope in old times was due less to the build or rig of the ships than to the course shaped: instead of steering southwest from Madeira across the Atlantic almost to the coast of Brazil at Cape San Roque, so as to get the north-east trade wind, and thence on another tack in a wide sweep round to the Cape with the south-east trade wind, the earlier navigators sailed past the Cape de Verde islands and along the Guinea coast, keeping within meridians 20 degrees to the eastward of the modern track, and so falling into the tropical calms at one part, and at another part of the voyage into the baffling south-east trades, varying in force according to the season.

[2] Purchas, I. 147.

which was laid out in the purchase and outfit of the ships, and in loading them with merchandise.   The crews were as follow :

Dragon,	600 tons,	202 men.
Hector,	300 ,,	108 ,,
Ascension,	260 ,,	82 ,,
Susan,	—- ,,	88 ,,
		480
Guest,	130 tons.	

Further, "in every of the said ships, three merchants to succeed one the other, if any of them should be taken away by death"— a sufficient indication of the risks of foreign trade.

The ships, having loaded in the Thames, sailed from Dartmouth on April 18, 1601, and got clear of Tor Bay on the 22nd. On July 24, two months from the Channel, they crossed the southern tropic. But they had been so long under the Line that "many of our men fell sick." On August 1, in 30° S., they met the south-west wind, "to the great comfort of all our people. For, by this time very many of our men were fallen sick of the scurvy in all our ships, and, unless it were in the general's ship only, the others were so weak of men that they could hardly handle the sails." Head-winds again hindered their course, and "now the few whole men we had began also to fall sick, so that our weakness of men was so great that in some of the ships the merchants took their turn at the helm and went into the top to take in the top sails, as the common mariners did." Lancaster at length made Saldanha Bay, where he had landed to refresh his crews on his first voyage round the Cape ten years before. The state of three of the ships "was such that they was hardly able to let fall an anchor to save themselves withall ;" but "the general went aboard of them and carried good store of men, and hoysed out their boats for them....And the reason why the general's men stood better in health than the men of other ships was this : he brought to sea with him certain bottles of the juice of lemons, which he gave to each one as long as it would last, three spoonfuls every morning fasting, not suffering them to eat anything after it till noon. This juice worketh much the better if the partie keepe short diet, and wholly refrain salt meat, which salt meat, and long being at the sea, is the only cause of the breeding of this disease. By this means the general cured many of his men and preserved the rest, so that in this ship (having the double of men that was in the rest of the ships) he had not so many sick, nor lost so many men as they did, which was the mercie of God to us all."

At Saldanha Bay they bartered with the natives for an abundant supply of fresh meat and other provisions, and in due time doubled the Cape of Good Hope. On Christmas day, eight months out from England, they put in to Antongil Bay, on the east side of Madagascar. On landing they found a writing on the rocks that five Dutch ships had sailed thence two months before, having "lost between 150 and 200 men while they roade in that place." The English had a similar experience in store for them : on board Lancaster's ship, the master's mate, the preacher, the surgeon and some ten others, died ; and, in the vice-admiral's ship, the master with other two. It was mostly the flux that they died of, brought on by the drinking-water, or by the excessive wetness of the season, or by "going open and cold in the stomacke, which our men would often do when they were hot" (Hawkins gives the latter reason for flux at the Cape de Verde islands).

The references to scurvy before reaching the Cape, and to dysentery in Madagascar, are all that is said of sickness in this first venture of the East India Company. But in the accounts of the voyages which regularly followed we hear a great deal of the loss of men at the factories, or in the country trade, or on the voyage home, as well as on the outward voyage[1]. The Directors in London were naturally well aware how greatly their ventures were imperilled and their profits reduced by the enormous loss of men. Under their own eyes ships would arrive in the mouth of the Channel with crews so weakened that they had to be met at Scilly with help to navigate them through the narrow seas to the Thames. By their correspondence from abroad, they were frequently hearing of artificers dying in their factories, of ships arriving out with so many men dead, and of other ships cast away, partly by stress of weather no doubt, but sometimes from inability of the crews to man them. Accordingly we find that they were alive to the best means of preventing " flux, scurvy, and fever." Lancaster, as we have seen, carried lime-juice on his first voyage for the Company in 1601. In the Court minutes of August 13, 1607, the following were ordered to be provided with expedition : "Lemon water, 'alligant' from Alicante, a wine very fit for beverage and good against the flux, and old corn, etc." At the Court of Directors on December 10,

---

[1] *Calendar of State Papers.* East Indies (under the respective dates).

1614, there was considered an "offer of Dr Burgis to present the Company with an antidote against poison, scurvy, and other diseases to which people are subject these long voyages : Sir Thomas Roe and Captain Keeling to confer with him and report their opinions." Trial was also to be made of baking fresh bread at sea, with the grinding of corn, "an exercise fit to preserve men in health." The offer of Dr Burgis was accepted ; and on January 26, 1615, the minutes of the Court mention "instructions in writing, and boxes of such things as are to be used, for prevention of the flux, scurvy, and fever, prepared by Dr Burgis, to be delivered to each ship ; the cost, about £23, to be paid." In the minutes of the Court, November 22, 1619, there is reference to another preventive of scurvy : "The fleet to be supplied with 15 tons of white wine, to be drunk at the Line, and the Cape, which is used by the Dutch to preserve men from scurvy, and will refresh the men and scour their maws, and open and cool as well as lemon water"—the latter having been in all probability disliked or refused by the men. In 1624, "the death of mariners" is a topic at the Court of Directors ; again, on October 15, 1626, the Court considers of the great mortality from scurvy in the 'Charles' and 'Hart,' homeward bound, and how to prevent it. Some were of opinion that lemon water was very good, but Mr Styles related that tamarind was the excellentest thing. However, there had been plenty of tamarinds aboard the ships ; and on Lieutenant Hill being called in, he testified that the crews had all got tamarind, but they were all debauched people.

John Woodall, surgeon to St Bartholomew's Hospital, was at this time surgeon-general to the East India Company, having medical charge of their dockyard at Blackwall; his name appears in the Court minutes as early as 1614. In 1617 he published his 'Surgion's Mate,' "chiefly for the benefit of young sea-surgions imployed in the East India companies affairs," and dedicated it to Sir Thomas Smith, himself a navigator, and then chairman of the Court of Directors. This practical manual is largely occupied with the management of fractures, dislocations, amputations, and the like, a part of his subject wherein Woodall was thoroughly competent ; but there appears also in the title, "the cure of the scurvie, the fluxes of the belly, of the collica and iliaca passio, tenasmus and exitus ani, the callenture." The section on scurvy, twenty-six pages long, is the one that here concerns us. This was what Sir Richard Hawkins had desired: "And I wish that some learned men would write of it, for it is the plague of the sea and the spoil of mariners." Woodall begins by disclaiming learning: "A learned treatise befits not my pen." But, at all events, his was the voice of the faculty, and he plunges boldly into pathology in the very first lines: "Scurvy is a disease of the spleen, whereby it is sometimes wholly stopped" etc. Being a man of much good sense, Woodall quickly leaves that line of remark, for a time at least. He repeats all the familiar experience of Hawkins, Lancaster, and the numerous captains of East Indiamen, with whom he must have conversed many times (it does not appear that he had himself sailed). He mentions the great benefit to the crews from landing at the Cape, with the fresh air and food, scurvy being thereby cured "without much other help." He enforces the need of changes of clothing, and other things in the regimen on board, just as Hawkins and others were wont to do in practice. He is as clear on the virtues of lime-juice as Lancaster, and copies somewhat closely the practice of the latter in 1601: "each morning two or three spoonfuls, and fast after it two hours"; his originality appearing in the rider, grateful to seamen: "and if you add one spoonful of aqua vitae thereto, to a cold stomach it is the better." He mentions that a "good quantity of juice of lemons is sent in each ship out of England, by the great care of the merchants, and intended only for the relief of every poor man in his need." The ship's surgeon is advised to lay in a store of fresh lemons and oranges where they were to be had on the voyage, and of tamarinds at Bantam.

So far, Woodall merely sets down what every shipmaster knew as to the things that bring on scurvy, the best regimen to keep it off, and the extraordinarily rapid curative effect of lime-juice and of change to land air and fresh food. But there was a certain professional doctrine of scurvy, and a treatment of it *secundum artem*, namely the wisdom of learned men which Hawkins had called for; and we have now to see what that

was, according to Woodall. His pathology is that of " obstructions," a curious fancy of the learned[1].

The spleen, said Woodall in his opening lines, is the chief
seat of obstruction ; but on resuming the pathology, he proceeds
to obstructions also of the liver and brain :

" But it is plain that this grief is a lazy foul disease with obstructions of
the liver, or spleen, or both ; as also it appeareth that the head is much
diseased, and that there is great obstructions in the brain, for that the eyes
not only look evil coloured, but also the gums putrefy, and the teeth grow
loose, and all the sinewy parts of the body bear their part in the disease, for
the shrinking and withering of the sinews, with the great pains the party
hath, declareth no less " (p. 180).

This theoretical pathology Woodall supports by an appeal
to morbid anatomy :

"Also it is manifest that divers of those which have been opened after
death have had their livers utterly rotted "—others having their livers much
swollen, and the spleen swollen, others full of water, others their lungs
putrefied and stunk while they have lived, (which last may have been an
incorrect inference from the foul state of the mouth).

Such being the pathology of the disease, he comes next to
the indications of cure ; and these he takes from " a famous
writer, Johannes Echthius." They are :

1. The opening of obstructions.
2. The evacuating of offending humours.
3. The altering the property of the humours.
4. The comforting and corroborating the parts late diseased.

The order of treatment, *lege artis,* is accordingly as follows :
the administration of a clyster or clysters ; the opening of a vein,
if strong ("but beware of taking too much blood away at once");

---

[1] It seems to have passed into common usage, as "to lie in cold obstruction and to
rot" (*Meas. for Meas.* III. 1), and to have been kept up therein after the faculty had
dropped it—if indeed Byron's line, " Where cold Obstruction's apathy " be a survival
of medical terminology. There is an instance of the same kind of survival in the use
of "scorbutic;" at one time land-scurvy was detected (under the influence of theory)
in many forms, and we find in the *Pickwick Papers* a late reminiscence of that
singular dogma in the "young gentleman with the scorbutic countenance."

next day after the bleeding, "if he can bear it," give him pills of euphorbium or gamboge ; and lastly, "if you see cause," certain days after you have given of any of your former laxatives, you may give a sweat to the patient in his bed. Thus the indications from the pathology would be fulfilled—opening of obstructions, evacuating of ill humours, and altering the property of the humours. It should be said for Woodall that his practice was better than his theory. Thus, he cautions the young dogmatists who sailed as surgeons in East Indiamen, not to carry their principles too far ; he has heard that they are somewhat fond of the lancet, and he cautions them not to take too much blood at sea, as excessive depletion "makes the disease worse ;" he cautions them also as to the use of gamboge.

We may now proceed with a few more illustrations of what the Company's ships were actually experiencing during the period that those questions were before the Court of Directors[1].

In the sixth voyage for the Company, under the command of Sir H. Middleton, the captain of the 'Darling' and three of his merchants died at Tecoa, and most of the men were ill. In the eighth voyage, when homeward bound between the Cape and St Helena in the month of June, many of the men fell ill with scurvy, and the ship had to come in to Waterford instead of the Thames. A similar experience befell Captain Thomas Best in the 'Dragon' and 'Hosiander,' carrying together 380 persons. Having left Gravesend on February 1, 1612, he completed his trading in the Indies, and arrived in the Thames on June 15, 1614, six months from Bantam. The scurvy in this voyage comes in towards the end. On March 4, 1614, "I did set sail in the roade of Saldanha ; yet notwithstanding our short passage, having been from Santa Helena but two monethes and nine days, the one half or more of our company are laid up [on June 4] of the scurvie and two dead of it. Yet we had plentie of victuals, as beef, bread, wine, rice, oil, vinegar, sugar ; and all these without allowance. Note that all our men that are sick have taken their sickness since we fell with Flores and Corvo. For since that time we have had it very cold, especially in two great storms....From the Cape of Good Hope to the islands of Flores and Corvo I had not one man sick." While in the Malay Archipelago they had buried twenty-five men at one place.

On November 3, 1618, the Directors have letters from two of their

---

[1] The three earlier instances from Purchas, I. 248, 466, the later from the *Cal. State Papers*, East Indies.

captains at the Cape, of July 6 and 7, with news of their arrival there on June 26, and the loss or sickness of many men, partly through the stinking beer, the tainted beef, the lack of fresh provisions at the Cape, and the want of warm clothes. A letter of February 25, 1619, announces the arrival of the 'Peppercorn' in Bantam roads : A great many men had died in the ten-months' voyage between England and Bantam ; putrefied beef and pork, "not man's meat," the chief cause of sickness. When they arrived at Bantam, not six men able to work ; the whole fleet in the like distress. Twenty-five men in all dead or drowned. A letter from Batavia, January 11, 1622, says the master of the 'Anne' and 14 men of the fleet were dead : "so many men are deceased that they have not enough to man all the ships now in the roads." The 'Diamond' sailed from England on October 8, 1621, and after a "long and tedious voyage" arrived at Jacatra previous to November 24, 1622 : enclosed are the accounts of those men who have died, and nine wills. Another letter from Batavia, sometime in 1623, covers an "abstract of the men deceased in the ships."

On March 28, 1624, the 'Royal James,' with five others, sailed from the Downs ; she called at Saldanha Bay, and arrived on or before November 15, at Swally bar, Batavia ; the bread had been very bad, the water too little, the beef not fit for men ; have enclosed the names of those deceased. The 'Jonas,' also arrived out at Batavia on November 15, appears to have been one of the five others ; she called at Saldanha Bay on July 19 ; "the wholesomeness of the air and the herb baths caused the most part of their sick men to recover in ten days from the scurbeck." In June, 1625, the 'Anne' had been at Mocha for eight months in great distress, with most part of her men dead and the ship ready to founder.

Writing on October 13, 1625, from Batavia to the East India Company in London, Governor Hawley says that the 'London' had arrived out on August 23, with loss of 36 men, and 80 sick. She reported the 'Discovery' to have left the Cape for St Helena, having lost 21 men ; two other ships, the 'Moon' and 'Ruby' had their crews "in remarkable health." On September 14, the 'Swallow' arrived out, having lost only 3 men. Of 46 men shipped in the 'Abigail' out of England, all were dead but 5, in her coasting voyages upon Sumatra. Most of the workmen and soldiers sent in the 'London' had arrived; "but since, by disorders, are dead, as are those in the 'Swallow.' The smiths are all dead ; of the armourers, only John Speed and a boy alive. Most other workmen dead or incapable. This is not remissness of government, but the newcomers, dreaming of nothing but sack and sugar-plums in India, are with much difficulty brought to obedience." A Dutch ship, the 'Leyden' arrived out in 1626, with loss of 22 men, having been twelve months on the passage.

In the end of October, 1628, the 'Morris' reached the mouth of the Channel from Bantam, "which was most happily met with near Scilly by Captain Bickly, who was sent out to relieve any ship from the Indies, she being in a very weak state by reason of an infectious disease." She reached the Downs safely with two other East Indiamen; but having been driven from her anchors in a great storm, was wrecked on the coast of Holland previous to November 19. Next year, about October 28, 1629, the 'Mary' of the East India Company was reported to have put into Scilly having lost most of her men by sickness. Therefore, Sir H. Mervyn, of H.M.S. 'Lyon,' in the Downs, having got early word of the 'Mary's' distress, writes to E. Nicholas, to say that if the Company desire a convoy for the 'Mary' from their lordships of the Admiralty, "she being rich," he (Mervyn) hopes that Nicholas will remember him.

But, although it was not unusual for ships to come home with crews weakened by scurvy, it was not invariable. The 'William' returned to England in 1628, as rich a ship as the Company ever had from the East Indies, with not a sick man in her, nor any dead on the way; her lading was computed to be worth £170,000[1].

In a despatch of February 6, 1626, Hawley gives an account of a truly disastrous sickness in the factory and among the Company's ships at Batavia during the previous year, which illustrates another risk than that of scurvy or flux, and an experience in the East Indies not altogether exceptional[2].

"On March 12, I dispeeded the 'Diamond' for Japan to fetch boards, planks, etc. [to repair the 'Bull' with]; but hardly had fourteen days passed when the 'Bull's' men fell sick and died daily; then the 'Reformation's' men died by five, six or more in a day; in a short time the 'Bull's' men all died but the master and one more, who were dangerously sick, and in the 'Reformation' the master and all the men lay at God's mercy. We were forced to relieve them by blacks, and hale the ships to the open bay [they would seem to have been careened] where they rode like wrecks without other help than some few to comfort their sick, for more from the other ships might not be spared. The contagion was so pestilent that their blood, being licked by dog or cat, caused them to swell, burst and die. It was more moderate on shore, and was least on the ships in the open bay, though they also were daily visited....The 'Diamond' returned on April 11, with planks etc.; also slaves and 44 Chinamen, which were with no small charge procured, and who all fell sick, and 10 or 12 died....Thinking the mortality was occasioned, not by pestiferous air or soil, nor by any noxious tree, but by surfeit and the wet monsoon, I enacted orders for government building, and cleansing the trees to get more air. Wanted no provisions of fresh victual; could at pleasure command neighbours to fish and fetch anything

---

[1] *Cal. S. P.* Colonial. East Indies. Dec. 24, 1628.
[2] *Ibid.* Feb. 6, 1626, p. 146.

needed, and the island itself furnished deer. On April 12, took general view of all people, as follows :

		English in health	English sick	Portuguese sick
On shore		40	58	5
In the	'Charles'	32	10	
,,	'Roebuck'	16	2	
,,	'Bull'	2	8	
,,	'Reformation'	23	14	12
,,	'Abigail'	8	3	
,,	'Rose'	7	2	5
		128	97	22

—leaving, of course, an immense proportion dead.

These are instances from the records of the East India Company during the first thirty years of its existence. It would be tedious, even if it were practicable, to follow the history continuously. But meanwhile to show that its experiences, good and bad, remained much the same until long after, let us take two voyages in the year 1682. Governor William Hedges, passenger on board one of the Company's ships, enters in his diary the 25th of May, 1682, being then off the Cape of Good Hope : " Not lost a man (except Mr Richards) either by sickness or any other accident, since we left England, which wants but three days of four months, and is just two months since we passed the Equinoctial Line," nothing being said of sickness in the rest of the voyage. But another of the Company's ships the same year fared worse : " December 9, 1682, ship 'Society' arrived at Balasore. She left the Downs on May 30, and, not touching at any place by the way, lost seventeen men of the scurvy[1]."

Sickness in the Colonizing of Virginia and New England.

Leaving now the long voyages of the English beyond the Line, and their factories in the East, let us see how they fared as regards health when they merely crossed the Atlantic in their own latitudes. The earliest series of voyages to Virginia, at Raleigh's instigation, from 1585 to 1590, have been already referred to. The continuous history of Atlantic voyages, and of

[1] *William Hedges' Diary.* Hakluyt Society, 1887, I. 24, 54.

the North American colonies, begins with the expedition of
1609 under Sir Thomas Gates and Sir George Somers[1].

Seven of the ships fitted out in the Thames, and sailed from
Woolwich on May 15, 1609. Having been joined at Plymouth
by two more, the fleet sailed thence on June 2, and from
Falmouth on June 8. The expedition included "many unruly
gallants, packed thither by their friends to escape ill destinies,"
with the proportion of women and children usual among emigrants, as well as horses, and probably other live stock. The
navigation, to reach Western land in 37° N., appears to have
been somewhat erratic :

"We ran a southerly course from the tropic of Cancer, where, having the
sun within six or seven degrees right over our head in July, we bore away
West ; so that by the fervent heat and loomes breezes, many of our men fell
sick of the calenture "—Noah Webster takes that to mean a spotted
pestilential fever—"and out of two ships was thrown overboard thirty-two
persons. The vice-admiral [the 'Diamond'] was said to have the plague in
her ; but in the 'Blessing' we had not any sick, albeit we had twenty women
and children."

A storm came on, in which the ships were scattered, the
admiral's ship being driven to the Bermudas and there wrecked[2].
In the storm "some lost their masts, some had their sails blown
from their yards; the seas over-raking our ships, much of our
provision was spoiled, our fleet separated, and our men sick,
and many died; and in this miserable state we arrived at
Virginia." The 'Blessing,' on board which was Gabriel Archer,
the principal narrator of events, seems to have fared better than
the rest : "The 'Unity' was sore distressed when she came up
with us; for, of seventy landmen [emigrants], she had not ten
found, and all her seamen were down, but only the master and
his boy, with one poor sailor ; but we relieved them, and we
four consorting, fell into the King's River [James River] haply
the 11th of August." They found the colony "all in health (for
the most part)." There were fourscore living 20 miles from the

[1] *A Letter of M. Gabriel Archar*, in Purchas, pt. IV. p. 1733 ; Smith's *Virginia*,
in Pinkerton, XIII. 99 ; W. Strachey, in Purchas, pt. IV. p. 1753.

[2] Theobald makes this the storm and shipwreck which Shakespeare brings into
the *Tempest*.

Fort, who fed upon nothing but oysters eight weeks' space. "After our four ships had been in harbour a few days, came in the vice-admiral, having cut her mainmast overboard, and had many of her men very sick and weak." This was the ship that was said to have the plague in her. The admiral and his ship's company, wrecked on the Bermudas, fared in health best of all ; the whole number of 150 persons reached Jamestown in due course, to find only 60 remaining alive of the 350 who had formed the complement of the other ships. Part of the mortality had happened on board ship, but probably the most of it after landing ; Jamestown "is in a marish ground, low, flat to the river, and hath no fresh water springs serving the town, but what we drew from a well six or seven fathom deep, fed by the brackish river oozing into it, from whence I verily believe the chief causes have proceeded of many diseases and sicknesses which have happened to our people, who are indeed strangely afflicted with fluxes and agues." Lord De La Warre, one of the early governors, had a succession of illnesses—hot and violent ague, followed by a relapse still more violent and lasting a month, "then the flux surprised me and kept me many days," then the cramp, with strong pains, afterwards the gout, and finally the scurvy—which last, however, might have been the eczema of gout, although it was said to have been cured by the oranges and lemons of the Western Islands, and by the voyage thither[1].

Much in these early ventures was put down to climate, which was really due to other causes. There are, of course, unhealthy climates ; but a great deal of the talk in the 17th and 18th centuries about the "tainted air" of "foreign climes" was mere confusion of ideas. A more correct view of events was that of the Governor and Council of Virginia, in a letter of January 30, 1624, to the Virginia Company in London :

"The mortality, which is imputed to the country alone, is chiefly caused by the pestilent ships, which reach Virginia victualled with musty bread and stinking beer, heretofore so earnestly complained of....Robert Benet in his lifetime boasted that the sale of four butts of wine would clear a voyage. Rotten wines destroy their bodies and empty their purses[2]."

[1] Purchas, IV. p. 1762.   [2] *Cal. S. P.* America and West Indies.

The letter then goes on to relate how sickness had brought down great numbers "since their last." According to Purchas, the emigration to Virginia in three years immediately preceding this, the years 1619, 1620 and 1621, had amounted to 3570 persons in 42 ships. Overcrowding, we may be sure, was the rule. We shall find particular evidence of it in speaking of West Indian colonization in the sequel; and for the present, it may suffice to quote a document of April 24, 1638, a list of 110 passengers for New England per 'Confidence' of 200 tons.

If Virginia was settled by a crew of broken gallants and their humbler followers, the New England colony was officered by strict Puritans, who were accompanied by men and women sharing, as nearly as might be, the same beliefs and principles of conduct. The records of the Massachusetts Bay settlements might be expected, therefore, to show less of sickness and failure than the Virginian; and so, indeed, they do, although they are by no means clear of it. The first voyage of the 'Mayflower' in 1620, carrying the small sect of Brownists who had tried Holland for a time as a place of refuge, presents nothing for our purpose. Like the settlers along the shores of Chesapeake Bay before them, these first New Englanders had to encounter famine and sickness. Famine appears to have been the cause also of the disastrous epidemics among the Indians along the whole coast from Cape Cod to Cape Charles, on two occasions, the one previous to 1614 and the other in 1619[1]. The emigration to New England really began in 1630, and of one of the expeditions of that year we have authentic particulars by the leader of it, John Winthrop[2]. On board the 'Arbella,' under date April 17, 1630, he enters in his journal:

"This day our captain told me that our landmen were very nasty and slovenly, and that the gun-deck, where they lodged, was so beastly and noisome with their victuals and beastliness as would much endanger the health of the ship. Hereupon, after prayer, we took order, and appointed four men to see to it, and to keep that room clean for three days, and then four others should succeed them, and so forth on."

[1] Dermer, in Purchas, IV. p. 1778: Belknap's *American Biography* ("Life of Gorges"), I. 355.
[2] John Winthrop's *Journal*, p. 11.

Nothing more is said of the health on board the 'Arbella.' The 'Mayflower' and 'Whale' had their passengers all in health, but most of their cattle and horses dead. The 'Success' lost — goats, and many of her passengers were near starved. The 'Talbot' lost fourteen passengers. The colony had various experiences of sickness in due course. In 1633, smallpox proved fatal to whole settlements of Indians: "the English came daily and ministered to them; and yet few, only two families, took any infection by it[1]." In 1646 an epidemic of influenza went among the Indians, English, French and Dutch, "not a family, nor but few persons, escaping it;" few died, not above 40 or 50 in Massachusetts, and near as many at Connecticut[2]. In the spring of 1654, a general fast was appointed by the government of Connecticut, one reason among others being "the mortality which had been among the people of Massachusetts." In 1655 there was another influenza, in 1658 "great sickness and mortality throughout New England," in 1659 "cynanche trachealis," croup perhaps, and in 1662 again general sickness, which, along with drought, called for a day of thanksgiving on their cessation in October[3]. It is beside the purpose to follow the epidemics in America minutely; but before quitting the subject, the following, from a Philadelphia letter of August 24, 1699, will suffice to keep in mind the conditions of emigration which prevailed long after the first voyages: "Arrived the 'Britannia' from Liverpool, which had been 13 weeks on her passage; she had 200 passengers on board,—had lost 50 by death, and others were sickly[4]."

West Indian Colonization: Yellow Fever and the Slave Trade.

The other field of English colonial enterprise that concerns us is the West Indies. The West Indian colonies of Britain play a great part in the commercial history, in the naval history,

---

[1] Winthrop, I. pp. 119, 123.   [2] *Ibid.* II. 310.
[3] Refs. in Noah Webster's *Hist. of Epid. and Pestil. Diseases.* Hartford, 1799, I. 189, 191, 193.
[4] Letter of Norris, in *Hist. of S. Carolina*, I. 142.

and in the legislative history in connexion with the negro slave-
trade and the institution of negro slavery. From the very first
they play a great part, also, in the history of epidemic sickness;
they and the Spanish, French and other colonies there were the
peculiar home of yellow fever for two centuries, having shared
that unenviable distinction, after a generation or two, with
certain ports of the North American continent. The larger
part of the history of yellow-fever epidemics falls outside the
period to which I here limit myself. But the beginnings fall
within it; and as the beginnings raise the whole question of
causation, this part of the subject resolves itself into a somewhat
comprehensive discussion of the circumstances of yellow fever
as illustrated by the first English colonizations in the Caribbean
Sea, and the tradings connected therewith.

By far the most important disease-producing conditions in
the West Indies arose out of the Guinea slave-trade. But, so
that we may set down to that no more than it deserves, we shall
have to review also the earlier experiences of English and
French emigrants, both on the voyage and in their settlements
in Barbados and St Christopher, and, at greatest length, the
disastrous first occupation of Jamaica in 1655 by the army of
the Commonwealth. It will be convenient to begin the history,
in which there is so much to disentangle, with a few facts about
the negro labour-traffic to the New World previous to the time
when the demands of the sugar-plantations caused it to be
established on a great scale.

African negroes were brought first to the West Indies by the
Spaniards to work in the mines of Hispaniola. They are heard
of as early as 1501, and are much in evidence after that date.
The Christian conscience appears to have been at first tender.
It was the high purpose of Isabella of Spain to convert the
Indies to the Christian faith; and the cruelties of the negro
importation and of the forced labour in the mines were obviously
inconsistent with the humanitarian teaching of the Gospels.
The remonstrances of missionaries were listened to at the
Spanish Court, and licences to trade in negroes were either
granted under strict conditions or withheld altogether. How-
ever, there were rapacious pro-consuls to deal with as well as

monarchs at home, and cargoes of slaves found their way to Cuba, to Hispaniola (St Domingo), and at length to the Spanish Main. Each importation as late as 1518 was still regulated by special licence; but soon after that date a powerful minister sold the privilege to the Genoese, so that it passed somewhat beyond control of the Spanish Court[1]. Connected with these importations in the first quarter of the 16th century, were the disastrous epidemics of two diseases with somewhat similar names and inextricably confused in the records—the great pox and the small pox; it is not easy to say which did the most harm among the native population of the islands and mainland occupied by Spain; but it is said that by disease of one kind or another Mexicans and Caribs on the main, in Hispaniola, and in Cuba, came near to being exterminated[2].

The first English share in the negro traffic over sea fell to John Hawkins and partners, who had not even the excuse of an open market for their wares in the Spanish colonies, and had sometimes to dispose of their negroes by stealth. It would appear that it was still in part for the mines that African negroes were in request. In Richard Hawkins' account of his voyage to the Pacific in 1593, he mentions that he captured a Portuguese ship of 100 tons shortly after leaving the coast of Brazil; she

---

[1] Saco, *History of African Slavery in the New World* (Spanish). Barcelona, 1879.

[2] Oviedo, in Purchas, III. 996 :—"Extract of Gonzalo Ferdinando de Oviedo :— 'I had acquaintance with divers which went in the first and second voyages of Columbus; of which was Peter Margarite, commendator in the second voyage, of most respect with the king and queen, who complained of those paines. [Syphilis was prevalent in Barcelona and Valencia previous to 1494. See Chapter VIII.] Soon after, in the year 1496, began the disease to arrest some courtiers; but in those beginnings it was only amongst baser persons of small authority; and it was thought that they got it by having to do with common women. But afterwards it extended to principal persons, and the physicians could not tell what to think of it, so that many died.'...But indeed it came from Hispaniola, where it is ordinary, and the remedy also [guaiacum]. *Our author* (*l.c.* civ.), and Ramusio in his preface to his third Tome, say that the souldiers of Pamfilo de Nuney, having the small pocks, infected the Indians which never before heard of that disease; in so much that of 1,600,000 soules in that island there are so few left, as by and by you shall hear...The covetousnesse of the mine-workers, neglect of diet, change of gouvernours growing worse and worse, caused them to poison, kill and hang themselves, besides those which were consumed by infectious or pestilentiall pocks (those before mentioned out of Ramusio) and other diseases."

was bound for Angola to load negroes to be carried to and sold in the River Plate: "It is a trade of great profit and much used. The negroes are carried to work in the mines of Potosi."

It is not until a generation after that we hear of the English as slave-owners. On February 16, 1624, there were 22 negroes on the English settlements in Virginia, the whites numbering 1253[1]. In somewhat greater numbers, negroes are next heard of in English possession in the Bahamas; but, from the correspondence between the Company of Providence Island in London and their agents in the colonies, it would appear that the policy of using forced labour was by no means admitted by all, or free from difficulties. Thus in 1635 the Company condemned as indiscreet and injurious Mr Rushworth's behaviour concerning the negroes who ran away, "arising, as it seems, from a groundless opinion [of Rushworth] that Christians may not lawfully keep such persons in a state of servitude during their strangeness from Christianity[2]."

Whatever negroes the English colonists possessed at this time they got either by capture or purchase from Dutch and other foreign traders. Thus, in the instructions to a ship-master sailing from London, dated March 19, 1636, captured negroes were to be conveyed to the Somers Islands, those who can dive for pearls to be employed at Providence. Again, the instructions to the captain of the 'Mary Hope,' bound for the West Indies, January 20, 1637, refer to the distribution of negroes "if a prize be taken." And, on June 7, 1643, the earl of Warwick instructs the captain of the 'Elias,' 400 tons, that captured negroes are "to be left at my island of Trinidad[3]." The negro carrying-trade was in those years mostly in the hands of the Dutch, who not only stocked their own colony of Surinam on the mainland but used their small island of Curaçoa as a slave-depot for the supply of colonies belonging to other nations. Thus the governor of Antigua, which had then no negroes, says in a despatch of about the year 1670: "At Curaçoa they [the Dutch] send a vast quantity of negroes to the Spaniard, and of late four ships from Jamaica for ready

---

[1] *Calendar of State Papers.* Amer. & W. I., I. 57.   [2] *Ibid.*
[3] *Cal. S. P.* Amer. & W. I., under the respective dates.

pieces-of-eight carried thence great store. They intend to settle a mart for negroes at Tortola to engross the trade of Porto Rico."

The direct share of England in the negro carrying-trade arose out of the monopoly of the Guinea Company. The history of English interests in Guinea and "Binney" need not detain us. When the first patent for sole trade was granted in 1624, it was felt to be a grievance, as "many had been there almost for fifty years since." The charter was renewed on November 22, 1631 ; but in course of time, some who had been ousted from their original share in the monopoly traded on their own account, the rivalries at home being aggravated by conflicts with Swedes (in 1653) and Dutch at the factories on the coast. The trade was ostensibly for gold dust and ivory, but live freight soon found a place in English bottoms as well as in Dutch, Swedish, Danish, French, Portuguese, Spanish and others. We may now return to our proper subject—the state of health in the first English and French plantations in the West Indies.

The English and French arrived in the West Indies almost at the same moment. Their experiences were probably not very different, but it happens that it is of the French emigrants that we have particulars, which it is important to introduce here.

In the year 1625, a Norman adventurer of good family, D'Enambuc, sailed from Dieppe in a brigantine armed with four pieces and manned with 35 or 40 men, on a roving cruise to the West Indies[1]. Having been battered by a Spanish galleon at the Kaymans, D'Enambuc made the island of St Christopher. He found it occupied by the native Caribs and a few stranded Frenchmen, who were on good terms with the natives. Shortly after, an English captain ("Waërnard") appears upon the scene, who joined D'Enambuc in the alleged murdering and poisoning of the natives and the plundering of the island. Loaded with his Carib spoils and a quantity of tobacco, D'Enambuc set sail for France, and having sold his tobacco and other things in Normandy, entered Paris with a

---

[1] The account that follows is taken from Father Dutertre's *Histoire generale des Antilles habitées par les François*, 4 vols., Paris, 1667–1671, which superseded his earlier work of 1654.

fine equipage, thus giving evidence to all men of the fortunes
that awaited them in the Indies. In a short time he had an
audience of Richelieu, and on the 31st October 1626 the charter
was signed of the Compagnie des Isles, granting a monopoly
of trade with " les isles situées à l'entreé du Perou "—namely
St Christopher and Barbados. The Company raised 45,000
livres, of which capital Richelieu held 10,000 livres in his own
name. The money was spent in fitting out and furnishing with
stores three ships—the 'Catholique' at Havre, a craft of 250
tons, and the 'Cardinal' and 'Victoire' at St Malo, two much
smaller vessels. Numerous poor peasants and artisans from
Brittany and Normandy were induced to go out as colonists,
the 'Catholique' (250 tons) carrying 322 souls, the 'Cardinal'
70, and the 'Victoire' 140. The two last sailed from St Malo
on February 24, 1627 under the command of Du Rossey. The
passage was long, the provisions both bad and insufficient, and
the mortality terrible. When the 'Cardinal' arrived at the
Pointe de Sable of St Christopher on May 8, only 16 of her 70
souls remained alive, and these were sick. In the other ships,
also, " most of the people died on the passage out."

The English experience can hardly have been so bad as
that. When the French colonists landed, they found four
hundred Englishmen settled near the chief anchorage, hale and
strong and well stocked with provisions, having lately come out
under Lord Carlisle's patent. Cordial to each other at first, the
two nationalities soon fell out. The French had rather the
worst of it, having lost many of their number by sickness, while
the English kept their health. Help came to the former from
home, and a victory over the English is claimed for them. But
they had also a Spanish fleet to reckon with, and eventually the
French colony fell into disorder and escaped to Antigua, while
its leader, Du Rossey, went home to France and was thrown
into the Bastille by Richelieu, one of the largest shareholders.
The refugees to Antigua soon returned to St Christopher, again
suffered from famine, and had the mortification of seeing all
the profits of their monopoly swallowed up by unlicensed
Dutch traders. In 1635 they obtained a new charter; at the
same time a fortunate capture of a ship-load of negroes from

the Spaniards gave them a supply of labour so that "the island began to change its face." English usurpation was kept within limits, and the French colony grew daily, by addition of European settlers and of "Moorish slaves whom the French and Dutch ships go to buy in Guinea, or capture from the Spaniards along the coasts of Brazil." The French on St Christopher were now strong enough to send branch colonies to Guadeloupe and Martinique (1635). It was then the turn of the English to have disastrous sickness among their immigrants. Sir Thomas Warner, who had planted the English colonies in Barbados and St Christopher, and was now governor of the latter, went to England in 1636 to bring over new settlers. On his arrival out on 10 September, he wrote home that one of his two ships, the 'Plough,' was given up for lost, and that in his own ship there had been "great sickness and mortality, not 20 out of 200 having escaped and 40 having died, some near to him in blood and many of especial quality and use."

Meanwhile Barbados had been the chief scene of English enterprise, from a date (1624–26) almost the same as that of the joint occupation of St Christopher by French and English. Its earliest annals contain little else than the accounts of rivalries under Lord Carlisle's patent and other patents. So far as regards sickness, the annals were probably uneventful. In 1643 the island had plantations stocked with no fewer than 6400 negro slaves, and its prosperity advanced so steadily, that by the year 1666, the slaves in the island numbered some 50,000 : "The buildings in 1643 were mean; but in 1666 [when Bridgetown was burned], plate, jewels and household stuff were estimated at £500,000[1]." It is a date intermediate between those two that directly concerns us—the year 1647. In that year, Ligon, the historian of the colony, arrived out from England about the beginning of September[2]. The ship in which he came to Barbados was consigned thence to Cutchew, on the African coast, to trade for negroes. On their arrival they found twenty-two good ships at anchor in Carlisle Bay (Bridgetown), a brisk trade going on, and plantations visible all along the shore. A

---

[1] *Cal. S. P.* Amer. & W. I., II. 529.
[2] Ligon, *Hist. of Barbadoes.* London, 1657.

plantation of 500 acres had 96 negroes and 28 Christians ; some plantations contained 10,000 acres. The population was difficult to estimate, so many ships were arriving with passengers daily ; and Ligon's estimate of 50,000, " besides negroes," is doubtless too much. About one hundred sail visit the island every year ; they bring " servants " and negro slaves, both men and women. The servants are bound for five years, and are worse treated than the negroes. The negroes are more than double the number of the Christians ; they come from different parts of Africa—Bonny, Cutchew, Angola and Gambia—and do not understand each other's language. They are bought out of the ship naked, being chosen as horses are in a market, the strongest, youthfullest and most beautiful yielding the highest price (man £30, woman £25 to £27, children at easier rates).

We have to note, also, Ligon's account of the colony's chief harbour—Bridgetown. The whole of Carlisle Bay is environed by high ground. Bridgetown is so-called " for that a long bridge was made at first over a little nook of the sea, which was rather a bog than sea." The stream which discharges there into the bay is like a lake for want of outfall. The spring tides fill it, but during the neap tides the salt water is kept stagnant behind the sea-banks, making a small lagoon. The spring tides seldom rise above four or five feet, but high enough to flow over the low ground in front of the houses, making the flat a kind of bog, which vents out a loathsome savour.

Ligon landed at Bridgetown about the beginning of September, 1647, in time to witness the ravages of a deadly epidemic :

"Yet, notwithstanding all this appearance of trade, the inhabitants of the island, and shipping too, were so grievously visited with the plague (or as killing a disease) that before a month was expired after our arrival, the living were hardly able to bury the dead. Whether it was brought thither by shipping, (for in long voyages diseases grow at sea and take away many passengers, and these diseases prove contagious), or by the distemper of the people of the island "—he leaves uncertain. For one woman that died, there were ten men. The ships at anchor in Carlisle Bay were, for the most part, infected with this disease.

What was the disease ? How came it there ? What sort of origin did its characters, symptoms, or type suggest ? On these questions we have some light thrown by other writings besides Ligon's, relating to the same epidemic.

John Winthrop, the Governor of Massachusetts, writes in his journal, under the year 1647[1]:

"It pleased the Lord to open to us a trade with Barbados and other islands in the West Indies, which as it proved gainful, so the commodities we had in exchange there for our cattle and provisions, as sugar, cotton, tobacco and indigo, were a good help to discharge our engagements in England. And this summer there was so great a drouth as their potatoes and corn, etc. were burnt up; and divers London ships which rode there were so short of provisions as, if our vessels had not supplied them, they could not have returned home....After the great dearth of victuals in these islands followed presently a great mortality (whether it were the plague, or pestilent fever, it killed in three days), that in Barbados there died six thousand, and in Christophers, of English and French, near as many, and in other islands proportionable."

The mention of the French on St Christopher brings us to the third source of information, the Jesuit father Dutertre, who was an eye-witness[2]:

"During this same year, 1648, the plague (*la peste*), hitherto unknown in the islands since they were inhabited by the French, was brought thither by certain ships. It began in St Christopher, and in the eighteen months that it lasted, it carried off nearly one-third of the inhabitants." This plague, or *peste*, was marked by violent pain in the head, general debility of all the muscles, and continual vomiting. It was contagious. A ship, the 'Bœuf' of Rochelle, carried it to Guadeloupe, the sailors and passengers dying on board of her. A priest went on board to administer the sacraments, and caught the infection; he recovered, but [had a relapse and] died on August 4. It was contagious at Guadeloupe also, and lasted twenty months.

This testimony of Dutertre is important for several things. He had arrived at Guadeloupe in 1640 in a small vessel of 100 to 120 tons, crowded with stores and carrying besides, 200 souls of both sexes and all ages. Much distress and sickness followed their arrival; he mentions nearly 100 sick in the quarters of M. de la Vernade, with only the ground to sleep on; more than three-fourths of the help for the struggling colony that arrived from St Christopher died, perhaps by infectious disease bred by

---

[1] Winthrop's *Journal*, II. 312.
[2] Dutertre, *Hist. gen. des Antilles habitées par les François.* 4 vols. Paris, 1667–1671.

the others. Now, with that personal experience in his mind, and with personal experience also of the epidemic of 1647–8, he describes the latter as a pestilence "hitherto unknown in the islands since they were inhabited by the French." Like Ligon and Winthrop, he is led to think of plague itself by the rapidity and fatality of the infection; but he mentions no signs of plague proper, and at the same time mentions continual vomiting. The disease was, in short, the Yellow Fever; and the epidemic in the end of 1647 at Bridgetown, and shortly after at St Christopher and Guadeloupe, was the first of it, so far as is known, in the West Indies.

But what then were the earlier epidemics spoken of by Dutertre? The branch colony to Guadeloupe from St Christopher in 1635 had been only two months in their new home, when, in September, their experiences of famine began. The famine or scarcity, says Dutertre, continued for five years, and was followed by "a mortality almost general." It was part of that mortality which Dutertre himself saw on his arrival at Guadeloupe in 1640. He calls the fever *coup de barre*—a name which in the sequel was sometimes given to yellow fever; and he mentions symptoms which agree, in part at least, with those of yellow fever—violent pains in the head, throbbing of the temporal arteries, great distress of breathing, lassitude, pains in the calf of the legs, as if they had been struck by a *coup de barre.* But in speaking of the sickness which he found prevalent on landing in 1640, he does not mention the irrepressible vomiting, which he puts in the first place when he describes the other fever of 1647–8; and, to repeat, he says that the latter was a pestilence hitherto unknown since the occupation of the French Antilles, and as fatal as the plague. It is tolerably certain, therefore, that the sickness on Guadeloupe sometime between 1635 and 1640, was of the usual kind incidental to the settlement of a new colony. We have had to notice it in Virginia ("from pestilent ships," the governor thought), in St Christopher, and in other new settlements. In a petition of the Governor and Company of the Somers Islands, July 28, 1639, it is said that about one hundred and thirty of their colonists had transplanted themselves last year to St Lucia, where they suffered so much from sickness that not one was in health[1]. Any one of those epidemics among new settlers might be diagnosed yellow fever with as much warrant as another; but the deadly infection of 1647–8 was something special, different from all that had preceded, and to be accounted the first appearance of yellow fever whether in the West Indies or anywhere else[2].

Yellow fever received much elucidation in after years, both as regards its symptoms and pathology, and as regards its circumstances and causation. To get a familiar view of what the disease was like, let us take the following graphic case recorded by Moseley at Jamaica more than a century after the date with which we are still engaged[3]:

"The last patient I saw, in the last stage of the yellow fever, was Captain Mawhood of the 85th regt. at Port Royal, in Jamaica on the 24th Sept., 1780. It was on the fourth day of his illness. He had been in the island seven weeks.

I arrived at the lodgings of this much esteemed young man about four hours before his death. When I entered the room, he was vomiting a black, muddy cruor; and was bleeding at the nose. A bloody ichor was oozing from the corners of his eyes, and from his mouth and gums. His face was besmeared with blood; and with the dulness of his eyes, it presented a most distressing contrast to his natural visage. His abdomen was swelled, and inflated prodigiously. His body was all over of a deep yellow, interspersed with livid spots. His hands and feet were of a livid hue. Every part of him was cold excepting about his heart. He had a deep, strong hiccup, but neither delirium nor coma; and was at my first seeing him, as I thought, in his perfect senses. He looked at the changed appearance of his skin, and expressed, though he could not speak, by his sad countenance, that he knew life was soon to yield up her citadel, now abandoning the rest of his body. Exhausted with vomiting, he at last was suffocated with the blood he was endeavouring to bring up, and expired."

One of the best summaries of its symptoms is that given by the Rev. Griffith Hughes, rector of one of the Barbados parishes[4]:

[1] *Cal. State Papers*, Amer. and W. I., 1. 301.

[2] The chronology of yellow-fever epidemics in Hirsch (1. 318) is made to begin with Guadeloupe, 1635 and 1640, on the authority of Dutertre (as above), the epidemic of 1647 at Bridgetown being the third in order.

[3] Benjamin Moseley, M.D., *Treatise on Tropical Diseases, and on the Climate of the West Indies*, 3rd ed. (1803), p. 476.

[4] Hughes, *The Natural History of Barbados*. London, 1750, p. 37.

" The attack begins with a feeling of chill lasting an hour or two. Then violent fever comes on, with excessive pain in the head, back, and limbs, loss of strength, great dejection of spirits, insatiable thirst, restlessness, sometimes vomiting, redness of the eyes, and that redness in a few days turning to yellow. If the patient turn yellow soon, he has scarce a chance for life, and, the sooner he does, the worse. After some days the pain in the head abates, as well as the fever. A sweat breaks out, and the patient appears to be better ; but on a narrow view a yellowness appears in his eyes and skin, and he becomes visibly worse. About this time he sometimes spits blood, and that by mouthfuls ; as this continues, he grows cold and his pulse abates till at last it is quite gone, and the patient becomes almost as cold as a stone, and continues in that state with a composed sedate mind. In this condition he may perhaps live twelve hours, without any sensible pulse or heat, and then expire. Such were the symptoms and progress of this fever in the year 1715." He adds that the hæmorrhage was sometimes from the nose or rectum. "A loose tooth being drawn from a person who had the fever very severely, there issued out from the hole a great quantity of black stinking blood, which still kept oozing till the third day, on which the patient died in great agonies and convulsions." The symptoms were not uniform in all, nor in every visitation. It was most commonly rife and fatal in May, June, July and August, and then mostly among strangers, though a great many of the inhabitants died of it in 1696 and a great many at different periods since. (The next Barbados epidemic after 1647 was in 1671.)

Now, of that remarkable disease, a pestilent fever with hæmorrhages, having a final stage of collapse not unlike the algid termination of cholera, and a mortality equalled only by that of plague itself, or, in after times, by that of cholera, it will be difficult to find instances in any part of the world previous to the Barbados, St Christopher, and Guadeloupe epidemics of 1647—48. Not only so, but these and other West Indian harbours were the distinctive seats of it for long after. From first to last yellow fever has been an infection of certain harbours—of the shipping anchored, moored, or careened in them, and of the houses nearest to the shore. In the Barbados epidemic of 1647, Ligon says, the ships at anchor in Carlisle Bay were for the most part infected ; Dutertre says that the crew and passengers died of it on board the ship which brought it to Guadeloupe ; he says, also, that it had come to St Christopher with certain ships ; and Ligon clearly suspects that it may have had an origin on board ship : "for in long voyages diseases grow at sea and take away many passengers, and these diseases prove contagious." We have had many instances of the sicknesses of voyages, not only scurvy but also fevers. But these ship-fevers were not yellow fever; we know more of them in later periods of the history, when they were recognized as ship-typhus. For yellow fever we must seek something more distinctive, and that distinctive thing we shall probably find in a kind of voyage which we have not hitherto considered from the point of view of its sicknesses—the Middle Passage, or the voyage with negroes from the African coast across the tropical belt to one part or another of the New World. Let us then take that particular kind of voyage, as we have already taken the voyages of the East India Company's ships, the voyages of emigrant ships from England to the North-American Colonies, and those from France and England to the West Indies.

Dutertre, our authority for the first yellow fever in St Christopher, is also a witness to the sicknesses and mortality of the Middle Passage. Of the negroes, he says, more die on the passage than land. He has known captains who have taken on board up to 700 in one ship and landed only 200; they died of misery and hunger, and the stifling monotony of tropical calms. Some of the slaves are of high degree; there was one negress, in particular, whom all the rest looked up to as a princess.

The African slave-trade was not altogether so reputable as to have had the incidents of the voyages recorded with anything approaching to scientific fulness. But within the period that now occupies us, there are four notices of arrivals of slavers in the West Indies from Guinea, in which the health of the voyage had called for remark[1]. In a letter from Barbados, March 20, 1664, it is said that the 'Speedwell' has arrived with 282 negroes, who have greatly lost in value owing to smallpox breaking out amongst them; the 'Success' brought 193 blacks; the 'Susan' 230, which were not allowed to be landed until the officers of the ship had proved that they had not collected them within the Royal African Company's limits. Another Barbados letter of March 31, 1664, says that "there has been a great mortality amongst the negroes [? on St Christopher and Nevis] which the African Company's physician at Barbados, De La Rouse, assures

[1] *Cal. S. P.* Amer. and W. I., under the dates.

C.   40

them is through a malignant distemper contracted, they think, through so many sick and decaying negroes being thronged together, and perhaps furthered by the smallpox in Captain Carteret's ships. Most men refused to receive any of them, and Philip Fusseires, a surgeon, to whom they sold twenty at a low rate, lost every one." This is a confused letter, but the reference to "sick and decaying negroes thronged together," appears to mean, not a sharp sickness soon over, but a general sickly state and loss of condition, which had come upon them during the voyage[1]. The third letter is from Barbados, June 25, 1667: from Guinea are arrived four ships, two of the African Company's, and two private; in which had happened a great mortality of negroes and of the ships' companies. Once more, to bring out the long imprisonment of negroes under decks while the slaver was filling up on the coast, T. Barrett writing from Port Royal on October 17, 1672, to James Littleton, "has heard that Capt. James Tallers bought the negroes for Littleton from another ship in Guinea which had them three months aboard, and that they were almost all starved and surfeycatted [surfeit had come to mean dysentery], he having fed them with little else but musty corn. There must have been something extraordinary that so many of them died."

In one of the letters we hear of sickness and mortality not only of slaves on the passage but also of the ships' companies. Long after, Clarkson showed from the muster-rolls of Liverpool slave-ships that the slave-trade, instead of being a "nursery" of British sailors, was their grave[2]. There are, however, few medical

[1] In Sir John Hawkins' second voyage as a slaver (1565), he was allowed to trade on the Spanish Main only for his "lean negroes," which were within the purchasing means of the poorer Spaniards. The voyage had been tedious, and the supply of water short "for so great a company of negroes......Many never thought to have reached to the Indies without great death of negroes and of themselves; but the Almighty God, who never suffereth His Elect to perish," etc. Hakluyt, III. 501.

[2] Clarkson, *History of the Abolition of the African Slave Trade.* New ed., Lond. 1839, pp. 307, 352. He showed his prepared document to Pitt:—

"Mr Pitt turned over leaf after leaf, in which the copies of the muster-rolls were contained, with great patience; and when he had looked over about a hundred pages accurately, and found the name of every seaman inserted, his former abode or service, the time of his entry, and what had become of him, either by death, discharge, or

particulars; doubtless many of the deaths among the crews occurred on the coast, from fever, dysentery and the like brought on by debauchery and during trading excursions up the rivers in the long-boat; but from the third of the letters quoted it appears that there had been also deaths on the voyage. Of the sicknesses among the negroes, more is said of smallpox than of any other malady in the foregoing records. But smallpox was not in ordinary circumstances a very fatal or very severe disease among negroes, although it was very common. An early medical writer on the diseases of the Guinea Coast, both of white men and negroes, Dr Aubrey, "who resided many years on the coast of Guinea," may pass as a credible witness in the matter, the more so as his book shows him to have been competent in his profession[1].

"Measles and smallpox," he says, "are no ways dangerous, nor so troublesome as in cold climates, neither are they so very sick e'er they come out, nor remains there any great sign of them after they recover. Abundance of these poor creatures are lost on board ships, to the great prejudice of the owners and scandal of the surgeon, merely through the surgeon's ignorance; because he knows not what they are afflicted with, but supposing it to be a fever, bleeds and purges or vomits them into an incurable diarrhœa, and in a very few days they become a feast for some hungry shark. When they are in the woods sick of these diseases, they take nothing but cold water, and suck oranges, and yet recover, as I myself have been an eye-witness many a time; and the grandy-men's children are treated no otherwise in their sickness, and are very well of the smallpox in less than half a moon," etc. It is conceivable, however, that smallpox left to itself would not have run so favourable a course in the hold of a slaver as in the native huts of the negroes. On board ship the subjects of smallpox died from a complication of diarrhœa; and, according to the same writer,

---

desertion, he expressed his surprise at the great pains which had been taken in this branch of the inquiry; and confessed, with some emotion, that his doubts were wholly removed with respect to the destructive nature of this employ." (p. 273.)

[1] T. Aubrey, M.D., *The Sea-Surgeon, or the Guinea Man's Vade Mecum.* London, 1729, p. 107.

diarrhœa or dysentery was the grand cause of mortality on the voyage, the most inveterate form of it, (according to his fixed belief), occurring in those who had been constitutionally affected by yaws: " This (the yawey flux) is the mortal disease that cuts off three parts in four of the negroes that are commonly lost on board ships." But the same writer reveals enough to let us understand the prevalence of flux as a primary malady. The food of the slaves on board ship, to say nothing of the regimen, was distasteful to them. They missed their palm oil and other accustomed articles of diet. They were fed, morning and evening, on pease, beans, and the like, mixed with " rotten salt herrings," with an occasional meal of salt beef or salt pork, and a stinted allowance of water.

"These are foods that very few of them will eat. Very often they are abused by sailors, who beat and kick them to that degree that sometimes they never recover ; and then the surgeon is blamed for letting the slaves die, when they are murthered, partly by strokes and partly famished ; for if they do not eat such salt things as are enough to destroy them, they must fast till supper ; and then they lose their appetites, and perhaps fall sick, partly through fasting and partly with grief to see themselves so treated ; and if once they take anything to heart, all the surgeon's art will never keep them alive ; for they never eat anything by fair means or foul, because they choose rather to die than be ill-treated...When they are costive and griped [by the salt food], they stay betwixt decks and will eat nothing ; but cry *yarry*, *yarry*, and perhaps creep under one of the platforms and hide themselves, and die there, and the surgeon can't think what is the meaning on't...I am very sensible that it is impossible to maintain the slaves on board, after one quits the Coast, without salt provisions ; but then care might be taken to water the beef and pork ere it be boiled, and also to bring a cruce of palm-oil round the deck from mess to mess, and also pepper, and let everyone take as he pleaseth....Another principal cause of their destruction is forcing them into a tub of cold water every day, and pouring the water on their heads by buckets-full "—doubtless for the sake of cleanliness, although they were too ill to stand such washings.

Whatever else the negroes died of on the voyage from Guinea, they did not die of yellow fever : there is hardly another generality of pathology so well based as that Africans of pure blood have been found immune from that infection in all circumstances ashore or afloat—protected not by acclimatisation but by some strange privilege of their race. And yet we have to think of yellow fever as somehow related to the over-sea traffic in negroes. Two instances from the later history will serve to bring the problem concretely before us. In 1815, a British transport, the 'Regalia,' was employed in carrying recruits from the West Coast of Africa to the black regiments in the West Indies. The health of the ship when on the African coast had been good; but on the voyage across with the newly-enlisted negroes, much sickness, chiefly dysenteric, occurred among the latter, whereupon yellow fever broke out with great malignancy, attacking all on board except the black soldiers, who were from first to last untouched by it. From such experiences as that, Sir Gilbert Blane formulated a somewhat vague doctrine that the causes which produced dysentery in the negro produced yellow fever in the white race. But it is more probable that the dysenteric matters of the negroes had themselves in turn bred an infection of yellow fever for the whites. To take another case: In 1795, after the capture of Martinique from the French, one of the frigates 'La Pique,' was manned by a British crew and sent to Barbados. On the voyage they rescued two hundred negroes from a ship which was about foundering. The negroes were confined in the hold of 'La Pique;' and in a short time yellow fever broke out among her English crew, killing one hundred and fifty of them, although it was not prevalent among the blacks at all. "Such a mixture of men," says Gillespie, "strangers to each other, has been often found to occasion sickness in ships; and, together with other causes, fatally operated here before the arrival of the ship at Barbados....This is a melancholy instance of the generation of a fatal epidemic on board ship at a time when the inhabitants of Barbados and the crews of the other ships in company remained free from any such disease[1]."

But such instances are comparatively rare, while epidemics of yellow fever on shore, or among the shipping in an anchorage, have been common. It is possible that the yellow fever experiences of the 'Regalia' and 'La Pique' had happened often to the white crews of slavers; we shall never know. What we do know is that the ports of debarkation of the slave-trade became

---

[1] Gillespie, *Obs. on the Diseases in H. M.'s Squadron on the Leeward Island Station in* 1794–6. Lond. 1800.

the endemic seats of yellow fever. The theory is that the matters productive of yellow fever were brought to the West Indian harbours, deposited there, left to ferment and accumulate, and so to taint the soil, the mud and the water as to become an enduring source of poisonous miasmata. The facts in support of that view are not far to seek.

Let us come back to the circumstances of Bridgetown, Barbados, when the yellow fever broke out first in 1647. A good many slavers had landed their cargoes at Bridgetown in the years preceding (in 1643 the island had at least 6400 negroes), and each of them had left behind a material quantity of the filth of the voyage, having probably been careened for the purpose of cleaning out and overhauling. There are traditions still extant that the cleaning of a slave-ship after a voyage from Africa was an exceptional task, to which Kroomen used to be set. Be that as it may, it needs only a little reflection to see that a crowd of some hundreds of negroes under gratings in the hold or 'tween decks of a brig or schooner, suffering at first from sickness of the sea and, as the voyage across the tropic belt progressed, from the more distressing flux, must have set all rules of cleanliness at defiance. The ship's bilges and ballast would be foul beyond measure: and it was just the contents of her bilges, with or without the ballast itself, that would be pumped out or thrown out when the ship was moored in the harbour or careened on the mud. At Bridgetown there were no plunging tides, such as we watch on our own shores, to carry the filth out to sea. The spring tides, says Ligon, rose only four or five feet; the flood tide carried the water over the banks into the lagoon, and the ebb carried it off; but at neap tides a quantity of water remained stagnant behind the sea-banks, according to the familiar experience in such circumstances. The flat shore, says Ligon, became "a kind of bog, which vents out so loathsome a savour as cannot but breed ill blood, and is (no doubt) the occasion of much sickness to those that live there." A brackish estuary, with an impeded outfall, will often smell badly, from rotting sea-wrack or other decomposing matters; but we have yet to learn that any so commonplace conditions can breed a deadly pestilence such as arose at Bridgetown for the first time in the autumn of 1647. Carlisle Bay was doubtless a leeward harbour, with high land all round it and a sluggish ebb and flow of the tide, subject to calms and a scorching sun ; but besides all that, the careenage at the head of the bay was the regular receptacle of the ordure of slave-ships year after year. Travellers and imaginative writers have sometimes pictured the bays and creeks of the islands and main of the Caribbean Sea as if the mere decay of tropical vegetation had made them pestilential[1]. Risk, of course, there is in such situations, but chiefly when men are exposed by turns to the noonday heat and the nocturnal chill. The ill repute of West Indian harbours, with their sweltering mud, mangrove swamps, and lazy tides, is a composite and confused idea. It is not so much Nature that has made them unwholesome, as man. Yellow fever, in particular, is not a miasm of remote and primeval bays or lagoons into which a boat's crew may come once and again ; it is not a fever of any and every part of the coast of a tropical island ; it is a fever of only a few inhabited spots on the wide shores of the globe ; and those seats of it, so far as it has been steady or periodic in its prevalence, are all of them harbours distinguished at one time or another as the resort of slave-ships, and distinguished from many other ports of either Hemisphere in no other way. Everything in the subsequent history of yellow fever pointed to its being a poison lurking in the mud or even in the water of slave-ports, and in the soil of their fore-shores, wharves and houses along the beach. Miasmata rose from the ground in the latter situations, to taint the air of the town at certain seasons ; the poison also entered the bilges of ships moored or careened in the harbour, and rose from the holds as a noxious vapour to infect the crews. The miasmata were deadly for the most part to new comers, especially to those from the colder latitudes, although acclimatised residents were not exempt in a time of epidemic; but there is very general agreement that they carried no risk for negroes of pure blood.

What was there special in the circumstances of 1647 to give rise to the first epidemic explosion of yellow fever? There was,

[1] For example, Mr R. L. Stevenson in a striking passage of *Treasure Island.*

in the first place, the accretion of the peculiar fermenting filth in the mud and soil, which had been going on for several years. Secondly, there was the brisk trade, as indicated by the large number of ships in the harbour, a great concourse of new arrivals having been often remarked in the later history as one of the conditions of an outbreak. But more particularly there were the peculiarities of the season : it was one of those seasons in which the regular rains of June and following months had failed. What we know on that head comes exclusively from Winthrop's 'Journal,' already quoted. There was so great a drouth, he says, that their potatoes, corn, &c., were burnt up ; and after the "great dearth of victuals in these islands followed presently a great mortality." But the mortality was certainly not from famine, nor from the effects of famine. It was the parching drought that the epidemic really followed, and not merely the scarcity, which was, indeed, relieved by the ships from New England, and was so little felt that Ligon does not mention it. The rainy season missed, or all but missed, in a tropical country means a great fall of the ground water ; it means the pores of the ground filled with air to an unusual extent ; and that is a state of any soil, if it be already full of fermenting organic matters, which breeds the most dangerous half-products of decomposition, or, in other words, the most poisonous miasmata. There needs always some such special determining thing to explain the epidemic outbursts of yellow fever ; in the later history we shall see that the first great epidemic of it at Jamaica followed immediately upon the earthquake that destroyed Port Royal.

Illustrations of the ordinary principle that seasonal and periodic infection is dependent on the state of the ground water, are given at greater length in the chapters upon the later epidemics of plague in London. What applies in that respect to one soil-poison applies to another ; and it will be shown in the proper place to apply with least ambiguity of all to Asiatic cholera, as well as to typhoid fever. Yellow fever is, in clinical characters, allied more to typhus than to typhoid ; but it is a typhus of the soil, whereas the common and much less fatal typhus of ordinary domestic life in colder latitudes is an infection above ground—of the air, walls, floors and furnishings of rooms. There is the same relation between yellow fever and ordinary typhus in that respect, as between plague and ordinary typhus. When ordinary typhus has passed into a soil-poison, by aggravation of conditions, as in the experience of Arab encampments in North Africa, it has become at the same time bubonic fever, or, approximately plague proper. Yellow fever had its habitat essentially in the soil, from the peculiar circumstances (importation of the crude materials of it by ships engaged in the slave-trade); and plague in ordinary, or in European experience, had also its habitat in the soil, from circumstances which have been elsewhere given as its probable conditions.

It is perhaps because they are soil-poisons that those two diseases rank so high in their fatality and quickness of execution, in which respects they resemble Asiatic cholera, and differ from most other infections. Winthrop says that the first yellow fever killed in three days, and was therefore comparable to the plague. Ligon says that it was as killing a disease as the plague (of which both he and Winthrop would have had old experience at home), and he uses the stock phrase, that the living were hardly able to bury the dead. Winthrop says that 6000 died in Barbados : and one of his correspondents in the island, Vines, writes that " in our parish there were buried twenty in a week, and many weeks together fifteen or sixteen." Dutertre says that nearly a third of the colonists of St Christopher died of it, and that it lingered there for eighteen months, and for twenty months in Guadeloupe, whither it was believed to have been brought in the ship ' Le Bœuf.'

Barbados, St Christopher and Guadeloupe (with minor settlements on Martinique, Nevis, &c.) were the earliest English and French colonies in the Caribbean Sea. The Spaniards had occupied the Greater Antilles (Hispaniola or San Domingo, Cuba, Porto Rico and Jamaica) long before. Nothing particular is known of the health of these colonies except for the earlier years of the 16th century, when the native populations were ravaged by the great pox and the smallpox. But when Jamaica was seized from the Spaniards by the army of the

Commonwealth in 1655 we begin to have authentic information, the state of health being perhaps the most prominent thing (although little noticed by historians) in the despatches. That incident in the expansion of England, relating as it does to the planting of what was for long our greatest island colony, and illustrating the risks of those early enterprises more fully than any other of the kind, may fitly come into this chapter and conclude it.

The Great Mortality in the occupying of Jamaica.

The Lord Protector's design in the year 1654, to acquire one or more of the Spanish Antilles for an English colony, was more methodically conceived and more strenuously supported by the resources of the State than any previous attempt at colonization. It was attended with disasters on a proportionate scale, and at first with ignominy and failure which must have added seriously to the burden of Cromwell's later years. The original design, in the admiral's sealed orders, was to seize upon the old Spanish colony of Hispaniola or San Domingo[1]. A fleet had been fitted out at Portsmouth, which sailed on 19th—21st December, 1654, carrying a land force of three thousand men. After a favourable voyage, the fleet of thirty sail, half of them victuallers, arrived at Barbados on February 1, where they lay until March 31, engaging settlers for the proposed new colony as well as campaigners, including a troop of cavalry, from the not very choice class of English subjects in that island. Some twenty Dutch ships were seized and made victuallers or transports. The expedition received a draft also from Nevis, and calling at St Christopher they took up 1300 more, making in all an addition of over 5000 colonial men, besides women and children, to their original force. On April 13 the fleet arrived off the harbour of St Domingo. It came out afterwards that the sight of so many English frigates and other ships had driven the townspeople to instantaneous flight, so that the capital would have fallen to the English

---

[1] Thurloe's *State Papers*, III. IV. and V.; *Harl. Miscell.* III. 513; Long's *History of Jamaica*, 3 vols. London, 1774; *Cal. S. P.*, Amer. and W. I.

without a blow.   But no landing was attempted in the harbour, owing to difficulties about piloting, ignorance of the depth of water, and the like.   It was decided to disembark the force in a bay at the mouth of a river some six or ten miles (two leagues) to the eastward, where Drake had landed in 1586.   Most of the ships, however, were carried past the appointed place, and came to anchor in another bay thirty miles (ten leagues) eastwards from St Domingo ; there a multitude of some 7000 soldiers and colonials, with their women and children, were landed on the beach with three days' rations.   Several of the ships landed their men at the original rendezvous two leagues from St Domingo, to the number of about 2000 in three regiments.   The larger and farther-off force began to advance on St Domingo through dense woods ; their presence in the country was soon known in all the plantations, whence the people fled to the capital for safety, so that the San Domingans were able to extemporise a considerable force for defence.   The advance of the English was hindered by the stifling heat ; distressed by thirst, they ate immoderately of oranges and other fruits, and in one way or another brought on dysentery.   General Venables, in a despatch to Cromwell, says that by these causes they "were troubled with violent fluxes, hundreds of our men having dropped down by the way, some sick, others dead."   Meanwhile the nearer and smaller force of some 2000 had advanced on St Domingo ; they got over one of the two leagues between them and the capital, but an old fort, manned for the occasion, barred the way, and the regiments fell back upon the river whence they had started, and rested there five days, the main body having meanwhile come up with them.   One attempt after another was made to pass the half-way fort, but the Spaniards held their ground, and actually inflicted defeat in the open and a disgraceful rout upon the English, some of whose gallant officers threw their lives away in a vain attempt to lead their men.   All the while this broken and demoralised mob was without proper supplies from the fleet, the officers of which were either unable to communicate with the land force or indifferent as to their duty. The state of health on the 25th of April, some ten or twelve days after landing, is thus described in a letter : " And the rains nightly pouring, with fogs and dews along the river, so soaked our bodies with flux, and none escaping that violence, that our freshment [by retreat to the river] proved a weakening instead of support." Another letter of two days' later date (April 27) says: "The rains increasing, our men weakening, all even to death fluxing, the seamen aboard neglecting,—that forced us to eat all our troop horses." An attempt was made to restore discipline; an officer of high rank was cashiered for a coward, his sword having been broken over his head; a soldier was shot for desertion; some loose women in men's clothes from Barbados were chastised, and a sharp look-out kept for other camp-followers of the kind. At length it was decided by Venables and his council that the attempt on San Domingo must be abandoned; probably it was seen that the Barbadian and St Christopher following was a fatal encumbrance at that stage, the more so as the rainy season was in progress. By the third of May the whole expedition was re-embarked, the Spaniards making no attempt to harass the operation. The number reshipped is said to have been seventeen hundred short of that which landed three weeks before: a good many had fallen fighting, others were slain by the Spaniards or negroes in the woods, and some appear to have died of the flux. The attempt on St Domingo having failed it was decided to make a descent on Jamaica, the least important of the Spanish Antilles. On the passage thither, Winslow, one of the three lay commissioners or "politicals" with the expedition, died "very suddenly of a fever."

On May 10 the ships entered the bay of Caguya. Admiral Penn, being resolved not to repeat the mistake they had made at St Domingo, kept sail on the 'Martin' galley until she was beached under the small fort of the Passage, at the head of the bay, so as to cover the debarkation with his guns. However, the few Spaniards living at the shore fled, and the whole force, to the number of some 7000, was landed by midnight. Venables then returned to his ship for his usual repose, leaving the men under arms all night. Not until nine next day, by which hour the cool of the morning was lost, did the march begin to the capital, St Jago de la Vega ("St James of the Plain"), situated on an elevation by the river Cobre, in the midst of an alluvial plain with an amphitheatre of hills behind it, some six miles from the place of landing. About two in the afternoon they came before the town, and marched in that night: they found it empty, "nothing but bare walls, bedsteads, chairs and cowhides." The town is said to have had some 1700 houses (too many for its population), two churches, two chapels, and an abbey; there all the Spaniards dwelt in ease and indolence, "having their slaves at their several small plantations, who constantly brought them store of provisions and fruits." In this great island there were but about 3000 inhabitants, half of them, if not more, being slaves. There were no manufactures or native commodities, except a very little sugar and cocoa. The four ships that came thither in a year traded generally for hides and tallow only.

The Spanish colony had removed as much of their property as they could in their first flight, and shortly sent their head men with their governor, "an old decrepid seignior full of the French disease" carried by two bearers in a hammock, to treat for their re-entry into the town. Venables was afterwards much blamed for returning the politeness of the Spaniards; he received their presents of fresh provisions and fruit, accepted their promises of a steady supply for his men, and gave them the free run of their own houses for a week or so, by which time they are said to have carried off all their personal belongings of value. They objected to leave the island, saying that Jamaica was their home, and that they had no friends either in New Spain or in Old Spain. At length they left their old settlement, with the avowed purpose of embarking for Cuba from a bay on the same side to the west. There were divided counsels among the English as to the treatment of the Spaniards, and Colonel Bullard was sent towards the bay with a large force to intercept them in their flight. They had, however, given a false direction, and had in reality crossed the mountains northwards to the other side of the island, clearing the country as they went of cattle and produce of every kind. Some of them, including eight families of the upper class, at length found their way to Cuba, but the larger number remained on the north of the island, where they were overtaken by famine and pestilence before a few months, and nearly exterminated.

Their negroes took to the mountains, and became the maroons, famous in the later history of Jamaica.

In pursuing the Spaniards, the English troops went roaming over the country, destroying the hogs and cattle in mere wantonness, and leaving their carcases to putrefy. In a short time the multitude of English at St Jago de la Vega (Spanish Town) were on short rations, and before long "dogs and cats the best part of their diet." The stores from the ships had been left on the beach exposed to the weather, and soon turned mouldy, the men refusing to carry them, in the absence of waggons, over the six miles between the shore and the head-quarters. Two or three victuallers besides had arrived from England within a week or two of the first landing, but, for all that, the expedition was starving. Many of the men were suffering from the flux which they had contracted in St Domingo. Venables, in a private letter of May 25, or a fortnight after landing, gives the number of the sick at near 3000; in a despatch to Cromwell, of June 4, he says:

"The want we have been in hitherto of bread (we not being able to be suddenly supplied therewith out of the fleet, or our stores, through want of waggons and other conveniences for the transportation thereof), joined with the drinking of water, hath already cast both officers and soldiers into such violent fluxes that they look more like dead men crept out of their graves than persons living; and this so generally that we have not above two colonels in health, three majors, some seven field officers in all; besides many have been already swept away with this disease. We lost Mr Winslow very suddenly, in our sailing towards this island, of a fever."

On June 9 there was a general muster of the land forces, "whose number was found to be much diminished of late, not so much by any pestilential or violent disease, as for mere want of natural sustenance; which, in common reason, may seem strange that of all men soldiers should starve in a cook's shop, as the saying is[1]."

In a despatch of June 13, Venables says that "about 2000 are sick. Our men die daily, eating roots and fresh fish (when any food is got), without bread or very little." He was himself ill, having had the flux for five weeks. Admiral Penn (father of

[1] *Harl. Miscel. l.c.*

the founder of Pennsylvania) had resolved to go home with two-thirds of the ships, thinking that his services were no longer needed, and having been advised that he could be of more service to Cromwell in England. He sailed on June 21, leaving the frigates and the Dutch prizes, under Goodson; and Venables followed in four days, with the surviving "political," leaving the settlement in charge of Fortescue, who wrote home, "I am left to act without book."

Meanwhile Cromwell had got ready reinforcements, sparing no trouble or expense at home. The expedition in aid left Plymouth on July 11, 1655, under the command of Sedgwick, and arrived at Barbados on August 26–31, after a fine passage; they left again on September 7, having trimmed their casks and taken in water with other refreshments. This force was in the best of health until after leaving Barbados. Sedgwick writes:

"I think never so many ships sailed together with less trouble, grief or danger than we did; only God did in a little visit us between this [Jamaica] and Barbados with some sickness, I apprehend caused by some distemper taken there [? yellow fever]; in which visitation, I think, in the whole fleet we lost between 20 and 30 seamen and soldiers."

Finding the Spanish flag flying at San Domingo, they came on to Jamaica on October 1, and there found a calamitous state of things.

"For the army, I found them in as sad and deplorable and distracted condition as can be thought of: commanders, some left them, some dead, some sick, and some in indifferent health; the soldiery many dead, their carcases lying unburied in the highways and among bushes, to and again; many of them that were alive walked like ghosts or dead men, who, as I went through the town, lay groaning and crying out, Bread, for God's sake!"

Sedgwick brought with him in four victuallers a thousand tons of provisions, which he secured in a store built for the occasion on the beach. Among his troops was Colonel Humphry's regiment of 831 "lusty, healthful, gallant men, who encouraged the whole army." But now we begin to see that the sickness at St Jago de la Vega had become infective or pestilential. The new-comers, healthy and well found as they were, began at once to sicken and to die. Of Humphry's regiment, on November 5 :

"There are at this day 50 of them dead, whereof two captains, a lieutenant, and two ensigns, the colonel himself very weak, the lieutenant-colonel at death's door. Soldiers die daily, I believe 140 every week, and so have done ever since I came hither. It is strange to see lusty men, in appearance well, and in three or four days in the grave, snatched away in a moment with fevers, agues, fluxes and dropsies, a confluence of many diseases. We furnished the army now with 60 butts of Madeira wine, and to every regiment a butt of brandy, and a hogshead or two of sweet oil. Our soldiers have destroyed all sorts of fruits, and provisions and cattle. Nothing but ruin attends them wherever they go." On January 24, 1656, Sedgwick again writes to Thurloe : "Did you but see the faces of this poor small army with us, how like skeletons they look, it would move pity ; and when I consider the thousands laid in the dust in such a way as God hath visited, my heart mourns. Here hath come down to us from many of the Windward Islands divers people with intentions of sitting down with us, but at their coming hither, either fall sick and die, or are so affrighted and dismayed as that, although to their much impoverishing, yet will not be persuaded to stay with us."

The men in the fleet were in better health ; but among them also "some die and some are sick, in so much that we need a good recruit fully to man our ships as men-of-war." On the same date (January 24, 1656) Admiral Goodson, writing to Thurloe, estimates the surviving officers and men at 2600, besides women and children ; and in another despatch of that date from Sedgwick and Goodson jointly to Cromwell it is stated :

"The numbers of the army are much lessened since our last letters [November 5]; the whole not extending to 3000, many of them sick and weak, the best and soundest much abated of their strength and vigor, and God goes on every day to shorten our number. We die daily, not less than fifty every week, which is much considering our small numbers."

As the season advanced the health of the troops on shore improved. A letter of March 12 says that the condition of the army is much mended ; the soldiers are far more healthful, but much dejected and averse to the place. The fleet was in good spirits, and impatient for action ; however, there was sickness also on board the ships ; they had lost some fourscore men since the last despatch ; and on April 30 the report is : "our seamen are indifferently well in health ; yet some few are sick, and God is daily shortening them, so that our fleet will want a recruit of men." Several of the frigates were wormeaten, and careened for repairs. Sickness is reported in the ships as late as October 10, 1656.

The sickness among all ranks had been so general and severe that it was hardly possible to find senior officers to undertake the government. Fortescue died in October, 1655, and was succeeded temporarily by D'Oyley and others, the sole government being at length given by Cromwell to Sedgwick, who died a few days after receiving his unwelcome commission. Brayne, transferred from Lochaber to Jamaica, also died, and it fell at length to D'Oyley, an effective person in whom all on the spot had confidence, to carry the colony through its troubles. Cromwell spared no effort at home. Immense quantities of provisions were shipped; planters, with their families, 'servants' and slaves, to the number of some 1700, were removed to Jamaica from Nevis, under Stokes, the governor of that island; the New Englanders were also encouraged to resort to the new colony; and a thousand or so of young men and marriageable young women were furnished from Ireland, together with pioneers, described as of a rougher kind, from Scotland. "And so at length," says Carlyle, "a West-Indian interest did take root; and bears spices and poisons, and other produce, to this day."

The sickness and mortality among the first English colonists of Jamaica gave the island a bad name, and must have added not a little to the confusion of ideas already existing as to the pestilent character of tropical climates[1]. The older sugar-colonies, such as Barbados, which saw in Jamaica a formidable competitor, would appear to have encouraged the notion that

---

[1] Sir Anthony Shirley touched at Jamaica in 1596, and reported, "we have not found in the Indies a more pleasant and wholesome place." Hakluyt, III. 601. Long (*History of Jamaica*, 1774, II. 221) states the case very fairly with reference to the unfortunate expedition of Venables in 1655 : "The climate of the island has unjustly been accused by many writers on the subject, the one copying from the other, and represented as almost pestilential, without an examination into the real sources of this mortality, which being fairly stated, it will appear that the same men carrying the like thoughtless conduct and vices into any other uninhabited quarter of the globe, must infallibly have involved themselves in the like calamitous situation."

climates varied much, that of Jamaica being bad. Soon after
the Restoration, Charles II. was urged to give back Jamaica to
Spain, and is said to have seriously entertained that purpose.
Among the state papers is a document, supposed to have been
written in November, 1660, which sets forth the natural advantages of Jamaica, together with two sets of reasons why
England should retain it[1]:

"The air here is more temperate than in any of the Caribee Islands,
being more northerly and as sufferable hot as in many places...The winds
here constantly all day blow easterly, so coolly that it renders any labour
sufferable at midday...We find here is not such antipathy between the
constitution of the English and the climate that sickness is not inevitable and
contingent ; for we have experimentally found that persons observing a good
diet and using moderate exercise, enjoy a somewhat (?) measure of health.
The said causes of the mortality of the Army at their first arrival were want
of provisions, unwillingness to labour or exercise, and inexcusable discontent
to be constrained to stay here.   The diseases that strangers are most incident to are dropsies (occasioned often by evil diet and slothfulness), calen-
tures (so frequently produced of surfeit), and fevers and agues, which,
although very troublesome, are never mortal....Cagway [Port Royal] is the
place where all the merchants reside, being the most healthy place in the
island ; whither resort all the men that frequent the Indies, which makes
houses so dear that an ordinary house in this town is worth £40 or £60 per
annum.   There are about 200 houses there, all built by the English.   About
50 houses have been built by the English at the fort of the Passage [at the
head of the harbour and the nearest point to Spanish Town]; of the houses in
the old capital, St Jago de la Vega, about 800 are ruinous.   As to the number
of English in the island, the relics of the six regiments do muster 2200, and
it is probable that the planters, merchants, sailors and others may be as
many."

The above statements about the healthiness of Jamaica in
1660 were repeated by Dr Trapham, in his work on the climate
and diseases of the colony in 1678[2]. This earliest medical
writer is, indeed, more optimist than those who followed him, as
to contagious or infective sickness ; there was no smallpox, or
very rarely, saving sometimes brought from Guinea by negroes ;
and "no depopulating plague that ere I have heard of," saving a

---

[1] *MS. State Papers, Colonial* (Record Office), Vol. XIV. No. 57 (1660).
[2] Thomas Trapham, M.D., *Discourse of the State of Health in Jamaica.*   Lond.
1679.

pestilential fever brought in by the victorious fleet returned from the signal Panama expedition in 1670. The experiences of yellow fever at Port Royal and Kingston were mostly, if not entirely, subsequent to these dates. But, as there had been yellow fever at Barbados, St Christopher, and Guadeloupe as early as 1647–48, it has been thought probable that the enormous mortality in Jamaica in 1655–56 was from the same endemic cause[1]. Undoubtedly the epidemic at Spanish Town became at length more than the dysentery which had been brought by some of the troops from San Domingo, or had been induced among others of them by bad food and water; it became a virulent specific infection, attacking the healthy and well-found reinforcements from England and the new arrivals from the Windward Islands, and destroying them quickly, "in three or four days." Fevers are specially named, as well as fluxes and dropsies; and the question arises whether the pestilential fever was not yellow fever.

There is certainly nothing said of the striking and ghastly symptoms of the *vomito negro.* Moreover the sickness was nearly all at the town of St Jago de la Vega, six miles from the bay, situated on a rising of the plain with a declivity to the Cobre river, a place which was only exceptionally the seat of yellow fever in after-experience. Thus Judge Long, the able historian of Jamaica, says[2]:

"After a series of hot, dry, and calm weather, eight days of continued rain succeeded in May, 1761. Spanish Town grew more sickly than ever I knew it, either before or since. From that period to August there were buried 29 white inhabitants, of whom 15 were soldiers. Their disorder had all the appearance of being the true yellow fever, and was supposed to have been communicated from some ship in Kingston harbour:"

—Kingston and Port Royal, or the ships moored near to them, being the common habitat of the disease, as in the corresponding circumstances at other West Indian islands.

But if the infective fever at Spanish Town in 1655—56 was almost certainly not yellow fever, it was probably allied to it in

---

[1] Moseley, *op. cit.* p. 421, without reasons given; followed by Hirsch. *Geog. and Hist. Pathol.* (English transl.), I. 318.

[2] *Hist. of Jamaica*, III. 615.

type. Dysentery had been almost universal; there was no care
of the sick, and, so far as one hears, no medical attendance, no
hospitals, no scavenging, no security taken to keep the water-
supply pure—nothing, in short, of what is now called sanitation.
Sedgwick, arriving on October 1, 1655, found even the dead unburied by the highways and among the bushes. The correlation
between dysentery and pestilential fever is no new hypothesis:
flux first and fever afterwards has been an experience both
in sieges and in ordinary domestic famines on many occasions.
The origin of the yellow fever at Barbados and elsewhere in
1647—8, which has been outlined in this chapter, is but a special
application of the same principle, the dysenteric matters which
represent the crude source of the infection having been brought
in the bilges and ballast of slave-ships, thrown into the mud
of almost tideless harbours, left to ferment amidst the heat and
moisture of the shore, and so made into a soil-poison which, in
due season, would give off emanations, fatal especially to new-
comers.   Port Royal and Kingston had full experience of that
endemic influence in after-years, for the first time in 1692, after
the earthquake and disturbance of soil which destroyed the
former town and occasioned the building of the latter on the
other side of the bay.   By that time there had been slavers
enough in the bay to bring all the ordure that the hypothesis
requires.   But, down to 1655, the Spaniards had traded only with
hides and tallow in some four ships every year, and had the
headquarters of their cultivation and stock-raising at the town in
the plain some six miles from the shore.   Four or five years after
their expulsion we find the whole aspect of the port changed, according to the description already given.   It does not appear
that Cromwell looked forward to negro labour in his colony,
although the Nevis planters brought their blacks with them.
Charles II. had not been many months on the throne when
James, earl of Marlborough, petitioned him to offer inducements
to the Royal African Company to make Jamaica the staple for
the sale of blacks, and to contract with that company for one
hundred negroes to be delivered at the island[1]. Negroes did
begin from that time to arrive in Jamaica, although Port Royal

[1] *Cal. S. P.* Amer. and W. I.

was at first rather a general centre of commerce and piracy than a slave-port like Bridgetown, perhaps because the Windward Islands were strong enough to keep their privileges undivided. As late as 1670 the negro slaves in Jamaica were reckoned at no more than 2500, not counting the old Spanish maroons[1]. On September 20 of that year, Sir Thomas Modyford, governor of Jamaica, sent to Secretary Arlington certain proposals for the improvement of the colony, of which the following bears upon our subject[2]:

"That they may have licence gratis or at moderate rates to trade for negroes in Africa. Did those honourable persons, which make that Royal [African] Company so glorious, but fall into considerations how much more it is his Majesty's interest to increase the number of his subjects than bullion of gold or silver (which by law all nations may import), they would not only freely consent to this proposal for us but for the whole nation and foreigners also. Mankind is the principal, gold the accessory: increase the first considerably, and the other must follow. Barbados had never risen to its late perfection had it not been lawful for Dutch, Hamburghers, and our whole nation, and any other, to bring and sell their blacks or any other servants in the colony's infancy."

The harbours of Port Royal and Kingston did, in the event, become the chief resort of slave-ships in the British West Indies, slaves having been landed there up to ten thousand in a year throughout the 18th century. They came also to be among the chief seats of yellow fever, and continued so until a recent date. The subsequent progress of yellow fever there, and in other West Indian harbours as well as in the ports of some of the North American colonies, is not the least important of the subjects that fall to the second period of this history.

---

[1] *Cal. S. P.* Amer. and W. I. 1669–74, § 144.   [2] *Ibid.* § 264, III.

CHAPTER XII.

THE GREAT PLAGUE OF LONDON, AND THE LAST OF
PLAGUE IN ENGLAND.

Literature of the Great Plague.

THE writings called forth directly by the London Plague of 1665 were hardly more numerous or of better quality than those of 1603 and 1625. At its beginning in June, or in August, there appeared a number of tracts by enterprising practitioners, containing a few commonplace remarks on causes and the like, and advertisements of nostrums—by G. Harvey, Kemp, Garrencieres ("Plague is one of the easiest diseases in the world to cure, if" etc.), and Gadbury, an astrologer. The directions drawn up by the College of Physicians in 1636, for the preservation of the sound and recovery of the sick were re-issued, and an excellent set of "cautionary rules" by H. Brooke was published by order of the mayor. The writings which contain accounts of the Great Plague fall under two periods—the years immediately following 1665, and the years 1720 to 1723 when there was a sudden revival of interest in the subject in London owing to the great plague of Marseilles in 1720. To the latter period belongs the most famous work on the plague of 1665, Defoe's *Journal of the Plague Year*, which embodied in a picturesque form the substance of various writings that preceded it, together with traditions known to Defoe. A brief account of those writings that preceded Defoe's in both periods will serve at the same time to show the sources of a great part of his information.

The weekly bills of mortality issued by Parish Clerks' Hall, which showed the number of deaths week by week in each of the one hundred and forty parishes of London, with a rough classification of the causes of death, were reprinted at the end of the year 1665 in a volume with the title *London's Dreadful Visitation*[1]. The bills thus collected in convenient form were made great use of by Defoe, and became, indeed, the backbone of his work. Next to them in importance, although it is not certain that Defoe used it, is a treatise on the medical aspects of the Great Plague, which has never had the fortune to be published. The author of it was William Boghurst, a young apothecary practising at the White Hart in St Giles's-in-the-Fields, who advertised in the *Intelligencer* on July 31, 1665, at the height of the plague in his parish, that he had treated forty, fifty or sixty patients in a day, that he was prepared to undertake the treatment of cases in the City, the suburbs, or the country, and that he had a water, a lozenge, and an electuary, as well as an antidote at eightpence an ounce[2].

After the epidemic was over he employed his spare half-hours in writing a book upon his experiences, "considering that none hath printed anything either since this plague, or that forty years since—which I something wonder at." He professes to have taken nothing from hearsay, or from books, or from the testimonies of others; he writes in English "for general readers and sale," and he had omitted many things "so as not to make the book too tedious and too dear to bie." The manuscript was completed for the press, with a title-page, at the foot of which is what appears to be a publisher's name (the surname now torn off); but it was never published, although the author lived until 1685. It is conceivable that the printed sheets, or the composed type, may have been destroyed in the fire of September, 1666, and the enterprise abandoned. The manuscript came into the possession of Sir Hans Sloane, and is

---

[1] With a preface by the Printer to the Reader, beginning "The reprinting of these sad sheets." Printed and are to be sold by E. Cotes, living in Aldersgate Street, printer to the said Company.

[2] The advertisement is cited in Brayley's edition of Defoe's *Journal of the Plague Year*.

now in the British Museum[1]. It gives much fuller clinical details of the plague than any other English work, although in somewhat aphoristic form; and it may be allowed the character of originality which the author claims for it, except in some of the more systematic chapters showing the influence of Diemerbroek.

Another medical essay following the plague was that of Dr Hodges, of Watling Street, first written in English in 1666 (May 8) under the title *A Letter to a Person of Quality*[2], and expanded in 1671 into a Latin treatise[3]. Besides a few pages at the beginning, giving some general facts of the London outbreak (which Defoe used), it is mostly a systematic disquisition, although a few cases are interspersed. One other medical piece of 1666 (June 16) is known, by Dr George Thomson, of Duke's Place near Aldgate, a Paracelsist or chemical physician; it contains the account of a dissection of a plague-body, but is mostly occupied with a polemic against the Galenists, which the author carried on for a number of years in numerous other writings[4].

Descriptive pieces, in prose or verse, such as the plagues of 1603 and 1625 elicited, are entirely wanting for that of 1665. But there was the usual crop of religious and moral exercises to improve the occasion. These appear to have come mostly, if not exclusively, from Dissenters. "Many useful and pious treatises," says a Dissenter in 1721, "were published upon the occasion of the last visitation, as by Mr Zach. Crofton, Mr Shaw, Mr Doolittle, and others." But the only one that attained popularity, having gone through five editions at once, and been often reprinted, even as late as 1851, was *God's Terrible Voice in the City*[5], by the Rev. Thomas Vincent, of Christ Church,

---

[1] Sloane MS. no. 349. Λοιμογραφια, *or, An experimental Relation of the Plague, of what happened remarkable in the last Plague in the City of London*, etc. By William Boghurst, Apothecary in St Giles' in the Fields. London, 1666.

[2] Reprinted in *A Collection of very Valuable and Scarce Pieces relating to the last Plague in the year 1665.* London, 1721.

[3] Λοιμολογια. London, 1671. Translation by Quincy, 1720.

[4] Λοιμοτομια, *or, the Pest Anatomized.* By George Thomson, M.D. London, 1666.

[5] London, 1667.

Oxford, who had been ejected from his living of St Mary Magdalen, Milk Street, and was then a leader of Dissent. Vincent preached in several parish churches (deserted by their parsons) all through the plague, and ministered constantly among the sick. His book, which moralizes also upon the great fire of 1666, will be drawn upon in the sequel.

We come next to the revival of interest in the Great Plague of London, which was occasioned by the Marseilles epidemic in the summer of 1720, an event that alarmed Western Europe as if the old recurrences of plague were about to begin afresh after a long interval. In London, in 1721, several books were published upon the Marseilles plague itself; and the years from 1720 to 1722 saw a whole crop of writings,—new essays and reprints of old ones,—upon the last London plague of 1665. Among the books reprinted were Hodges' *Loimologia*, in an English translation by Quincy, his *Letter to a Person of Quality*, the *Necessary Directions* of the College of Physicians, the *Orders drawn up by the Lord Mayor and Aldermen of the City* (these three in 1721 in a *Collection of very Valuable and Scarce Pieces relating to the last Plague in* 1665), and Vincent's *God's Terrible Voice in the City*. The new medical books on the Great Plague were by Scarborough, Hancock and Browne.

When Defoe in 1722 wrote his *Journal of the Plague Year*, he had these recent reprints and original books convenient to his hand. He had to go back to 1665 for the collection of the weekly bills of mortality in the plague-year (in a volume called *London's Dreadful Visitation*), and he may have consulted Boghurst's manuscript, which was probably then in the possession of Sir Hans Sloane. But it is impossible to trace all his copious narrative of the Great Plague to these sources, even if we make due allowance for his legitimate construction of incidents out of the generalities of contemporary writers. It is possible that he may have had some unknown manuscript, less technical than Boghurst's, to draw from. At all events, he was a likely person to have had many stories of the plague in his memory. He was a child of four when the plague was in London, the son of a butcher named Foe in St Giles's, Cripplegate, which was one of the most severely visited parishes. The most graphic parts of his *Journal* are those which contain such tales as he might have been told in boyhood concerning the plague in Cripplegate, the scene of them being carried round to Aldgate, opposite to the Butchers' Row (still there) in Whitechapel High Street. He must have had some testimony from which to construct the visit to Blackwall, the view of the shipping moored all up and down the Thames, and the other particulars of the river-side population in the plague-time. The rough experiences of the three Stepney men in the country near London are in the manner of *Robinson Crusoe,* and needed only a few hints from Dekker's stories, or from the writers of 1625. His account of the burials by the cart-load in plague-pits is also suggestive of Dekker. The somewhat meagre references by Hodges might have sufficed him for his frequent theme of the hardships and horrors of shut-up houses, even if he had not seen two other tracts, of 1665, on the same. The accounts of the Marseilles plague, one of the worst in history, would have kept him right in picturing that of London.

Whatever materials Defoe took from Hodges, Vincent, or the writers on other plagues, he enlarged them by his power of circumstantial construction into a narrative which must be accounted on the whole veracious. He based upon figures, whenever he could get them ; he seems even to have sought among the archives of the City for accounts of monies distributed to the poor. He prints in full the orders of the Mayor and Aldermen, and professes to give the text of a formal resolution which they passed to remain at their posts throughout the crisis. His table of the number of plague-deaths in each of twenty-six towns or villages near London does not, indeed, agree with the figures in the parish registers, as the table on a later page will show ; but it can hardly have been drawn up at a guess.

The best instance of Defoe's skilful use of authentic documents is his description of how the infection invaded one part of London after another from the western suburbs to the eastern, so that its intensity was nearly over in one place before it had begun in another. That is the most interesting epidemiological fact in the whole outbreak ; and Defoe has done ample justice to it. Boghurst had stated it with equal clearness and emphasis in his manuscript of 1666, which Defoe may or may not have seen[1]; however the latter deduced it afresh, and illustrated it by numerous tables from the bills of mortality, which showed the incidence of plague upon each of the one hundred and forty parishes from week to week.

Antecedents, Beginnings and Progress of the Plague of 1665.

When the London plague of 1665 had given indications that it would grow to be one of the great outbreaks of that infection, much was made, in the retrospect, of a single death from plague which had occurred towards the end of December, 1664, in a house in or near Long Acre. Connected with that case was one of those trivial chains of evidence which are so often produced as the easy solution of a difficult problem. A bale of silks had come to the house from Holland, and that bale of silks could be traced to the Levant; therefore the seeds of the great plague of London were imported Levantine seeds. This was pretty well for a city which had a continuous record of plague-infection in its soil ever since the Black Death of 1348. But credulity could ignore facts more recent than the history for three centuries. The death in Long Acre in December was a solitary one, and

---

[1] Among the crop of books brought up by the Plague of Marseilles, in 1720 (the immediate cause of Defoe's book also) was one by Richard Bradley, F.R.S., a writer upon botany, on *The Plague of Marseilles. Also Observations taken from an original Manuscript of a graduate physician, who resided in London during the whole time of the late plague, anno* 1665. London 1721 (and two more editions the same year). The title-page of this astute gentleman is of the catch-penny order. All that is said of the original manuscript occupies about the same number of lines in the text as in the title, and might have been extracted in the course of five minutes' research; it consists merely of a list of a few things supposed to be distinctive signs of plague— extraordinary inward heat, difficulty of breathing, pain and heaviness in the head, inclination to sleep, frequent vomiting, immoderate thirst, dryness of the tongue and palate, and then the risings, swellings, or buboes. Boghurst's third chapter is occupied with twenty-one such signs, and his fourth chapter with a hundred more signs and circumstances, in numbered paragraphs. It is possible that his was the manuscript out of which the botanist made capital in his title-page; but his meagre list of signs might have been got from almost any work on almost any febrile disorder, and is not sufficient to identify Boghurst by, although a word or phrase here and there is the same. However, Defoe would have seen Bradley's title-page, and might have inquired after the Sloane MS.

was of no more import for what followed than any of the five other sporadic plague-deaths in 1664[1]. Only one more death from plague occurred in the bills (in the middle of February), until the last week of April, 1665 ; even then the progress of the infection was slower for the next two months than it had been in many former seasons of moderate plague, such as the five years 1606—1610 and the eight years 1640—1647, or than it had been in the great plague-years of 1603, 1625 and 1636. An importation from abroad had been alleged as early as the great plague of 1563, namely from Havre, which was then held by an English garrison. But on that occasion the epidemic in London was gaining ground before the sickness at Havre had declared itself plague, and was of the bubonic type while the latter was still a malignant fever. The return of the whole English garrison from Havre, with the seeds of sickness among them, might well have introduced infection ; but that return was not until the end of July, by which time the mortality in London had been progressing for two months. There is equally little reason for Stow's statement that the plague of 1603 was brought to London from Ostend, or for the corresponding theory of origin for the plague of 1625. A foreign source was not thought of unless the plague became one of the greater degree. Year after year in London there were a few cases of plague, and sometimes for a succession of years the plague-deaths kept steadily at a level of from one thousand to three thousand. There are, indeed, few years from 1348 to 1666 in which the infection did not declare its presence in London. Whether the few threatening cases in the spring were to rise to a plague of the greater degree depended upon a concurrence of circumstances—upon the interval since the last great plague, upon the number of strangers crowding to the capital, and upon the kind of weather preceding. In 1665 the various determining things did chance to come together, and a plague of the first degree ensued. The one singular thing in the history is that such a concurrence never happened again, or that the conditions had so far cllanged (certainly not for the

---

[1] Of the six plague-deaths in 1664, three were in Whitechapel parish, and one each in Aldgate, Cripplegate and St Giles's-in-the-Fields.

better), that the type of epidemic disease was no longer the bubo-plague.

According to precedent, a great plague was somewhat overdue in the year 1665. Its two great predecessors (not reckoning the smaller plague of 1636) had happened each at the beginning of a new reign—in 1603 on the accession of James I., and in 1625 on the accession of Charles I. The Restoration of 1660 was the time for the next great outburst; but that was delayed for five years. Those five years were occupied with a good deal of fever and other infective disease in London, and the fever in the beginning of 1665 was, according to Sydenham, of a marked pestilential type. It may be said to have led up to the plague ; but the bubonic disease itself needed something in addition to the determining causes of spotted fever. It is generally admitted that London was unusually crowded with the poorer classes whose work is required by the luxury of the rich (Defoe says that an enumeration for the Lord Mayor had made out 100,000 ribbon-weavers in the eastern suburbs, although the number is incredible). There was also a general relaxation of morals, which may have predisposed many constitutions to receive the seeds of infection. Another element in the case was the weather.

The summer before had been remarkable for the immense number of house-flies, and of other insects and frogs. From November to the end of March the earth was held in almost continual black frost. Boghurst says the wind was westerly for seven months. No rain fell all the time except a slight sprinkling in the end of April. The dry cold continued after the frost broke, and produced, says Sydenham, an unusual number of cases of pleurisy, pneumonia and angina. Richard Baxter says of the seasons preceding the great plague, that they were " the driest winter, spring and summer that ever man alive knew, or our forefathers ever heard of; so that the grounds were burnt like the highways, the meadow ground where I lived [Acton] having but four loads of hay which before bare forty[1]." The hay crop was "pitiful," says Boghurst, in consequence of the long cold and drought. But the summer was made pleasant

---

[1] *Reliquiae Baxterianae.* London, 1696, I. 448. This entry in his journal is dated September 28, 1665, at Hampden, Bucks.

by refreshing breezes, and there was abundance of all kinds of grain, vegetables and fruit.

It was not until the beginning of June that the deaths from plague in all London, according to the bills of mortality, reached the sum of 43 in the week. But the mortality had been excessive from the beginning of the year, and it was suspected, as in the like circumstances in 1625, that the searchers had been concealing the existence of plague, or calling cases of it by other names, so as to save the infected houses from being shut up. The motive for bribery and concealment doubtless existed; it had been kept in view by the authorities from the first institution of searchers, who were solemnly sworn before the Dean of the Arches to make a true return of the cause of death. In all the great plagues, less so in 1563 and 1603 than in other years, there was reason to suppose that a large proportion of deaths put down to other causes than plague were really cases of plague. However there is no doubt that, in the early months of 1665, just as in the beginning of 1625, there was a great deal of spotted fever in London, not to mention smallpox and dysentery. The season was a sickly one, such a sickly season as often occurred in the latter part of the seventeenth century and throughout the whole of the eighteenth, when there could be no longer any question of plague. The weekly bills contain numerous deaths in the several parishes from "fever" and from "spotted fever" for months before they contain more than an occasional plague-death. There was no reason why these and other maladies should not have swelled the bills to three or four hundred in a week; in the year 1739, when London was probably not a third larger than in 1665, Strother says that fever brought the weekly bill up to near a thousand. It is remarkable, however, that Boghurst claims to have been treating cases of plague from the month of November, 1664; Hodges also says that he was called in the middle of the Christmas holidays to a young man in a fever who acquired, two days after, a plague-botch in each groin as large as a nutmeg, and recovered. Boghurst admits that "tokens," by which he means the marks of plague other than the botch or bubo, "appeared not much till about the middle of June, and carbuncles not till the latter end of July." He suspects that the

bills of mortality did not tell the whole truth ; and, as an instance
of evasion, he says that there had been plague in St Giles's, St
Martin's, St Clement's, and St Paul's, Covent Garden, for three
or four years before (the bills of mortality give only 12, 9, and 5
deaths respectively for all London in the years 1662, 1663 and
1664), "as I have been certainly informed by the people themselves that had it in their houses in those parishes."

But, in claiming an earlier beginning for the plague than
the bills recognize, and in setting aside the diagnosis of fever
as insufficient, Boghurst takes what is known, in the controversies
upon the nature and affinities of plague, as the "ontological"
view : that is to say, he sees in plague a fixed and uniform
entity, and he sees the same in fever. The other view is the
developmental, which recognizes transitions from the one type
of pestilential disease into the other. The great writers of the
time, Willis, Sydenham, and Morton, were none of them "onto-
logists." They all taught the scale of malignity, which had
simple continued fever at one end, then a severer fever with
spots and "parotids," then a fever with buboes, and at the
farthest end of the scale the true plague, with its buboes,
carbuncles, and tokens. Nor is it denied by competent observers, such as Boghurst himself, that an epidemic of plague
declined as a whole in malignity towards the end, so that
the buboes suppurated, and three out of four, or three out of
five, patients recovered. If that were the case in the descent
of the curve, why should there not have been something corresponding in the ascent ? If certain cases of the prevailing
fever in the beginning of the year developed buboes which
suppurated (as in the case treated by Hodges at Christmas,
1664), should they be called plague or fever ? Willis would
have answered in favour of fever, until such time, at least, as
the "epidemic constitution" of the season changed definitely
to plague[1] ; he does in effect answer so in the particular

---

[1] *Ed. cit.* Chap. XIV. p. 131 :—"Diseases which seem to be nearest like its
(plague's) nature ; which chiefly are fevers, called pestilent and malignant ; for 'tis
commonly noted that fevers sometimes reign popularly, which for the vehemency of
symptoms, the great slaughter of the sick, and the great force of contagion, scarce
give place to the pestilence ; which, however, because they imitate the type of

instance of the Oxford fever of 1643, which in some cases was bubonic, whereas, in 1645, he makes no doubt that the disease prevailing in Oxford and Wallingford was true plague.

The more general discussion of this theme will be found in the concluding section of the chapter on the Black Death, where illustrations are given of typhus fever turning to bubonic fever and to plague, from recent and anomalous outbreaks of plague in Arab villages or encampments, in some Indian villages, and elsewhere. The conclusion there come to was that the type of plague, or the bubonic type, prevailed when the infection of the filthy habitations began with change of season to rise from the soil, whereas the form of sickness was typhus fever so long as the infection was primarily in the atmosphere of the dwellings.

We may admit, then, that there was some ambiguity in the naming and classifying of pestilential cases in the early months of 1665. If we follow the bills—and there is nothing else to follow—the plague-deaths in all the parishes of London for the seven weeks from April 18 to June 6 were respectively no more than 2, 0, 9, 3, 14, 17 and 43, the deaths from "fever" and "spotted fever" being much more numerous.

Having thus far determined the date of beginning, we come next to the line of advance of the plague of 1665. It was from the western and northern suburbs towards the City, the eastern suburbs, and Southwark. Boghurst, who practised in St Giles's-in-the-Fields, says:

"The plague fell first upon the highest ground, for our parish is the highest ground about London, and the best air, and was first infected. Highgate, Hampstead and Acton also all shared in it." From the west end of the town, Boghurst continues, "it gradually insinuated and crept down Holborn and the Strand, and then into the City, and at last to the east end of the suburbs, so that it was half a year at the west end of the city [in his experience] before the east end and Stepney was infected, which was about the middle of July. Southwark, being the south suburb, was infected almost as soon as the west end." But the same writer farther explains that "it fell upon several places of the city and suburbs like rain—at the first at St Giles',

putrid fevers, and do not so certainly kill the sick as the plague, or so certainly infect others, they deserve the name, not of the plague, but by a more minute appellation of a pestilential fever."

St Martin's, Chancery-lane, Southwark, Houndsditch, and some places within the City, as at Proctor's-houses."

The slow progress from west to east has been made much of by Defoe, who used the bills of mortality to ascertain the rise of the infection in the several districts. His conclusion is the same in the main as Boghurst's contemporary observation ; only that he makes the infection of Southwark later, and with reason so far as the bills show :—

"It was now mid-July, and the plague which had chiefly raged at the other end of the town, and as I said before, in the parishes of St Giles's, St Andrew's, Holbourn, and towards Westminster, began now to come eastward towards the part where I lived. It was to be observed, indeed, that it did not come straight on toward us ; for the City, that is to say within the walls, was indifferent healthy still; nor was it got then very much over the water into Southwark; for though there died that week 1268 of all distempers, whereof it might be supposed above 900 died of the plague [only 725 in the bill], yet there was but 28 in the whole City within the walls, and but 19 in Southwark, Lambeth included ; whereas in the parishes of St Giles' and St Martin's in the Fields alone, there died 421...We perceived, I say, the distemper to draw our way ; viz. by the parishes of Clerkenwell, Cripplegate, Shoreditch, and Bishopsgate ; which last two parishes joining to Aldgate, Whitechapel and Stepney, the infection came at length to spread its utmost rage and violence in those parts, even when it abated at the western parishes where it began. It was very strange to observe that in this particular week, from the 4th to the 13th July, when, as I have observed, there died near 400 of the plague in the two parishes of St Martin's and St Giles' in the Fields only, there died in the parish of Aldgate but four, in the parish of Whitechapel three, and in the parish of Stepney but one." In the following week of July, with a total of 1761 deaths, whereof of the plague 1089, only 16 occurred on the Southwark side. Soon, however, Cripplegate had the infection at its hottest, and at the same time Clerkenwell, St Sepulchre's parish, St Bride's and Aldersgate. "While it was in all these parishes, the City and the parishes of the Southwark side of the water, and all Stepney, Whitechapel, Aldgate, Wapping and Ratcliff were very little touched ; so that people went about their business unconcerned, carried on their trades, kept open their shops, and conversed freely with one another in all the City, the east and north-east suburbs, and in Southwark, almost as if the plague had not been among us."

In another passage Defoe brings out the moral of its gradual advance. He had shown

"how it began at one end of the town, and proceeded gradually and slowly from one part to another; and like a dark cloud that passes over our

C. 42

heads, which as it thickens and overcasts the air at one end, clears up at
the other end: so while the plague went on raging from west to east, as it
went forwards east it abated in the west, by which means those parts of the
town which were not seized, or who were left, and where it had spent its
fury were, as it were, spared to help and assist the other ; whereas had the
distemper spread itself all over the City and suburbs at once, raging in all
places alike, as it has done since in some places abroad, the whole body
of the people must have been overwhelmed" etc.

That is how Defoe constructs a concrete picture from the dry
statistics of the weekly bills. He has defined the stages, and
pointed the moral, with a firmer hand than the reality would
most likely have warranted. But no scientific writer could have
apprehended more correctly the general fact of a gradual
invasion from the west end of the town.

These striking facts of the gradual advance of the Great
Plague of London from west to east will be found to suit that
theory of the plague-virus which has been illustrated in various
parts of this volume. The virus of plague is a soil-poison, or the
ground is its habitat; its quiescence or activity depends upon
whether or not the state of the soil favours the fermentation
of the special organic matters therein, which special organic
matters we here take to be the products of cadaveric decomposition. The conclusion that the poison of plague lay in the
soil, and that it rose into the air in emanations or effluvia,
was forced upon all those who thought much about the matter
from the medieval period onwards. Thus, the apothecary
Boghurst, says in his first chapter : " And therefore my opinion
falls in wholly with those who make the earth the seminary
and seed-plot of these venomous vapours and pestiferous
effluvia, which vitiate and corrupt the air, and consequently
induce the pestilence." And again: "The plague is a most
subtle, insinuating, venomous, deleterious exhalation, arising
from the maturation of the ferment of the forces (?) of the earth,
extracted into the air by the heat of the sun." It is true that
Boghurst, like the sixteenth-century writers abroad, such as
Ambroise Parè, locates the venom in mysterious cavities and
bowels of the earth, and dwells upon the agency of earthquakes
in setting it free. But he comes to more ordinary causes in
his enumeration of favouring things—" dunghills, excrements,

dead bodies lying unburied, putrefying churchyards too full," and again "breaking up tombs and graves where dead bodies have been long buried." As telling against the last, however, he adds : "When the charnel-house at St Paul's was demolished, there was a thousand cart-loads of dead men's bones carried away to Finsbury, yet no plague followed it."

The activity of this soil-poison depends upon processes in the soil which go on so slowly that the link of cause and effect is easily overlooked. In the last resort, they are dependent on the rise and fall of the ground-water. It was observed beyond all doubt as the law in Lower Egypt, that the plague came forth annually after the Nile had begun to fall, and that it reached its height in the months of March, April and May, when the soil was driest, or the pores of the ground occupied solely by air after having been full of water. It was observed, also, that the plague-area and the inundation-area were co-extensive. Lower Egypt is, of course, somewhat peculiar (Lower Bengal coming near to it) in these regular alternations of air alone and water alone in the pores of the ground. But other countries have the same sharp contrast occasionally, and London had the contrast very decidedly in the years 1664 and 1665. The months from November 1664 to June 1665, some of which ought to have brought snow or rain to raise the wells and springs to their highest periodic water-mark early in the year, were quite remarkable for drought: Richard Baxter says that no one remembered the like. The ground-water, instead of rising all through the winter, must have fallen lower and lower as the spring and summer advanced. The pores of the ground had been occupied with air to an unusual depth of the subsoil, and the presence of air in these circumstances had given occasion to that ferment-activity in the special organic matters of an old-inhabited soil which produced the virus of plague. The stratum of subsoil would become dry first in the more elevated parts; and as the ground-water continued to fall, the air would reach in due course an unwonted stratum in the lower situations. Defoe says that they came to water at eighteen feet in digging the Whitechapel plague-pits. The same seasonal march of a soil-infection from the higher ground to the lower has been observed in modern times in other cities, and in other diseases than plague. The drought for seven months from November to June would not, of itself, have caused a great plague. But it was an essential member of the co-operating group of things; and it probably determined of itself the season when the great plague was once more to come and take away the enormous increase of poor people.

Mortality and Incidents of the Great Plague.

The plague of 1665 was justly called the Great Plague, and is sometimes spoken of as "the plague of London," as if it were unique. But it was not much more severe than those of 1603 and 1625 had been for the London of their generation; and there had been many plagues when London was a small capital, such as those of 1407, 1479, 1500, 1513 and 1563, which had cut off as large a proportion (one-fifth to one-sixth) of the population. The inhabitants in 1665 were not far short of half a million, nearly twice as many as in 1603, and about a third more than in 1625. The increased mortality in 1665 was somewhat more than proportionate to the increase of inhabitants, as the following table shows :—

Year	Estimated population	Total deaths	Plague deaths	Highest mortality in a week	Worst week
1603	250,000	42,940	33,347	3385	25 Aug.—1 Sept.
1625	320,000	63,001	41,313	5205	11—18 Aug.
1665	460,000	97,306	68,596	8297	12—19 Sept.

Reckoned from the christenings and burials in the bills of Parish Clerks' Hall, the population in 1605 would have been 224,275, and in 1622, 272,207. But in those years (and until after 1636) certain of the newer parishes (known as the Seven Parishes), including Stepney and Westminster, kept separate bills, of which some figures for 1603 and 1625 are given at p. 477 and p. 511. The population of the Seven Parishes appears to have been about one-ninth of the whole metropolis in 1603, and about one-seventh in 1625, while Graunt, a contemporary, makes it one-fifth in 1662. These fractions have been added in the table, so as to make 1603 and 1625 comparable with 1665. In 1603 and 1625, the highest mortality in a week does not show the deaths in those parishes (Westminster, Stepney &c.) which did not send their returns to the general bill until 1636, but their figures have been included in the totals for those years. It will be seen that the plague of 1665 fully kept pace with the increase of population. The old City within the walls had 15,207 deaths in the year from all causes. It had become crowded since the beginning of Elizabeth's reign by its gardens and church-yards being built upon, and its mansions turned into tenement-houses for a poorer class; and yet in 1563 the mortality from plague and other causes in the City and its Liberties, with a population hardly exceeding that of the City alone in 1665, was 20,372. The enormous total of 1665 was largely made up from the populous suburbs of Cripplegate, Whitechapel, Stepney, St Martin's in the Fields, St Giles's in the Fields, Southwark and Westminster, which would have contributed but little to the total down to the middle third of the sixteenth century.

The following tables will show the progress of the epidemic from week to week, the weekly deaths from all causes and from plague, and the incidence upon the several parts of London. The so-called ordinary deaths are much in excess of the average, and must have included many that were really cases of plague. Part of the excess, however, was due to the great prevalence of fever and spotted fever, which made a heavy mortality in the early months before the plague began. Bowel complaint also is credited with a good many deaths. The other more important items in the bills are consumption and infantile troubles. Boghurst, however, says : "Almost all other diseases turned into the plague. For five or six months together there was hardly any other disease seen but the plague and a few casualties, whatever the Bills say; and Thucydides says the same of the plague at Athens." As to the total of deaths in the year from all causes (97,306), Hodges thinks that it does not show the whole mortality. The largest number of burials in one week is 8297; but he thinks that 12,000 were buried in that week, and that 4000 were buried in one day and night. But there seems to be no reason to set aside the tally of the sextons to that extent; the returns were made weekly from one hundred and forty parishes, and might easily have been exact to within a few in each.

Bill of Mortality of the Plague-year 1665 *in London.*

Week ending	Christened	Buried	Plague	Week ending	Christened	Buried	Plague
Dec. 27	229	291	1	June 27	199	684	267
Jan. 3	239	349	0	July 4	207	1006	470
10	235	394	0	11	197	1268	725
17	223	415	0	18	194	1761	1089
24	237	474	0	25	193	2785	1843
31	216	409	0	Aug. 1	215	3014	2010
Feb. 7	221	393	0	8	178	4030	2817
14	224	462	1	15	166	5319	3880
21	232	393	0	22	171	5568	4237
28	233	396	0	29	169	7496	6102
Mar. 7	236	441	0	Sept. 5	167	8252	6988
14	236	433	0	12	168	7690	6544
21	221	363	0	19	176	8297	7165
28	238	353	0	26	146	6460	5533
Apr. 4	242	344	0	Oct. 3	142	5720	4929
11	245	382	0	10	141	5068	4327
18	287	344	0	17	147	3219	2665
25	229	398	2	24	104	1806	1421
May 2	237	388	0	31	104	1388	1031
9	211	347	9	Nov. 7	95	1787	1414
16	227	353	3	14	113	1359	1050
23	231	385	14	21	108	905	652
30	229	400	17	28	112	544	333
June 6	234	405	43	Dec. 5	123	428	210
13	206	558	112	12	133	442	243
20	204	615	168	19	147	525	281
					9,967	97,306	68,596

Incidence on Parishes of the Plague in 1665.

Ninety-seven Parishes within the Walls.

	All deaths	Plague deaths
97 City parishes	15,207	9,877

(The parishes with heaviest mortalities were St Anne's, Blackfriars ; Christ Church, Newgate; St Stephen's, Coleman St; St Martin's, Vintry; Allhallows Barking, the Great, and in-the-Wall ; St Andrew's, Wardrobe).

Sixteen Parishes without the Walls and in the Liberties.

St Giles's, Cripplegate	8069	4838	St George's, Southwark	1613	1260
St Botolph's, Aldgate	4926	4051	St Botolph's, Aldersgate	997	755
St Olave's, Southwark	4793	2785	St Dunstan's in the West	958	665
St Sepulchre's	4509	2746	St Bartholomew the Great	493	344
St Saviour's, Southwark	4235	3446	St Thomas's, Southwark	475	371
St Andrew's, Holborn	3958	3103	Bridewell Precinct	230	179
St Botolph's, Bishopsgate	3464	2500	St Bartholomew the Less	193	139
St Bride's, Fleet Street	2111	1427	Trinity, Minories	168	123
			Pesthouse	159	

Twelve Out-parishes in Middlesex and Surrey.

Stepney	8598	6583	St Mary's, Newington	1272	1004
Whitechapel	4766	3855	St Katharine's, Tower	956	601
St Giles's in the Fields	4457	3216	Lambeth	798	537
St Leonard's, Shoreditch	2669	949	Islington	696	593
St Magdalen's, Bermond-			Rotherhithe	304	210
sey	1943	1362	Hackney	232	132
St James's, Clerkenwell	1863	1377			

Five Parishes in the City and Liberties of Westminster.

St Martin's in the Fields	4804	2883	St Paul's, Covent Garden	408	281
St Margaret's	4710	3742	St Mary's, Savoy	303	198
St Clement's Danes	1969	1319			
		Pesthouse	156		

The Great Plague brought back all the familiar incidents of 1603 and 1625, and revealed no new feature. As before, all that could afford to do so made their escape at the outset. Sydenham, who fled with the rest, says that two-thirds of the population left; which may be true of the City proper, but certainly not of the populous Liberties and suburbs on both sides of the water, as Defoe points out. The poorer classes were left stranded, and bore the brunt of the calamity, as they had always done. Flight was, doubtless, the best step to take, the motive being to get "into clean air," as cardinal Wolsey expressed it in 1515. Those that were left behind knew that they were in bad air, and knew that it mattered little whether they came into contact with the sick or not[1]. Their employments and wages mostly ceased as the plague extended from suburb to suburb and to the City, so that with starvation on the one side and plague on the other, they held their lives cheaply and bore themselves with an unconcern which was strange to the rich. Their desperate case explains, as Defoe correctly saw, the ease with which the mayor could always get men to undertake for pay the disagreeable and risky work of day and night watchmen to the multitude of shut-up houses, of bearers of the dead, of buriers, of nurses, and distributors of the public charity. As soon as any fell in these humble ranks, others were willing to take their place; so that at no period of the

[1] In a letter from London, 9 May, 1637 (Gawdy MSS. at Norwich, *Hist. MSS. Commis.* X. pt. 2. p. 163) it is said: "There is a strange opinion here amongst the poorer sort of people, who hold it a matter of conscience to visit their neighbours in any sickness, yea though they know it to be the infection."

epidemic was there any break-down in the work of expeditious burial or any failure in good order and decency. To carry the poor through the great crisis much money was needed ; Defoe says that it was forthcoming from all parts of England and he estimates the distribution of relief at thousands of pounds weekly, although he failed to find the exact accounts, which, he thinks, had been destroyed in the fire of 1666. A thousand pounds a week, he says, was given from the king's purse. The whole of this great system of relief was under the direction of the Lord Mayor, Sir John Lawrence, who proved himself worthy of the best traditions of his office. In the out-parishes there were Justices of the Peace who discharged the like duties.

The regular clergy for the most part left the town, but two are honourably mentioned as having stayed with the plague-stricken people, Dr Anthony Walker, of St Mary Aldermanbury, and Mr Meriton[1].

Sometime in August Lord Arlington wrote to the bishop of London that the king was informed of many ministers and lecturers being absent from their posts during this time of contagion, and that nonconformists had thrust themselves into their pulpits to preach seditions and doctrines contrary to the Church. His majesty wishes the bishop to prevent such mischiefs to Church and State[2]. The bishop replied, from Fulham, 19 August, that the sober clergy remain, that he had refused some that offered to supply vacancies, suspecting them to be of the factious party, though they promised to conform, that most of his officers had deserted him and gone into the country, but he could not learn that any nonconformists had invaded the pulpit[3]. The bishop, however, was not likely to hear much within his garden walls at Fulham of what was passing at Aldgate. There can be no question that Church pulpits were occupied during the plague by ministers who had been ejected in 1662. Chief among them was Thomas Vincent, formerly minister of St Magdalen's, Milk Street, who preached in St Botolph's, Aldgate, Great St Helen's, and Allhallows Staining[4]. Vincent says that it was the opportunity of irregular practitioners both in the Church and in medicine,

---

[1] Evans, in preface to 1721 edition of Vincent's book.
[2] *Cal. State Papers.*   [3] *Ibid.*   [4] Evans, *l. c.*

and he is disposed to say a good word for the latter from a fellow feeling with them. Besides Vincent, says Richard Baxter[1], there were " some strangers that came thither since they were silenced, as Mr Chester, Mr Janeway, Mr Turner, Mr Grimes, Mr Franklin, and some others." These all became prominent in London Nonconformity ; and Baxter clearly traces their subsequent power to the opportunity that the plague gave them :

> " But one great benefit the plague brought to the city, that is, it occasioned the silenced ministers more openly and laboriously to preach the Gospel to the exceeding comfort and profit of the people; in so much that to this day [1670] the freedom of preaching which this occasioned, cannot, by the daily guards of soldiers, nor by the imprisonments of multitudes be restrained. The ministers that were silenced for Nonconformity had ever since 1662 done their work privately."

Baxter knew of none among the Nonconformist ministers remaining in London who fell victims to the plague, except " Mr Grunman, a German, a very humble, holy, able minister, but being a silenced Nonconformist, was so poor that he was not able to remove his family." Two others of the sect, who fled, lost their lives—" Mr Cross, flying from the plague into the country died with his wife and some children as soon as he came thither, in the house of that learned worthy man, Mr Shaw, another silenced minister," and Mr Roberts, " a godly Welsh minister, who also flying from the plague, fell sick as far off as between Shrewsbury and Oswestry and died in a little straw, but none durst entertain him." Baxter himself found refuge in the house of the Hampdens, in Bucks[2], leaving his family, as he says,

---

[1] *Reliquiae Baxterianae.* London, 1696, II. 1. 2.

[2] Milton, with his wife and daughters, spent the summer and autumn in the same quiet neighbourhood, at Chalfont St Giles, in a cottage which Ellwood had secured for him, still remaining with its low ceilings and diamond window-panes. He there showed Ellwood the manuscript of *Paradise Lost*, which was published in 1667. The poem contains no reference to the plague, unless, indeed, the flight to the country had given point to the lines in the 9th book :

> " As one who long in populous city pent,
> Where houses thick and sewers annoy the air,
> Forth issuing on a summer's morn, to breathe
> Among the pleasant villages and farms,"—

An opportunity arises in the 12th book, where the Plagues of Egypt come into the

in the midst of plague at Acton.   Defoe draws from the incident
of the Nonconformists in Church pulpits a somewhat sentimental
moral; he sees nothing aggressive in it, but merely the levelling
of differences by affliction, and a short-lived prospect of recon-
ciliation.

The irregular practitioners of physic would appear to have
been in great force, just as in former plagues, when their bills
were on every post.   Defoe professes to give specimens of their
advertisements, which he might have adapted from actual advertisements in the news-sheets, the ' Intelligencer' and the ' Newes.'
The empirics were of both sexes, and of foreign extraction as
well as native.

Among the regular physicians who practised for a time, at
least, in the plague were the famous Professor Glisson, Dr Nathan
Paget (an intimate friend of Milton and cousin of Elizabeth
Minshull whom the poet, in 1664, had married for his third wife),
Dr Wharton, of St Thomas's Hospital, a distinguished anatomist,
Dr Berwick or Barwick, Dr Brooke, Dr Hodges, and Dr
Conyers.   The last was one of two of his order who died of
the plague.   Two Paracelsist or chemical physicians, Dr Dey
and Dr Starkey, died of it: and Dr George Thomson says that
he survived three several attacks of the buboes, the first sore
lasting for four months.   A considerable number of chirurgeons
and apothecaries are said (by Defoe) to have fallen victims.
Pepys says that at the first meeting of Gresham College (the

prophetic vision of events after the Fall ; but the movement is too rapid to allow of
delay, and we have no more than—

> " Botches and blains must all his flesh emboss,
>   And all his people."

Gibbon thought that the comet of 1664 (which was generally remarked upon as
a portent of the plague that followed) might have suggested the lines, II. 708—11

> " and like a comet burn'd,
>   That fires the length of Ophiuchus huge
>   In the arctic sky, and from his horrid hair
>   Shakes pestilence and war."

Gibbon seems to make a slip in taking these as "the famous lines which startled
the licenser;" those are usually taken to have been I. 598–9, the figure of the sun's
eclipse, which

> "with fear of change
>   Perplexes monarchs."

Royal Society) since the plague, held on January 22, 1666, Dr Goddard "did fill us with talk in defence of his and his fellow physicians' going out of town in the plague-time," his plea being that their particular patients were out of town, and they left at liberty. But that excuse ignores the fact that the time was a great emergency, and puts the defence upon the wrong ground.

Goddard had attended Cromwell in the Irish and Scottish campaigns as physician to the army. For a short time he had been a member of the Council of State, and for several years was master of a College at Oxford. He was Gresham professor of physic, and one of the original council of the Royal Society. This eminent man of science was the inventor and proprietor of " Goddard's drop," the secret of which he sold to Charles II. for a large sum, said to have been £6000. Dr Martin Lister says that the king showed him the receipt, and that the drops were nothing more than the volatile spirit of raw silk rectified with oil of cinnamon, and no better than ordinary spirit of hartshorn. Another writer says that the drops contained also skull of a person hanged and dried viper. According to Sydenham, Goddard's drops were preferable to other volatile spirits for the particular purpose, namely, the recovery of people from faintings of various kinds. Even if Dr Goddard had remained in town, he would have been a trafficker in nostrums as much as the empirics; nor is it probable, from all that we know, that he could have brought epidemiological principles to bear upon the management of the epidemic among the poor. The best teaching of the time counselled that which he himself practised, namely, flight.

Defoe says that the Lord Mayor (Sir John Lawrence), the Sheriffs (Sir George Waterman and Sir Charles Doe), the Court of Aldermen and certain of the Common Council, or their deputies, came to a resolution and published it, viz. :

"That they would not quit the City themselves, but that they would be always at hand for the preserving of good order in every place, and for the doing justice on all occasions ; as also for the distributing the public charity to the poor ; and, in a word, for the doing the duty and discharging the trust reposed in them by the citizens to the utmost of their power."

The minutes are extant of numerous meetings of the Mayor

and Council, with the orders made (on May 11, June 17, 19, and 27, July 12, and at short intervals thereafter)[1]. Two of the Aldermen died of plague.

It appears to be admitted by all, that good order was kept, the dead buried expeditiously, day and night watchmen provided for an immense number of infected houses (until, as Vincent says, the infected houses became so many that there was no use shutting them up), bearers of the dead and grave-diggers engaged to fill the places of those who died, and applications heard for relief. One of the things that justly excited the admiration of Defoe was the abundant supply of all the markets, and the almost unvarying weight of the penny wheaten loaf, which is given every week at the foot of the bill of mortality. The Parish Clerks brought out their bill regularly, although Hodges says that the sextons failed at length to keep an accurate account of the number of corpses. All the dead were buried at first in coffins and with full ceremony; but when the infection became hottest in August and September, especially in the crowded East-end and in Southwark, the bodies are said to have been brought to the pits in cartloads and thrown in, sometimes without even a covering[2]. That is alleged by the writers on the plagues of 1603 and 1625, and the same must have happened to some extent in 1665, but whether to the extent that Defoe's graphic account implies may be doubted.

The burials took place over night until, as Vincent says, "now the nights are too short to bury the dead." This was a reversal of the order, first issued in 1547 and probably carried out in the plague of 1603, that no burial was to take place between six in the evening and six in the morning. Even at

---

[1] *Brit. Mus. Addit. MS.* 4376 (8). "Abstract of several orders relating to the Plague," from 35 Hen. VIII. to 1665.

[2] In excavating the foundations of the Broad Street terminus of the North London Railway, the workmen came upon a stratum four feet below the surface and descending eight or ten feet lower, which was full of uncoffined skeletons. Some hundreds of them were collected and re-interred. (*Notes and Queries,* 3rd Ser. IV. 85.) The ground was part of the old enclosure of Bethlem Hospital (St Mary's Spital outside Bishopsgate), and was acquired for a cemetery, to the extent of an acre, by Sir Thomas Roe, in 1569. Probably there were plague-pits dug in it during more than one of the great epidemics, from 1593 to 1665.

the worst time, coffins would seem to have been got for most. Vincent says, "Now we could hardly go forth but we should meet many coffins," and he mentions one woman whom he met with a little coffin under her arm. Evelyn enters in his diary on September 7, the worst week of the epidemic : "I went all along the City and suburbs from Kent Street to St James's, a dismal passage and dangerous, to see so many coffins exposed in the streets now thin of people." Defoe's weird description of the Aldgate plague-pit at midnight, with seven or eight lanterns set on the heaps of earth round the edge, and of the constant journeys to and fro of the dead-carts, has probably made the most of the realities of the case.

A letter of Pepys to Lady Carteret, written from Woolwich on September 4, gives us a glimpse of the state of the City :

"I having stayed in the city till about 7400 died in one week, and of them above 6000 of the plague, and little noise heard day nor night but tolling of bells ; till I could walk Lumber-Street and not meet twenty persons from one end to the other, and not fifty upon the Exchange; till whole families, 10 and 12 together, have been swept away ; till my very physician, Dr Burnet, who undertook to secure me against any infection, having survived the month of his own being shut up, died himself of the plague ; till the nights, though much lengthened, are grown too short to conceal the burials of those that died the day before, people being thereby constrained to borrow daylight for that service." The butcheries are everywhere visited, his brewer is shut up, and his baker dead with his whole family.

On September 20, he writes in his diary :

"But Lord ! what a sad time it is to all : no boats upon the river, and grass grows all up and down Whitehall Court, and nobody but poor wretches in the streets."

Some three weeks later (October 11) Evelyn writes in his diary : "Went through the whole city, having occasion to alight out of the coach in several places about business of money, when I was environed with multitudes of poor pestiferous creatures begging alms. The shops universally shut up." Vincent says that he would meet "many with sores and limping in the streets," (from the suppurating buboes in the groins). Again :

"It would be endless to speak what we have seen and heard of :—some in their frenzy rising out of their beds and leaping about their rooms ; others crying and roaring at their windows ; some coming forth almost naked into the streets"

—the delirium being sometimes of the gentle or foolish kind, and sometimes violent. These incidents are much enlarged upon by Defoe, who makes out the cries and groans (mentioned by Dekker and others for the earlier plagues) to have been from the pain of the hard and tense buboes. Boghurst says that the treatment by actual cautery and other escharotics caused more pain than the buboes.

As a set-off to the more horrible picture given by Defoe of the inmates of a house all dying together, their bodies being found by the watchmen and taken away in the dead-cart, we may turn to Vincent's plain account of what happened in the house where he lodged, probably in the neighbourhood of Aldgate or Bishopsgate, when he came up from Islington to minister to the sick.

" We were eight in the family—three men, three youths, an old woman and a maid ; all which came to me, hearing of my stay in town, some to accompany me, others to help me [he was a celebrity in the religious world with a large following]. It was the latter end of September before any of us were touched...But at last we were visited...At first our maid was smitten ; it began with a shivering and trembling in her flesh, and quickly seized on her spirits...I came home and the maid was on her death-bed ; and another crying out for help, being left alone in a sweating fainting-fit. It was on Monday when the maid was smitten ; on Thursday she died full of tokens. On Friday one of the youths had a swelling in his groin, and on the Lord's day died with the marks of the distemper upon him. On the same day another youth did sicken, and on the Wednesday following he died. On the Thursday night his master fell sick of the disease, and within a day or two was full of spots, but strangely recovered...The rest were preserved."

The two boys appear to have been conscious to the end, and to have died in the placid mood that often came on in the last hours of plague, as in other prostrating infections such as yellow fever and cholera. In those two weeks at the end of September and beginning of October the burials in all London were 6460 (of plague 5533) and 5720 (of plague 4929).

The chief preventive measure which the mayor had to give effect to was the shutting-up of infected houses. Defoe says that he carried out that odious policy considerately. The policy was a traditional one, and may or may not have had its origin in medical prescription. It was practised, as we have seen in a former chapter, early in the reign of Henry VIII., if not even before that. The doctrine underlying it was the contagiousness of plague, which was much more a doctrine of the faculty than of the people, and was most of all a doctrine of the Court. Originally the dogma of contagiousness, in all its rigour, had been made for the persons of the Tudor monarchs, and as late as 1665 it was in the atmosphere of the Court that the contagion of plague was invested with the most powerful properties. The common people of London gave no heed to it, because they saw every hour that it was a matter of indifference; the middle classes held it in a qualified way, knowing that there was less to fear from plague-bodies than from plague-infected ground ; but kings took the comprehensive view of it, allowing no exceptions or scientific reservations, and the Court doctors, such as Mead in the 18th century, at length succeeded in making the high doctrine of plague-contagion to pass current. Two instances are known from extant petitions, of its rigorous application upon Court servants in 1665: one in the case of a trumpeter of the king, and the other in the case of the barber to the household. In the latter case, apparently when the Court was at Salisbury in the autumn, a stranger supposed to be visited with the sickness ran into the barber's tent in his absence ; whereon the tent and all his goods and instruments of livelihood were burnt, he himself confined, and his servants sent away, according to the orders for the preservation of the Court, "so that he lost his trade and was utterly ruined[1]."

The more discriminating of the profession knew and taught that the seeds of plague could lurk in a bundle of clothes, or of bedding, or in other effects, or in bales of goods, and that they became the more virulent through the fermentation that goes on in these circumstances. The contagion was understood to be *per fomitem* and *per distans*; on the other hand, experience was rather against a contagion from the exhalations of the sick: the immunity of nurses was as striking as it has been in many other contagions. The people were instinctively right in their

[1] *Cal. State Papers*, Domestic, 1665, p. 579.

belief that they mostly caught the plague because the infection was in the air of the place; so long as they were living on a plague-stricken spot, they were exposed to the risk; and if there were any difference in safety between dwelling-houses, and the streets, markets or shops, the preference seemed to lie with the former. The traditional or official doctrine, however, was that the plague-stricken were the sources of contagion, that all who had come near them were suspect, and that the safety of the well depended upon the rigorous shutting-up of the sick and the suspected together. The experience of epidemic after epidemic might have shown that this theoretical reasoning, so attractive to the "thorough" order of mind, was worthless in practice. A great plague pursued its course until the infected houses became too many for shutting up; if many plague-years did not develop epidemics of the first degree, that was in accordance with some epidemiological law, and not because the preventive measures were one year effective and another year ineffective. However, a traditional doctrine will always survive a good deal of adverse experience; and the shutting-up of houses, which had signally failed in 1563, 1593, 1603, 1625 and 1636, was resorted to once more in 1665, and perhaps with more rigour than ever so as to give it a fair chance. Defoe has stated with great fairness the hardships of it, and he follows Hodges and Boghurst in pronouncing it a mistake and a failure. Most of the horrible incidents of the plague came from the shutting-up of houses; those which Defoe introduces in that connexion do not exceed probability. It is hard to say whether the condemnation of shutting-up, which found wide currency during and immediately after the plague of 1665, would have at length made any difference to the traditional doctrine and practice. The occasion did not arise again in London except for a few months in 1666, when the old practice seems to have been enforced. The corresponding doctrine and practice that arose in its place, was quarantine against foreign importation; that rested firstly upon the sophistical assertion of the all-powerful Mead, that plague had been an exotic to England, and secondly upon the doctrine of plague-contagion in its most comprehensive and least discriminating form. But the quarantine law dates really from the Queen Anne period, and the curious history of its rise, progress, and overthrow belongs to another part of this work.

The other general preventive measure besides the shutting-up of " visited " houses was the burning of fires in the streets, which was also a tradition from Tudor times. The mayor loyally carried out that also; until in the beginning of autumn a concurrence of things made an end of the practice. These adverse influences were first, the heavy showers of rain, which put the fires out; secondly, the differences in medical opinion whether coal-fires or wood-fires were the better, and whether fires were to be recommended at all; and thirdly the popular perception that the fires made no difference to the progress of the epidemic.

In the way of individual protection and treatment, the College of Physicians issued a tract full of directions and prescriptions, which Boghurst says were all old, being taken from De Vigo († 1520). It is not necessarily against methods of practice that they are old; but one cannot fail to observe how closely the medieval teaching about plague, cause and cure together, was followed to the last in England : for two centuries the writers on plague reproduced the chapters and paragraphs almost without change that we find in the treatise of the bishop of Aarhus, which circulated in manuscript in England in the 15th century and was first printed about 1480. The most popular preventive was something " to smell to," not sweet but *aigre.* Hence the use of civet-boxes, pouncet-boxes, and pomanders, which were made to suit all purses. There were also plague-waters, one of which, "the plague-water of Matthias," figures among the prescriptions of the College of Physicians both in a cheap and in an expensive form. The College's prescription " to break the tumour " is as follows :

"Take a great onion, hollow it, put into it a fig, rue cut small, and a dram of Venice treacle ; put it close stopt in a wet paper, and roast it in the embers ; apply it hot unto the tumour ; lay three or four, one after another ; let one lie three hours."

The Paracelsist or chemical physician, Thomson, gives a prescription which brings out the mystical tendencies of that

C.

43

otherwise meritorious sect.   It relates to a method of curing plague by means of a toad.

"The great difficulty to bring this animal to a true Zenexton lies in an exquisite preparation of it, the manner whereof that great investigator of verity, Van Helmont, hath thus delivered, as he received instructions from Butler, an Irishman who (to Helmont's knowledge) had cured some thousands of the pest in London.   He gave directions that a large Bufo, taken in the afternoon in the month of June, should be hung up by the legs, nigh the fire, over a vessel of yellow wax" etc.

Tobacco, smoked or chewed, came into great vogue in 1665 as a preservative from the plague.   Hearne, the antiquary, says:

"I have been told that in the last great plague at London [1665] none that kept tobacconists shops had the plague.   It is certain that smoking it was looked upon as a most excellent preservative; in so much that even children were obliged to smoak.   And I remember that I heard formerly Tom Rogers, who was yeoman beadle, say that when he was that year, when the plague raged, a schoolboy at Eaton, all the boys of that school were obliged to smoak in the school every morning, and that he was never whipped so much in his life as he was one morning for not smoaking[1]."

The best medical details of the Great Plague come from Boghurst, who claims that the observations were all his own.

With regard to its incidence he says: "About the beginning most men got it with fuddling, surfeiting, over heating themselves, and disorderly living."   Again: "Those that married in the heat of the disease (if they had not had the disease before) almost all fell into it in a week or a fortnight after it, both in the city and in the country, of which most died, especially the men."   One of Dekker's stories of the year 1603 is an illustration of the same thing.   "It usually went through a whole kindred, though living in several places; which was the cause it swept away many whole families... In some houses ten out of twelve died, and sixteen out of twenty."   Melancholy for the loss of friends predisposed to it, while cheerfulness and courage fortified some against it.   Old people that had many sores upon them, especially carbuncles, almost all died.   The natural constitution, disposition, or complexion "did much to make or mar the disease."   People with hollow eyes commonly died.   Those who drank brandy and strong waters grew mad, looked about them wildly, and died quickly in two days.   "All that I saw that were let blood, if they had been sick two, three, four or five days or more, died the same day."   Teeming women fared miserably; they were not more subject than others: but scarce one in forty lived (this is enlarged

[1] *Reliquiae Hearnianae.*   Ed. Bliss, 1869, II. 117 (under the date of Jan. 21,

upon by Defoe). Many people had the spotted fever and the plague both together, and many the French pox and the plague both together, and yet both sorts commonly lived (someone says that men caught the French pox of purpose[1]). All sorts died, but more of the good than the bad, more men than women, more of dull complexion than fair. "Of all the common hackney prostitutes of Luteners-lane, Dog-yard, Cross-lane, Baldwin-gardens, Hatton-garden and other places, the common criers of oranges, oysters, fruits etc., all the impudent drunken drabbing bayles and fellows, and many others of the *rouge route*, there is but few missing—verifying the testimony of Diemerbroeck that the plague left the rotten bodies and took the sound[2]." It fell not very thick upon old people till about the middle or slake of the disease, and most in the decrease and declining of the disease. Cats, dogs, cattle, poultry, etc., were free from infection.

Some died in twelve or twenty days, but most in five or six. In summer about one-half that were sick, died; but towards winter, three of four lived. None died suddenly as stricken by lightning: "I saw none die under twenty or twenty-four hours." After one rising, or bubo, was broke and run, commonly another and another would rise in several parts of the body, so that many had the disease upon them half a year; some risings would not break under half a year, being so deep in the flesh.

This explains Dekker's statement in 1603 that some had buboes repeatedly, and that one person had eighteen sores. Dr Thomson himself had buboes thrice. Hodges, also, knew of many cases fatal at the third seizure, the later attacks being not relapses but new infections; some even fell at the fifth or sixth time, being before well recovered. In one of the earlier London plagues, that of 1563, Jones saw a case of a woman near Temple Bar that ended fatally at the third attack, the buboes having suppurated twice, but not at the third time. Boghurst goes on:

Of evil omen was "a white, soft, sudden, puffed up tumour on the neck behind the ears, in the armpit, or in the flank;" also a "large extended hard tumour under the chin, swelling downwards upon the throat and fetching a

---

[1] *The City Remembrancer*. London, 1769 (professing to be Gideon Harvey's notes).

[2] Procopius (*De Bello Persico*, II. cap. 23, Latin Translation) says the same of the great Justinian plague in A.D. 543 at Byzantium: "ut vere quis possit dicere, pestem illam, seu casu aliquo seu providentia, quasi delectu diligenter habito, sceleratissimos quosque reliquisse. Sed haec postea clarius patuerunt." On this Gibbon remarks: "Philosophy must disdain the observation of Procopius, that the lives of such men were guarded by the peculiar favour of fortune or Providence;" and most men will agree with Gibbon. But, if we could be sure of the fact of immunity (and Boghurst's testimony is a little weakened by his deference to Diemerbroek, who knew the classical traditions of plague), it might be possible to explain it on merely pathological grounds.

great compass" (the brawny swelling of the submaxillary salivary glands and surrounding tissues). Tokens came out after a violent sweat, which was often induced of purpose by nurses, who said, 'Cochineal is a fine thing to bring out the tokens.' Nurses often killed their patients by giving them cold drinks. Many also were killed by the shutting-up of houses, by wickedness (of nurses?), by confident and ignorant mountebanks, by over-hasty cutting and burning of buboes. Servants and poor people removed to the pest-house or to other houses in their sickness, took harm therefrom. People using corrosives, actual cauteries and many intolerable applications put their patients to more pain than the disease did.

The botches, or buboes (swollen lymph-glands in the neck, armpits or groins), were the most distinctive sign of the plague, having given to it the old name of "the botch." Besides these, there were the "tokens" (specially limited in meaning to livid spots on the skin), carbuncles and blains. Carbuncles, says Boghurst, commonly rose upon the most substantial, gross, firm flesh, as the thighs, legs, backside, buttock; they never occurred, that he saw, on the head among the hair, or on the belly. They were not seen until the end of July, were most rife in September and October, commonly in old people, never in children.

Hodges saw one carbuncle on the thigh, the size of two handbreadths, with a large blister on it, "which being opened by the chirurgeon and scarification made where the mortification did begin, the patient expired under the operation." But most commonly carbuncles did not exceed the breadth of three or four fingers. Boghurst continues :

"Blains are a kind of diminutive carbuncle, but are not so hard, black, and fiery; sometimes there is a little core in them. Generally they are no bigger than a two-penny piece, or a groat at the biggest, with a bladder full of liquor on the top of them, which, if you open but a little, will come out whitish or of a lemon or straw colour." "Besides a blain there is a thing you may call a blister, puffing up the skin, long like one's finger in figure, like a blister raised with cantharides; and such usually die." The following experience is remarkable, but it is doubtful whether Boghurst has not taken it from Diemerbroek : "Towards the latter end of a plague, many people that stayed, and others that returned, have little angry pustules and blains rising upon them, especially upon the hands, without being sick at all. But such never die, nor infect others ; and I remember Diemerbroeck saith, etc." Can this be the meaning of "smallpox" following the plague, as in the 16th century books by Alphanus, Kellwaye and others?

The tokens proper, according to Hodges, were spots on the skin "proceeding from extravasated blood." The body of the youth dissected by Thomson was "beset with spots, black and blue," some of which when opened "contained a coagulated matter." The tokens, as the name implies, were made the most distinctive sign of the plague; but they were far from being so constant as the botches or buboes. Boghurst says that "tokens appeared not much until about the middle of June;" and, according to a letter of September 14, they must have been very variable even at the height of the plague: "The practitioners in physic stand amazed to meet with so many various symptoms which they find among their patients; one week the general distempers are blotches and boils, the next week as clear-skinned as may be, but death spares neither; one week full of spots and tokens, and perhaps the succeeding bill none at all[1]."

The account of the dissection by Thomson, of a youth dead of the plague, is perhaps all the morbid anatomy that has come down to us. He found what appear to have been infarcts in the lungs; the surface was "stigmatised with several large ill-favoured marks, much tumified and distended," from which, on section, there issued "sanious, dreggy corruption and a pale ichor destitute of any blood." The stomach contained a black, tenacious matter, like ink. The spleen gave out on section an ichorish matter. The liver was pallid and the kidneys exsanguine. There were "obscure large marks" on the inner surface of the intestines and stomach. The peritoneal cavity contained a "virulent ichor or thin liquor, yellowish, or greenish." There was a decoloured clot in the right ventricle, but "not one spoonful of that ruddy liquor properly called blood could be obtained in this pestilential body." In all other cadavers that he ever dissected he had found that the right ventricle had blackish blood condensed, but this one had a pale clot "like a lamb-stone cut in twain," which puzzled him greatly; perhaps it came, he conjectures, from a sumption of mere crude milk which an indiscreet nurse had given the boy not long before he died.

---

[1] John Tillison to Dr Sancroft, September 14, 1665. Harl. MSS. cited by Heberden, *Increase and Decrease of Diseases.* London, 1801. Woodall, writing in 1639, and basing on his experience of London plague in 1603, 1625, and 1636, is in like manner emphatic that the symptoms varied much in individuals and in seasons.

Among the symptoms of a fatal issue, Boghurst mentions the following: Hiccough, continual vomiting, sudden looseness, or two or three stools in succession, shortness of breath, stopping of urine, great inward burning and outward cold, continual great thirst, faltering in the voice, speaking in the throat and occasionally sighing, with a slight pulling-in one side of the mouth when they speak, sleeping with the eyes half-open, trembling of the lips and hands and shaking of the head, staggering in going about rooms, unwillingness to speak, hoarseness preventing speech, cramp in the legs, stiffness of one side of the neck, contraction of the jaws, the vomit running out from the side of the mouth, prolonged bleeding at the nose, the sores decreasing and turning black on a sudden.

It is to be remarked that Boghurst says very little of the gentle or the violent delirium, on which Defoe enlarges picturesquely; nor does he emphasize the extreme pain of the hard and tense buboes, which is another of Defoe's themes. Hodges, however, says that "some of the infected run about staggering like drunken men, and fall and expire in the streets; while others lie half-dead and comatous...Some lie vomiting as if they had drunk poison."

The progress of the epidemic would seem to have been little influenced by the weather or by what was done, unless the shutting-up of houses had helped to intensify the virus. Boghurst says: "If very hot weather followed a shower of rain, the disease increased much;" and again: "If, in the heat of the disease the wind blew very sharp and cold, people died very quickly, many lying sick but one day." We are told, however, by Hodges that "the whole summer was refreshed with moderate breezes," and that "the heat was too mild to encourage corruption and fermentation." The air itself, he says, "remained uninfected." Rain fell from time to time in the end of summer, copious enough to put out the fires in the streets. There was at least one very hot day, near the beginning of the epidemic, the 5th of June, which Pepys says was "the hottest day that I ever felt in my life." On September 20, however, he says that the increase of the plague could not have been expected "from the coldness of the late season."

The plague lingered in London throughout the year 1666, causing 1998 deaths in all. In January 1666 it was still at as high a figure as 158 deaths in a week, and in the week ending September 18 it rose again to the exceptional height of 104 deaths. In the first three weeks of December, the deaths were 2, 4, and 3; and from that low level the plague never rose again in London. A few annual deaths continued to appear in the bills down to 1679, when they finally disappeared.

Plague near London in 1665.

Meanwhile various parts of England were affected with plague during and after the great epidemic, and in one or two instances a little before it. In the immediate neighbourhood of the capital all the towns and villages usually implicated by the exodus from the City had cases of plague, as the following table shows. It has been compiled from the parish registers, as extracted in Lysons' *Environs of London*, Defoe's widely discrepant figures being given for comparison in the third column.

	All causes	Plague	Defoe's list.		All causes	Plague	Defoe's list.
Barking	230		200	Hertford			90
Barnes	27			Hornsey	53	43	85
Barnet and Hadley			43	Isleworth	195	149	
Battersea	113			Kensington	62	25	
Beckenham	18			Kingston			122
Brentford	103		432	Lewisham	56		
Brentwood			70	Mortlake	197	170	
Bromley	27	7		Newington, Stoke			17
Camberwell	133			Norwood	12	2	
Charlton	7	3		Putney		74	
Chertsey			18	Romford	90		109
Chiselhurst	21			St Albans			121
Clapham	28			Stratford-Bow	139		
Croydon		141	61	Staines			82
Deptford	548	374	623	Tottenham	no entries		42
Ealing	286	244		Twickenham		21	
Edmonton			19	Uxbridge			117
Eltham	44	32	85	Waltham Abbey			23
Enfield	176		32	Walthamstow	68		
Epping			26	Wandsworth		245	
Finchley	38			Ware			160
Greenwich	416		231	Watford			45
Hampstead	214			Windsor			103
Heston	48	13		Woodford	33		
Hodsdon			30				

The most striking fact that comes out is that most of the parishes around London had actually fewer deaths from plague in 1665 than in 1603. The exceptions to this rule in 1665 are the villages on or near the Thames above London—Battersea, Wandsworth, Putney, Mortlake, Brentford, Isleworth, and Ealing, which had all a very high mortality, Barnes being almost exempt. On the lower reaches of the Thames, Barking on the Essex shore, and Deptford, Greenwich and Lewisham on the other side, had the infection in them very severely; but these three places in Kent had a still more severe visitation in 1666, along with other towns in that county.

On September 9, Evelyn wrote from his Deptford house, Sayes Court, that "near thirty houses are visited in this miserable village." The infection got also among the ships of the navy; on August 29, on board the 'Loyal Subject' at Deal, Captain Fortescue and six men died suddenly, it was feared of the plague.

Plague in the Provinces in 1665-6.

The earliest accounts of plague in the provinces come from Yarmouth in November, 1664. On the 18th it is said to have been brought in a vessel from Rotterdam; three died in one house, of whom one had the plague. On November 30, the plague was spreading, if the searchers (drunken women, however) were to be credited. On February 8, 1665, there was another death from plague, and as the summer wore on the mortality increased rapidly. On June 16, thirty had died in the week, the inhabitants had fled, the town was like a country village, and the poor left behind were lamenting at once the lack of work and of charity. On August 21, the king wrote from Salisbury to the bailiffs of Yarmouth concerning the plague. In the weeks ending August 30 and September 6, there were 117 deaths (96 from plague) and 110 deaths (100 from plague), and as late as November 6, there had been 22 plague-deaths in the week. In March, 1666, the epidemic came to an end[1]. Smaller outbreaks occurred in the autumn of 1665 and spring of

---

[1] *Cal. State Papers. Hist. MSS. Com.* IX. 321.

1666 at Lynn, Norwich, Ipswich and Harwich.   The great
epidemic at Colchester began in summer, 1665, but fell mostly
in 1666, at a time when there was little plague elsewhere, so
that it practically closes the history of plague in England, and
will come naturally at the end of the chapter.

Most of the provincial outbreaks in 1665 were of small
extent, and were probably due to introduction of the virus from
London.   The valley of the Tyne, which had often experienced
severe plagues, had a slight epidemic, said to have originated
from the colliers returned from the Thames.   On July 18, there
were seven houses shut up at Sunderland, one at Wearmouth
and one at Durham[1].   A paragraph in the 'Newes,' from
Durham, October 13, says that the sickness in the north is now
much assuaged.   Newcastle remained almost free (although
Defoe says different), two houses being shut up on January 30,
1666, and two at Gateshead.   The whole north-west and west of
England, which had suffered most during the last plague-period,
in the Civil Wars, appears to have escaped altogether.

In the south, there was a good deal of the infection at
Southampton in the summer and autumn of 1665 ; on July 6,
" the poor will not suffer the rich to quit the town and leave
them to starve[2]."   It is heard of, also, at Poole and Sherborne
in Dorset (in November), at Salisbury, where the Court lay for
some weeks, and at Battle[3] in Sussex; but in none of these places
to any great extent.   Various places in Kent had cases in 1665
—Rochester, Chatham, Sandwich, Eastry, Westwell, Deal, Dover
and Canterbury[4]; but it was only the naval stations that had
more than a few cases in 1665 ; while all of them had it far
worse in 1666.   Other centres in 1665 were in Northamptonshire
and Cambridgeshire.

At Peterborough, Oundle and Newport Pagnell, there was a
visitation of the severer kind, with flight of the richer inhabitants,
and the usual arrest of work and trade.   The parish register of
Yardley, Hastings, records that 60 persons died of plague in that

---

[1] *Cal. State Papers.   Cal. Le Fleming MSS.* p. 37 (also for Cockermouth).
[2] *Ibid.*
[3] Mead seems to have known that there were plague-cases at Battle in 1665.
[4] *Cal. S. P.*

town from June 5, 1665, to January 3, 1666.   There was also a sharp epidemic in Cambridge and in the country around, of which we get a glimpse in a letter of October 19, 1665, written from Clare Hall to one of the fellows of Clare[1]:

> "Alderman Mynell the brewer and one of his children died of the plague this last Monday ; he hath had four children in all dead of it.   Clayton, the barber in Petty Cury, and one of his children, died last Saturday of the sickness.   It is newly broken out sadly by Christ's (though they are all fled from the Colledge upon Mr Bunchly, their manciple, dying of the plague)— where Nicholson the smith, his wife and two children are dead within three days, his other children being deadly sick in the house.   But it most rageth in St Clement's parish, where seldom a day passeth without one dead of the sickness…Poor Mr Brown, the old man that is one of the University musicians, and Mr Saunders that sings the deep bass, are shut up in Mr Saunders' house in Green Street, whose child died last week suspected. Two houses at Barton are infected by two of Alderman Mynell's children, that are dead there.   Ditton is broke out just by the butcher, from whom we had our meat, which made us hastily remove to Grantchester.   H. Glenton, the carrier, fled from this town to Shelford, where he died within two or three days, suspected…Royston is sadly in two or three places, the last of which is just in the middle of the town.   The infection, they say, was brought thither by a Cambridge man, whom they caught, and shut him up ; but he hath since made his escape."

The Epidemic of Plague at Eyam, 1665–6.

Another of the English towns visited by plague in 1665 was Derby ; whether the cases were many or few, they caused great alarm, the town being forsaken, the streets grass-grown, and the market set up on a new stance, to which the farmers and traders came primed with a plug of tobacco in their mouths as a preservative.   But the epidemic in Derby itself was totally eclipsed in interest by an extraordinary outbreak of plague in the small village of Eyam, at the opposite end of the county, in the North Peak, some twelve miles to the west of Sheffield. The plague of Eyam is, indeed, the most famous of all English plagues ; the story of it has been told many times in prose and verse, its traditional incidents being well suited to minor poets and moral writers, and the whole action of the drama con-

---

[1] *Hist. MSS. Com.* II. 115.

veniently centered within a circuit of half a mile in a cup of the heathy hills[1].

Eyam was a village of some three hundred and fifty inhabitants, standing among meadows around which the hills towered. It had no resident doctor, but it had two ministers. The one was the rector, the Rev. William Mompesson, a young man of twenty-seven, with a wife and two children, who had been settled in Eyam only a year and did not like it; the other was the former rector, the Rev. Thomas Stanley, who had been ejected for nonconformity in 1662, and had remained to carry on his ministrations as a Dissenter among such of his old flock as adhered to him. The wealthier householders resided at the western and higher end of the village, on the other side of a brook which crossed under the road; as we shall see, they escaped the infection almost if not altogether. The annual village wake had been held in August, 1665, with more than the usual concourse of people from villages near. On the 2nd or 3rd September a box arrived from London to the village tailor, who lived in a small house at the western end of the churchyard; it contained old clothes which someone in London is supposed to have bought for him cheap, and some tailors' patterns of cloth. This box is assumed to have been opened by one George Vicars, a servant, who was certainly the first victim of plague. He found the contents to be damp and hung them up at the fire to dry. He was quickly seized with violent sickness, became delirious, developed buboes in his neck and groin, a plague-token on his breast the third day, and died in a wretched state on September 6. His body, which is said to have become soon putrid, was buried in the churchyard on the 7th. Nearly a fortnight passed before another case occurred, that of a youth supposed to have been the tailor's son, who was buried on the 22nd September. Before the 30th four more had died, and in

---

[1] *The History and Antiquities of Eyam, with a full and particular account of the Great Plague which desolated that village* A.D. 1666. By William Wood, London, 1842. This small volume, which owes its interest solely to the plague-incident, has gone through at least five editions. Among those who have written, in prose or verse, upon the same theme, Wood mentions Dr Mead, Miss Seward, Allan Cunningham, E. Rhodes, S. T. Hall, William and Mary Howitt, S. Roberts, and J. Holland. The story is also in the *Book of Golden Deeds*.

the course of October twenty-two more were buried of the plague. The deaths in November declined to seven, and in December they were nine.   There was now snow on the ground, with hard frost, and at the beginning of January, 1666, the plague was confined to two houses.   Four died in January, eight in February, six in March, nine in April, and only three in May.   On June 2, another burial occurred, and then there was another pause. But in a week or more the epidemic broke out with renewed power, three having been buried on the 12th of June, three on the 15th, one on the 16th, three on the 17th, and so on until the total for June reached nineteen.   The wealthier villagers at the west end had taken the alarm before and had mostly fled in the spring; those who stayed kept within their houses or at least did not cross the stream.   Now that the infection was revived in the hot weather of June, the rector's wife also proposed flight, but on her husband's refusal, she resolved to remain with him, and to send her two children to a relative in Yorkshire.   At the same time the villagers in general were instinctively moved to escape from the tainted spot ; but Mompesson used his authority to prevent them, and a boundary line was drawn round the village, about half a mile in circuit and marked by various familiar objects, beyond which no one was to go.   Mompesson's motive appears to have been to prevent the spread of the infection to the country around, and his parishioners submitted passively.   After the end of June the villagers would have found it difficult to escape, owing to the terror which the very name of their village caused in all the country round.   Some of them quitted their cottages and took up their abode in shelters built along the side of a rocky glen within the cordon.   The earl of Devonshire, then at Chatsworth, promised Mompesson that the village should not be left without supplies ; and people from the villages near brought their market produce to certain stated points on the boundary, where the Eyam people came to fetch it, the money paid being dropped into water.   Thus shut up in their narrow valley, the villagers perished helplessly like a stricken flock of sheep.   By the end of June ceremonial burials came to an end, the church and the churchyard were closed, the dead were carried out wrapped in sheets by one of the villagers noted for his herculean strength, and laid in shallow graves in the meadows or on the hill-sides.   In July the deaths mounted up to five or six on some days, and the total for the month to fifty-seven.   In August the dead numbered seventy-eight, among them the rector's wife on the 25th, after a walk with her husband through the meadows, during which she is said to have made the ominous remark that the air smelled sweet[1].   September added twenty-four to the total, and there were now only about forty-five left alive in the place.   Of these, fifteen died to the 11th October, when the mortality ceased.   Some of the survivors had passed through an attack of the plague, among them the rector's man, whose buboes suppurated.   Mompesson himself, who had an issue open in his leg all the time, escaped the infection, as well as his maid-servant.   A young woman of Eyam, married in the village of Corbor, two miles off, came one day to see her mother, whom she found sick of the plague; on her return home she took the sickness and died, but no one else in Corbor had it.   A man was also at large in the neighbourhood suspected of plague, to whom the earl of Devonshire sent a doctor.   The doctor and patient met by appointment on the opposite banks of a stream, and the diagnosis made across the water acquitted the man of plague; even in these unconventional circumstances the consultation did not end without a prescription (still extant) for a bottle of " stuff."   Seventy-six households in Eyam were infected, and out of these two hundred and fifty-nine persons were buried of the plague.   During the time that the infection lasted eight more died from other causes.   When the sickness had ceased Mompesson set about burning the infected articles in the empty cottages.   Three years after, in 1669, he was presented to the better living of Eakring, in Notts; but on arriving to enter on his duties he was refused admission by the villagers, and had to take up his residence in a temporary hut in Rufford Park, until such time as the preju-

---

[1] Bacon (*Sylva Sylvarum,* Cent. x. § 912. Spedding 11. 643) says : " The plague is many times taken without a manifest sense, as hath been said. And they report that, where it is found, it hath a scent of the smell of a mellow apple ; and (as some say) of May-flowers ; and it is also received that smells of flowers that are mellow and luscious are ill for the plague : as white lilies, cowslips and hyacinths."

dices of his new parishioners had been overcome. He married another wife, and for thirty-nine years held the living of Eakring, where he died on March 7, 1708. Stanley, his Dissenting colleague at Eyam, died there a few years after the plague.

Several things combined to magnify the disaster at Eyam. The story of the box of clothes from London is entirely credible, and can be matched by many other instances in the history of plague and of cholera[1]. Nothing intensifies the virus of such diseases so much as fermentation without air in the textures of clothes or linen; a whiff from the opened box or bundle suffices soon to prostrate the person who breathes it. The poison at Eyam was a powerful one from the first, and it is credible that the body of the earliest victim did become quickly putrid. The heavy mortality, with few recoveries, which followed after a fortnight's interval, and continued all through the winter, also shows a virus raised to no ordinary potency. But, for the revival of the infection in June, 1666, we must seek other causes. Eyam was one of those basins which, on a large scale or on a small, have often been observed to keep infection in their soil. The virus must have passed into the pores of the ground after the first sixty or more burials in the churchyard down to the lull of the epidemic in winter; with the rise of the ground-water in spring, it would be comparatively inactive; but in June, when the water was again sinking in the soil and the great heat was raising emanations from the dry ground, it broke forth with an intensity which poisoned the whole air of the valley. The burials, after the end of June, without coffins and in shallow graves in the meadows or on the hill-side, were so much ferment added to a soil already permeated by it. Flight from such a place was the only safety, and the rector, with the best motives, counselled the people to remain. Mompesson's conduct has always been held up as a pattern of heroism, as if the circumstances had been desperate like those of the Trojans when the Greeks were in their streets and houses:

Una salus victis nullam sperare salutem.

---

[1] Sir Thomas Elyot, in *The Castle of Health* (1541), says that "infected stuff lying in a coffer fast shut for two years, then opened, has infected those that stood nigh it, who soon after died." (Cited by Brasbridge, *Poor Man's Jewel*, 1578, Chapter VIII.)

No word of detraction should be spoken of anyone who does manfully what he conceives to be his duty to his neighbours; but the villagers of Eyam were sacrificed, all the same, to an idea, and to an idea which we may now say was not scientifically sound. When the impulse came upon them to flee, they might have left their tainted soil without much risk to the country around so long as they did not collect in one spot or carry with them bedding or the like susceptible articles: those who did flee from the houses at the upper end of the village are not known to have carried the infection to other places, and the young woman who brought it to Corbor gave it to no one else. But the wisdom of flight may be regarded by some as still disputable; while it will be admitted by all that Mompesson acted for the best according to his lights.

The plague in 1666 raged severely in a number of towns, while it lingered on in London. The information from Winchester is vague; it is said that the dead were carried out in carts and buried on the downs to the eastward[1]; the epidemic was over by the 1st of December, so that the College resumed[2]. Pepys enters in his Diary (April 4, 1667): "One at the table [the duke of Albemarle's] told an odd passage in the late plague, that at Petersfield (I think he said), one side of the street had every house almost infected through the town, and the other not one shut up." There may have been other such centres of plague, and equally interesting observations made on them; but it appears to be the merest chance whether anything is recorded of them at all, or whether one has the luck to come across the record.

The great centres of plague in 1666 had some connexion with the fleet, and were mostly in Kent and Essex. Deptford and Greenwich had more plague that year than the year before, the total deaths at the former having been 715 (of plague 522) and at the latter 423. Eltham and Lewisham were also visited

[1] Milner's *Hist. of Winchester.*
[2] *The City Remembrancer*, Lond. 1769, vol. I.—an account of the plague, fire, storm of 1703, etc., said to have been "collected from curious and authentic papers originally compiled by the late learned Dr [Gideon] Harvey." But the section on the plague is almost purely Defoe and Vincent, with a few things from Mead.

in proportion.   The other intense centre of infection in Kent was Deal.   On the 26th August, seven died of the plague, and twenty in the whole week.   At that date there were said to be only 16 houses which had not had plague in them.   On December 9, all the houses were clear, although the crews of ships still avoided the town.   Next to Deal, Sandwich, Dover, Canterbury and Maidstone had considerable outbreaks in the autumn.   At Portsmouth also there was a sharp outbreak in the summer of 1666, twenty-one having died of plague in a week at the beginning of July.

In the Eastern Counties, plague revived to a considerable extent in 1666 at Norwich, Ipswich, Harwich and Woodbridge, the Yarmouth outbreak, which had been the great one in that quarter the year before, having come to an end in the spring. But it was at Colchester that the epidemic engrossed attention in 1666.   Colchester had, indeed, two successive seasons of plague, or rather a continuous prevalence of it from the summer of 1665 to December, 1666.   The plague at Colchester in 1665–66 was the greatest of all provincial plagues since the Black Death, unless, indeed, we credit the numbers (11,000 or 12,000) given for a plague at York in 1390.   It reproduced the mortality of the Great Plague of London on a scale more than proportionate to its size, and it doubtless called forth the same class of incidents—flight of the wealthier classes, and almost total extermination of the poor.   No documents remain, however, of this plague except the oaths administered to searchers and bearers of the dead (printed below) and the weekly totals of deaths from plague and from other causes[1].   The weekly

---

[1] These figures, with the two oaths, had been copied by the antiquary Morant for his *History of Essex*, and are preserved in No. 87. ff. 55 and 56, of the Stowe MSS. in the British Museum, where Mr J. A. Herbert, of the Manuscript Department, pointed them out to me.   In his printed *History* Morant has summarized the plague-deaths in monthly periods.

The Bearers' Oath, fol. 57 :—

" Ye shall swear, that ye shall bear to the ground and bury the bodies of all such persons as, during these infectious times, shall dye of the pestilence within this Towne or the Liberties thereof, or so many of them as ye shall have notice of, and may be permitted to bury, carrying them to burials always in the night time, unless it be otherwise ordered by the Mayor of this Towne ; And ye shall be always in readiness for that purpose at your abode, where you shall be appointed, keeping apart from

bills are, indeed, as eloquent a testimony as any detailed description could have been ; and as they are the most complete of the kind for a provincial town, I have transcribed them from the manuscript record in full. The small number of deaths from ordinary causes points to the emptiness of the better quarters of the town; the total deaths in seventeen months, 5345, including 4817 plague-deaths and 528 from other causes, must have meant an enormous clearance of the poorer classes. Colchester was then a place of considerable wealth, with a thriving Dutch trade and a considerable Dutch colony. Perhaps the connexion with Holland, where plague had been rife in the years just before, may explain the origin of the outbreak ; but local conditions of soil, overcrowding, and the

your families together with the searchers, and not to be absent from thence more than your office of Bearers requires. Ye shall always in your walk, as much as may be, avoid the society of people, keeping as far distant from them as may bee, and carrying openly in your hands a white wand, by which people may know you, and shun and avoid you. And shall do all other things belonging to the office of Bearers, and therein shall demean yourselves honestly and faithfully, discharging a good conscience ; So etc.

August 1665. JAMES BARTON and
JOHN COOKE :—sworn, who are to have for their pains 10 sh. a week a piece ; and 2d for every one to be buried, taking the 2d out of the estate of the deceased. If there be not wherewithal, the parish to bear it.

Oath 6. p. 44.
The Oath for the Searchers of the Plague, 1665.

" Yee and either of You shall sweare, that ye shall diligently view and search the corps of all such persons, as during these infectious times, shall dye within this Towne or the Liberties thereof, or so many of them as you shall or may have access unto, or have notice of ; And shall according to the best of your skill, determine of what disease every such dead corps came to its death. And shall immediately give your judgment thereof to the Constables of the parish where such corps shall be found, and to the Bearers appointed for the burial of such infected corps. You shall not make report of the cause of any one's death better or worse than the nature of the disease shall deserve. Yee shall live together where you shall be appointed, and not walk abroad more than necessity requires, and that only in the execution of your office of Searchers. Ye shall decline and absent yourselves from your families, and always avoid the society of people. And in your walk shall keep as far distant from men as may be, always carrying in your hands a white wand, by which the people may know you, and shun and avoid you. And ye shall well and truly do all other things belonging to the office of Searchers, according to the best of your skill, wisdom, knowledge, and power, in all things dealing faithfully, honestly, unfeignedly and impartially. So help " etc.

C.   44

like must be looked to for the cause of its extraordinary persistence and fatality.

Weekly mortalities in Colchester, August 14, 1665, *to December* 14, 1666, *from plague and other diseases.*

1665 Week ending	Plague	Other	1666 Week ending	Plague	Other
Aug. 21	26	2	Apr. 27	90	4
28	62	2	May 4	169	8
Sept. 8	122	4	11	167	7
15	153	22	18	150	11
22	159	25	25	98	12
29	100	25	June 1	89	10
Oct. 6	161	27	8	110	10
13	122	23	15	139	3
20	106	15	22	195	6
27	60	41	29	176	4
Nov. 3	104	13	July 6	167	8
10	88	22	13	160	9
17	88	18	20	175	3
24	62	8	27	109	4
Dec. 1	38	10	Aug. 3	109	2
8	39	6	10	85	4
15	67	4	17	70	1
22	53	7	24	51	1
29	21	3	31	53	4
1666			Sept. 7	31	6
Jan. 5	23	6	14	22	2
12	46	8	21	16	2
19	36	13	28	10	2
26	26	10	Oct. 5	7	2
Feb. 2	34	9	12	7	0
9	25	3	19	7	2
16	23	7	26	4	2
23	33	6	Nov. 2	4	2
Mar. 2	53	2	9	4	2
9	26	11	16	2	6
16	37	5	23	1	4
23	48	4	30	1	8
30	66	1	Dec. 7	1	7
Apr. 6	73	2	14	0	0
13	90	2			
20	68	4		4817	528

To relieve the poverty caused by this great disaster a tax was levied on various other parts of the county of Essex, and contributions were made by private individuals, the London churches collecting £1311. 10s. in the breathing-time between the plague and the fire. Colchester had so far recovered in the end of 1666 as to be able to contribute in turn about a hundred pounds for the relief of London after the fire[1].

The Last of Plague in England.

The history of plague in England must be made to end with a solitary epidemic at Nottingham in 1667, but not without some misgivings as to the correctness of the date. Dr Deering, the historian of the town in 1751, paid little heed to epidemics, although medicine was his business; but he mentions one of smallpox in 1736, which had probably come within his own experience, and proceeds:

"I question much whether there has been the like since the plague which visited the town in 1667, and made a cruel desolation in the higher part of Nottingham, for very few died in the lower; especially in a street called Narrow Marsh, it was observed that the infection had no power, and that during the whole time the plague raged, not one who lived in that street died of it, which induced many of the richer sort of people to crowd thither and hire lodgings at any price; the preservation of the people was attributed to the effluvia of the tanners' ouze (for there were then 47 tanners' yards in that place), besides which they caused a smoak to be made by burning moist tanners' knobs[2]."

If there had been any reference to the parish registers or to the corporation minutes, we should have had no reason to doubt that this epidemic had been correctly assigned to 1667. The last Winchester epidemic had been given under the year 1668, first by one local historian, and then by another who copied him; but when a third went to the manuscript records, he found that the year was 1666, as indeed an incidental reference to the re-opening of Winchester School on 1st December, 1666, "the sickness being in all appearance extinguished," might have warranted one in concluding. It is a singular experience to have brought the history of plague down through several centuries, not without particulars of times and numbers,

---

[1] Morant, *Hist. of Essex*, I. 74.

[2] Deering, *Nottingham*, vetus et nova, 1751, pp. 82—83. Copied in Thoresby's edition of Thoroton's *History of Nottingham*, II. 60.

and to be obliged to end it in the latter half of the 17th century with an unauthenticated date.   The Nottingham epidemic may have been an exception to the generality that all England was finally delivered from the plague in 1666; it is due, at least, to the local historian, in the absence of evidence against, to record his date of 1667.   The difficulty of confirming so simple a fact at so late a period may dispose the readers of this work to be tolerant of any lack of certainty and precision that they may discover in its history of more remote times.

INDEX.

at Cambridge 375, at Oxford 376–382, at Exeter 383–386, referred to in Act 388, in the Queen's Bench, Southwark 395, 539, Bacon on 332

Garter, Order of the 178

Gascoigne T., cases of syphilis 74, Henry IV's "leprosy" 77 *note*, "legists" after Black Death 189

Gaubil, abbé, on the Chinese annals 154

Geynes, Dr 307

Gibbon, on the Justinian plague 2, on a remark by Procopius 675 *note*

Gibbons, Orlando 465, 524

Gilbertus Anglicus, on leprosy 70–72, morphaea 76, diet to keep off leprosy 113, on smallpox 446, 447

Glasgow, leper-house 99, keeps out plague 366, 369, plague 370, 563, syphilis 418

Gloucester, Black Death 116, 117, plague in 1580 348, in 1638 545, a quack at 426, relief of siege 549

Goddard, Dr, his excuse for leaving London in the plague 667

Gordonio, Bernard, on leprosy 70, case at Montpellier 72, on morphaea 76, on smallpox 447

Grandgore, in Scotland 417–18, derivation of 418

Grantham, plague near 500, sickness at 502

Graunt, John, syphilis in London 428, London mortality 532

Gravesend, plague 287, 293, 531

Greaves, Sir E., fever at Oxford 547, 551

Greenwich, sweat at 244, 251, plague at 293, plague in 1666 687

Gregory, W. ref. to "pokkes" 454

Gruner, on the sweat 258, collections on medieval smallpox 446 *note*

Grünbeck, Jos. on syphilis 432

Guignes, Des, on origin of Black Death 143, 152

Guinea, voyages to in 16th cent. 581–3, slave trade from 583, 625–9

Guy, Dr W., on "parish infection" 396 *note*

Hackney, leper-hospital 97, 98 *note*,

plague in 1535 301, in 1603 492, in 1625 511

Haddington, *pestilentia volatilis* 234, plague during siege 303

Hall, his Chronicle on the sweat of 1517 250, on the mercenaries of Henry VII. 274, on the Cambridge Black Assizes 375

Hampshire, parish in, statistics of 411, 541

Harrison, W. English houses 330 *note*, fever of 1557-8 401

Hartlepool, plague 349

Harwich, plague at in 1665-6

Havre de Grace (or "Newhaven"), plague during siege 307

Hawkins, Sir John, in the slave trade 583

Hawkins, Sir Richard, on health of Cape de Verde islands 589 *note*, scurvy in his voyage of 1593 594–6

Hecker, antecedents of Black Death 143–4, on fecundity after Black Death 200, sweating sickness 240, 244 *note*, 258, 263, 265, 271 *note*, 277 *note*

Hendon, sends help in 1625 plague 518

Henry I., taxation under 31

Henry II., charities of 33–34

Henry III., famine under 43

Henry IV., "leprosy" of 77

Henry V., vigorous sanitation under 325

Henry VII., his expedition of 1485 237, 240, 265, 270, 275, in the sweat of 1508 244, reception of Catharine of Arragon 288, sanitation under 325–6

Henry VIII., in the sweat of 1517 247–8, in plague of 1517–18 290, in sweat of 1528 250–53, in plague of 1535 297, 300, measures to check plague 291, 312, 313–14, repression of vagrancy &c. 390, his illness in 1514 456

Henry of Huntingdon, poem by 18

Hensler, his history of syphilis 416 *note*

Hensley, plague 309

Hereford, plague 348

Hereford, bishop of, case of morphaea 76

Herefordshire, plague 500

C.